# Wilkins'
# Clinical Assessment in Respiratory Care

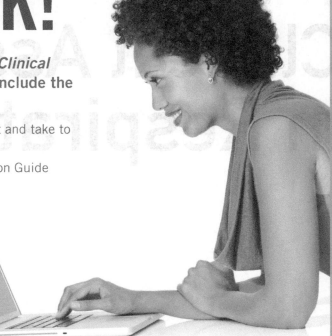

# Eighth Edition

# Wilkins'
# Clinical Assessment
# in Respiratory Care

## Albert J. Heuer

PhD, MBA, RRT, RPFT, FAARC
Professor & Program Director
School of Health Professions
Rutgers University
Newark, New Jersey

Adjunct Professor
Respiratory Care Program
County College of Morris
Randolph, New Jersey

Respiratory Therapist (Per Diem)
Morristown Medical Center
Morristown, New Jersey

## Craig L. Scanlan

EdD, RRT, FAARC
Professor Emeritus
School of Health Professions
Rutgers University
Newark, New Jersey

ELSEVIER

## ELSEVIER

3251 Riverport Lane
St. Louis, Missouri 63043

WILKINS' CLINICAL ASSESSMENT IN RESPIRATORY CARE, EIGHTH EDITION      ISBN: 9780323416351

---

**Notices**

---

International Standard Book Number: 978-0-323416351

*Senior Content Strategist:* Yvonne Alexopoulos
*Senior Content Development Manager:* Laurie Gower
*Publishing Services Manager:* Deepthi Unni
*Project Manager:* Manchu Mohan
*Design Direction:* Ryan Cook

Printed in the United States of America

Last digit is the print number:   9   8   7   6   5   4   3

Working together
to grow libraries in
developing countries

www.elsevier.com • www.bookaid.org

To fate, fortune and persistence, which have given me the opportunity to purse my passion as an educator and clinician; to my faculty mentors, Drs. Craig Scanlan and Robert Wilkins, who helped me develop the skills to do so; and to my wife, Laurel, family, friends and colleagues who continue to support me on the journey.

**AJH**

## Eighth Edition Contributors

**Zaza Cohen, MD, FCCP**
ICU Director
Department of Medicine
Hackensack University Medical Center at
    Mountainside
Montclair, New Jersey

**Tracy Davis, PhD, MA**
Assistant Professor
Interdisciplinary Studies
School of Health Professions
Rutgers, The State University of New Jersey
Newark, New Jersey

**Nadine A. Fydryszewski, PhD,
MLS(ASCP)$^{CM}$**
Professor
Department of Clinical Laboratory Sciences
School of Health Professions
Rutgers, The State University of New Jersey
Newark, New Jersey

**David A. Gourley, MHA**
Adjunct Professor
Department of Interprofessional Health
    Services and Health Administration
Seton Hall University
South Orange, New Jersey

**Laurel A. Heuer, RN**
Registered Nurse
Morristown Medical Center
Morristown, New Jersey

**Elaine M. Keohane, PhD, CLS**
Professor and Chair
Department of Clinical Laboratory Sciences
School of Health Professions
Rutgers, The State University of New Jersey
Newark, New Jersey

**Norman Mcleod**
Assistant Professor
School of Health Professions
Rutgers, The State University of New Jersey
Newark, New Jersey

**Charlyn K. Moellers**
Instructor, Program Director Respiratory
    Therapy Program
School of Health Professions
Rutgers, The State University of New Jersey
Newark, New Jersey

**Samone T. Norsworthy, EdD, MSLBE**
Adjunct Instructor
School of Health Professions
Rutgers, The State University of New Jersey
Newark, New Jersey

**Pooja Raju, MD, BSe**
Temple University
Doctor
Pulmonary, Corneal Care and Sleep
St. Luke's University Warren Campus
Phillipsburg, New Jersey
Central Care
Hackenback University Mountainade
Montclair, New Jersey

**Janet Reid-Hector, EdD, RD**
Assistant Professor
Healthcare Management–Interdisciplinary
    Studies
School of Health Professions
Rutgers, The State University of New Jersey
Newark, New Jersey

**Ruben Restrepo, MD, RRT, FAARC**
Professor of Respiratory Care
The University of Texas Health Science
    Center at San Antonio
San Antonio, Texas

**Narciso E. Rodriguez, BS, RRT-ACCS,
NPS, RPFT**
Adjunct Assistant Professor
School of Health Professions
Rutgers, The State University of New Jersey
Newark, New Jersey

**Kathleen Smith-Wenning, MA, RRT-
NPS, CPFT**
Assistant Professor and Program Director
Respiratory Care
School of Health Professions
Rutgers, The State University of New Jersey
Newark, New Jersey

**Richard Wettstein, MMEd, RRT,
FAARC**
Associate Professor; Director of Admissions
Division of Respiratory Care
UT Health San Antonio
San Antonio, Texas

**David Vines, MHS, RRT, FAARC, FCCP**
Chairman and Respiratory Care Program
    Director
Department of Cardiopulmonary Sciences
Rush University Medical Center
Chicago, Illinois

**Jane Ziegler, DCN, RDN, LDN**
Associate Professor and Program Director
Doctorate of Clinical Nutrition Program
School of Health Professions
Rutgers, The State University of New Jersey
Newark, New Jersey

## Seventh Edition Editors/
Contributors

**Robert F. Allen III, MA, RPSGT**
Manager, Sleep Wake Disorder Lab
St. Mary's Medical Center
Langhorne, Pennsylvania

**Cara DeNunzio, MPH, RRT, CTTS**
Adjunct Assistant Professor
Respiratory Care Program—North
School of Health Related Professions
University of Medicine and Dentistry of
    New Jersey
Newark, New Jersey

**Kenneth Miller, MEd, RRT-NPS, AE-C**
Educational Coordinator, Dean of Wellness
Respiratory Care Services
Lehigh Valley Health Network
Allentown, Pennsylvania

**Donna Davis, BS, RRT**
Program Director
Butte College
Oroville, California

**Allan Gonzales, MEd, RRT-NPS, RCP**
Director of Clinical Education
Platt College, Los Angeles
Alhambra, California

**Anne Marie Hilse, RRT-ACCS**
Lead Therapist, Adult ICU
Respiratory Care, Morristown Medical Center
Atlantic Health System
Morristown, New Jersey

**Tim Op't Holt, EdD, RRT, AE-C, FAARC**
Professor of Cardiorespiratory Care
University of South Alabama
Mobile, Alabama

Our continued thanks go out to our previous edition reviewers: Georgine Bills, Craig P. Black, Hele Schaar Corning, Erin Ellis Davis, Dale Bruce Dearing, Lindsay Fox, Laurie A Freshwater, Christine A Hamilton, Sharon L Hatfield, Robert L. Joyner, Chris Kallus, Kevin Shane Keene, Tammy Kurszewski, J. Kenneth LeJeune, Stacy Lewis-Sells, Cory E. Martin, Michael McLeland, Harley R Metcalfe, Michell Oki, Sara Parker, Jose D. Rojas, Paula Denise Silver, Helen M. Sorenson, Shawna L. Strickland, Cam Twarog, and Michael D. Werner.

# PREFACE

The primary purpose of the eighth edition is similar to the previous ones: to provide relevant information related to the knowledge and skills needed for respiratory therapists (RTs) to be competent and to trust in their patient assessment skills. The eighth edition is based on the assumption that every patient is an interactive, complex person who is more than a collection of his or her parts. The health status of patients depends on many internal and external environmental interactions. These interactions occur within their physical environments and include what they eat, drink, and breathe; how they sleep; and if and when they exercise. External or social environments also affect their health status and include what kind of activity and work they participate in and where they live. Other factors, such as when, why, and how often patients seek health care, can also affect their overall well-being.

Although the language of this text continues to be aimed primarily at students and the faculty who teach them, experienced therapists or other health care clinicians may benefit from its content as well. We hope that this book helps students and clinicians gain important insight into the value, purpose, and skills associated with patient assessment. The important tools provided in these pages can assist you to inspect and examine the patient's body. However, learning to listen to the patient's explanation of what is wrong and right is often the most valuable practice in meeting a patient's health needs.

Assisting physicians in assessing patients for the treatment needed, the complications that may arise, and when a treatment regimen should be changed or discontinued is a competency expected of almost all health care professionals.

We have seen firsthand the difference in patient care when clinicians are competent at patient assessment. Identifying the early signs of atelectasis through the use of a stethoscope and evaluation of breathing pattern, identifying the potential misplacement of an endotracheal tube through the use of a stethoscope and the chest radiograph, and recognizing serious abnormalities based on the arterial blood gas are all scenarios in which you could find yourself.

Application of such skills can favorably affect the outcomes experienced by patients both in and outside the hospital. On the other hand, those clinicians who lack good assessment skills generally are relegated to following the orders of others, which is not always the best way to serve the patient. Although we believe that high-tech equipment can be smart and sophisticated, it can never replace the well-honed bedside assessment skills of the experienced clinician. We hope that the knowledge in this book will help develop and refine your clinical skills and inspire you to develop a passion for patient assessment.

## NEW TO THIS EDITION

The eighth edition retains the strengths of the first seven editions: a clear, concise, and understandable writing style; an attractive and user-friendly format; and the inclusion of relevant clinical case studies and helpful hints for practice. However, this new edition ushers in many significant changes:

- With the passing of coeditor Craig L. Scanlan in 2016, Albert J. Heuer has now assumed sole responsibility for editing the eighth edition of this book. Dr. Scanlan was a Professor Emeritus at the University of Medicine and Dentistry of New Jersey (now Rutgers University) with over 40 years of experience in respiratory care. He was a coeditor for four editions of *Egan's Fundamentals of Respiratory Care*, two in collaboration with Dr. Robert Wilkins. Albert J. Heuer is a long-time respiratory educator and is Professor for the Respiratory Care Program at the School of Health Professions, Rutgers University, Newark, New Jersey. Dr. Heuer served as coeditor on the seventh edition of this textbook, was a contributor and consulting editor on the sixth edition, and is also a coeditor of *Egan's Fundamentals of Respiratory Care* for the 10th and 11th editions. Dr. Heuer is a practicing respiratory therapist who continues to work regularly in acute care at a major medical center in New Jersey. It was because of his expertise as a respiratory educator, scholar, and clinician, coupled with their professional relationship, that Robert Wilkins requested to have Dr. Heuer succeed him as lead editor for this project. Dr. Heuer is continuing Wilkins' legacy in maintaining the high standards of this text set into motion seven editions ago.
- Each chapter has been carefully updated to reflect the latest standards of practice and credentialing examination content.
- All chapters also have been peer reviewed, and the content is reflective of reviewer input and expertise.
- The latest technologic advancements, including those related to the assessment of critical care and non–critical care patients, have been included.
- This edition includes a renewed focus on providing a reading level that is appropriate for any respiratory care student.
- A full-color illustration program has been implemented to enhance student understanding of key concepts.
- Along with the inclusion of color illustrations, this edition has also adopted a color design intended to enhance learning by making content easier to read and elements of the text easier to locate.

## FEATURES

We continue to use learning features to help guide the student to mastery of the content. This edition features the following:

- Chapter outlines introduce students to chapter content and progression to enhance note taking
- Content that is focused on relevant, measurable, and attainable chapter learning objectives that help with mastery of information

- Key terms are bolded and defined within the text to enhance terminology comprehension.
- Simply Stated boxes are scattered throughout each chapter to succinctly summarize and highlight key points within the text.
- Bulleted Key Points at the end of each chapter emphasize the topics identified in the learning objectives and provide the student with an overview of chapter content for easy review.
- Select chapters include Case Studies that feature realistic clinical scenarios for student practice and/or classroom discussion.
- Questions to Ask boxes are also included in select chapters. They provide lists of questions that practitioners should ask when confronted with certain pathologies.
- Assessment Questions conclude each chapter to easily assess mastery of the content. Answers for the assessment questions are located on the Evolve site.

## LEARNING AIDS

Evolve Resources—http://evolve.elsevier.com/Heuer/Wilkins

Evolve is an interactive learning environment designed to work in coordination with this text. Instructors may use Evolve to provide an Internet-based course component that reinforces and expands the concepts presented in class. Evolve may be used to publish the class syllabus, outlines, and lecture notes; set up "virtual office hours" and e-mail communication; share important dates and information through the online class calendar; and encourage student participation through chat rooms and discussion boards. Evolve allows instructors to post examinations and manage their grade books online.

## FOR THE INSTRUCTOR

Evolve offers valuable resources to help instructors prepare their courses, including the following:
- A test bank of approximately 800 questions in ExamView
- An image collection of the figures from the book and Comprehensive PowerPoint presentations for each chapter
- NBRC CRT/RRT Summary Content Outline Correlation Guide mapping the text to the content outlines

## FOR STUDENTS

Evolve offers valuable resources to help students succeed in their courses, including the following:
- Student Lecture Notes in PowerPoint format for students to print and take to lectures for enhanced note taking
- NBRC CRT/RRT Summary Content Outline Correlation Guide mapping the text to the content outlines
- Answers to the textbook assessment questions

For more information, visit http://evolve.elsevier.com/Heuer/Wilkins/ or contact an Elsevier sales representative.

# CONTENTS

# Preparing for the Patient Encounter

*Craig L. Scanlan and Charlyn Moellers*

## LEARNING OBJECTIVES

*After reading this chapter, you will be able to:*

1. Define patient-centered care and identify its key elements.
2. Identify the major factors affecting communication between the patient and clinician.
3. Differentiate among the stages of the clinical encounter and the communication strategies appropriate to each stage.
4. Incorporate patients' needs and preferences into your assessment and care planning.
5. Apply concepts of personal space and territoriality to support patients' privacy needs.
6. Employ basic rules to ensure the confidentiality and security of all patient health information.
7. Identify the key abilities required for culturally competent communication with patients.
8. Specify ways to involve patients and their families in the provision of health care.
9. Identify the steps in assessing a patient's learning needs, including how to overcome any documented barriers to learning.
10. Explain the use of patient action plans in facilitating goal setting and patient self-care.
11. Specify steps the patient and family can take to enhance safety and reduce medical errors.
12. Identify standard infection control procedures needed during patient encounters.
13. Outline ways to ensure effective communication with other providers when receiving orders and reporting on your patient's clinical status.
14. Specify how to coordinate your patient's care with that provided by others, as well as when transferring responsibilities to others and planning for patient discharge.
15. Identify examples of how the respiratory therapist can participate effectively as a team member to enhance outcomes in caring for patients with both acute and chronic cardiopulmonary disorders.

## OUTLINE

## KEY TERMS

action plan
closed-loop communication
culturally competent
  communication
intimate space
nonverbal communication

patient-centered care
personal space
Protected Health Information (PHI)
return demonstration
SBAR
social space

Speak Up initiative
standard precautions
teach-back method
territoriality

Patient-centered care (Fig. 1.1) depicts three main elements: individualized care, patient involvement, and provider collaboration. Patient-centered care is founded on a two-way partnership between providers and patients (and their families) designed to ensure that (1) the care given is consistent with each individual's values, needs, and preferences, and (2) patients become active participants in their own care. The core of patient-centered care is the quality of interactions between patients and care providers. Additionally, patient-centered care helps minimize medical errors and contributes to enhanced patient safety.

The patient-provider encounter is at the heart of effective patient-centered care. Such encounters are so commonplace in the daily routine of the respiratory therapist (RT) that we often forget how important these short interactions can be in determining the effectiveness of the care we provide. This chapter focuses on how RTs can use these encounters to promote high-quality care that is attentive to the needs and expectations of each individual patient.

## INDIVIDUALIZED CARE

Individualized care requires empathetic, two-way communication; respect for each patient's values and privacy; and sensitivity to cultural values.

**Individualized Care**
Empathetic communication
Respect for patient values/privacy
Sensitivity to cultural values

**Patient Involvement**
Patient education
Shared decision making
Patient participation in care

**Provider Collaboration**
Communication
Coordination
Shared responsibility

**FIG. 1.1** The essential elements of patient-centered care.

### Providing Empathetic Two-Way Communication

Underlying patient-centered communication is empathetic and effective communication. Communication, a two-way process, involves both sending and receiving meaningful messages. *If the receiver does not fully understand the message, effective communication has not occurred.* Multiple personal and environmental factors influence the effectiveness of communication during clinical encounters (Fig. 1.2). Attending to how each of these components may affect communication can make the difference between an effective and ineffective clinical encounter.

Each party to a clinical encounter brings attitudes and values developed by prior experiences, cultural heritage, religious beliefs, level of education, and self-concept. These personal factors affect the way a message is sent, as well as how it is interpreted and received. Messages can be sent many different ways and at times without awareness. Body movement, facial expression, touch, and eye movement are all types of nonverbal communication. Combined with voice tone, nonverbal cues frequently say more than words. Because one of the purposes of the encounter is to establish a trusting relationship with the patient, the clinician must make a conscious effort to send signals of genuine concern, to show compassion and empathize with the patient's circumstances. Techniques useful for this purpose are facing the patient squarely, using appropriate eye contact, maintaining an open posture, using touch, and actively listening. It also may be helpful to treat the patient as you would expect to be treated if in the patient's situation (the "golden rule" applied to bedside care).

One of the most common mistakes made by clinicians during patient encounters is failing to listen carefully to the patient. Good listening skills require concentration on the task at hand. Active listening also calls for replying to the patient's comments and questions with appropriate responses. Patients are quick to identify the clinician who is not listening and will often interpret this as a lack

INTERNAL FACTORS
Previous experiences
Attitudes, values
Cultural heritage
Religious beliefs
Self-concept
Listening habits
Preoccupations, feelings

SENSORY/EMOTIONAL FACTORS
Fear
Stress, anxiety
Pain
Mental acuity, brain damage, hypoxia
Sight, hearing, speech impairment

INTERNAL FACTORS
Previous experiences
Attitudes, values
Cultural heritage
Religious beliefs
Self-concept
Listening habits
Preoccupations, feelings
Illness

ENVIRONMENTAL FACTORS
Lighting
Noise
Privacy
Distance
Temperature

VERBAL EXPRESSION
Language barrier
Jargon
Choice of words/questions
Feedback, voice tone

NONVERBAL EXPRESSION
Body movement
Facial expression
Dress, professionalism
Warmth, interest

**FIG. 1.2** Factors influencing the effectiveness of communication during clinical encounters.

of empathy or concern. If the patient says something you do not understand, ask the patient to clarify what was said rather than replying with the response you think is right. Asking for clarification tells the patient that you want to make sure you get it right.

Messages are also altered by feelings, language differences, listening habits, comfort with the situation, and preoccupation. Patients experiencing pain or difficulty breathing will have a hard time concentrating on what you are communicating until their comfort is restored. The temperature, lighting, noise, and privacy of the environment also may affect comfort. Look for nonverbal cues of discomfort such as sighing, restlessness, looking into space, and avoiding eye contact.

Your use of communication techniques may differ according to the stage of interaction with a patient. Generally, a patient encounter begins with a chart review and then progresses through four additional stages: introductory, initial assessment, treatment and monitoring, and follow-up. Table 1.1 outlines the purpose of these stages and provides example strategies to help ensure effective communication during each major aspect of the patient encounter.

## Respecting Patient Needs and Preferences

Individualized care requires that providers respect each patient's needs, preferences, and privacy. Within this framework, we do not, for example, treat "the COPD patient in room 345," but a *patient with COPD*, whose ability to cope with its full range of physical and psychosocial consequences is unique. Effective therapy requires that the individual patient's response to disease be determined as part of the initial patient encounter. For patients with chronic afflictions regularly assess responses and adapt care plans accordingly.

Whenever possible, care plans also should reflect each individual patient's preferences. For example, after their urgent situation is resolved, patients with asthma should be allowed to participate in deciding which aerosol drug delivery system is best for them. Likewise, a patient with cystic fibrosis should be allowed to participate in selecting from a variety of equally effective airway clearance techniques. An individual's needs *during* treatment may involve modifying the therapy based on the patient's response.

## Ensuring Privacy and Confidentiality

We address privacy concerns in part by respecting personal space. Respecting patients' privacy rights is both a legal and a moral obligation for health care professionals.

To respect patients' personal space, understand both the general and cultural effects of proximity and direct contact.

| TABLE 1.1 | Stages of the Clinical Encounter | |
| --- | --- | --- |
| **Stage** | **Purpose** | **Communication Strategies** |
| Chart review (preinteraction) | Identifying key patient information | Apply this information in the introductory and initial assessment stages |
| Introductory | Introducing oneself<br>Confirming patient identity<br>Clarifying purpose/your role<br>Acknowledging family presence<br>Building rapport<br>Inspecting the patient (initial) | Look and act in professional manner<br>Refer to patient using formal last name<br>Avoid encroaching on personal space<br>Pay attention to nonverbal cues<br>Identify patient emotions<br>Express support and empathy (compassion)<br>React in nonjudgmental way |
| Initial assessment | Determining patient's status (interview and physical examination)<br>Determining learning needs<br>Assessing cultural differences<br>Determining appropriateness of orders (new Rx) | Use active listening<br>• Avoid interrupting the patient<br>• Use body position to indicate interest<br>• Avoid writing while patient is talking<br>• Make eye contact but do not stare<br>• Encourage open expression<br>Reflect what the patient shares<br>Summarize/request feedback<br>Make facilitative responses, e.g., nodding |
| Treatment and monitoring | Demonstrating/teaching treatment technique<br>Implementing and modifying treatment based on patient's preferences, monitored responses | Explain therapy in understandable terms<br>Invite questions about the treatment<br>Confirm acceptance of the treatment<br>Assess patient's concerns, expectations<br>Attend to patient discomfort |
| Follow-up | Confirming patient response<br>Developing shared goals<br>Ensuring follow-up<br>Restoring environment | Invite questions from patient and family<br>Determine information preferences<br>Check the patient's ability to follow the plan<br>Discuss follow-up (e.g., treatment schedule, what to do if symptoms worsen) |

*Rx*, Prescription.

**FIG. 1.3** Illustration of the social, personal, and intimate spaces characterizing the clinical encounter.

Fig. 1.3 shows the three zones of space commonly associated with the bedside patient encounter.

The social space (4 to 12 feet) is mainly used in the introductory stage of the encounter when you begin to establish rapport. At this distance, you can see the "big picture" and gain awareness of the whole patient and the patient's environment. Discussion is limited to the more formal issues. Avoid personal questions in this space because others in the room may overhear the conversation.

The personal space (18 inches to 4 feet) is used primarily during the interview component of the initial assessment, usually after establishing rapport with the patient. This enhanced proximity is generally needed to collect sensitive patient information, such as questions about daily sputum production or smoking habits. Pulling the bedside curtain may help the patient feel more comfortable about sharing personal information. Most patients also feel more comfortable and confident when your appearance is neat, clean, and professional. Patient trust can be enhanced by making appropriate eye contact while in the patient's personal space.

Intimate space (0 to 18 inches) is reserved primarily for the physical examination component and the treatment and monitoring stage of the encounter. Generally, moving into

such proximity and touching the patient should be done only after establishing rapport and being given permission to do so. Permission often is obtained by simply asking permission to listen to breath sounds or check vital signs. Doing this before moving into the intimate space communicates both your respect for patient privacy and your willingness to collaborate on decision making. *Minimal eye contact is used in this space.* Limit verbal communication to simple questions or brief requests, such as, "Please take a deep breath."

Some patients may respond poorly to encroachment into their space. Gender, age, race, physical appearance, health status, and cultural background are among the many factors that may influence a patient's comfort level when you enter the intimate space. If the patient's words or nonverbal responses indicate hesitancy with your actions, move more slowly and communicate your intent very carefully.

Related to the concept of proximity is that of territoriality. Removing items from the patient's "territory" should occur only after permission has been obtained. For example, when borrowing a chair from the bedside of Mr. Jones for use at the bedside of Mr. Smith, you should ask Mr. Jones for permission, being sure to replace any items temporarily removed from the patient's territory.

**SIMPLY STATED**

The social space (4 to 12 feet) is for introductions, the personal space (18 inches to 4 feet) is for interviewing, and the intimate space (0 to 18 inches) is for physical examination.

In regard to maintaining confidentiality, all health professionals manage sensitive patient information. For example, your chart review may reveal that a patient under your care has a history of drug abuse or has been diagnosed with a sexually transmitted disease. This information is private and not for public knowledge. You have both a legal and a moral obligation to keep this information in strictest confidence and share it only with other health professionals who have a need to know, such as the patient's nurse or attending physician. Most often, violations of patient confidentiality occur in public spaces while discussing patient information between caregivers and being overheard by visitors. *Discuss your patient's health status only with other members of the health care team who need to know such information and only in a private area where visitors are not allowed.*

Family members and visitors who ask about the patient's diagnosis should be referred to the health care provider. Most people will appreciate a polite and honest response in which you tell them that privacy rights prevent you from discussing the patient's diagnosis with others.

Your legal obligations regarding patient information are specified under the privacy and security rules of the Health Insurance Portability and Accountability Act (HIPAA). These rules establish regulations for the use and disclosure of Protected Health Information (PHI). PHI is any information about health status, provision of health care, or payment for health care services that can be linked to an individual. Examples of PHI include names and addresses, phone numbers, email addresses, Social Security and medical record numbers, and health insurance information. Under the law, patients control access to their PHI. For this reason, use or disclosure of PHI for purposes *other than* treatment, payment, health care operations, or public health requires patient permission (Table 1.2).

## Being Sensitive to Cultural Values

Individualized care requires sensitivity toward patients' cultural values and expectations. To establish collaboration with your patient, you'll need to identify and respond appropriately to the many cultural cues that can affect the clinical encounter and thus the success of therapy. Failure to do so can result in patient dissatisfaction, poor adherence to treatment regimens, and unsatisfactory health outcomes.

Some knowledge about specific cultural issues is helpful and can grow with experience. Aim to achieve at least a basic understanding of various cultures' beliefs. The growing diversity of the U.S. population makes it impossible to master all the nuances characterizing the many cultures now represented. Instead, one needs to develop culturally competent communication skills.

**TABLE 1.2  HIPAA-Related Privacy and Security Considerations**

| Do's | Don'ts |
|---|---|
| Do access only that information needed to perform your job | Don't discuss a patient's PHI with people with no need to know |
| Do keep voices low when discussing patient issues in joint treatment areas | Don't share your computer passwords and log-on information |
| Do provide only the minimal needed information on request | Don't leave a computer unattended without logging off |
| Do position workstations so that the screens are not visible to prying eyes | Don't discuss a patient's PHI in public settings where you can be overheard |
| Do keep patient information on whiteboards to a minimum | Don't communicate PHI by methods that the patient has not approved |
| Do place fax machines used to receive PHI in secure locations | Don't leave a patient's paper records open and available for prying eyes |

*PHI*, Protected Health Information.

Strategies for **culturally competent communication** are active listening, attending to individual needs, eliciting patient concerns, and expressing genuine concern. Apply these strategies during the initial assessment stage to briefly explore the patient's key cultural beliefs, especially those related to gender and family roles, responses to authority, personal space, religious values, and concepts of health and disease. For example, in some cultures it is normal to always defer to the authority of a doctor or health care provider when deciding what is best, so the provider's efforts to involve the patient in decision making may be difficult. Likewise, patients who believe that fate determines disease outcomes may be reluctant to participate in their own care. Reflecting on what the patient shares in a nonjudgmental way can help foster rapport and enhance one's ability to adapt to cultural differences.

Three additional abilities that enhance cultural competence are self-awareness, situational awareness, and adaptability. Self-awareness involves knowledge of one's own cultural beliefs, as well as any potential stereotypes one might hold about particular groups. By being self-aware, you can recognize in advance possible cultural prejudices or emotions you might have toward certain patients that might negate the impact on the care you provide. Situational awareness is the ability to recognize misunderstandings associated with patient-provider cultural differences as they occur during a patient encounter. For example, a woman who is constantly looking toward her husband for approval during a clinical interaction may be signaling a cultural tendency to defer to the man for all major decision making. The culturally competent clinician should be able to adapt to the specific situation by individualizing the communication approach in a manner consistent with the patient's (and family's) values and beliefs. In this case, consider reorienting the encounter by making the husband a major partner in the conversation.

## PATIENT INVOLVEMENT

Patient-centered care is a two-way street. To be successful, patient-centered care must involve the patient and family as partners in setting goals, making decisions, participating in the treatment regimen, providing appropriate self-care, and helping ensure safety. To meet these expectations, patients—especially those with chronic conditions—must understand the basics about their disease process and how to effectively manage it. This level of involvement can only occur when the clinician includes needed educational activities in each clinical encounter.

### Assessing Learning Needs and Providing Patient Education

Patient and caregiver education aims to promote healthy behaviors and increase patients' involvement in their health care and safety, resulting in outcomes that satisfy both patient and provider. Full achievement of this goal requires a comprehensive approach, and RTs are part of the interdisciplinary team that plays a key role in achievement of successful outcomes by providing appropriate patient education. The first step is to assess the patient's learning needs. In most hospitals, the initial assessment of learning needs is conducted by nursing staff, occurs after the patient is admitted to a care unit, and is documented in the patient's chart. For this reason, during your chart review you should access and evaluate this record for any important information helpful in planning the respiratory care of your patient.

Briefly conduct your own assessment, focusing on learning needs specific to the patient's disorder and the planned therapy. In general, learning needs assessment progresses through the following key steps:
1. Identify and accommodate barriers to patient learning
2. Assess the patient's preferred learning method
3. Evaluate the patient's readiness to learn
4. Determine the patient's specific learning needs

Table 1.3 identifies several of the barriers to learning commonly encountered by RTs in the clinical setting and various ways to accommodate them.

**TABLE 1.3 Barriers to Learning and Their Accommodation**

| Barrier to Learning | Accommodation |
|---|---|
| Age (young child) | Keep teaching/learning episodes short |
| | Use fun-and-games approach |
| | Enlist family assistance |
| Reduced level of consciousness | Postpone until patient becomes alert |
| | Apply methods that don't require cooperation |
| Presence of pain | Recommend analgesia |
| | Postpone until pain management is effective |
| Presence of anxiety | Take time to calm the patient and explain your actions |
| | Postpone until anxiety management is effective |
| | Enlist family assistance |
| | Recommend anxiolytic therapy |
| Physical limitations | Ascertain specific limitations |
| | Apply methods that circumvent limitation |
| | Enlist family assistance |
| Educational level (low) | Emphasize oral (vs. written) instruction |
| | Adjust language level as appropriate |
| | Provide written materials at fifth- to eighth-grade level |
| Potential language barrier | Enlist family assistance |
| | Secure translator |
| | Use an approved translation service |
| Cultural or religious factors | Ascertain key factors affecting care |
| | Modify to accommodate |
| | Enlist family assistance |
| Vision difficulty | Have patient wear glasses |
| | Emphasize sound and touch |
| | Enlist family assistance |
| Hearing difficulty | Speak slowly and clearly while facing the patient |
| | Have patient use hearing aid |
| | Emphasize visualization and touch |
| | Enlist family assistance |

From Scanlan CL, Heuer AJ: *Comprehensive respiratory therapy exam preparation guide,* Sudbury, MA, 2014, Jones & Bartlett Learning (www.jblearning.com). Reprinted with permission.

To assess a patient's preferred way of learning, first observe the environment for clues such as the presence of reading materials, use of television, or (for children) use of toys and games. You also should ask the patient about any recent learning efforts. Sometimes, preferred methods of learning can be determined from questions about the patient's work or hobbies.

Evaluating the patient's readiness to learn is the next step in assessing learning needs. Patients' spontaneous questions about their condition, its management, or their respiratory care indicate a desire to learn, as do expressions of discomfort with their current abilities or situation.

After you have addressed any barriers to learning and confirmed the patient's desire to progress, you should determine what the patient knows about the care you will provide. Ask relevant questions, using terms and language appropriate to

---

**BOX 1.1 Example Questions Assessing a Patient's Knowledge about a Medication**

Which medicine are you currently taking? How often?
Do you know why you are taking this medicine?
Who is responsible for administering the medicine?
Please show me how you take the medicine.
How many times a week do you miss taking the medicine?
What problems have you had taking the medicine (cost, time, lack of need)?
What concerns do you have about your medicine?

---

**BOX 1.2 Example Action Plan Developed by a Patient with Asthma**

**Action Plan**

1. **Goals** (something you *want* to do): cut school absences in half

   **How:** make sure I take my controller medicine as prescribed; avoid my triggers (pet hair and tobacco smoke); monitor my symptoms (cough, wheeze, chest tightness, shortness of breath); take my reliever if symptoms develop/worsen

   **Where:** administer meds at home (controller) and at home/school if reliever is needed

   **What:** controller: Pulmicort Flexhaler (b.i.d.); reliever: Proventil canister

   **When:** Pulmicort: AM/PM; Proventil puffs as needed; monitor symptoms

   **Frequency:** medications as prescribed; symptom monitoring daily using diary

2. **Barriers:** many friends smoke or have house pets; hate diary keeping

3. **Plans to overcome barriers:** avoid spending time indoors with smokers or pets; use Twitter to keep my diary entries

4. **Conviction:** 7/10 (being pushed by parents!); **confidence:** 9 (I'm stubborn)

5. **Follow-up:** track absences for the coming semester (goal is less than 5)

*b.i.d.,* Twice a day.

---

the patient's level of understanding. Questions in this phase of the assessment should address the following areas:

- Understanding of the current condition or disease process
- Knowledge of prescribed medications
- Familiarity with the procedures you will implement
- Familiarity with the equipment needed for care

Box 1.1 provides example questions focusing on a patient's knowledge about a prescribed medication.

A specific learning need is identified when any of the patient's answers indicates a knowledge deficit. In addition to assessing needs, you also should focus on determining "wants," meaning anything the patient wishes to learn more about. Together, these needs and wants can help establish education goals acceptable to both the patient and family.

After conducting any learning activity, evaluate the results. To evaluate a desired change in knowledge, have the patients repeat in their own words the information you are trying to communicate (the teach-back method). To confirm that your patients have learned how to perform a particular skill, have them perform a return demonstration—that is, going through the motions of the procedure shown to them.

## Sharing Goal-Setting and Decision-Making Responsibilities

Effective patient education is a requirement of shared responsibility for goal setting and decision making and collaboration between the patient and the health care interprofessional team, which is usually headed by the attending physician. In this regard, good communication within the team is essential. The RT's function within the team is to assess learning needs and also to help the patient set tangible goals related to the patient's respiratory care. Such goals may be as simple as a patient with cystic fibrosis selecting an airway clearance technique, or as complex as reaching agreement with the patient on an action plan for routine self-care of asthma and proper management of its exacerbations.

Written action plans are particularly useful for involving patients in goal-setting and self-care activities. Action plan goals should be *SMART,* that is, *s*pecific, *m*easurable, *a*ction oriented, *r*ealistic, and *t*ime limited. The action plan itself should address the following elements:

- Exactly what is the goal?
- How will the goal be achieved (e.g., how, how much, how often)?
- What barriers might prevent achieving the goal?
- How can barriers be overcome?
- By what mechanism will follow-up occur?
- How much confidence does the patient have in achieving the goal?

Box 1.2 provides an example of a simple action plan for an adolescent with moderate asthma who has a recent history of exacerbations causing frequent absences from school.

## Encouraging Patient and Family Participation in Care and Safety

Joint goal setting provides the basis for patient and family involvement in treatment regimens and ongoing self-care for those with chronic conditions. Given that the effectiveness of most respiratory care treatments requires patient cooperation and follow-through, you must constantly reiterate how better participation can result in better outcomes. A case in point is the daily tracking of symptoms that the patient with asthma included in her action plan (see Box 1.2). An acute care example is a patient with cystic fibrosis monitoring sputum production after self-administered positive airway pressure therapy. An illustration involving the family would be preparing a patient requiring long-term mechanical ventilation for discharge to home.

Involvement of the patient and family in care delivery also has been shown to enhance safety and reduce medical errors. The Joint Commission's Speak Up initiative provides excellent

Everyone has a role in making health care safe. The Joint Commission's Speak Up program gives simple advice on how you can help make health care a good experience. Research shows that patients who take part in decisions about their own health care are more likely to get better faster. To help prevent health care mistakes, patients are urged to "Speak Up."

S | Speak up if you have questions or concerns. If you still don't understand, ask again. It's your body and you have a right to know.

P | Pay attention to the care you get. Always make sure you're getting the right treatments and medicines by the right health care professionals. Don't assume anything.

E | Educate yourself about your illness. Learn about the medical tests you get, and your treatment plan.

A | Ask a trusted family member or friend to be your advocate (advisor or supporter).

K | Know what medicines you take and why you take them. Medicine errors are the most common health care mistakes.

U | Use a hospital, clinic, surgery center, or other type of health care organization that has been carefully checked out. For example, The Joint Commission visits hospitals to see if they are meeting The Joint Commission's quality standards.

P | Participate in all decisions about your treatment. You are the center of the health care team.

The Joint Commission, Oakbrook Terrace, IL, www.jointcommission.org/speakup.aspx

guidance in this regard (Box 1.3). Although most hospitals orient patients to this initiative on admission, RTs should use the clinical encounter to reinforce this important role.

To further promote infection control, instruct all patients, family members, and visitors with signs or symptoms of a respiratory infection to follow the Centers for Disease Control and Prevention (CDC) guidance on respiratory hygiene and cough etiquette:

- Cover the nose and mouth when coughing or sneezing
- Use tissues to contain respiratory secretions
- Dispose of tissues in the nearest hands-free waste receptacle after use
- Perform hand hygiene after contacting secretions or contaminated objects

**SIMPLY STATED**

Involve the patient and family in care delivery to enhance safety and reduce medical errors. RTs should orient patients and their families to their role in helping ensure safety using strategies such as The Joint Commission's Speak Up initiative and sharing the CDC guidance on respiratory hygiene and cough etiquette.

Clinicians themselves should implement infection control procedures before, during, and after all patient encounters.

At a minimum, this involves application of standard precautions (Box 1.4). Proper hand hygiene is the single most important element in preventing spread of infection. Alcohol-based rubs are the preferred method, except when one's hands become visibly soiled with dirt, blood, or body fluids or when caring for patients with infectious diarrhea (e.g., *Clostridium difficile*, norovirus). In these cases, one should proceed with a vigorous soap and water handwashing for at least 15 seconds.

## PROVIDER COLLABORATION

Medicine is now too complex and far too evolved for any one individual to have the whole picture. Quality patient-centered care requires that all patient providers work together as a team. When health care professionals fail to collaborate effectively, patient safety becomes at risk. Ineffective provider collaboration can result in increased length of stay, wasted resources, and poor patient outcomes.

Collaboration occurs when health care providers assume complementary roles and cooperatively work together, sharing responsibility for patient care. To maximize their impact on patient outcomes, RTs must integrate their services with other providers' services by participating in interprofessional communication, interdisciplinary coordination, and sharing of responsibilities.

### Enhancing Interprofessional Communication

The Joint Commission defines *effective communication* as being timely, accurate, complete, unambiguous, and understood by the recipient. Because good interprofessional communication is essential to quality care, all RTs must exhibit these skills, particularly when receiving orders, coordinating the patient's care, reporting the patient's clinical status, and helping plan for patient discharge.

Often, a clinical encounter begins with receipt of an order from an authorized health care provider, such as a physician, physician's assistant, or nurse practitioner. In general, clinicians should not accept orders transmitted to you by unauthorized third parties, such as registered nurses. If an order is transmitted to you by a third party, you must verify the order in the patient's medical record before proceeding unless it follows an institutional protocol. If the order is transmitted orally and you are authorized to take it, you should repeat the order back to verify its accuracy, which is known as closed-loop communication. The following actions should be taken to avoid such errors:

- Record the complete order in the medical record as it is being transmitted.
- Read the order back to the originator to verify its accuracy.
- Time and date the order with the name and credentials of the originator, specify "read back and confirmed," and provide your signature and credentials.

All respiratory care orders must be verified as accurate and complete. Should any element of an order be missing

## BOX 1.4 CDC Standard Precautions

### Hand Hygiene
Always perform hand hygiene in the following situations:
- Before touching a patient, even if gloves will be worn
- After contact with a patient and before leaving the patient care area
- After contact with blood, body fluids, excretions, or wound dressings
- Before performing an aseptic task (e.g., accessing a vascular port)
- Whenever hands move from a contaminated body area to a clean area
- After glove removal

### Gloves
Wear gloves when there is potential contact with blood, body fluids, mucous membranes, nonintact skin, or contaminated equipment.
- Wear gloves that fit appropriately (select gloves according to hand size)
- Do not wear the same pair of gloves for the care of more than one patient
- Do not wash gloves for the purpose of reuse
- Perform hand hygiene before and immediately after removing gloves

### Gowns
Wear a gown to protect skin and clothing during procedures or activities in which contact with blood or body fluids is anticipated.
- Do not wear the same gown for the care of more than one patient
- Remove gown and perform hand hygiene before leaving the patient's environment (e.g., examination room)

### Facemasks, Eye Protection, Respirators
Use a facemask during patient care activities likely to generate splashes or sprays of blood, body fluids, or secretions—especially during airway suctioning (using a standard catheter), endotracheal intubation, catheter insertion, and encounters with any patient under droplet precautions.
- Personal eyeglasses and contact lenses do not provide adequate eye protection
- Use goggles with facemasks, or face shield alone, to protect the mouth, nose, and eyes
- Wear an N95 or higher respirator when there is potential exposure to infectious agents transmitted by the airborne route (e.g., tuberculosis)

### Soiled Patient Care Equipment
Handle in a manner to prevent contact with skin or mucous membranes and to prevent contamination of clothing or the environment.
- Wear gloves
- Perform hand hygiene after handling

### Needles and Other Sharps
- Receive training on how to use sharps safety devices; assess hazards
- Keep exposed sharp in view; be aware of others around you
- Avoid hand passing sharps and use verbal alerts when moving sharps
- Activate safety features after use
- Place used sharps in puncture-resistant container; keep fingers away from openings (Centers for Disease Control and Prevention, http://www.cdc.gov/sharpssafety/)

### Patient Resuscitation
- Use mouthpiece with one-way valve, resuscitation bag, and other ventilation devices to prevent contact with mouth and oral secretions (Centers for Disease Control and Prevention, http://cdc.gov.)

---

or unclear, contact the prescriber for clarification before implementing the request. The same procedure applies if the order falls outside one's institutional standards. For example, if the order specifies an abnormally high drug dosage or includes a ventilator setting not normally applied in similar cases, you contact the prescriber and request an explanation before proceeding. More detail on standards for order writing and order taking is provided in Chapter 21.

After most patient encounters, communicate your findings to other members of the health care team. Written documentation in the patient's chart may suffice if the patient is stable after routine treatment. Whenever a patient's condition changes or a procedure is poorly tolerated, in addition to providing written documentation, you *must* communicate your findings orally to the patient's nurse and physician. In this case, your chart documentation should include not only your findings but also who was notified about the change in the patient's condition.

For example, on entering the room of Mr. Jones to provide treatment for his asthma, you note that he appears much more short of breath than usual. The treatment you give him does not appear to help. Document and communicate your findings. Oral discussion with the patient's nurse is a good place to start. Notify the patient's physician of the change in Mr. Jones' condition when warranted. Next, you must document the patient's condition in his chart and note whom you communicated with about the patient and what was said. If there is evidence of deteriorating vital signs, you should activate the Medical Emergency or Rapid Response Team and support the patient until the team arrives.

### SIMPLY STATED

Whenever you observe a change in a patient's condition, note your observations in the chart, orally report your findings to the patient's nurse, and document in writing whom you notified about the situation.

## Coordinating Patient Care

RTs also need to help coordinate their patients' care. To do so, you need to communicate with the interdisciplinary team to schedule procedures at times least likely to conflict with other essential patient activity and most likely to coincide with any relevant drug regimen. For example, you would communicate with nursing to ensure that before implementing a ventilator-weaning trial, sedation has been appropriately lowered or held back from the patient.

Another key aspect related to good communication and coordinating patient care is the patient "handoff." Common patient handoffs occur when delivering a patient to or receiving a patient from a care unit or diagnostic facility, when providing patient reports at shift change, or when having a colleague take over in an emergency situation. Ideally, communication during such handoffs should be short but precise, giving the essential information needed by the recipient. One method for standardizing these brief episodes is the SBAR format. Using this format, communication about your patient should address the following four essential elements: *situation, background, assessment, recommendation*. The same format also can be used when making recommendations to the patient's physician for a change in therapy or when documenting a patient encounter in the medical record. Chapter 21 provides more detail on the appropriate use of this communication tool, including an example.

Patient care should not end abruptly at hospital discharge. Ideally, an interdisciplinary posthospitalization care plan should be developed based on each patient's individual needs and consistent with current guidelines for managing the patient's condition. Such plans normally are ordered by the patient's primary care provider and coordinated by a nurse practitioner or case manager. As identified by the American Association for Respiratory Care (AARC), patient discharge plans should include the following:

- A time frame for implementation
- Clearly defined responsibilities of team members for daily care
- Mechanisms for communication among members of the health care team
- Arrangements for patient integration back into the community
- Plans for medication administration
- Strategies for patient self-care as appropriate
- Mechanisms for securing and training caregivers
- Plans for monitoring and responding to changes in the patient's condition
- Alternative emergency and contingency plans
- Plans for use, maintenance, and troubleshooting of equipment
- Methods for ongoing assessment of outcomes
- Specification of follow-up mechanisms

RTs should participate in discharge planning for patients with respiratory-related diagnoses. For example, to help prevent exacerbations and readmission of a patient with asthma, RTs help coordinate plans for aerosol drug therapy (based on assessment of learning needs), develop strategies for patient self-care, participate as appropriate in caregiver training, establish action plans for responding to changes in the patient's condition, plan for equipment needs, and specify approaches for assessing patient progress. More detail on the role of the RT in assessing the patient and planning for care at home is provided in Chapter 20.

## Sharing Responsibility

Truly integrated care requires that all the clinicians involved in a patient's management share a common set of goals and assume joint responsibility for their achievement. Ideally, each team member should be tasked with addressing a particular patient problem. For example, an RT working in the intensive care unit may be given primary responsibility for implementing a ventilator-weaning protocol. However, the team as a whole must coordinate these individual efforts and evaluate their overall success.

Team membership depends on each patient's unique set of problems. As experts on respiratory care, RTs function as vital members of teams supporting management of patients with both chronic and acute cardiopulmonary disorders. In terms of sharing responsibility for the management of chronic disorders such as chronic obstructive pulmonary disease (COPD), respiratory therapists should assume responsibility for providing patient education about the nature of the disease process, train patients in applicable self-care techniques (such as aerosol drug administration), and help patients develop good action plans to deal with exacerbations. In regard to shared responsibility for management of patients with acute care needs, working as a team member to prevent ventilator-associated pneumonia and weaning a patient from ventilatory support are good examples.

The best-documented approach to sharing responsibility for patients in acute care settings is to combine interdisciplinary intensive care unit rounds with a daily goals form (Fig. 1.4). The form facilitates communication during rounds by requiring team members, including RTs, to state their goals, the tasks needed to achieve them, and how they will communicate with the patient, family, and other caregivers. All members of the team then review the goals during each shift and modify or update them as needed. For example, an RT sets a goal for a newly intubated patient with acute respiratory distress syndrome (ARDS) of reducing the patient's plateau pressure below 30 cm $H_2O$ while maintaining adequate ventilation. Tasks involved might include making incremental adjustments in the tidal volume and rate according to the ARDSNet protocol while monitoring changes in arterial pH. As the patient's status improves, the therapist would recommend new goals, such as reducing the fraction of inspired oxygen ($Fio_2$) or positive end-expiratory pressure levels, with the ultimate aim being extubation and removal of ventilatory support. With the therapist being a key contributor to the management team, the full potential of the patient clinical encounter can be realized.

| DAILY GOALS | | | |
|---|---|---|---|
| **Room Number:** | | **Date:** | |
| **Attending initials:** | | **Initial as Goals Are Reviewed** | |
| **Goals+** | **0700-1500** | **1500-2300** | **2300-0700** |
| What needs to be done to discharge the patient from the ICU? | | | |
| What is this patient's greatest safety risk? How can we reduce that risk? | | | |
| Pain management/sedation | | | |
| Cardiac/volume status | | | |
| Pulmonary/ventilator (PP, VAP bundle) | | | |
| Mobilization | | | |
| Infectious disease, cultures, drug levels | | | |
| GI/nutrition | | | |
| Medication changes (can any be discontinued?) | | | |
| Tests/procedures | | | |
| Review scheduled labs; morning labs and CXR | | | |
| Consultations | | | |
| Communication with primary service | | | |
| Family communication | | | |
| Can catheters/tubes be removed? | | | |
| Is this patient receiving DVT/PUD prophylaxis? | | | |
| +PP, plateau pressure; HOB, head of bed; GI, gastrointestinal; labs, laboratory tests; CXR, chest radiograph; DVT, deep venous thrombosis; PUD, peptic ulcer disease | | | |

**FIG. 1.4** Daily goals form. (Adapted from Pronovost P, Berenholtz S, Dorman T, et al: Improving communication in the ICU using daily goals. *J Crit Care* 18(2):71–75, 2003.)

## KEY POINTS

- Patient-centered care involves three key elements: individualized care, patient involvement, and provider collaboration.
- Communication during a clinical encounter is affected by the attitudes and values of the clinician and patient, one's choice of words, nonverbal expressions, and environmental factors.
- A patient encounter generally begins with a chart review and then progresses through four stages: introductory, initial assessment, treatment and monitoring, and follow-up; communication strategies vary according to the purpose of each stage.
- Whenever possible, respiratory care plans should reflect each patient's preferences.
- Use the social space (4 to 12 feet) during the introductory stage of the clinical encounter to establish rapport, the personal space (18 inches to 4 feet) for the interview, and the intimate space (0 to 18 inches) to conduct the physical examination and apply and monitor therapy; enter the intimate space only after gaining patient permission.
- Discuss your patient's health status only with other members of the health care team who need to know such information and only in private locations where others cannot overhear; always refer questions about your patient's diagnosis to the attending physician.

- The culturally competent clinician is a good communicator who is aware of his or her own cultural beliefs and can recognize and adapt to differences in values and beliefs during the clinical encounter.
- Patients and their families should be engaged as partners in setting health care goals, making decisions, participating in the treatment regimen, providing appropriate self-care, and helping ensure safety.
- To assess a patient's learning needs, (1) identify and accommodate any barriers to learning, (2) assess the patient's preferred learning method, (3) evaluate the patient's readiness to learn, and (4) determine the patient's specific learning needs.
- Involve patients in goal-setting and self-care activities using a written action plan that specifies a measurable goal, the actions needed to achieve the goal (including barriers to overcome), and an appropriate follow-up mechanism.
- During clinical encounters, orient patients and their families to their role in helping ensure safety using strategies such as The Joint Commission's Speak Up initiative and sharing the CDC guidance on respiratory hygiene and cough etiquette.
- Proper hand hygiene is the single most important element in preventing spread of infection in the hospital.

- If any element of a respiratory care order is missing, is unclear, or falls outside institutional protocols, you must contact the prescriber for clarification before implementing the request.
- To coordinate your patient's care with that provided by others, communicate with the patient's nurse or team to schedule therapy at times least likely to conflict with other essential activities and most likely to coincide with any relevant drug regimen.
- Whenever you observe a change in a patient's condition or judge that a procedure was poorly tolerated, you must communicate your findings orally to the patient's nurse and physician and document in writing whom you notified about the situation; if the change involves deteriorating vital signs, call for the Medical Emergency or Rapid Response Team, and support the patient until the team arrives.
- To effectively communicate relevant information about your patient during handoffs to others, use the SBAR format (*situation, background, assessment, recommendation*).
- To enhance outcomes in critical care settings, RTs should participate in interdisciplinary rounds and be responsible for communicating the essential respiratory-related daily goals and tasks needed to achieve them, as well as coordinating these efforts with other members of the team.

## ASSESSMENT QUESTIONS

1. Which of the following are key elements in the provision of patient-centered care?
   1. Patient involvement
   2. Individualized care
   3. Legal representation
   4. Provider collaboration
      a. 1 and 2
      b. 1, 2, and 4
      c. 3 and 4
      d. 1, 2, 3, and 4
2. After a postoperative patient you are interviewing grimaces while holding her abdomen, you note some confusion about her responses. Which of the following factors likely is affecting communication?
   a. Self-concept
   b. Listening habits
   c. Pain and anxiety
   d. Hearing impairment
3. Active listening is most essential during what stage of the clinical encounter?
   a. Introductory stage
   b. Initial assessment stage
   c. Treatment and monitoring stage
   d. Follow-up stage
4. After several attempts to instruct a patient with COPD on the proper use of a metered-dose inhaler, the patient complains of the inability to master the correct technique. Applying patient-centered principles, you should:
   a. Request permission from the patient's doctor to find a more acceptable delivery system
   b. Cease trying to train the patient and recommend discontinuing the therapy
   c. Push the patient to keep practicing until a return demonstration indicates competency
   d. Chart the treatment as not given and return for another try on second rounds
5. In which of the following spaces is patient rapport best established?
   a. Social
   b. Personal

   c. Intimate
   d. Territorial
6. Which of the following violates HIPAA-related privacy and security rules?
   a. Providing the minimal needed patient information on request
   b. Never keeping patient information on a white board near the hallway or other public place
   c. Discussing a patient's health status with the nurse at the bedside
   d. Leaving a computer unattended without logging off
7. Which of the following cultural beliefs should be explored with your patients during the initial assessment stage of the clinical encounter?
   1. Concepts of health and disease
   2. Responses to authority
   3. Gender and family roles
   4. Religious values
      a. 1 and 2
      b. 3 and 4
      c. 1, 2, and 3
      d. 1, 2, 3, and 4
8. For most respiratory care to succeed, patients need to:
   a. Have at least a high-school education
   b. Actively participate in the treatment regimen
   c. Demonstrate good hand-eye coordination
   d. Be at least somewhat fluent in English
9. During an initial patient encounter, you note that the patient's acute anxiety appears to be affecting your ability to help her learn more about her disease process. To overcome this problem, you would consider all of the following *except:*
   a. Recommending that the doctor prescribe an analgesic
   b. Enlisting family assistance to calm the patient down
   c. Recommending that the doctor prescribe an anxiolytic
   d. Postponing further efforts until anxiety management is effective
10. A good patient action plan should include which of the following elements?
    1. Actions needed to achieve the goal
    2. Barriers to goal achievement

3. A specific, measurable goal
4. A follow-up mechanism
   a. 3 and 4
   b. 1 and 2
   c. 1, 2, and 3
   d. 1, 2, 3, and 4

11. While supervising a respiratory therapy student, you observe that an anxious patient asks her if the aerosol bronchodilator she is about to deliver has any bad effects. The student replies, "None to worry about." After the treatment session is over, you should explain to the student that:
    a. Only the patient's doctor should be discussing medication effects with the patient
    b. Her reply was consistent with what the patient needs to know
    c. Patients should be encouraged to ask questions about their medications
    d. Her reply was good—no need to further worry an anxious patient

12. For a clinical encounter with a patient on airborne precautions, you should:
    a. Wear goggles or an eye shield
    b. Wear a properly fitting N95 respirator
    c. Perform a surgical hand scrub
    d. Don sterile gloves

13. A patient responds poorly to a treatment you have given. After ensuring that the patient is stable, you should:
    a. Carefully note the patient's response to treatment in the patient's chart
    b. Speak with the patient's nurse, chart the response, and chart whom you notified
    c. Orally notify the patient's nurse of his poor response to treatment
    d. Request that the patient's physician discontinue the therapy

14. SBAR stands for:
    a. Situation, Background, Ailments, Requests
    b. Situation, Background, Assessment, Recommendation
    c. Scenario, Background, Assessment, Room Number
    d. Situation, Blood type, Assessment, Recommendation

15. All of the following are appropriate roles for a respiratory therapist serving on a team managing a patient with COPD *except*:
    a. Helping the patient develop good action plans
    b. Training the patient in self-care techniques
    c. Recommending changes in diet and nutrition
    d. Providing patient education about the disease

## BIBLIOGRAPHY

Bernacki RE, Block SD. American College of Physicians High Value Care Task Force: Communication about serious illness care goals: a review and synthesis of best practices. *JAMA Intern Med* 2014;**174**(12):1994–2003.

Betancourt JR. Cultural competence and medical education: many names, many perspectives, one goal. *Acad Med* 2006;**81**(6):499–501.

Engebretson J, Mahoney J, Carlson ED. Cultural competence in the era of evidence-based practice. *J Prof Nurs* 2008;**24**(3):172–8.

Jayadevappa R, Chhatre S. Patient centered care—a conceptual model and review of the state of the art. *Open Health Serv Policy J* 2011;**4**:15–25.

The Joint Commission. *Advancing effective communication, cultural competence, and patient- and family-centered care: a roadmap for hospitals.* Oakbrook Terrace, IL: The Joint Commission; 2014.

Kacmarek RM, Stoller JK, Heuer AJ. *Egan's fundamentals of respiratory care.* 11th ed. St. Louis: Mosby-Elsevier; 2017.

Lein C, Wills CE. Using patient-centered interviewing skills to manage complex patient encounters in primary care. *J Am Acad Nurse Pract* 2007;**19**(5):215–20.

Makoul G. Essential elements of communication in medical encounters: the Kalamazoo consensus statement. *Acad Med* 2001;**76**(4):390–3.

Mochan E, Nash D. Weaving quality improvement and patient safety skills into all levels of medical training: an annotated bibliography. *Am J Med Qual* 2015;**30**(3):232–47.

Pronovost P, Berenholtz S, Dorman T, et al. Improving communication in the ICU using daily goals. *J Crit Care* 2003;**18**(2):71–5.

Purkaple BA, Mold JW, Chen S. Encouraging patient-centered care by including quality-of-life questions on pre-encounter forms. *Ann Fam Med* 2016;**14**(3):221–6.

Robinson JH, Callister LC, Berry JA, et al. Patient-centered care and adherence: definitions and applications to improve outcomes. *J Am Acad Nurse Pract* 2008;**20**(12):600–7.

Scanlan CL, Heuer AJ. *Comprehensive respiratory therapy exam preparation guide.* 2nd ed. Sudbury, MA: Jones & Bartlett; 2015.

Siegel JD, Rhinehart E, Jackson M, et al. *Guideline for isolation precautions: preventing transmission of infectious agents in healthcare settings.* Atlanta, GA: Centers for Disease Control and Prevention; 2007.

Teal CR, Street RL. Critical elements of culturally competent communication in the medical encounter: a review and model. *Soc Sci Med* 2009;**68**(3):533–43.

# The Medical History and the Interview

*Albert J. Heuer*

## LEARNING OBJECTIVES

*After reading this chapter, you will be able to:*

1. Recognize the importance of properly obtaining and recording a patient history.
2. Describe the techniques for structuring the interview.
3. Summarize the techniques used in interviewing.
4. Identify alternative sources available for the patient history.
5. Define the difference between objective and subjective data and the difference between signs and symptoms.
6. Describe the components of a complete health history and the type of information found in each section of the history.
7. Describe the value in reviewing the following parts of a patient's chart: (1) admission notes, (2) physician orders, (3) progress notes.
8. Summarize what is indicated by a DNR order and label on the patient's chart, as well as an advance directive.

## OUTLINE

## KEY TERMS

advance directive
do not attempt to resuscitate (DNAR)/do not resuscitate (DNR)

electronic medical record (EMR)
objective data
pack-years
pertinent negatives

pertinent positives
signs
subjective data
symptoms

The history is the foundation of patient assessment. It is a recorded picture of the patient's perception of his or her past and present health status and how health problems have affected both personal and family lifestyle. Properly performed, it generally provides an organized, unbiased, and detailed sequence of symptom development causing the patient to seek health care. The history guides the rest of the assessment process: physical examination, x-ray and laboratory studies, and special diagnostic procedures. When skillfully obtained, the history often contributes in a significant way to an accurate diagnosis. It is believed by many clinicians that an accurate diagnosis can often be made after the history has been obtained and before the physical examination begins.

Traditionally, the task of obtaining a patient's complete history has belonged to the physician, and only sections of the history were taken by other members of the health care team. Today, however, complete health histories are taken by nurses and physician assistants. In addition, physical therapists, social workers, dietitians, and respiratory therapists (RTs) obtain medical histories from patients, with an emphasis on information pertaining to their specialty.

Regardless of whether a student or clinician is expected to obtain and write a comprehensive history, each must be able to locate and interpret historical information recorded in the patient's medical record. The information is used with other assessment data and provides the foundation for communication to enable many medical disciplines to collectively develop or alter a plan of care. In addition, identifying the patient's symptoms and changes in those symptoms permits the patient care team to assess the effect of therapeutic interventions and overall progress.

This chapter highlights interviewing principles and describes the types of questions used in history taking and the content of the comprehensive health history, emphasizing specific information needed for assessment of the patient with cardiopulmonary complaints. Chapter 3 discusses the most common cardiopulmonary symptoms.

### SIMPLY STATED

The history is the foundation of comprehensive assessment—a recorded picture of the patient's perception of his or her health status, current problem, and effectiveness of treatment. It comprises subjective data—information that the patient reports, feels, or experiences that cannot be perceived by an observer.

## PATIENT INTERVIEW

### Principles of Communication

Communication is a process of imparting a meaningful message. The principles and practices of effective communication, which are outlined in Chapter 1, help form the basis for a properly conducted patient interview. Multiple personal, cultural, and environmental factors affect the way both patients and health care professionals communicate during an interview. As a result, attention to the effects each of these components may have on communication makes the difference between an effective and an ineffective interview.

### Structuring the Interview

The ideal interview, whether a 5-minute assessment of therapy or a 50-minute history, is one in which the patient feels secure and free to talk about important personal things. Interviewing is an art that takes time and experience to develop. It is a skill as useful in daily patient care as it is to the person obtaining a comprehensive history. Your ability to project a sense of undivided interest in the patient is the key to a successful interview and patient rapport. As such, it is generally best to review records or new information and prepare equipment and charting materials before entering the room. When practical, the RT or other clinician should know all available details of the patient case before the interview is started.

1. Your introduction establishes your professional role, asks permission to be involved in the patient's care, and conveys your interest in the patient.
   - Identify any language barriers, and make appropriate accommodation (translator services).
   - Dress and groom professionally.
   - Enter with a smile and an unhurried manner.
   - Make immediate eye contact, and if the patient is well enough, introduce yourself with a firm handshake or other appropriate greeting.
   - State your role and the purpose of your visit, and define the patient's involvement in the interaction.
   - Call the patient by name. A person's name is one of the most important things in the world to that person; use it to identify the patient and establish the fact that you are concerned with the patient as an individual. Address adult patients by title—Mr., Mrs., Miss, or Ms.—and their last name. Occasionally, patients will ask to be called by their first name or nickname, but that is the patient's choice and not an assumption to be made by the health care professional. Keep in mind that by using the more formal terms of address, you alert the patient to the importance of the interaction.
2. Professional conduct shows your respect for the patient's beliefs, attitudes, and rights and enhances patient rapport.
   - Be sure the patient is appropriately covered.
   - Position yourself so that eye contact is comfortable for the patient. Ideally, patients should be sitting up with their eye level with or slightly above yours, which suggests that their opinion is important, too. Avoid positions that require the patient to look directly into the light.
   - Avoid standing at the foot of the bed or with your hand on the door while you talk with the patient. This may send the nonverbal message that you do not have time for the patient.
   - Ask the patient's permission before moving any personal items or making adjustments in the room (see Chapter 1).
   - Remember, the patient's dialogue with you and the patient's medical record are confidential. The patient expects and the law demands that this information be shared only with other professionals directly involved in the patient's care. When a case is discussed for teaching purposes, the patient's identity should be protected.
   - Be honest. Never guess at an answer or information you do not know. Remember, too, that you have no right to provide information beyond your scope of practice. Providing new information to the patient is the privilege and responsibility of the attending physician.
   - Make no moral judgments about the patient. Set your values for patient care according to the patient's values, beliefs, and priorities.
   - Be mindful and respectful of cultural, ethnic, religious, and other forms of diversity (see Chapter 1).

- Expect a patient to have an emotional response to illness and the health care environment, and accept that response. Listen, then clarify and teach, but never argue. If you are not prepared to explore the issues with the patient, ask another clinician to do so.
- Adjust the time, length, and content of the interaction to your patient's needs. If the patient is in distress, obtain only the information necessary to clarify immediate needs. It may be necessary to repeat some questions later, to schedule several short interviews, or to obtain the information from other sources.

3. A relaxed, conversational style on the part of the health care professional with questions and statements that communicate empathy encourages patients to express their concerns.

- Expect and accept some periods of silence in a long or first interview. Both you and the patient need short periods to think out the correct responses.
- Close even the briefest interview by asking if there is anything else the patient needs or wants to discuss and telling the patient when you will return.

### SIMPLY STATED

A patient interview, whether a short assessment of therapy or an extended history, must allow the patient to feel secure and free to discuss personal things. Based on the material in this and the Chapter 01, be mindful of the following best practices:

- Identify language barriers before the patient encounter, and take appropriate action (translator services).
- Dress and act professionally.
- Prepare by reviewing relevant records in advance.
- Project a sense of undivided interest.
- Use a relaxed conversational style.
- Respect your patients' beliefs and attitudes.
- Remember to reassure your patients that their conversations with you, as well as their medical records, are confidential.

### Questions and Statements Used to Facilitate Conversational Interviewing

An interview made up of one direct question followed by an answer and another direct question is mechanical, monotonous, and anxiety producing. Frankly, such an approach can make patients feel as though they are being interrogated. In addition, this type of interview usually takes longer and acquires less pertinent information than a more casual, conversational interview. A rambling discussion is also inefficient and frustrating. Therefore a conversational style that combines the types of questions and responses as described in the following list encourages open and honest descriptions by the patient, family member, or other historian while giving enough direction to clarify, quantify, and qualify details.

1. Open-ended questions encourage patients to describe events and priorities as they see them and thereby help bring out concerns and attitudes and promote understanding. Questions such as "What prompted you to come to the hospital?" or "What happened next?" encourage conversational flow and rapport while giving patients enough direction to know where to start.

2. Closed questions such as "When did your cough start?" or "How long did the pain last?" focus on specific information and provide clarification.

3. Direct questions can be either open-ended or closed questions and always end in a question mark. Although they are used to obtain specific information, a series of direct questions or frequent use of "Why?" can sound intimidating.

4. Indirect questions are less threatening because they sound like statements: "I gather your doctor told you to monitor your peak expiratory flow rates every day." Inquiries of this type also work well to confront discrepancies in the patient's statements: "If I understood you correctly, it is harder for you to breathe now than it was yesterday."

5. Neutral questions and statements are preferred for all interactions with the patient. "What happened next?" and "Tell me more about . . ." are neutral open-ended questions. A neutral closed question might give a patient a choice of responses while focusing on the type of information desired: "Would you say there was a teaspoon, a tablespoon, or a half-cup?" By contrast, leading questions such as "You didn't cough up blood, did you?" should be avoided because they imply a desired response.

6. Reflecting (echoing) is repeating words, thoughts, or feelings the patient has just stated and is a successful way to clarify and stimulate the patient to elaborate on a particular point. For example, saying to the patient, "So you just said that you could not breathe well and your cough was getting worse for about a week," might encourage the patient to relay more information. However, overuse of reflecting can make the interviewer sound like a parrot.

7. Facilitating phrases, such as "yes" or "umm" or "I see," used while establishing eye contact and perhaps nodding your head, show interest and encourage patients to continue their story, but this type of phrase should not be overused.

8. Communicating support (empathy) with statements such as "That must have been very hard for you" shows your concern for the patient as a human being. Showing the patient that you really care about how life situations have caused stress, hurt, or unhappiness tells the patient it is safe to risk being honest about real concerns. Other techniques for showing empathy are described in Chapter 1.

### Alternative Sources for a Patient History

Various factors affect the patient's ability or willingness to provide an accurate history. Age, alterations in level of consciousness, language and cultural barriers, emotional state, medications, inability to breathe comfortably, and the acuteness of the disease process may alter a patient's ability to communicate. For instance, the patient suffering an acute asthma attack or someone just admitted to an intensive care unit may be unable to give even a brief history. Patients with long-standing chronic disease may have become so accustomed to the accompanying symptoms, or their lives may have changed so gradually, that they may minimize and even deny symptoms. In addition, some aspects of the history may be embarrassing to the patient, such as smoking history or alcohol use. In such cases, family members, friends, work associates, previous physicians, and past medical records often can provide a more accurate picture of the history and progression of symptoms. Keeping these possibilities in mind, most hospital histories begin with a one- or two-sentence description of the current state of the patient, the source of the history, and a statement of the estimated reliability of the historian.

## CARDIOPULMONARY HISTORY AND COMPREHENSIVE HEALTH HISTORY

Abnormalities of the respiratory system frequently reflect other systemic disease processes. In addition, alterations in pulmonary function may affect other body systems. Therefore cardiopulmonary assessment cannot be limited to the chest, and a complete evaluation of the patient's entire health status is essential. A detailed discussion of all aspects of obtaining and recording such a health history is beyond the scope of this text but has been well covered by other authors (see the Bibliography). This section provides an overview of the content of complete health histories and discusses specifically (in their classic order) chief complaint, history of present illness, past history, family history, and occupational and environmental history.

### Variations in Health Histories

Health (medical) histories vary in length, organization, and content, depending on the preparation and experience of the interviewer, the patient's age, the reason for obtaining the history, and the circumstances surrounding the visit or admission. A history taken for a 60-year-old person complaining of chronic and debilitating symptoms is much more detailed and complex than that obtained for a summer camp application or a school physical examination. Histories recorded in emergency situations are usually limited to describing events surrounding the patient's immediate condition. In such situations it is often difficult to get a thorough history, unless the patient is accompanied by someone who can speak on his or her behalf. Nursing histories emphasize the effect of the symptoms on activities of daily living and the identification of the unique care, teaching, and emotional support needs of the patient and family. Histories performed by physicians often focus on making a diagnosis. Because diagnosis and initial treatment may be done before there is time to dictate or record the history, the experienced physician may record data obtained from a combination of the history, physical examination, laboratory tests, and x-ray films rather than the more traditional history outlined in Box 2.1.

### General Content of Health Histories

Although variations in recording styles exist, all histories contain the following same types of information:
- General background information
- Screening information
- Descriptions of present health status or illness

---

**BOX 2.1   Outline of a Complete Health History**

1. Demographic data (usually found on first page of chart): name, address, age, birth date, birthplace, race, nationality, marital status, religion, occupation, source of referral
2. Date and source of history, estimate of historian's reliability ("the patient seems to be a good/fair/poor historian")
3. Brief description of patient's condition at time of history or patient profile
4. Chief complaint: reason for seeking health care
5. History of present illness (chronologic description of each symptom)
   Onset: time, type, source, setting
   Frequency and duration
   Location and radiation
   Severity (quantity)
   Quality (character)
   Aggravating/alleviating factors
   Associated manifestations
6. Past history or past medical history
   Childhood diseases and development
   Hospitalizations, surgeries, injuries, accidents, major illnesses
   Allergies
   Medications
   Immunizations
   General health and sources of previous health care
7. Family history
   Familial disease history
   Family history
   Marital history
   Family relationships
8. Social and environmental history
   Education
   Military experience
   Occupational history
   Religious and social activities
   Living arrangements
   Hobbies, recreation, and travel
   Habits, including smoking and vaping
   Alcohol or drug use
   Exposure to friends or family who are ill
   Satisfaction/stress with life situation, finances, relationships
   Recent travel or other event that might affect health
9. Review of systems (see Fig. 2.1)
10. Signature

---

### Background Information

Background information tells the interviewer who the patient is and what types of diseases are likely to develop. It also provides a basic understanding of the patient's previous experiences with illness and health care and the patient's current life situation, including the effect of culture, attitudes, relationships, and finances on health. Knowing the level of education, patterns of health-related learning, past health care practices, and reasons for compliance or lack of compliance with past therapy gives insight into patients' ability to understand their current health status. This may predict their willingness or ability to participate in learning and therapy. From the free discussion used to obtain background information, the interviewer may also get clues about patients' reliability and possible psychosocial implications of their disease.

### Screening Information

Screening information is designed to uncover problem areas the patient forgot to mention or omitted. This information is classically obtained by a head-to-toe review of all body systems but may also be obtained by a review of common diseases or from a description of body functions.

### Description of Present Health Status or Illness

A description of present health status or illness is included in even the briefest histories. Chief Complaint (CC) and History of Present Illness (HPI) are the most commonly used headings, although Reason for Visit and Current Health Status may be seen in some outpatient records. Because this is the information that most concerns the patient, the interview and recording of the history begin with this information.

## Review of Systems

Review of systems (ROS) is a recording of past and present information that may be relevant to the present problem but might otherwise have been overlooked. It is grouped by body or physiologic systems to guarantee completeness and to assist the examiner in arriving at a diagnosis. Fig. 2.1 is an example of an ROS checklist that may be completed by a patient before an interview or by a clinician. It provides for recording both positive and negative responses so that when the documentation is later reviewed, there is no doubt as to which questions were asked. Negative responses to important questions asked at any time during the interview are termed pertinent negatives; affirmative responses are termed pertinent positives. For example, if a patient complains of acute coughing but denies any fever, the fever would represent a pertinent negative, whereas the cough is a pertinent positive.

Experienced examiners usually elicit the ROS information in conjunction with the system-by-system physical examination; however, the two must not be confused. The physical examination provides objective data, or that which can be seen, felt, smelled, or heard by the examiner, commonly referred to as signs. On the other hand, the ROS provides subjective data, or that which is evident only to the patient and cannot be perceived by an observer or is no longer present for the observer to see and therefore can only be described by the patient. Subjective manifestations of disease are termed symptoms, several of which are detailed in Chapter 3.

## Chief Complaint

The CC relates to why the patient sought health care. It is the answer to such open-ended questions as "What caused you to come to the hospital?" or "What is bothering you the most?" Each symptom is recorded separately with its duration or date of initial occurrence. Ideally, symptom descriptions are written in the patient's own words. They should not be diagnostic statements, someone else's opinion, or vague generalities. At times, more directed questions such as "Could you describe what you mean by 'not enough air'?" or "In what ways don't you feel well?" are necessary to clarify the changes in perceptions or body functions experienced by the patient.

Asking the patient to recount the sequence of symptoms and then closing this section of the interview with a question such as "What else is bothering you?" often elicit problems the patient forgot to mention or was too uncomfortable to mention earlier. Now the interviewer is left with two types of problems: (1) those related to the CC and (2) those that are important to the patient but may have little or no relationship to the present illness. The interviewer must now group the problems and decide how to proceed with the interview. Problems not related to the illness are usually incorporated with an appropriate section of background data when the history is written.

The symptoms relating to the current illness are listed as the CC and then investigated one by one and described in detail under HPI. Once written, the CC should express the patient's, not the examiner's, priorities; provide a capsule account of the patient's illness; and guide the collection of the HPI.

The symptoms most commonly associated with problems of the cardiopulmonary system include coughing with or without sputum production (expectoration), breathlessness (dyspnea), chest pain, and wheezing, commonly described as chest tightness. Other symptoms associated with cardiopulmonary problems include coughing up blood (hemoptysis), hoarseness, voice changes, dizziness and fainting (syncope), headache, altered mental status, and ankle swelling. These symptoms are discussed in Chapter 3. Some symptoms, such as ankle swelling, can also be seen by the examiner and can therefore be both a sign and a symptom. Common cardiopulmonary signs are also discussed in Chapter 5.

Patients with cardiopulmonary problems may also have any of the so-called constitutional symptoms, which are those commonly occurring with problems in any of the body systems. Constitutional symptoms include chills and fever, excessive sweating, loss of appetite (anorexia), nausea, vomiting, weight loss, fatigue, weakness, exercise intolerance, and altered sleep patterns. Hay fever, allergies, acute sinusitis, postnasal discharge, and frequent bouts of colds or flu are upper respiratory tract symptoms commonly associated with pulmonary disease.

---

**SIMPLY STATED**

Cardiopulmonary symptoms are subjective (known only to the patient), so information about symptoms can be obtained only from the patient. Although initial information can be obtained by having the patient complete a questionnaire, a complete history can be obtained only through questioning the patient.

---

## History of Present Illness

The HPI is the narrative portion of the history that describes chronologically and in detail each symptom listed in the CC and its effect on the patient's life. It is the most difficult portion of the history to obtain and record accurately, but it is the information that guides the physical examination and diagnostic testing to follow. All caregivers should be familiar with the HPI for each of their patients.

**Have you recently had the following?** (Circle "yes" or "no"; if in doubt, leave blank)

**General**

| | | |
|---|---|---|
| Tire easily, weakness | yes | no |
| Marked weight change | yes | no |
| Night sweats | yes | no |
| Persistent fever | yes | no |
| Sensitivity to heat | yes | no |
| Sensitivity to cold | yes | no |

**Skin**

| | | |
|---|---|---|
| Eruptions (rash) | yes | no |
| Change in color | yes | no |
| Change in hair | yes | no |
| Change in fingernails | yes | no |

**Eyes**

| | | |
|---|---|---|
| Trouble seeing | yes | no |
| Eye pain | yes | no |
| Inflamed eyes | yes | no |
| Double vision | yes | no |
| Wear corrective lenses | yes | no |

**Ears**

| | | |
|---|---|---|
| Loss of hearing | yes | no |
| Ringing in ears | yes | no |
| Discharge | yes | no |

**Nose**

| | | |
|---|---|---|
| Loss of smell | yes | no |
| Frequent colds | yes | no |
| Obstruction | yes | no |
| Excess drainage | yes | no |
| Nosebleeds | yes | no |

**Mouth**

| | | |
|---|---|---|
| Sore gums | yes | no |
| Soreness of tongue | yes | no |
| Dental problems | yes | no |

**Throat**

| | | |
|---|---|---|
| Postnasal drainage | yes | no |
| Soreness | yes | no |
| Hoarseness | yes | no |

**Breasts**

| | | |
|---|---|---|
| Lumps | yes | no |
| Discharge | yes | no |

**Cardiorespiratory system**

| | | |
|---|---|---|
| Cough, persistent | yes | no |
| Sputum (phlegm) | yes | no |
| Bloody sputum | yes | no |
| Wheezing | yes | no |
| Chest pain or discomfort | yes | no |
| Pain on breathing | yes | no |
| Shortness of breath | yes | no |
| Difficulty breathing while lying down | yes | no |
| Swelling of ankles | yes | no |
| Bluish fingers or lips | yes | no |
| High blood pressure | yes | no |
| Palpitations | yes | no |
| Vein trouble | yes | no |

**Digestive system**

List average food selection each meal
Breakfast:

Lunch:

Dinner:

**Digestive system (cont.)**

| | | |
|---|---|---|
| Change in appetite | yes | no |
| Difficulty swallowing | yes | no |
| Heartburn | yes | no |
| Abdominal distress | yes | no |
| Belching or excess gas | yes | no |
| Abdominal enlargement | yes | no |
| Nausea | yes | no |
| Vomiting | yes | no |
| Vomiting of blood | yes | no |
| Rectal bleeding | yes | no |
| Tarry stools | yes | no |
| Dark urine | yes | no |
| Jaundice | yes | no |
| Constipation | yes | no |
| Diarrhea | yes | no |
| Hemorrhoids | yes | no |
| Need for laxatives | yes | no |

**Genitourinary system**

| | | |
|---|---|---|
| Increase in frequency of urination (day) | yes | no |
| Increase in frequency of urination (night) | yes | no |
| Feel need to urinate without much urine | yes | no |
| Unable to hold urine | yes | no |
| Pain or burning | yes | no |
| Blood in urine | yes | no |
| Albuminuria | yes | no |
| Impotence | yes | no |
| Lack of sex drive | yes | no |
| Pain with intercourse | yes | no |

**Endocrine system**

| | | |
|---|---|---|
| Thyroid trouble | yes | no |
| Adrenal trouble | yes | no |
| Cortisone treatment | yes | no |
| Diabetes | yes | no |

**Motor system**

| | | |
|---|---|---|
| Muscle cramps | yes | no |
| Muscle weakness | yes | no |
| Pain in joints | yes | no |
| Swollen joints | yes | no |
| Stiffness | yes | no |
| Deformity of joints | yes | no |

**Nervous system**

| | | |
|---|---|---|
| Headache | yes | no |
| Dizziness | yes | no |
| Fainting | yes | no |
| Convulsions or fits | yes | no |
| Nervousness | yes | no |
| Sleeplessness | yes | no |
| Depression | yes | no |
| Change in sensation | yes | no |
| Memory loss | yes | no |
| Poor coordination | yes | no |
| Weakness or paralysis | yes | no |

**GYN-OB**

Age started menstruating _____
Interval between periods _____
Duration of periods _____
Flow: light   normal   heavy
Pain with periods? _____
Date of last period _____
Pregnancies _____ Births _____
Weight of babies at birth _____

**FIG. 2.1** Review-of-systems form that can be completed by patient or examiner.

Encouraging the patient to talk freely about each problem allows maximal information to be obtained. The patient is initially asked to describe the progression of symptoms from the first occurrence to the present. On occasion, patients are unable to recall the first occurrence of the symptom, and the chronologic picture must then be developed by working backward from the most recent event.

Once a rough chronologic picture is outlined, the interviewer obtains a description of each symptom by using an open-ended approach such as "Now tell me about your (cough, chest pain, and so on)." Using silence, nonverbal clues (such as leaning forward expectantly), and facilitative expressions such as "Yes," "Hmm," and "Tell me more about . . . ," or restating or summarizing what the patient just said shows interest and encourages the patient to continue talking. When the patient exhausts the spontaneous description of each symptom, directed questions are used to elicit whatever additional information is necessary. Questions that can be answered with "yes" or "no" and leading questions are avoided. For example, "What brings on your cough?" encourages more accurate information than a question such as "The only time you cough is when you first get up in the morning, isn't it?" Because most patients want to please the interviewer, they are likely to agree with a leading question rather than report the specific information needed.

### SIMPLY STATED

All clinicians who care for patients should be familiar with the history of present illness for each patient treated.

### Describing Symptoms

When the patient's descriptions and the interviewer's clarifying questions are complete, it is often appropriate to gather additional information for each symptom. As an example, it is not unusual to ask patients to rate their pain on a scale of 1 to 10 (highest) or to ask nonverbal patients to point to the best visual descriptor, such as a happy or sad face. To accomplish this, the following information should be gathered for each symptom:

1. Description of onset: date, time, and type (sudden or gradual)
2. Setting: cause, circumstance, or activity surrounding onset
3. Location: where on the body the problem is located and whether it radiates
4. Severity: how bad it is and how it affects activities of daily living
5. Quantity: how much, how large an area, or how many
6. Quality: what it is like and character or unique properties, such as color, texture, odor, composition, sharp, viselike, or throbbing
7. Frequency: how often it occurs
8. Duration: how long it lasts and whether it is constant or intermittent
9. Course: is it getting better, getting worse, or staying the same?
10. Associated symptoms: symptoms from the same body system or other systems that occur before, with, or after the problem

### BOX 2.2   PQRST Mnemonic

P | Provocative/palliative: What is the cause? What makes it better? What makes it worse?
Q | Quality/quantity: How much is involved? How does it look, feel, sound?
R | Region/radiation: Where is it? Does it spread?
S | Severity scale: Does it interfere with activities? (Rate on scale of 1 to 10.)
T | Timing: When did it begin? How often does it occur? Is it sudden or gradual?

11. Aggravating factors: things that make it worse such as a certain position, weather, temperature, anxiety, exercise, and so on
12. Alleviating factors: things that make it better such as a change in position, hot, cold, rest, and so on

Various listings and mnemonic devices have been suggested to help the novice remember all of the information necessary to fully describe a symptom. One such mnemonic device is PQRST (Box 2.2).

Once all of the information is collected, it is written in narrative form, with a paragraph given to each time division in the chronologic progression of the symptoms. The left-hand margin of the page or the first few words of each paragraph are used to identify the applicable date or the time period (days, weeks, months, or years) before admission.

By the time each symptom is reviewed in detail, even a novice is usually able to assign the majority of the symptoms to one body system. The pertinent points of the ROS, personal history, and family history are reviewed for the applicable body systems. The pertinent negatives, as well as positives, are recorded. Usually, when writing the ROS, the interviewer puts "see HPI" behind the applicable body system rather than restating data previously recorded.

### Past History

The past history, also called the past medical history, is a written description of the patient's past medical problems. It may include previous experiences with health care and personal attitudes and habits that may affect both health and compliance with medical treatment plans. Information recorded in the past history includes a chronologic listing of the following:

1. Illnesses and development since birth
2. Surgeries and hospitalizations
3. Injuries and accidents
4. Immunizations
5. Allergies, including a description of the allergic reactions and effective treatment
6. Medications (both prescribed by a physician and over-the-counter drugs), vitamins, herbs, and "home remedies"
7. Names of physicians and sources and types of previous health care
8. Habits, including diet, sleep, exercise, and the use of alcohol, coffee, tobacco, and illicit drugs
9. Description of general health

Forms (Fig. 2.2) may be used by either the patient or the interviewer to concisely record much of the information just

PERSONAL HISTORY

Birthplace _____ Date _____

Nationality _____ Religion _____

Marital status _____ Health of spouse _____

Occupations _____

_____

Residence past 5 years: _____

Education through _____ grade    Sleep (usual hrs.) _____ Aids to sleep _____

Recreation _____

Exercise _____

Average per day: _____

  Alcohol (type) _____

  Tobacco (type) _____

  Tea, coffee _____

| Medicines taken regularly | Reason | Last Dose |
|---|---|---|
| | | |
| | | |
| | | |
| | | |
| | | |

PERSONAL PAST HISTORY

Circle "yes" or "no"                Circle "yes" or "no"

| Have you ever had: | | | Year | Operations | | | Year |
|---|---|---|---|---|---|---|---|
| Measles | yes | no | | Tonsils | yes | no | |
| Mumps | yes | no | | Appendix | yes | no | |
| Whooping cough | yes | no | | Gallbladder | yes | no | |
| Polio | yes | no | | Stomach | yes | no | |
| Scarlet fever | yes | no | | Breast | yes | no | |
| Diphtheria | yes | no | | Uterus and/or ovary | yes | no | |
| Meningitis | yes | no | | Prostate | yes | no | |
| Infectious mono | yes | no | | Hernia | yes | no | |
| Valley fever | yes | no | | Thyroid | yes | no | |
| Tuberculosis (TB) | yes | no | | Varicose veins | yes | no | |
| Exposure to TB | yes | no | | Hemorrhoids | yes | no | |
| Malaria | yes | no | | Heart | yes | no | |
| Hives | yes | no | | Other | yes | no | |
| Cancer | yes | no | | | | | |
| Venereal disease | yes | no | | **Injuries** | | | |
| Arthritis | yes | no | | Head | yes | no | |
| Back trouble | yes | no | | Chest | yes | no | |
| Bronchitis | yes | no | | Abdomen | yes | no | |
| Pneumonia | yes | no | | Broken bones | yes | no | |
| Pleurisy | yes | no | | Back | yes | no | |
| Asthma | yes | no | | Other | yes | no | |
| Emphysema | yes | no | | | | | |
| Rheumatic fever | yes | no | | **Allergies (are you allergic to)** | | | |
| High blood pressure | yes | no | | Tetanus antitoxin | yes | no | |
| Heart disease | yes | no | | Penicillin | yes | no | |
| Anemia | yes | no | | Sulfa | yes | no | |
| Bleeding tendency | yes | no | | Other drugs | yes | no | |
| Blood transfusion | yes | no | |   List _____ | | | |
| Hepatitis | yes | no | | _____ | | | |
|   (yellow jaundice) | | | | Foods | yes | no | |
| Ulcer | yes | no | | Cosmetics | yes | no | |
| Hemorrhoids | yes | no | | Other | yes | no | |
| Bladder infections | yes | no | | **Immunizations** | | | |
| Kidney disease | yes | no | | Smallpox | yes | no | |
| Hay fever/sinusitis | yes | no | | Tetanus | yes | no | |
| Glaucoma | yes | no | | Polio, shots | yes | no | |
| Nosebleeds | yes | no | | Polio, oral | yes | no | |
| | | | | Other | yes | no | |

FIG. 2.2 Form for recording personal history and personal past history (past medical history).

listed. It is important to record the dates of accidents, major illnesses, hospitalizations, and immunizations. If past medical records are needed during the patient's hospitalization, the names and addresses of hospitals and physicians that have provided care to the patient in the past should be recorded.

## Disease and Procedure History

For patients with cardiopulmonary complaints, it is important to ask about the frequency and treatment of each of the following diseases: pneumonia, pleurisy, fungal diseases, tuberculosis, colds, sinus infections, bronchiectasis, asthma, allergies, pneumothorax, bronchitis, or emphysema. Because of the close relationship between the heart and the lungs, it is also important to know whether the patient has a history of heart attack, hypertension (high blood pressure), heart failure, or congenital heart disease.

Dates and types of heart or chest surgeries and traumas should be recorded. Dates and results of tests that assess pulmonary status, including chest x-ray films, bronchoscopy, pulmonary function tests, and skin tests, should also be documented. This respiratory-specific past history information is summarized in the portion of a pulmonary history questionnaire shown in Fig. 2.3. A patient's discussion of previous diseases, tests, and treatments gives a good indication of his

---

Please answer by circling "yes" or "no" and provide the specific information.

PAST MEDICAL HISTORY

**Have you ever had the following?**      If "yes" give year/specifics

| | | |
|---|---|---|
| Asthma | yes no | _____ |
| Allergies | yes no | _____ |
| Frequent colds | yes no | _____ |
| Sinus infections | yes no | _____ |
| Chronic bronchitis | yes no | _____ |
| Emphysema | yes no | _____ |
| Pleurisy | yes no | _____ |
| Pneumonia | yes no | _____ |
| Pneumothorax | yes no | _____ |
| Tuberculosis | yes no | _____ |
| Other lung problems | yes no | _____ |
| Heart trouble of any type | yes no | _____ |
| Chest trauma | yes no | _____ |
| Chest, lung, or heart surgery | yes no | List: _____ |

**Have you ever had any of the following?**    If "yes" give month/year last performed

Chest x-ray: ever abnormal?   yes   no      _____ / _____
TB skin test: ever positive?    yes   no      _____ / _____

**Have you had any of the following?**

Other skin tests      yes   no      _____ / _____
Pulmonary function test   yes   no      _____ / _____
Bronchoscopy        yes   no      _____ / _____
Other pulmonary tests    yes   no      _____ / _____

SMOKING HISTORY

**Do you currently smoke or use tobacco regularly?**      yes   no
1. How old were you when you started smoking?    _____
2. For how many years have you smoked regularly?    _____
3. How many cigarettes do you now smoke each day?    _____
4. How many cigars do you now smoke each day?    _____
5. How much pipe tobacco do you now smoke each week?    _____
6. Were there periods when you stopped smoking?    _____
7. How long did you stop smoking?    _____

**Have you ever smoked regularly?**      yes   no
1. How old were you when you started smoking?    _____
2. How many years did you smoke regularly?    _____
3. When did you quit smoking? (month/year)    _____ / _____
4. How many cigarettes did you usually smoke per day?    _____
5. How many cigars did you usually smoke per day?    _____
6. How much pipe tobacco did you smoke per week?    _____

**Did you smoke anything other than tobacco?**      yes   no
What, how much, how often? _____

**Does someone smoke in your home or office?**      yes   no
1. How many years has someone smoked in your home?    _____
2. How many years has someone smoked in your office?    _____

**FIG. 2.3** Past medical history and smoking sections from a pulmonary history questionnaire.

or her understanding of the disease process and compliance with medical therapy.

### Drug and Smoking History

There is a strong link between the use of illicit drugs and cardiopulmonary problems; however, an honest history of drug abuse is extremely difficult for even the most experienced examiner to obtain. It is often the bedside clinician, such as the RT, who first learns that drug abuse may be related to the patient's complaints. The patient should be encouraged to share this information honestly with the primary physician so that the best treatment can be obtained as early as possible. Patients should be reassured of the confidential nature related to such disclosures. In addition, clinicians and students must remember that a breach of this confidentiality is illegal and may result in losing the patient's trust. Also, concluding too quickly that a drug history is the cause of the patient's problem may result in a missed diagnosis and an improper treatment program.

Because of the strong relationship between smoking and chronic pulmonary diseases, respiratory infections, lung cancer, and cardiovascular diseases, a careful and accurate smoking history is important. It is preferable to ask a patient "What types of tobacco have you used or at what age did you begin smoking?" rather than "Do you smoke?" Use of pipes, cigars, marijuana, chewing tobacco, or snuff is usually recorded in terms of the amount used daily. Because many substances used in vaping devices and electronic cigarettes contain nicotine and other potentially harmful chemicals, their use should be investigated and recorded in the medical record.

The use of cigarettes should be recorded in pack-years. The term **pack-years** refers to the number of years the patient has smoked times the number of packs smoked each day. It is also important to record the age when the patient began to smoke, variations in smoking habits over the years, the type and length of the cigarettes smoked, the habit of inhaling, the number and success of attempts to quit, and the date when the

### SIMPLY STATED

The term *pack-years* is the number of years the patient has smoked multiplied by the number of packs per day. If a patient smoked three packs a day for 10 years, it would be recorded as a 30 pack-year smoking history.

patient last smoked (see Fig. 2.3). Similar information should be gathered on the use of vaping devices and electronic cigarettes. Members of the health care team have a professional responsibility to educate patients and their family about the harmful effects of smoking and vaping to guide them to programs designed to help people stop.

### Family History

The purpose of the family history is to learn about the health status of the patient's blood relatives. This is where the interviewer records the presence of diseases in immediate family members with hereditary tendencies. Sources of physical, emotional, or economic support or stress within the family structure are also documented here when important.

To assess the current health status of the extended family, the patient is asked to describe the present age and state of health of blood relatives for three generations: siblings; parents, aunts, and uncles; and grandparents. The resulting information may be recorded in narrative style, drawn schematically as a family tree, or written on a form such as the one shown in Fig. 2.4. When patients are asked to complete a form before an interview, the responses should be reviewed and notations added as necessary to capture the age and cause of death or current health status for each family member. A notation such as "18 A/W" indicates that the person listed was 18 years old and alive and well on the day the history was recorded.

The health of the current family of a patient who was adopted is important for identification of communicable and environmentally related diseases; however, a history of

| Has any blood relative had any of the following? | Circle "yes" or "no" | If "yes," what relationship? |
|---|---|---|
| Anemia | yes    no | _____ |
| Bleeding tendency | yes    no | _____ |
| Leukemia | yes    no | _____ |
| Repeated infections | yes    no | _____ |
| Crippling infections | yes    no | _____ |
| Heart disease | yes    no | _____ |
| Chronic lung disease | yes    no | _____ |
| Tuberculosis | yes    no | _____ |
| High blood pressure | yes    no | _____ |
| Kidney disease | yes    no | _____ |
| Asthma | yes    no | _____ |
| Severe allergies | yes    no | _____ |
| Mental illness | yes    no | _____ |
| Convulsions or fits | yes    no | _____ |
| Migraine headaches | yes    no | _____ |
| Diabetes | yes    no | _____ |
| Gout | yes    no | _____ |
| Obesity | yes    no | _____ |
| Thyroid trouble | yes    no | _____ |
| Peptic ulcer | yes    no | _____ |
| Chronic diarrhea | yes    no | _____ |
| Cancer | yes    no | _____ |

|  | Present Age, or Age at Death | If living, health (good, fair, poor) if deceased, cause of death |
|---|---|---|
| Father |  |  |
| Mother |  |  |
| Brothers or Sisters |  |  |
| 1. |  |  |
| 2. |  |  |
| 3. |  |  |
| 4. |  |  |
| 5. |  |  |
| 6. |  |  |
| 7. |  |  |
| Children |  |  |
| 1. |  |  |
| 2. |  |  |
| 3. |  |  |
| 4. |  |  |
| 5. |  |  |
| 6. |  |  |
| 7. |  |  |

**FIG. 2.4** Form for recording family history.

the patient's true blood relatives is needed to assess genetically transmitted diseases or illnesses with strong familial relationships.

In addition to documenting the current health status of the family members, a review of diseases with strong hereditary or familial tendencies is also performed. Fig. 2.4 shows a form that permits either the patient or examiner to record the presence or absence of the most frequently reviewed diseases known to occur in the patient's family (pertinent positives) and those denied by the patient (pertinent negatives).

Patients with cardiopulmonary complaints are asked specifically about the following diseases or problems that have been shown to have a hereditary link with pulmonary disease: chronic allergies, asthma, lung cancer, cystic fibrosis, emphysema, neuromuscular disorders, kyphosis, scoliosis, sleep disturbances and sleep apnea, collagen vascular diseases (e.g., lupus erythematosus), $\alpha_1$-antitrypsin deficiency, cardiovascular disorders (e.g., hypertension, heart attack, heart failure, and congenital abnormalities), diabetes, and obesity. Because exposure to family and friends

with infections can also result in pulmonary symptoms, the patient is asked about contact with or family history of frequent colds, tuberculosis, influenza, pneumonia, and fungal infections.

## Occupational and Environmental History

An occupational and environmental history is particularly important in patients with pulmonary symptoms. The purpose is to elicit information concerning exposure to potential disease-producing substances or environments. Most occupational pulmonary diseases result from workers inhaling particles, dusts, fumes, or gases during the extraction, manufacture, transfer, storage, or disposal of industrial substances (Table 2.1). However, the hazards of an industrial society are not limited to those working directly with the toxic substances. Other employees working in or near an industrial plant, as well as people living in the surrounding areas, are subject to breathing toxic fumes and dusts. Family members come in contact with contaminated clothing, such as asbestos from clothing being laundered and may develop pulmonary disease years later. Accidental spills of toxic chemicals

### TABLE 2.1 Occupational Lung Disease

| Inhaled Substance | Occupation or Source | Usual Symptoms and Course | Disease Names |
|---|---|---|---|
| **Acute Airway or Lung Reactions** | | | |
| **Irritant Gases** | | | |
| Chlorine, ammonia, sulfur dioxide | Various industries<br>Accidental exposure | Short exposure<br>Eye and airway irritation, dry cough<br>Prolonged exposure<br>Dyspnea, wheezing, pulmonary edema | |
| **Insoluble Gases and Metal Fumes** | | | |
| Nitrogen dioxide | Filled silos, closed welding spaces, chemical laboratories | Very little airway irritation<br>Headache, shortness of breath, cough, chest tightness, pulmonary edema | Silo-filler's disease |
| Phosgene | Chemical warfare, heating metals treated with production chlorine | Acute pulmonary edema, pneumonitis | |
| Copper, zinc, iron, nickel, tin, antimony, manganese, magnesium | Welders in closed spaces, mining, electroplating | Fever, malaise, nausea, aching muscles, lasting 2-3 days | Metal fume fever<br>Galvanization<br>Polymer fume fever |
| Cadmium, mercury, beryllium | | Above with acute pulmonary edema and pneumonia | |
| **Acute or Subacute Allergic Reactions** | | | |
| Toluene diisocyanate (TDI) | Plastic and foam production | Immediate or delayed asthma-like reactions usually occur in sensitive persons but | Hypersensitivity pneumonitis<br>Extrinsic allergic alveolitis |
| Proteolytic enzymes (detergents) | Industrial accidents<br>Manufacture of detergents | may occur in others; fever, chills, malaise, weight loss, nocturnal wheezing, cough, cyanosis, dyspnea at rest | Occupational asthma |
| **Droppings/Feathers** | | | |
| Pigeons, parakeets, chickens, turkeys | Bird handlers | Acute reactions within 4-8 hours<br>Delayed reactions occur at night after leaving work environment<br>In some cases, chronic disease with fibrosis may develop if repeated exposure continues | Bird-fancier's lung, ornithosis<br>Pigeon-breeder's lung |

## TABLE 2.1    Occupational Lung Disease—cont'd

| Inhaled Substance | Occupation or Source | Usual Symptoms and Course | Disease Names |
|---|---|---|---|
| **Pituitary Extract/Organic Dusts** | | | |
| Paprika, fishmeal, coffee bean, weevil-infested flour<br>Cotton, hemp, flax<br>Fungal spores from moldy hay, straw, grains, malt or barley, sugar cane (bagasse), mushroom compost, maple bark, logs, wood pulp (Western red cedar) | Workers with specific products<br>Textile and farm workers<br>Agriculture and farm workers<br>Wood and paper mill workers<br>Lumbering | "Monday fever"<br>Repeated bouts of pneumonia with fever and weight loss | Pituitary snuff-taker's lung<br>Wheat-weevil lung<br>Byssinosis (brown lung)<br>Farmer's lung<br>Malt-worker's lung<br>Bagassosis<br>Mushroom-handler's lung<br>Wood/paper mill–worker's lung<br>Maple bark–stripper's lung |
| Contaminated water<br>Drugs and chemicals | Air conditioners, humidifiers<br>Antibiotic, pharmaceutical, chemical manufacture | | Air-conditioner (humidifier) lung |
| **Chronic Occupational Lung Diseases** | | | |
| Crystalline-free silica | Sandblasters in enclosed spaces, manufacture of ceramics and abrasive agents, construction, mines, quarries, foundries: gold, copper, lead, zinc, iron, coal, granite | Acute (1-3 years of intense exposure): shortness of breath, fever, frequent pulmonary infections<br>Chronic (20 years or more of exposure): no symptoms to exertional dyspnea, obstructed breathing, productive cough, reduced exercise tolerance, chest pain, weight loss, hemoptysis with fibrosis; 40+ years: infection, cor pulmonale | Silicosis<br>Associated in unknown way with rheumatoid arthritis and scleroderma<br>High incidence of associated tuberculosis and bronchogenic cancer |
| Coal | Coal miners | Simple: asymptomatic, cough with smoking<br>Complicated with fibrosis: as just listed with black sputum | Coal-worker's pneumoconiosis<br>Coal-miner's lung |
| Asbestos | Manufacture of fire-proofing and insulation, shipbuilding, automobile mechanics (clutch and brake), demolition workers, firefighters, living/working near dumps or high-use areas | Exertional dyspnea, clubbing, restricted breathing, crackles at lung bases usually appear before x-ray film changes and cancer symptoms about 20 years after exposure | Asbestosis |
| **Other Mineral Dusts** | | | |
| Fuller's earth, kaolin (China clay), graphite, tin, iron, mixed dusts, tungsten | Quarrying, mining, milling, drying, bagging, and loading minerals<br>Welding and foundries<br>Manufacture of industrial precision instruments | Vary from asymptomatic with dust retention to same as complicated silicosis | Pneumoconiosis<br><br>Stannosis<br>Siderosis |
| Beryllium | Nuclear physics, manufacture of electronics, ceramics, x-ray tube windows (in past: fluorescent lights) | Acute pulmonary edema, pneumonia<br>Chronic granulomatous disease appears years after exposure<br>Dyspnea, dry cough, weakness, weight loss, skin lesions, crackles | Pulmonary granuloma |
| Paraquat | Agriculture | Inhalation or ingestion may lead to pulmonary fibrosis | |

and gases can endanger and even necessitate evacuation and treatment of large numbers of people.

Although there have been dramatic decreases in exposure to some hazardous materials, exposures to dusts, fumes, and chemicals from indoor and outdoor air pollutants continue to increase. Outbreaks of work-related illnesses in buildings not contaminated by industrial processes can be traced to these pollutants or simply to an inadequate provision of fresh air with no identifiable contaminant. The terms *tight-building syndrome* and *sick-building syndrome* are now used to describe these epidemics in which large numbers of employees complain of symptoms, including runny or stuffy nose, eye irritation, cough, chest tightness, fatigue, headache, and malaise.

Reactions to inhalation of toxic substances can occur within minutes to hours (acute) or may take weeks, months, or years to develop. Inhalation of soluble gases, such as ammonia, chlorine, or sulfur dioxide, causes sufficient upper airway irritation to warn workers of immediate danger. However, metal fumes and insoluble gases, such as phosgene and nitrogen dioxide, are less irritating to the upper airways. Because they may be inhaled for long periods of time with little discomfort, workers are not warned to escape, and more severe pulmonary damage results.

Hypersensitivity reactions may be acute or delayed and often occur in patterns. Shortness of breath, wheezes, or flu-like symptoms usually occur within 4 to 8 hours of exposure. However, symptoms may occur only at night and may recur for several nights after a single exposure. In some cases the most severe symptoms occur at the start of the workweek, and tolerance develops as the week progresses. Such a pattern, often termed *Monday fever*, is commonly seen with inhalation of cotton dust. More commonly, allergic reactions worsen with reexposure and decrease during days off. In subacute forms of hypersensitivity pneumonitis, symptoms occur insidiously over weeks. Most of the chronic occupational pulmonary diseases (pneumoconioses) take 20 years or more to become symptomatic. Whenever there is a delay in the development of pulmonary symptoms, their relationship to occupational and environmental exposure becomes obscure.

The occupational and environmental history must therefore be more than just a chronologic listing of job titles. Questioning may include the occupation of the patient's father and descriptions of childhood residences. Lung disease caused by the inhalation of asbestos fibers (asbestosis) has been seen in people who lived near shipyards or asbestos dump sites as children and in people whose fathers were asbestos workers. The patient should be queried about location of schools, summer jobs, dates and types of military service, and all subsequent full- and part-time jobs. The precise dates, duration, and activities of each job must be delineated. These include materials and processes involved, amount of workspace and type of ventilation, use of protective devices, cleanup practices, and work going on in adjacent areas.

Work or residence near mines, farms, mills, shipyards, or foundries should be clarified. Sources of possible irritants within the home, such as humidifiers, air-conditioning systems, woodpiles, insulation, smoking, paints and glues used for hobbies, and household pets, must also be reviewed.

It is important to review the various places a patient has lived or visited for any period of time. Certain fungal infections that involve the respiratory system have strong geographic relationships. Histoplasmosis is particularly common in Ohio, Maryland, the central Mississippi Valley, and the Appalachian Mountains; blastomycosis is found in the southwestern United States, especially Arizona, Texas, and the San Joaquin Valley in California, as well as sections of South America.

When the pulmonary history is written, occupational and environmental histories are usually given specific headings because of the detail recorded. However, in most routine histories this information may be found under general headings such as personal history, social history, psychosocial history, or social-environmental history.

## REVIEWING THE PATIENT'S MEDICAL RECORD

The RT often prepares to visit the patient by first reviewing the patient's medical record. This record may be brief on admission but builds if the patient is admitted for more than a couple of days. It is the RT's responsibility to become familiar with pertinent information recorded in the chart and overall medical record.

In the past this generally meant reviewing only a hard copy of the patient's chart. However, with the advent of electronic medical records (EMRs), many such records, including admitting information, history and assessment notes, laboratory tests, and imaging studies (radiographs and computed tomography scans), are stored in computerized databases. Therefore it is essential for the RT to confirm the review of both the hard copy and relevant EMR data to ensure a comprehensive review of pertinent records. EMRs and overall documentation of the patient assessment and care plan are detailed in Chapter 21. The following information represents aspects of the patient's medical record that are generally most useful.

### Admission Note

The admission note is written by the admitting physician and is a narrative description of important facts related to the patient's need to be hospitalized. The physician documents the patient's baseline status on admission in the admission note. The RT should review this important notation before seeing the patient for the initial visit to identify whom the patient is, why the patient was admitted, what the patient's current clinical condition is, and the overall treatment plan.

### Physician Orders

The admitting physician lists the treatment plan and monitoring techniques that he or she believes are needed to best care for the patient. The RT should carefully review all orders related to the treatment and monitoring of cardiopulmonary disorders and specifically review the orders pertaining to respiratory care.

## Progress Notes

Each day the attending physician will visit the patient at least once. During this visit the physician will interview and examine the patient to identify the patient's progress and response to treatment. The physician will follow up by documenting progress notes in the patient's chart. RTs should review these notes daily to identify the physician's perception of the patient's progress toward treatment goals.

In addition to the physician, other health care providers will document progress notes in the patient's chart. The nurse, physical therapist, occupational therapist, nutritionist, social worker, and other health care providers may record their findings and treatment plan in a progress note, often using a SOAP (*subjective*, *objective*, *assessment*, *plan*) format (see Chapter 21).

## DNAR/DNR Status and Advance Directives

Some patients will have a do not attempt to resuscitate (DNAR) or do not resuscitate (DNR) label on their chart to alert the patient care team that there is a concurrent physician's order in the chart. A DNAR/DNR is usually instituted when resuscitation would not alter the ultimate outcome of a disease. In such cases resuscitation should not be attempted if the patient experiences respiratory or cardiac arrest. The DNAR/DNR may be initiated by someone entitled to make decisions on a patient's behalf. Alternatively, it can be instituted on the basis of a physician's own initiative, in consultation with the patient and/or family members, when it is determined that the patient is in the end stages of a terminal illness that is not reversible.

It is important to remember that there are variations of DNAR/DNR orders. One such variation, which prohibits intubation but may allow the administration of certain cardiopulmonary resuscitative medications such as epinephrine or atropine, is known as a do not intubate (DNI) order. It should also be noted that the increasingly popular alternative term for a DNAR is an *allow natural death* (AND) order.

An advance directive is a legal document in which individuals specify what actions should be taken for their health if they are no longer able to make decisions for themselves because of illness or incapacity. In the United States an advance directive has a legal status, and many states require that patients be asked and/or informed about whether they have or want such a document on admission to a hospital or other health care facility. A living will is one form of advance directive, leaving instructions for treatment. Another form is a specific type of power of attorney or health care proxy, in which the person authorizes someone to make decisions on his or her behalf when the person is incapacitated. Associated procedures generally require one or more trained medical professionals to determine that patients are not competent to make their own health decisions before the advance directive takes effect and clinical decisions are made on their behalf. Most medical records have a separate section for DNAR/DNR and advance directives.

## ASSESSMENT STANDARDS FOR PATIENTS WITH PULMONARY DYSFUNCTION

The beginning student may be confused by the fact that the patient's medical record contains more than one style of history recorded on or about the same date. This occurs in teaching institutions because students and residents, as well as the attending physician, see the patient. It also occurs because each of the health care professions is responsible for specifying the scope of practice for its practitioners and monitoring the quality of their performance. As a result, there may be patient histories completed by nursing and several allied health professions in addition to those done by physicians. Some hospitals are moving toward what is termed the *patient history*—one history per patient per admission—which is used and augmented by all the allied health professionals involved in the patient's care, as well as by physicians.

The American Thoracic Society adopted specific standards for assessment of adult patients with actual or potential pulmonary dysfunction. These process and outcome standards are used with assessment, goal setting, intervention, and evaluation to ensure that the patient receives an acceptable level of care. The pulmonary history assessment guide from these standards is shown in Box 2.3. Note that in addition to gathering and analyzing the traditional pulmonary history, this assessment includes additional categories that focus on the

---

### BOX 2.3   American Thoracic Society's Nursing Assessment Guide for Adult Patients with Pulmonary Dysfunction

**History and Symptoms**
***Pulmonary Symptoms*[a]**
Dyspnea
Cough
Sputum
Hemoptysis
Wheeze
Chest pain (e.g., pleuritic)

***Extrapulmonary Symptoms*[a]**
Night sweats
Headaches on awakening
Weight changes

Fluid retention
Nasal stuffiness, discharge
Fatigue
Orthopnea, paroxysmal nocturnal dyspnea
Snoring, sleep disturbances, daytime drowsiness
Sinus problems

***Pulmonary Risk Factors***
Smoking, vaping, and tobacco history
Type (cigarettes, cigar, pipe, vaping device or smokeless tobacco)
Amount per day
Duration (years)

*Continued*

---

**BOX 2.3    American Thoracic Society's Nursing Assessment Guide for Adult Patients with Pulmonary Dysfunction—cont'd**

Childhood respiratory diseases/symptoms
Family history of respiratory disease
Alcohol and chemical substance abuse (e.g., heroin, marijuana, cocaine)
Environmental exposures
Location (e.g., home, work, region)
Type (e.g., asbestos, silica, gases, aerosols)
Duration
Obesity or nutritional depletion
Compromised immune system function (e.g., immunoglobulin G deficiency, HIV infection, $\alpha_1$-antitrypsin deficiency)

**Previous History**
Pulmonary problems
Treatments
Number of hospitalizations
Medical diagnoses
Immunizations

**Self-Management Capacity**
**Physical Ability (0-to-4 scale, 0 = independent, 4 = dependent)**
Lower extremity (e.g., walking, stair climbing)
Upper extremity (e.g., shampooing, meal preparation)
Activities of daily living
  Toileting
  Hygiene
  Feeding
  Dressing
Activity pattern during a typical day
Patient statement about management of problems
Sensory-perceptual factors (e.g., vision, hearing)

**Cognitive Ability**
Mental age
Memory

Knowledge about diagnosis, end treatment of pulmonary problems, or risk factors of pulmonary disease
Judgment

**Psychosocial-Cultural Factors**
Self-concept
Self-esteem
Body image
Roles, changes
Value system (e.g., spiritual and health beliefs)
Coping mechanisms
Displaced anger
Anxiety
Hostility
Dependency
Withdrawal, isolation
Avoidance
Denial
Noncompliance
Acceptance

**Socioeconomic Factors**
Social support system
Family
Significant others
Friends
Community resources
Government resources
Financial situation/health insurance
Employment/disability

**Environmental Factors**
Home
Community
Worksite
Health care setting (e.g., hospital, nursing home)

[a]Consider onset, duration, precipitating factors, aggravating factors, and relieving factors of symptoms.
Modified from American Thoracic Society Medical Section of the American Lung Association: Standards of nursing care for adult patients with pulmonary dysfunction, *Am Rev Respir Dis* 144(1):231–6, 1991.

---

patient's response to interferences with normal respiratory function, self-management capacity, resources, and knowledge of respiratory medications and treatments. The student will find this document helpful as a tool to review the multiple variables that affect both the quality of care and quality of life for a patient with pulmonary dysfunction.

## KEY POINTS

- The medical history of the patient is most often obtained by the patient's physician. RTs often interview the patient to identify changes in the patient's health status in response to therapy.
- Interviewing skills require practice and are an important part of patient assessment for all health care providers.
- Communicating with the patient to obtain information about his or her health status requires the interviewer to be skilled at verbal and nonverbal communication.
- Body movement, facial expression, touch, and eye movement are all types of nonverbal communication.

- One of the most common mistakes made by the interviewer is failing to listen carefully to the patient's answers and questions.
- The ability of the interviewer to project a sense of undivided interest in the patient is the key to a successful interview and the development of good patient rapport.
- Open-ended questions encourage patients to describe events and priorities as they see them and thereby help bring out concerns and attitudes and promote understanding.

- Closed questions such as "When did your cough start?" or "How long did the pain last?" focus on specific information and provide clarification.
- Neutral questions and statements, as opposed to leading questions, are preferred for all interactions with the patient. Leading questions prompt the patient to provide a certain answer and therefore may lead to inaccurate information.
- ROS is a recording of past and present information that may be relevant to the present problem but might otherwise have been overlooked.
- The CC is documentation in the patient's current medical history explaining why he or she sought health care. It is the answer to such open-ended questions as "What brought you to the hospital?"
- The HPI is the narrative portion of the history that describes chronologically and in detail each symptom listed in the CC and its effect on the patient's life.
- Because of the strong relationship between smoking and chronic pulmonary diseases, respiratory infections, lung cancer, and cardiovascular diseases, a careful and accurate smoking history is important.
- Because many substances used in vaping devices and electronic cigarettes contain nicotine and other potentially harmful chemicals, their use should be investigated and recorded in the medical record.

- The purpose of the family history is to learn about the health status of the patient's blood relatives. The interviewer records the presence of diseases in immediate family members with hereditary tendencies.
- The purpose of the occupational history is to elicit information concerning exposure to potential disease-producing substances or environments. Most occupational pulmonary diseases are the result of workers inhaling particles, dusts, fumes, or gases during the extraction, manufacture, transfer, storage, or disposal of industrial substances.
- It is important to document in the history the various places a patient has lived or visited for any period of time. Certain fungal infections that involve the respiratory system have strong geographic relationships.
- It is the RT's responsibility to become familiar with pertinent information recorded in the chart before caring for the patient with respiratory illness.
- A DNAR/DNR order is usually instituted for very ill patients when resuscitation would likely not alter the ultimate outcome of a disease.
- An advance directive is a legal document that specifies what medical actions should be taken (or not taken) if the patient is no longer able to make decisions for himself or herself.

## ASSESSMENT QUESTIONS

1. T/F Proper diagnosis and treatment are determined to a great extent by the accuracy and detail of the patient's history.
2. During the interview, if the therapist responds to the information provided by the patient with appropriate comments, this is evidence of which of the following?
   1. Nonverbal communication
   2. Active listening
   3. Pertinent positives
   4. Reflecting
      a. 1 and 3
      b. 2 and 4
      c. 3 and 4
      d. All of the above
3. Proper introduction of yourself to the patient before the interview is useful for all the following *except:*
   a. Establishing your role
   b. Asking permission to be involved
   c. Conveying your sincere interest in the patient
   d. Identifying diagnostic information
4. Which of the following would be examples of techniques used in conversational interviewing?
   a. Using questions such as "What happened next?"
   b. Saying things such as "You feel better now, don't you?"
   c. Asking for clarification of a symptom
   d. a and c

5. A patient cannot provide a medical history, and it is obtained from a close relative. This is an example of which of the following?
   a. Family history
   b. Background information
   c. Screening information
   d. Alternative source
6. In what section of the patient history can a detailed description of the patient's current symptoms be found?
   a. Chief complaint
   b. History of present illness
   c. Past medical history
   d. Occupational history
7. Information that is evident only to the patient and cannot be perceived by the observer is known as which of the following?
   a. Subjective data
   b. Objective data
   c. Clinical signs
   d. Pertinent negatives
8. In what section of the patient's history would you find information about a possible history of exposure to asbestos?
   a. History of present illness
   b. Family history
   c. Occupational history
   d. Past medical history

9. Your patient has a 50 pack-year smoking history. Which of the following is consistent with this history?
   a. He has smoked 2 packs/day for 25 years
   b. He has smoked 1 pack/day for 50 years
   c. He has smoked 5 packs/day for 10 years
   d. All of the above

10. Subjective manifestations of disease are termed:
    a. Symptoms
    b. Clinical findings
    c. Objective data
    d. Pertinent negatives

11. Your patient has pneumonia and complains of chest pain and cough but denies fever. How would you classify the lack of fever in this case?
    a. Objective data
    b. Pertinent positive
    c. Pertinent negative
    d. Physical examination finding

12. Which of the following is not considered a constitutional symptom?
    a. Nausea
    b. Weakness
    c. Chills and fever
    d. Dyspnea

13. The family history may be helpful in diagnosing a patient with which of the following problems?
    a. Acute bronchitis
    b. Cystic fibrosis
    c. Pneumothorax
    d. Pulmonary edema

14. Which of the following illnesses may be related to visiting or living in certain geographic locations?
    a. Congestive heart failure
    b. Fungal pneumonia
    c. Cystic fibrosis
    d. Emphysema

15. Your patient has a DNR label on his chart and at the head of his bed. This indicates which of the following?
    a. The patient is not responsive
    b. The patient is not oriented to time, place, and person
    c. The patient should not be resuscitated if cardiac arrest occurs
    d. The patient has psychiatric problems and needs close supervision

## BIBLIOGRAPHY

Airpuru F, Latorre A, Ibanez B, et al. Variability in the detection and monitoring of chronic patients in primary care according to what is registered in the electronic health record. *Fam Pract* 2013;**29**:696.

Ball J, Dains E, Flynn J, et al. *Seidel's guide to physical examination.* 8th ed. St. Louis: Mosby-Elsevier; 2015.

Cullinan S, O'Mahony, Byrne S. Application of the structured history taking of medication use tool to optimise prescribing for older patients and reduce adverse events. *Int J Clin Pharm* 2016;**1**:21.

Edwards K, Chiweda D, Oyinka A, et al. Assessing the value of electronic records. *Nurs Times* 2011;**107**:12.

Ferreir-Valente MA, Pais-Rabeiro JL, Jensen MP. Validity of four pain intensity rating scales. *Pain* 2011;**152**:2399.

Gupta A, Harris S, Naina H. To sit or stand during the medical interview: a poll of Caucasian patients. *J Med Pract Manage* 2015;**31**:110.

Heuer AJ, Geisler SL, Kamiensk M, et al. Introducing medical students to the interdisciplinary health care team: piloting a case-based approach. *J Allied Health* 2010;**39**:76.

Jarvis C. *Physical exam and health assessment.* 7th ed. St. Louis: Mosby-Elsevier; 2016.

Kacmarek RM, Stoller JK, Heuer AJ. *Egan's fundamentals of respiratory care.* 11th ed. St. Louis: Mosby-Elsevier; 2017.

Norlyk A, Haahr A, Hall E. Interviewing with or without the partner present? An underexposed dilemma between ethics and methodology in nursing research. *J Adv Nurs* 2015;**12**:871.

Roscoe L, Eisenberg E, Forde C. The role of patients' stories in emergency medicine triage. *Health Commun* 2016;**16**:1.

Topal E, Celiksoy M, Catal F, et al. The value of the clinical history for the diagnosis of immediate nonsteroidal anti-inflammatory drug hypersensitivity and safe alternative drugs in children. *Allergy Asthma Proc* 2016;**37**:57.

Venneman SS, Narnor-Harris P, Perish M, Hamilton M. "Allow natural death" versus "do not resuscitate": three words that can change a life. *J Med Ethics* 2008;**34**:2.

# 3

# Cardiopulmonary Symptoms

*Albert J. Heuer*

## LEARNING OBJECTIVES

*After reading this chapter, you will be able to:*

1. Describe the causes and common characteristics of the following symptoms:
   - Cough
   - Sputum production
   - Hemoptysis
   - Dyspnea
   - Chest pain

   - Dizziness and fainting
   - Swelling of the ankles
   - Fever, chills, and night sweats
   - Headache, altered mental status, and personality changes
   - Snoring
   - Gastroesophageal reflux
   - Daytime somnolence (sleepiness)

## OUTLINE

## KEY TERMS

angina
bronchorrhea
cough
daytime somnolence
diaphoresis
dyspnea
edema
fetid
fever

frothy
gastroesophageal reflux disease
    (GERD)
hematemesis
hemoptysis
night sweats
obstructive sleep apnea (OSA)
orthodeoxia
orthopnea

orthostatic hypotension
paroxysmal nocturnal dyspnea (PND)
phlegm
platypnea
sleep disordered breathing
sputum
syncope
tenacious
trepopnea

Symptoms are subjective clinical findings generally reported by the patient during or shortly after the initial interview (described in Chapter 2). Clinical signs, on the other hand, are objective and measurable, such as the vital signs and laboratory studies detailed in subsequent chapters of this text. Respiratory therapists (RTs) will encounter patients with a variety of symptoms. The primary symptoms associated with cardiopulmonary disorders are cough, sputum production, hemoptysis, shortness of breath (dyspnea), and chest pain. Other less specific complaints include dizziness and fainting; ankle swelling (peripheral edema); fever, chills, and night sweats; snoring; personality changes; daytime somnolence (sleepiness); and gastric reflux. This chapter defines the terms associated with these symptoms, briefly discusses their causes (etiology), and describes how these symptoms relate to commonly associated diseases. The more familiar RTs are with these symptoms and their characteristics, the better they can ask relevant questions, assist the patient care team in making a correct diagnosis, and help design an appropriate interdisciplinary treatment plan.

### SIMPLY STATED

Cardiopulmonary symptoms are assessed to determine the following:
- The seriousness of the patient's problem
- The potential underlying cause of the problem
- The effectiveness of treatment

## COUGH

Cough is one of the most common, though nonspecific, symptoms seen in patients with pulmonary disease. It is the powerful protective reflex arising from stimulation of receptors located in the pharynx, larynx, trachea, large bronchi, and even the lung and the visceral pleura. Coughing can be caused by inflammatory, mechanical, chemical, or thermal stimulation of cough receptors found anywhere from the oropharynx to the terminal bronchioles or simply by tactile pressure in the ear canal. There are many conditions that can make a patient cough. The key to determining the cause in many cases can be found in a careful review of the history, physical examination, and chest radiograph (Table 3.1).

Stimulation of the cough receptors is carried by afferent pathways of the reflex, primarily the vagus, phrenic, glossopharyngeal, and trigeminal nerves, to the cough center located diffusely in the medulla, separate from the respiratory center. Conduction of the impulses down the efferent pathway of the reflex stimulates the smooth muscles of the larynx and tracheobronchial tree, the diaphragm and other respiratory muscles through the phrenic and other spinal motor nerves. The cough mechanism can be divided into the following three phases:

**TABLE 3.1    Possible Causes of Cough Receptor Stimulation**

| Types of Stimulation | Possible Causes |
|---|---|
| Inflammatory | Infection, lung abscess, drug reaction, allergy, edema, hyperemia, collagen vascular disease, radiotherapy, pneumoconiosis, tuberculosis |
| Mechanical Obstructive | Inhaled dusts, suction catheter, food Foreign bodies, aspirations of nasal secretions, tumor or granulomas within or around the lung, aortic aneurysm |
| Airway wall tension | Pulmonary edema, atelectasis, fibrosis, chronic interstitial pneumonitis |
| Chemical | Inhaled irritant gases, fumes, smoke |
| Temperature | Inhaled hot or cold air |
| Ear | Tactile pressure in the ear canal (Arnold nerve response) or from otitis media |

1. *Inspiratory phase:* reflex opening of the glottis and contraction of the diaphragm, thoracic, and abdominal muscles cause a deep inspiration with a concomitant increase in lung volume accompanied by an increase in the caliber and length of the bronchi.
2. *Compression phase:* closure of the glottis and relaxation of the diaphragm while the expiratory muscles contract against the closed glottis can generate very high intrathoracic pressures and narrowing of the trachea and bronchi.
3. *Expiratory phase:* opening of the glottis, explosive release of trapped intrathoracic air, and vibration of the vocal cords and mucosal lining of the posterior laryngeal wall shake secretions loose from the larynx and move undesired material out of the respiratory tract.

The cough reflex may be voluntary or involuntary and normally occurs in everyone from time to time. The quality of a cough (force of the airflow) is determined by the depth of the inspiration and amount of pressure that can be generated in the airways. The effectiveness of a cough is reduced if one or more of the following conditions exist:

1. Weakness of either the inspiratory or expiratory muscles
2. Inability of the glottis to open or close correctly
3. Neurologic abnormalities that inhibit normal airway reflexes
4. Obstruction, collapsibility, or alteration in shape or contours of the airways
5. Decrease in lung recoil as occurs with emphysema
6. Abnormal quantity or quality of mucus production (e.g., thick sputum)

### Causes and Clinical Presentation

Most patients will have a single cause for their cough; however, in some patients two or three simultaneous causes (comorbidities) may be present. Cough may be acute (sudden onset, usually severe with a short course, self-limited),

## TABLE 3.2   Terms Used to Describe Cough

| Description | Possible Causes |
| --- | --- |
| Acute (<3 wk) or recurrent (adults) productive | Postnasal drip, allergies, infections, especially viral URI, bronchitis |
| Acute or recurrent (adults) and nonproductive | Laryngitis, inhalation of irritant gases |
| Chronic productive | Bronchiectasis, chronic bronchitis, lung abscess, asthma, fungal infections, bacterial pneumonias, tuberculosis |
| Chronic (>3 wk) or recurrent (adults) and nonproductive | Postnasal drip, asthma, gastroesophageal reflux, bronchiectasis, COPD, lung tumor, sarcoidosis, ACE inhibitors, left-sided heart failure |
| Recurrent (children) | Viral bronchitis, asthma, allergies |
| Dry | Viral infections, inhalation of irritant gases, interstitial lung diseases, pleural effusion, cardiac condition, nervous habit, tumor, radiation therapy, chemotherapy |
| Dry, progressing to productive | Atypical and mycoplasmal pneumonia, AIDS, Legionnaires' disease, asthma, silicosis, pulmonary embolus and edema, lung abscess, emphysema (late in disease), smoking |
| Inadequate, weak | Debility, weakness, oversedation, pain, poor motivation, emphysema |
| Paroxysmal (especially night) | Aspiration, asthma, left-sided heart failure |
| Barking | Epiglottal disease, croup, influenza, laryngotracheal bronchitis |
| Brassy or hoarse | Laryngitis, laryngotracheal bronchitis, laryngeal paralysis, pressure on recurrent laryngeal nerve: mediastinal tumor, aortic aneurysm, left atrial enlargement |
| Inspiratory stridor | Tracheal or main stem bronchial obstruction, croup, epiglottitis |
| Wheezy | Bronchospasm, asthma, bronchitis, cystic fibrosis |
| Morning | Chronic bronchitis, smoking |
| Associated with position change or lying down | Bronchiectasis, left-sided heart failure, chronic postnasal drip or sinusitis, gastroesophageal reflux with aspiration |
| Associated with eating or drinking | Neuromuscular disease of the upper airway, esophageal problems, aspiration |

*ACE,* Angiotensin-converting enzyme; *AIDS,* acquired immunodeficiency syndrome; *COPD,* chronic obstructive pulmonary disease; *URI,* upper respiratory infection (common cold).

chronic (persistent and troublesome for more than 3 weeks), or paroxysmal (periodic, prolonged, and forceful episodes). An acute self-limited cough is usually due to a viral infection involving the upper airway, which usually resolves in a few days. A chronic persistent cough is most commonly caused by postnasal drip syndrome, followed by acute asthma, acute exacerbation of chronic obstructive pulmonary disease (COPD), allergic rhinitis, gastroesophageal reflux disease (see discussion later in this chapter), chronic bronchitis, bronchiectasis, and other conditions such as left-sided heart failure, bronchogenic cancer, and sarcoidosis. In long-term smokers, chronic cough is usually due to chronic bronchitis ("smoker's cough"). Still other chronic coughs may result from certain medications, such as angiotensin-converting enzyme (ACE) inhibitors (e.g., lisinopril and ramipril), which are commonly prescribed for congestive heart failure and other cardiac conditions. Though not fully understood, patients taking ACE inhibitors may develop a chronic dry cough, possibly as a result of an increase in cough mediators that accumulate in the upper airway. Hence the medication history described in Chapter 2 can provide vital clues to the underlying cause. Aggravating, painful, or persistent cough or cough equivalent, such as throat clearing, is not normal and warrants further clinical investigation.

Cough may occur with other pulmonary symptoms such as wheezing, stridor, chest pain, and dyspnea. In addition, cough may cause problems. The intense muscular activity and high intrathoracic pressures created by forceful coughing may produce a number of complications, such as torn chest muscles, rib fractures, disruption of surgical wounds, pneumothorax or pneumomediastinum, syncope (fainting), arrhythmia, esophageal rupture, and urinary incontinence.

### Descriptions

Cough should be described as effective (strong enough to clear the airway) or inadequate (audible but too weak to mobilize the secretions), productive (mucus or other material is expelled by the cough), or dry and nonproductive (moisture or secretions are not produced). Because dry coughs often become productive, a chronologic report of the circumstances surrounding the change and a description of the sputum should be recorded.

The quality, time, and setting in which a cough occurs may also provide some clues to the location and type of disorder (Table 3.2). Barking (like a seal), brassy (harsh, dry), and hoarse coughs, as well as those associated with inspiratory stridor, are usually heard when there is a problem with the larynx (e.g., infection or tumor). Wheezy coughs (accompanied by whistling or sighing sounds) suggest bronchial disorders. Acute productive coughs are most often seen with allergic asthma, as well as bacterial or viral respiratory infections, and chronic productive coughs are generally indicative of significant bronchopulmonary disease (e.g., chronic bronchitis). Hacking (frequent brief periods of coughing or clearing the throat) may be dry and the result of smoking, a viral infection, a nervous habit, or difficult-to-move secretions, which may occur with postnasal drip.

Acute onset or change in a cough is often obvious to the patient and family and is therefore often reported to the interviewer recording the clinical history. However, careful inquiry is often required to identify the characteristics of a chronic cough. Because coughing and sputum production are generally not socially acceptable, patients may deny or minimize the presence of the cough or learn to adapt to the extent that they may even be unaware of coughing chronically. Questioning family members or close friends may provide valuable information about the presence and characteristics of a cough.

---

**QUESTIONS TO ASK**

**Cough**

*Ask the patient to describe the cough in his or her own words; if unable to give a description, use suggestions of descriptive words.*

- Can you describe your cough? How long have you had the cough?
- When did the cough start? Did the cough start suddenly? What were you doing when the cough started?
- Do you smoke? If so, what do you smoke? How much and for how many years?
- Do you have postnasal drip? Do you wheeze? Do you have heartburn? Do you notice an acid or bitter taste in your mouth?
- Do you cough up sputum or mucus and, if so, what is the amount, color, thickness, and odor?
- Is your cough better or worse at certain times of the day and does it wake you up?
- Do you cough on most days? Do you cough more during a particular day of the week? A particular season of the year?
- Is the cough worse in any position or when you are in a certain location?
- Is the cough associated with eating, drinking, or medications?
- Are there any other symptoms associated with the cough like chest pain? Wheezing? Fever? Runny nose? Hoarseness? Night sweats? Weight loss? Headache? Dizziness? Loss of consciousness?
- What relieves the cough?
- Have you had the flu or a "cold" with a cough recently?
- Have you ever been exposed to anyone with tuberculosis, the flu, or a "cold"?
- Do you have contact with animals? If so, what type, when, and how often?
- Are you taking ACE inhibitors? Have you taken ACE inhibitors in the past?
- Are you under stress?
- Is your cough dry? Do you clear your throat frequently?
- Have you been diagnosed with nasal allergies or allergic rhinitis?
- Do you have chronic bad breath (halitosis)? Do you have facial pain?
- Do you sleep with more than one pillow?
- Do you cough after exercise or physical exertion?
- What is your occupation? Is your cough worse during or immediately after work?

---

## SPUTUM PRODUCTION

Sputum is the substance expelled from the airways, mouth, sinuses, and nose by coughing or clearing the throat. The term phlegm refers strictly to secretions from the lungs and tracheobronchial tree. These respiratory tract secretions may contain a variety of materials, including mucus, cellular debris, microorganisms, blood, pus, and foreign particles and should not be confused with saliva. Up to 100 mL of sputum is produced each day. Sputum is moved upward by the wavelike motion of the cilia (tiny hairlike structures) lining the larynx, trachea, and bronchi, and it is usually swallowed unnoticed. As previously mentioned, sputum may be difficult or impossible for the patient to describe accurately because of the social stigma and lack of awareness. Thus collection and inspection of a sputum sample is often necessary to evaluate the patient's pulmonary status.

### Causes and Descriptions

Excessive sputum production is most often caused by inflammation of the mucous glands. Inflammation of these glands occurs most often with infection, cigarette smoking, and allergies.

Sputum should be described as to the color, consistency, odor, taste, quantity, time of day, and presence of blood or other features. The amount may vary from scanty (a few teaspoons) to copious (as much as a pint or more), as seen in certain chronic bronchial infections and bronchiectasis. Excessive bronchial secretion production of more than 100 mL per day associated with these and other conditions is also known as bronchorrhea. The amount and other characteristics of the sputum may be highly indicative of the underlying disorder (Table 3.3). Though sputum culture and sensitivity tests described in Chapter 7 provide for a more in-depth microbiologic examination of sputum, bedside examination can be helpful as an initial screening tool.

The consistency of sputum may be described as thin, thick, viscous (gelatinous), tenacious (extremely sticky), or frothy. Color depends on the origin and cause of the sputum production. Descriptions for the color of sputum include mucoid (clear, thin, and may be somewhat viscous as a result of oversecretion of bronchial mucus), mucopurulent (thick, viscous, colored, and often in globs with an offensive odor), and blood tinged. Large amounts of foul-smelling, or fetid, sputum that separates into layers when standing often occurs with bronchiectasis and lung abscess.

Excessive morning secretions are often due to the accumulation of secretions during the night, as seen with bronchitis. Nonpurulent, silicone-like bronchial secretions that assume the shape of the airway are called *casts* and are seen with severe cases of asthma. Sudden large amounts of sputum production may be indicative of a bronchopleural fistula.

## QUESTIONS TO ASK

**Sputum**

*Ask the patient to describe the sputum in his or her own words; if unable to give a description, use suggestions of descriptive words (e.g., green, yellow, white, clear, teaspoon, tablespoon, cup).*

- Do you usually bring up phlegm or mucus from your chest first thing in the morning?
- Do you usually bring up phlegm or mucus at other times of the day?
- Can you estimate the amount you bring up? About a cup? About a tablespoon? Has this amount changed?
- What color is it? Does it have a foul odor or taste?
- Has the sputum changed color recently?

## SIMPLY STATED

Chronic sputum production is most often related to irritation or disease of the airways (e.g., asthma or chronic bronchitis).

## TABLE 3.3   Presumptive Sputum Analysis

| Appearance of Sputum | Possible Cause |
| --- | --- |
| Clear, colorless, like egg white | Normal |
| Black | Smoke or coal dust inhalation |
| Brownish | Cigarette smoker |
| Frothy white or pink | Pulmonary edema |
| Sand or small stone | Aspiration of foreign material, broncholithiasis |
| Purulent (contains pus) | Infection, pneumonia caused by: |
| Apple-green, thick | *Haemophilus influenzae* |
| Pink, thin, blood-streaked | Streptococci or staphylococci |
| Red currant jelly | *Klebsiella* species |
| Rusty | Pneumococci |
| Yellow or green, copious | *Pseudomonas* species pneumonia, advanced chronic bronchitis, bronchiectasis (separates into layers) |
| Foul odor (fetid) | Lung abscess, aspiration, anaerobic infections, bronchiectasis |
| Mucoid (white-gray and thick) | Emphysema, pulmonary tuberculosis, early chronic bronchitis, neoplasms, asthma |
| Grayish | Legionnaires' disease |
| Silicone-like casts | Bronchial asthma |
| Mucopurulent | As above with infection, pneumonia, cystic fibrosis |
| Blood-streaked or hemoptysis (frankly bloody) | Bronchogenic carcinoma, tuberculosis, chronic bronchitis, coagulopathy, pulmonary contusion or abscess (see discussion of causes of hemoptysis) |

## BOX 3.1   Notable Causes of Hemoptysis

**Frequent Causes of Hemoptysis**
Acute bronchitis with severe coughing
Bronchogenic carcinoma
Bronchiectasis[a]
Chronic bronchitis[a]
Tuberculosis[a]

**Less Frequent Causes of Hemoptysis**
*Pulmonary*
Aspiration of a foreign body
Bronchoarterial fistula[a]
Broncholithiasis
Deep mycotic infection[a]
Metastatic carcinoma
Pulmonary abscess[a]
Pulmonary embolism, infarction
Trauma, pulmonary contusion

*Cardiopulmonary*
Arteriovenous malformation
Mitral stenosis
Cardiac pulmonary edema
Pulmonary hypertension

*Systemic*
Coagulation disorders[a]
Goodpasture syndrome
Sarcoidosis, Wegener granulomatosis

*Other Pseudohemoptyses*
Emesis
Oropharyngeal or nosebleed

[a]Potential causes of massive hemoptysis.

## HEMOPTYSIS

### Definition

Hemoptysis, expectoration of sputum containing blood, varies in severity from slight streaking to frank bleeding. It can be an alarming symptom that may suggest serious disease and massive hemorrhage. In more severe forms, it is a frightening experience for both the patient and the RT or other member of the health care team.

### Causes

Differential diagnosis is complex and includes bronchopulmonary, cardiovascular, hematologic, and other systemic disorders (Box 3.1). A history of pulmonary or cardiovascular disease; cigarette smoking, vaping, or e-cigarette use and tobacco use; trauma; aspiration of a foreign body; repeated and severe lung infections; bleeding disorder; use of anticoagulant agents (warfarin or heparin), aspirin, nonsteroidal antiinflammatory agents, or chemotherapeutic agents; or inhaling crack cocaine suggests the possible cause of hemoptysis. A history of travel to places where tuberculosis or fungal infections, such as coccidioidomycosis or histoplasmosis, are prevalent, including central Africa (tuberculosis) and the San Joaquin Valley of California (coccidioidomycosis), may also help identify the underlying disorder.

The site of bleeding may be anywhere in the respiratory tract, including the nose or mouth. The amount and mechanisms of bleeding are varied. Tissues engorged by inflammation or back pressure from heart failure or other cardiac problems may bleed easily and cause frothy pink sputum. Trauma bruises tissue or may tear a vessel. Chronic or repeated respiratory infections resulting in bronchiectasis can predispose the patient to bleeding. A tumor or granuloma can erode surrounding tissue or the bronchial wall. An acute infective process can create an abscess in the bronchial tree or lung parenchyma, which can erode into another structure (e.g., bronchopleural fistula) or completely through a vessel wall. If the vessel is an artery, hemorrhage can be sudden and massive and may lead to death due to excessive blood loss.

Historically, tuberculosis and bronchiectasis were the most common causes of hemoptysis. Erosive bronchitis in smokers with chronic bronchitis and bronchogenic carcinoma are now also recognized as frequent causes of hemoptysis. In fact, blood-streaked sputum may be the only hint that bronchogenic cancer has developed in the smoker.

## Descriptions

Obtaining a description of the amount, odor, color, and appearance of blood produced, as well as the acuteness or chronicity of the bleeding, may provide a clue to the source of bleeding. The most common causes of streaky hemoptysis are pulmonary infection (chronic bronchitis, bronchiectasis, or bacterial pneumonias), lung cancer, and thromboemboli.

Careful evaluation and description of hemoptysis production are crucial because it can include clots of blood as well as blood-tinged sputum. Coughing up clots of blood is a symptom of extreme importance that suggests serious illness. Massive hemoptysis (400 mL in 3 hours or more than 600 mL in 24 hours) is seen with lung cancers, tuberculosis, bronchiectasis, and trauma. It is an emergency condition associated with possible mortality. Immediate action is required to maintain an adequate airway, and emergency bronchoscopy and surgery may be necessary.

Associated symptoms may also provide a clue to the source of bleeding. Sometimes patients can describe a sensation, often warmth, in the area where the blood originates. Others perceive a bubbling sensation in the airways followed by expectoration of blood. Hemoptysis associated with sudden onset of chest pain and dyspnea in a patient at risk for venous stasis of the legs must prompt evaluation for pulmonary embolism and possible infarction. Frothy, blood-tinged sputum associated with nighttime cough accompanies cardiac-induced pulmonary edema.

Hemoptysis without severe coughing is sometimes associated with a bronchial tumor.

## Hemoptysis versus Hematemesis

"Spitting up blood," as patients frequently call it, may be confused with blood originating in the oropharynx, esophagus, or stomach. The patient with a nosebleed at night could cough up blood in the morning. The presence of symptoms, such as nausea and vomiting, especially with a history of alcoholism or cirrhosis of the liver, may suggest the esophagus or stomach as the source. Conversely, vomiting of blood may sometimes manifest from bronchopulmonary bleeding. When bleeding occurs during the night and the blood reaches the oropharynx, it may be swallowed without the patient waking. The swallowed blood may act as an irritant, and the patient may vomit early in the morning. Careful questioning and often examination of the bloody sputum are required to distinguish hemoptysis from hematemesis (vomited blood) (Table 3.4). It is important to try to determine whether the blood originated in the respiratory tract and was swallowed and then vomited, or the blood was vomited, aspirated, and later expectorated, to help ensure an accurate differential diagnosis.

---

### QUESTIONS TO ASK

**Hemoptysis**

*Ask the patient the following questions to help obtain an accurate and impartial history:*

- Do you smoke? If so, how much and what do you smoke?
- Do you use a vaping device or electronic cigarettes? If so, how much and how often?
- Do you use smokeless tobacco? If so, how much and what do you use?
- Did you start coughing up blood suddenly?
- How long have you noticed the blood?
- Do you have a fever? Do you have a cough?
- Do you cough up anything else with the blood? Can you describe what it looks like?
- Is the sputum blood tinged or are there actual clots of blood?
- Have there been recurrent episodes of coughing up blood?
- Do you have chest pain?
- What seems to bring on the coughing up of blood? Is it brought on by vomiting, coughing, or nausea?
- Have you felt any unusual sensations in your chest after you cough up the blood? Before you cough up the blood? If yes, where? Can you tell me how it feels?
- Have you had a recent nosebleed?
- Have you been involved in a recent accident or had an injury to your chest, side, or back?
- Have you traveled lately?
- Have you ever had tuberculosis? Have you been exposed to anyone who has had tuberculosis?
- Are you human immunodeficiency virus (HIV) positive? Do you have a history of cancer?
- Have you had recent surgery?
- Have you had night sweats? Shortness of breath? Irregular heartbeats? Hoarseness? Weight loss? Swelling or pain in your legs?
- Is there a family history of coughing up blood? Are you aware of any bleeding tendency in you or your family?
- Have you been exposed to anything at work or hobbies?
- Do you take any blood thinners or aspirin? If yes, how much and how often? Do you take oral contraceptives? Do you use injection drugs?

# SHORTNESS OF BREATH (DYSPNEA)

Shortness of breath (SOB, as it is commonly abbreviated in the medical record) or difficult breathing as perceived by the patient is the most distressing symptom of respiratory disease and is also a cardinal symptom of cardiac disease. Dyspnea may also be associated with metabolic diseases (such as diabetic ketoacidosis), hematologic disorders, toxic ingestion, or psychiatric conditions. Difficult breathing impairs the ability to work or exercise and may interfere with the simplest activities of daily living such as walking, eating, bathing, speaking, and sleeping. In patients with pulmonary disease, it is the single most important factor limiting their ability to function on a day-to-day basis and is frequently the reason the patient seeks medical care.

Dyspnea (*dys,* difficult; *pnea,* breathing) is defined as a subjective experience of breathing discomfort that consists of qualitatively distinct sensations that vary in intensity. The sensations associated with dyspnea range from a slight awareness of breathing to severe respiratory distress and may be mixed with anxiety in severe cases. The sensations experienced by the patient are a product of various factors such as the severity of the physiologic impairment and the psychological makeup of the patient.

## Subjectiveness of Dyspnea

Dyspnea may be difficult to evaluate because it is so subjective. The sensation of dyspnea is made up of the following components:

1. *Sensory input to the cerebral cortex.* Multiple sources of sensory information from mechanoreceptors in the upper airway, thorax, and muscles are integrated in the central nervous system and sent to the sensorimotor cortex in the brain. In general, the sensation of dyspnea is related to the intensity of the input from the thoracic structures and from chemoreceptors. It varies directly with ventilatory demand such as exercise and inversely with ventilatory capacity (ability to move gas in and out of the lung). The more stimulation of the drive to breathe when ventilatory abnormalities exist, the greater the dyspnea.
2. *Perception of the sensation.* Perception relies on interpretation of the information arriving at the sensorimotor cortex, and interpretation is highly dependent on the psychological makeup of the person. The emotional state, distraction, and belief of significance can influence the perception of dyspnea.

A patient's perception of dyspnea may have no relation to the patient's breathing appearance. Remember, dyspnea is subjective—a symptom—and what the patient feels. A patient may have labored and rapid breathing and deny feeling short of breath. Conversely, a patient may appear to be breathing comfortably and slowly but may feel breathless. You can never assume that a patient with a rapid respiratory rate is dyspneic. In addition, a patient's complaint of dyspnea must be considered a symptom of a medical problem and must be taken seriously until proved otherwise. In fact, the onset of dyspnea may be the first clue to identifying serious problems.

Patients' perceptions of dyspnea vary greatly. A healthy person notices the increased ventilatory demand required to climb stairs or to exercise but expects it and does not interpret it as unpleasant. In fact, the athlete may consider the breathlessness occurring after a sprint to be exhilarating and even a necessary aspect of physical conditioning. Patients, on the other hand, may describe the feeling as "breathless," "short winded," "feeling of suffocation," or a sensation of "air hunger" at rest or during minimal exercise.

## Dyspnea Scoring Systems

A variety of methods have been devised to help quantify dyspnea at a single point in time or to help track changes in dyspnea over time or with treatment. In the clinical setting, patients are frequently asked to rate the severity of a symptom, such as dyspnea or pain, using a severity scale of 0 to 10. The patient is asked a question such as "On a scale of 0 to 10, how would you rate your shortness of breath when you are resting? Using this scale, 0 means no shortness of breath, and 10 means the worst or maximum shortness of breath." The patient's response may be recorded simply as "SOB at rest 7/10."

Visual analog scales are straight lines, "usually 10 cm long," with the words "Not Breathless" at one end and "Extremely Breathless" at the other end. The patient marks the line to indicate his or her level of respiratory discomfort. The score is measured as the length of the line between "Not Breathless" and the mark made by the patient. The score may be recorded as 5.5/10 or simply as 5.5 (the 10 is implied).

A Modified Borg Scale, such as shown in Table 3.5, also uses a 0-to-10 scoring system with descriptive terms to depict the perceived intensity of a symptom such as dyspnea after a specified task. In addition, there are questionnaires that attempt to quantify the severity of dyspnea by asking patients to rate their shortness of breath while performing a variety of activities of daily living.

## TABLE 3.4 Distinguishing Characteristics of Hemoptysis and Hematemesis

| Characteristic | Hemoptysis | Hematemesis |
|---|---|---|
| History | Cardiopulmonary disease | Gastrointestinal disease |
| As stated by the patient | Coughed up from lungs/chest | Vomited from stomach |
| Associated symptoms | Dyspnea, pain or tickling sensation in chest | Nausea, pain referred to stomach |
| Blood: pH | Alkaline | Acid |
| Mixed with | Sputum | Food |
| Froth | May be present | Absent |
| Color | Bright red | Dark, clotted, "coffee grounds" |

More recently, other scales have emerged for rating dyspnea in cardiopulmonary disease. One such scale is the Dyspnea-12 Survey, or "D-12," which quantifies a patient's level of breathlessness using 12 physical and psychosocial descriptors. This rating scale is showing particular promise in determining the severity of dyspnea in patients who have asthma. Another even simpler such scale often used for COPD patients is the Modified Medical Research Council (MMRC) Dyspnea Scale. This scale classifies the grade of

dyspnea based on which one of five choices best describes the patient's breathlessness. The MMRC ranges from a grade of "0" for patients who *only get breathless with strenuous exercise* to a grade of "4" for those who claim to be *too breathless to leave the course* or become *breathless when dressing.*

## Causes, Types, and Clinical Presentations of Dyspnea

Dyspnea is most often related to pulmonary or cardiac disease, but it is also seen with hematologic, metabolic, chemical, neurologic, psychogenic, and mechanical disorders. Dyspnea may be described by clinical type as shown in Table 3.6, or the causes of dyspnea may be grouped by body system as listed in Table 3.7.

Attempts to understand the physiologic bases of dyspnea have evolved around several separate concepts, including mechanics of breathing, ventilatory performance, work and efficiency of breathing, oxygen cost, length-tension inappropriateness, chemoreception, and exercise testing. The discussion of each concept and its related disorders is beyond the scope of this text. However, it is helpful to remember that patients with respiratory disorders will complain of dyspnea when any of the following are present alone or in combination:

1. The work of breathing is abnormally high for the given level of exertion. This is common with narrowed airways as in asthma and when the lung is stiff as in pneumonia.

### TABLE 3.5  Modified Borg Scale for Estimation of Subjective Symptoms

| Rating | Intensity of Sensation |
|--------|------------------------|
| 0 | Nothing at all |
| 0.5 | Very, very mild/weak |
| 1 | Very mild/weak |
| 2 | Mild/weak |
| 3 | Moderate |
| 4 | Somewhat severe/strong |
| 5 | |
| 6 | |
| 7 | Very severe/strong |
| 8 | |
| 9 | Very, very severe/strong |
| 10 | MAXIMAL |

### TABLE 3.6  Clinical Types of Dyspneas

| Dyspnea | Associated with | Associated Signs and Symptoms |
|---------|-----------------|-------------------------------|
| Physiologic | Exercise, acute hypoxia (e.g., high altitude) | Awareness of increased ventilation |
| | Breathing high concentration of $CO_2$ in a closed space | If space is also devoid of $O_2$, confusion and unconsciousness may occur before dyspnea warns of danger |
| **Pulmonary** | | |
| Restrictive | Pulmonary fibrosis | Comfortable at rest |
| | Chest deformities | Intensely dyspneic when exertion nears patient's limited breathing capacity |
| | Pleural effusion | |
| | Pneumothorax | |
| Obstructive | Asthma | Increased ventilatory effort |
| | Obstructive emphysema | Dyspnea at rest |
| | | Breathing labored and retarded, especially during expiration |
| Cardiac | Heart failure | Orthopnea, paroxysmal nocturnal dyspnea, "cardiac asthma," periodic respiration |
| Circulatory | Chronic anemia | Dyspnea only with exertion unless anemia is extreme |
| | Exsanguinating hemorrhage | "Air hunger" a grave sign |
| Chemical | Uremia (kidney failure) | Dyspnea with severe panting caused by acidosis, heart failure, pulmonary edema, and anemia |
| Central | Head injury | Hyperventilation |
| | Cerebral lesion | Intense hyperventilation |
| | | Sometimes noisy and stertorous |
| | | Biot respiration |
| Psychogenic | Pain-related dyspnea | Continuous hyperventilation or deep sighing respirations at maximal depth |
| | Hysterical overbreathing | |
| | Sighing dyspnea | |

2. The ventilatory capacity is reduced. This is common when the vital capacity is abnormally low as seen in patients with neuromuscular disease.
3. The drive to breathe is elevated beyond normal (e.g., hypoxemia, acidosis, or exercise).

### Clinical Types of Dyspneas

The physiologic cause of a patient's dyspnea often results in the patient using unique terms to describe his or her discomfort. The patient with asthma frequently describes dyspnea as "tightness in the chest." Patients with congestive heart failure (CHF) often describe a sensation of "suffocation" or "air hunger." Patients with COPD and interstitial lung disease often complain of "increased effort to breathe," probably because of the increased work of breathing associated with these disorders. These results suggest that dyspnea may vary from patient to patient according to the underlying pathophysiology.

Cardiac- and circulatory-related dyspnea occurs primarily when there is an inadequate supply of oxygen to the tissues. In early heart failure, dyspnea is seen primarily during exercise when the decreased pumping power of the heart cannot keep up with the demands created by exercise. The shortness of breath may be accompanied by hyperventilation and be associated with fatigue or a feeling of smothering or sternal compression. In later stages, the lungs become congested with blood and edema, causing an increase in the work of breathing and dyspnea at rest and when lying down. Dyspnea is also associated with anemia and occurs primarily with exertion unless the anemia is extreme. "Air hunger" is a grave sign indicating the need for immediate transfusion in the anemic patient.

Psychogenic dyspnea, or *panic disorder* as it is sometimes called, is a hysterical type of overbreathing that usually presents as breathlessness. A precipitating event other than a stress can rarely be identified. The event is not related to exertion; testing and physical examination are negative. Hyperventilation is common in patients with panic disorder.

Hyperventilating is breathing at a rate and depth in excess of the body's metabolic need, which causes a decrease in arterial carbon dioxide ($Paco_2$) and results in a decrease in cerebral blood flow. Patients with psychogenic dyspnea are usually very anxious and may describe feeling faint or lightheaded, with numbness and tingling around their mouth and in their extremities. They may report having visual disturbances. If they continue to hyperventilate, they may lose consciousness.

### Acute and Chronic Dyspnea

Dyspnea may be acute or chronic, progressive, recurrent, paroxysmal, or episodic. Acute dyspnea in children is most frequently associated with asthma, bronchiolitis, croup, and epiglottitis. In adults the causes are more varied (Box 3.2). Pulmonary embolism should be suspected if a patient is in the postoperative

| TABLE 3.7 Causes of Dyspnea by Body System | |
|---|---|
| **System** | **Common Causes of Dyspnea** |
| Respiratory | Airway obstruction, asthma, COPD, pneumonia, pulmonary embolus, pneumothorax, pulmonary fibrosis, pleural effusion |
| Cardiac | Congestive heart failure, pericardial effusion, cardiac shunts, valvular lesions |
| Hematologic | Severe anemia, carbon monoxide poisoning, hemoglobinopathies |
| Neurologic | Brain tumor, CNS inflammation, increased intracranial pressure, hypertensive encephalopathy, CVA |
| Metabolic and endocrine | Toxins, uremia, hepatic coma, thyrotoxicosis, myxedema |
| Psychiatric | Pain-related dyspnea, severe anxiety, hyperventilation syndrome |
| Mechanical factors | Chest wall deformities, diaphragmatic paralysis, hepatosplenomegaly, massive ascites, tumors, pregnancy, obesity |

*CNS*, Central nervous system; *COPD*, chronic obstructive pulmonary disease; *CVA*, cerebrovascular accident.

### BOX 3.2 Common Causes of Acute and Chronic Dyspnea

**Acute Dyspnea**
Asthma[a]
Chest trauma
Physical exertion
Pleural effusion
Pneumonia
Pulmonary edema
Pulmonary embolism
Pulmonary hemorrhage
Spontaneous pneumothorax
Cardiac pulmonary edema
Acute interstitial lung disease (e.g., hemorrhage, ARDS)
Upper airway obstruction (e.g., aspirated foreign body, laryngospasm)

**Chronic Dyspnea**
*(usually progressive)*
Asthma[a]
CHF, left ventricular failure[a]
Cystic fibrosis
Pleural effusion
Interstitial lung diseases
Pulmonary vascular disease
Pulmonary thromboembolic disease
COPD
Severe anemia
Psychogenic dyspnea
Hypersensitivity disorders
Chest wall abnormalities (e.g., neuromuscular disease, kyphoscoliosis, diaphragm paralysis)

*ARDS*, Acute respiratory distress syndrome; *CHF*, congestive heart failure; *COPD*, chronic obstructive pulmonary disease.

[a]Asthma and left ventricular failure represent chronic causes of dyspnea with paroxysmal exacerbations.

period or has a history of prolonged bed rest, phlebitis, or cardiac arrhythmia. Women who are pregnant or taking birth control pills are also at higher risk for pulmonary embolism. Asthma, upper airway obstruction, foreign body aspiration, pneumonia, pneumothorax, pulmonary edema, hyperventilation, and panic disorder may also cause acute dyspnea.

Chronic dyspnea is almost always progressive. It begins with dyspnea on exertion and over time progresses to dyspnea at rest. Most patients with chronic dyspnea do not seek medical help until their lung disease is advanced and treatment options are limited. Instead, as their lung disease progresses, they adopt a sedentary lifestyle that requires very little exertion to avoid feeling short of breath.

COPD and CHF are the most common causes of chronic dyspnea in adults. Determining whether the dyspnea is related to the lungs versus the heart can be difficult, especially in older patients. Pulmonary function testing, electrocardiogram, and chest radiographs often prove helpful.

## Descriptions

Patients may complain of dyspnea occurring at certain times of the day, in association with a position, or during a specific phase of the respiratory cycle. Inspiratory dyspnea is usually associated with upper airway obstruction, whereas expiratory dyspnea occurs with obstruction of smaller bronchi and bronchioles.

Paroxysmal nocturnal dyspnea (PND) is the sudden onset of difficult breathing that occurs when a sleeping patient is in the recumbent position. It is often associated with coughing and is relieved when the patient assumes an upright position. In patients with CHF, PND usually occurs 1 to 2 hours after lying down and is caused by the gradual transfer of fluid in the lower extremities to the lungs.

Orthopnea is the inability to breathe when lying down. It is often described as two- or three-pillow orthopnea, depending on the number of pillows the patient must use to elevate the upper portion of the body and obtain relief. PND and orthopnea are most commonly associated with left-sided heart failure and occur when reclining causes fluid to collect in the lungs.

Trepopnea is dyspnea caused by lying on one side that does not occur when the patient turns to the other side. Trepopnea is most often associated with disorders of the chest that occur on only one side such as unilateral lung disease, unilateral pleural effusion, or unilateral airway obstruction.

Platypnea, the opposite of orthopnea, is dyspnea caused by upright posture and relieved by a recumbent position. Orthodeoxia (ortho, positional; deoxia, decrease of oxygen) is arterial oxygen desaturation (hypoxemia) that is produced by assuming an upright position and relieved by returning to a recumbent position. Orthodeoxia and platypnea are seen in patients with right-to-left intracardiac shunts from congenital heart disease and in patients with venous-to-arterial shunts in the lung related to severe lung disease or chronic liver diseases such as cirrhosis. Simply stated, when these patients are upright there is an increased amount of blood being shunted from the right side of the heart to the left without

being adequately oxygenated. When orthodeoxia is severe, patients experience increasing dyspnea (platypnea) while standing. Orthodeoxia also may occur after a pneumonectomy (removal of a lung). Terms commonly used to describe dyspnea are listed in Table 3.8.

Occurrences of dyspnea should be chronologically recorded, including related symptoms such as coughing, wheezing, pain, position, and exertion. Coughing in conjunction with dyspnea occurs with acute or chronic infection, asthma, aspiration, CHF, COPD, and many of the diffuse lung diseases. Dyspnea with minimal exertion is frequently associated with poor conditioning, inactivity, obesity, and heavy smoking. Shortness of breath during exercise or excitement is also a common complaint associated with chronic severe anemia (e.g., hemoglobin concentration less than 6 to 7 g/dL). Table 3.9 lists associated symptoms, precipitating and relieving factors, and characteristics of the dyspnea-related disorders.

The effects of dyspnea on activities of daily living (dressing, eating, sleeping, or walking) must be reviewed. Patients with COPD tend to decrease their exercise progressively to prevent being short of breath until their activities of daily living are compromised out of proportion to their actual cardiorespiratory potential. It is essential to gain a picture of the patient's daily habits and routines, as well as the physical, emotional,

| TABLE 3.8 | Terms Commonly Used to Describe Breathing |
|---|---|
| **Medical Term** | **Definition** |
| Apnea | Absence of spontaneous ventilation |
| Dyspnea | Unpleasant awareness of difficulty breathing, shortness of breath, or breathlessness |
| Eupnea | Normal rate and depth of breathing |
| Bradypnea | Less than normal rate of breathing |
| Tachypnea | Rapid rate of breathing |
| Hypopnea | Decreased depth of breathing |
| Hyperpnea | Increased depth of breathing with or without an increased rate |
| Orthopnea | Dyspnea in the recumbent position but not in the upright or semivertical position |
| Trepopnea | Dyspnea in one lateral position but not in the other lateral position |
| Platypnea | Dyspnea caused by upright posture and relieved by a recumbent position |
| Orthodeoxia | Arterial oxygen desaturation (hypoxemia) that is produced by assuming an upright position and relieved by returning to a recumbent position |
| Hyperventilation | Increased alveolar ventilation caused by an increased rate or increased depth of breathing or both |
| Hypoventilation | Decreased alveolar ventilation caused by a decreased rate or decreased depth of breathing or both |
| Air hunger | A grave sign associated with extreme shortness of breath, indicating the need for immediate treatment |

familial, and occupational environment. The potential for relief of the factors contributing to dyspnea should be assessed and recorded.

## CHEST PAIN

The causes of chest pain vary greatly and can range from a self-limiting orthopedic injury such as a pulled chest muscle to much more serious conditions, including cardiac ischemia (low blood supply to the myocardium) or inflammatory disorders affecting thoracic or abdominal structures or organs. As a result, it is important to promptly and correctly determine the cause of a patient's chest pain. However, uncovering the root cause can be challenging for many reasons, including the complexity of the nerve structure of the chest, which can result in pain from other locations being referred to the chest and pain from the chest being referred to other sites. For example, pain from indigestion is often referred to the chest. Pain from a dissecting aneurysm of the thoracic aorta may start just below the sternum (anterior substernal location) but then migrates or tears toward the back. Despite such challenges, by investigating the characteristics of a patient's chest pain, the RT can assist in making a correct diagnosis and optimizing patient care.

Chest pain can also occur from musculoskeletal disorders, trauma, drug therapy, indigestion, and anxiety. It can range in character from sharp or stabbing to a vague feeling of heaviness or discomfort. It may be steady or intermittent, mild or acute. It may be caused or aggravated by stress, exertion, deep breathing, coughing, moving, or eating certain foods. The precise cause of chest pain cannot always be determined by taking a history, but it is usually possible to determine whether the origin is from the chest wall, the pleurae, or viscera and whether emergency care is needed. *History taking and the patient interview are key to evaluating chest pain.*

For example, chest pain is the cardinal symptom of heart disease. In its classic presentation, a patient may report "viselike" chest pain radiating down the arms, most often the left, which may spread to the shoulders, neck, jaw, or back. This type of chest pain is known as angina and signals a medical emergency. Intervention to open a clogged coronary artery and reestablish blood flow to the heart muscle should occur within about 90 minutes from the onset of pain, or else irreversible damage to the heart muscle is likely. Unfortunately, not all heart pain presents with this classic picture. In fact, in some people there is only a weak relationship between the severity of the chest pain and the importance of the underlying cause. Therefore *all chest pain must be taken seriously.*

### SIMPLY STATED

Cardiac chest pain in men is most often located in the center of the chest and may radiate to the arm, jaw, or back; in women it is located across the center of the chest, may radiate to the back and down the legs, and may be accompanied by nausea and dizziness.

The characteristics of the more common causes of chest pain are summarized in Table 3.10.

### Pulmonary Causes of Chest Pain

Chest pain caused by pulmonary disease is usually the result of involvement of the chest wall or parietal pleura (the serous membrane that lines the inner chest wall), both of which are well supplied with pain fibers. The lung parenchyma has no pain receptors. However, acute pulmonary diseases such as

**TABLE 3.9    Causes and Characteristics of Shortness of Breath**

| Cause | Type of Dyspnea | Associated Symptoms | Precipitating and Aggravating Factors | Patient Characteristics | Usual Physical Findings |
|---|---|---|---|---|---|
| **Acute or Recurrent Dyspnea** | | | | | |
| Asthma | Acute dyspnea Periodic | Cough indicates asthmatic bronchitis | Allergies, noxious fumes, exercise, respiratory tract infection | Most common cause of recurrent dyspnea in children | Bilateral wheezing, prolonged expiration |
| | | Dyspnea may be exertional and/or worse at night | Exposure to cold or use of certain types of β-blockers | | |
| Pneumothorax | Acute onset | Sudden, sharp pleuritic pain | Spontaneous, COPD, trauma, cystic fibrosis | Often a prior history of similar episode | Decreased or absent breath sounds Tracheal shift if tension pneumothorax |
| Foreign-body aspiration | Acute dyspnea | | | Most common in children and intoxicated or semiconscious people during eating | Tachypnea, inspiratory stridor, localized or unilateral wheeze, suprasternal retraction with respiration |
| Pulmonary emboli | Acute onset | Chest pain, faintness, loss of consciousness | Prolonged lying down; women using birth control pills, especially those who smoke | Postoperative, phlebitis, postpartum, arrhythmia (atrial fibrillation and flutter) | Tachypnea, crackles, low blood pressure, wheezing → pleural friction rub |
| Pulmonary edema | Acute onset Episodic | Dyspnea on exertion Orthopnea, PND | | | Gallop rhythm crackles at bases |
| Hyperventilation and anxiety | Acute dyspnea, "sighing" respiration | Lightheaded, palpitations, tingling (especially around mouth and extremities) | Stress, panic | Usually anxious | Signs of anxiety but no signs of dyspnea |
| Poor physical conditioning | Dyspnea on minimal exertion | | | Obese, physically inactive | After exercise, pulse slows very gradually |
| **Chronic Dyspnea** | | | | | |
| Congestive heart failure | Chronic dyspnea with gradual onset, PND | Edema, dyspnea remains long after exercise is stopped | Exercise, lying down, trauma, anesthesia, shock, hemorrhage, calcium channel blockers or β-blockers | Older patients, nocturnal dyspnea relieved by sitting | Shallow respirations but not necessarily rapid, basilar crackles, jugular venous distention, edema, third heart sound, hepatomegaly |
| Chronic bronchitis | Dyspnea not necessarily presenting symptom | Persistent, productive cough | Infection, exertion | Overweight | Coarse crackles, cyanosis |
| Emphysema | Progressive, usually no dyspnea at rest | Weak cough | Exertion | Malnourished | Hyperinflated lungs, decreased breath sounds, increased resonance, increased AP chest diameter, use of accessory muscles at rest |

*AP,* Anteroposterior; *COPD,* chronic obstructive pulmonary disease; *PND,* paroxysmal nocturnal dyspnea.

## TABLE 3.10   Causes and Characteristics of Chest Pain

| Condition | Location and Characteristics | Etiology/Precipitating Factors | Associated Findings |
|---|---|---|---|
| **Chest Wall Pain** | | | |
| Myalgia | Intercostal and pectoralis muscles | Trauma, seizure, nonisometric and isometric exercise, COPD, steroid therapy | Usually no visible erythema or ecchymosis with occult trauma |
| | Localized dull aching Increases with movement Usually long-lasting | Persistent severe cough | |
| Chondro-ostealgia | Ribs and cartilages, precisely located (chondral pain in sternal area) | Trauma (e.g., steering wheel, cardiopulmonary resuscitation), severe coughing, osteoporosis, tumor, myelocytic leukemia, systemic autoimmune disease, COPD | Rib fractures, chondral dislocations, periostitis, fever with some systemic causes |
| | Increases with pressure to area, movement, respiration, coughing Can be severe and disabling | | |
| Neuralgia | Dermatome distribution Superficial tingling to deep burning pain | Thoracic spine disease, metastatic tumor, blunt trauma, herpes zoster (shingles) | Specific changes on x-ray films, fever with infection |
| **Pleuritic and Pulmonary Pain** | | | |
| Pleuritis (pleurisy) | Pleura, usually well localized Sharp, stabbing, raw, burning Often rapid onset, increased by inspiration, coughing, laughing, hiccupping | Infection/inflammation of pleura, trauma, autoimmune and connective tissue disease | Fever, productive cough, tachypnea, splinting of affected side |
| Pulmonary embolus, pulmonary infarction | Usually at base of lung, may radiate to abdomen or costal margins | Immobilization, obesity, pelvic surgery | Symptoms vary with size of embolus |
| | Stabbing, sudden onset, increased by inspiration | | Anxiety to panic Dyspnea, tachypnea, tachycardia, coughing with blood-tinged to hemoptoic sputum |
| Pneumothorax | Lateral thorax, well localized | Interstitial lung disease, bullous emphysema, asthma, idiopathic | Dyspnea, tachypnea, decreased breath sounds on affected side |
| | Sharp, tearing Sudden onset Increased by inspiration | May follow deep inspiration, Valsalva maneuver, or exercise or occur at rest | Mediastinal shift and jugular venous distention if tension pneumothorax develops |
| Tumors | May be localized or diffuse | Invasion of primary or metastatic tumor through parenchyma to parietal pleura, mesothelioma | Symptoms vary with type and location |
| | Constant, sharp, boring, or dull | | Evidence from x-ray films History of asbestos exposure |
| Pulmonary hypertension (primary) | Substernal, dull, aching, similar to angina | Unknown | Dyspnea, tachypnea, anxiety, syncope, jugular venous distention |
| | Related to stress and exertion | Seen most commonly in young women | |
| **Cardiac Pain** | | | |
| Angina pectoris | Substernal, may radiate to arms, shoulders, neck, jaw, and back | Coronary artery blockage or spasm | Anxiety, feeling of impending doom, dyspnea, sweating, nausea |
| | Tightness or dull, heavy pressure-like pain not related to respiration | Hot, humid weather, large meals, intense emotion, exercise | Relieved by nitroglycerin and rest |
| Myocardial infarction | Substernal, radiating like angina | | As above, diaphoresis, vomiting |
| | Sudden crushing, viselike pain lasting minutes to hours | | Not relieved by nitroglycerin or rest |

*Continued*

### TABLE 3.10   Causes and Characteristics of Chest Pain—cont'd

| Condition | Location and Characteristics | Etiology/Precipitating Factors | Associated Findings |
|---|---|---|---|
| Pericardial pain | Substernal or parasternal radiating to neck, shoulder, and epigastrium (rarely to arms) | Inflammation of pericardium, infection, metastatic tumor, trauma, irradiation, autoimmune diseases | Pericardial friction rub |
| | Sharp, stabbing, intermittent | | Tachycardia, distended neck veins, paradoxic pulse with tamponade, dyspnea |
| | Intensified by respiration and lying on left side | | |
| **Mediastinal Pain** | | | |
| Esophageal | Substernal, retrosternal, epigastric | Esophagitis aggravated by bending over, lying down, smoking, ingestion of coffee, fats, large meals | Regurgitation of sour-tasting acid secretions relieved by antacids or may be relieved by nitroglycerin |
| | Radiates toward shoulders | Esophageal spasm | Hematemesis, shock |
| | Deep burning pain | Esophageal tear | |
| | Sudden tearing pain | | |
| Dissecting aortic aneurysm | Tearing midline chest or posterior thoracic pain | Blunt trauma, hypertension, inflammatory or degenerative diseases | May have lower blood pressure in legs or one arm, paralysis, murmur of aortic insufficiency, paradoxic pulse, hypertension, shock, death |
| | Sudden onset, may last hours | | |
| Tracheobronchitis | Substernal burning discomfort | Acute viral infections, prolonged cigarette smoking | Cough may or may not be productive |
| | May have fever with infection | | May be referred to anterior chest |
| Other causes | Substernal, retrosternal, epigastric pain or burning | Referred abdominal pain: hiatal hernia, peptic ulcer, gallbladder, acute pancreatitis | Symptoms vary with disease |
| | Vague tightness to severe crushing | | Respiratory distress, tachypnea, diaphoresis, numbness of fingers and around mouth |
| | | Hyperventilation syndrome | Respiratory alkalosis |

pneumonia, lung abscess, and pulmonary infarction often involve the overlying pleura and may induce pleuritic pain. Mediastinitis (inflammation of mediastinal structures) causes aching, oppressive retrosternal sensations that may be severe. Chronic disorders of the large airway, such as tracheal or bronchial tumors or ulcers, usually do not cause pain. The inflammation of bronchitis may, however, induce substernal discomfort that changes to a tearing, rasping, and sharp substernal pain with coughing.

Pleuritic pain, often described as inspiratory pain, is the most common symptom of disease causing inflammation of the pleura (pleurisy). It is sharp, often abrupt in onset, and severe enough to cause the patient to seek medical help (often within hours of onset). It increases with inspiration, a cough, a sneeze, a hiccup, or laughing. Pleuritic pain is usually localized to one side of the chest, frequently the lower, lateral aspect. It may be only partially relieved by splinting and pain medication. Pleuritic pain increases with pressure and movement but not to the same degree as pain originating from the outer chest wall. In contrast, the lung parenchyma and the visceral pleura that cover the lungs are relatively insensitive to pain; therefore pain with breathing usually indicates involvement of the parietal pleura.

Chest wall pain may originate from the intercostal and pectoral muscles, ribs, and cartilages or from stimulation of a neural pathway (neuralgia) anywhere along a dermatome (skin area innervated by a particular spinal cord segment). It is usually described as a well-localized, constant aching soreness that increases with direct pressure on the area of tenderness and with any arm movement that stretches the thoracic muscles.

## Descriptions

The patient's body language, as well as his or her descriptive terms, gives clues about the cause of chest pain. Patients with pleuritic pain may be bent to the side, taking shallow breaths, and holding their chest to decrease the amount of movement. They describe their pain as "sharp," "stabbing," "raw," or "burning," progressing to "excruciating" when they breathe or laugh. A patient with chest wall pain may complain of aching pain or soreness at a specific site and will pull away from being touched. Esophageal pain may be described as "knotlike," "like a big bubble trapped inside," or "burning." Patients with spontaneous pneumothorax or dissecting aortic aneurysm may describe the pain as excruciating "tearing" or "knifelike."

Patients with heart pain (angina) will frequently hold a clenched fist over their sternum as they describe the pain as "aching," "squeezing," "pressing," or "viselike." Their pain is worse with exercise and may prevent them from performing physical activity. The pain may diminish with rest. Patients with this type of chest pain must be evaluated by a physician.

Pain is a purely subjective symptom. The perception of pain varies not only with the source of pain but also with previous experience, culture, personality traits, amount of rest, and emotional implications of the pain. Because chest pain varies from relatively benign neuromuscular skeletal pain (the most common) to life-threatening angina (caused by a decreased blood supply to the heart muscle), the interviewer must be careful to obtain an accurate and impartial history. The following characteristics must be reviewed in detail: onset, location, radiation, frequency, duration, severity (a 0-to-10 scale is often used, with 10 being the worst), precipitating and relieving factors, and specific descriptions (e.g., tearing, stabbing, dull, sharp, crushing, or burning). Clues to locating the source of chest pain include a history of trauma, surgery, or muscle strain; local tenderness; swelling; and relationship to inhaling, coughing, position, and activity.

## QUESTIONS TO ASK

**Chest Pain**

*Ask the patient the following questions to help obtain an accurate and impartial history:*

- Where is the pain?
- Did the pain start suddenly or gradually? Is it more severe now than when it started?
- Have you ever had a pain like this before? What did you do to relieve the pain? Did you take medication to relieve the pain? What medicine did you take?
- How would you describe the pain? (Let the patient describe the character of the pain in his or her own words; if unable to give a description, suggest descriptive words.) Would you describe the pain as aching? Throbbing? Knifelike? Sharp? Constricting? Sticking? Burning? Dull? Shooting? Tearing?
- Can you rate your pain on a scale of 0 to 10, with 10 being the worst pain you have ever felt?
- How long have you had the pain?
- Do you have recurrent episodes of pain? How often do you get the pain? How long does the pain last?
- What makes the pain worse? Breathing? Lying flat? Moving your arms or neck?
- Is the pain associated with coughing? Shortness of breath? Palpitations? Coughing up blood? Nausea or vomiting? Leg pain? Dizziness? Weakness? Headache? Muscle fatigue?
- Does the pain occur at rest? Exercise? While sleeping? With stress? After eating?
- What do you do to make it better?
- Have you ever had a heart attack? Has anyone in your family had heart disease? At what age?
- Have you had a recent respiratory infection? Do you have pulmonary disease?
- Have you had trauma to your chest? A hip or leg fracture? Been involved in an accident?
- What medications are you taking? Have you recently changed the dose or how you take them?
- Do you take any other types of legal or illegal drugs? If so, what are the drugs, and how much and how often do you take such drugs?

## DIZZINESS AND FAINTING (SYNCOPE)

### Definition

Syncope is a temporary loss of consciousness caused by reduced blood flow and therefore a reduced supply of oxygen and nutrients to the brain. Reduced cerebral blood flow may be localized (as in cerebral thrombosis, embolism, or atherosclerotic obstruction) or generalized, as occurs with obstruction to blood flow from the heart, cardiac arrhythmias, and hypovolemia (decreased available blood volume).

### Causes

Pulmonary causes of syncope include pulmonary embolism (obstruction of blood flow from the right side of the heart into the left side of the heart), prolonged bouts of coughing (tussive syncope), and hypoxia (low levels of blood oxygen) or hypocapnia (low levels of carbon dioxide). Holding one's breath after a deep inspiration (Valsalva maneuver) results in high intrathoracic pressure and decreased venous return to the heart. Excessively low blood pressure can also predispose patients to syncope. Causes of syncope are listed in Box 3.3. Although some of these causes of syncope are not associated with poor long-term outcomes, others can be serious problems.

The activity that preceded syncope and the position of the patient give clues to the causes of syncope. Primary pulmonary hypertension and some cardiac causes are associated with syncope during exercise. An irregular heart rhythm or palpitations before syncope suggest cardiac arrhythmia as the cause.

Vasovagal syncope, or "common dizziness and fainting," is the most common type of syncope and results from a loss of peripheral venous tone. It can occur with all forms of physical and emotional stress, including (but not limited to) pain; venipuncture; prolonged standing, especially in hot weather; and anxiety. Special attention must be given to careful review of all parts of the history and to the physical examination to rule out the organic causes of syncope.

Orthostatic hypotension is an excessive drop (>20 torr drop in systolic blood pressure) in blood pressure when a person stands up. In normal individuals, standing suddenly causes pooling of blood in the venous capacitance vessels of the legs and trunk, but compensatory mechanisms in the autonomic system maintain blood pressure and the blood supply to the brain. When portions of the reflex arc are impaired by disease processes, drugs, or an inadequate blood volume, these homeostatic mechanisms may be inadequate for restoring the lowered blood pressure. If the patient stands suddenly, the adaptive reflexes do not compensate fast enough, and there is a sudden drop in blood pressure. The patient will experience dizziness, blurring vision, profound weakness, and syncope. Orthostatic hypotension is suggested when a patient reports fainting after suddenly getting up from a chair or after rising suddenly from bed in the middle of the night to run to answer the telephone. Drugs that affect vascular tone or vascular volume can lead to orthostatic hypotension. Elderly patients are more prone to orthostatic hypotension because of dehydration.

---

**BOX 3.3    Causes of Syncope**

**Circulatory Control Abnormalities**
Drugs (very common)
Vasovagal syncope
Orthostatic hypotension
Severe systemic hypotension
Hypovolemia
Carotid sinus hypersensitivity
Autonomic failure

**Cardiopulmonary Abnormalities**
*Valvular and Myocardial Disease*
Prosthetic valve dysfunction
Aortic stenosis
Mitral valve prolapse
Pulmonary stenosis
Pulmonary embolism
Hypertrophic obstructive cardiomyopathy
Acute myocardial ischemia/infarction

*Inadequate Cardiac Filling*
Coughing, Valsalva maneuver
Atrial myxoma

*Cardiac Arrhythmias*
Sick sinus syndrome
Atrioventricular block
Supraventricular tachycardia
Ventricular tachycardia
Wolff-Parkinson-White syndrome
Long QT syndrome

**Metabolic Conditions**
Hypoxia
Hypocapnia
Hypoglycemia
Intoxication

**Neurologic Conditions**
Neurovascular disease
Convulsive disorders
Generalized seizures
Transient ischemic attack

**Psychological Conditions**
Hysterical fainting
Panic attacks

---

Carotid sinus syncope is associated with a hypersensitive carotid sinus and is seen more commonly in elderly people. Whenever a patient with carotid sinus syncope wears a tight shirt collar or turns the neck in a certain way, there is an increased stimulation of the carotid sinus. This slows the pulse rate and causes a sudden fall in systemic pressure, resulting in syncope.

Cough (tussive) syncope is the transient loss of consciousness after severe coughing. It occurs most commonly in middle-aged men with underlying COPD who are outgoing and moderately obese and have a great appetite for food, alcohol, and smoking. It rarely occurs in women. The cough may be chronic and is usually dry and unproductive. Typically, there is a "tickle" in the patient's throat precipitating a coughing paroxysm; then the patient's face becomes red, vision dims, the eyes become fixed, and the patient suddenly loses consciousness. The attacks usually last only a few seconds, but the patient may fall or slump in a chair as the muscles relax completely. Some patients have reported more than 20 episodes a day. Cough syncope is usually a benign symptom, and patients return to their previous activity with little recall of the episode. However, deaths and serious injury have been reported when the syncope occurred while driving.

## Descriptions

A precise description of the syncopal event should include a description of the preceding events and the coexisting symptoms, including dyspnea, nausea, neurologic events, angina (chest pain), and palpitations or irregular heartbeat. A careful interview of witnesses (if available) and ambulance personnel can be extremely helpful. In addition, a detailed review of medications and medical history, including known neurologic or heart disease, arrhythmia, pacemaker placement, or known sudden death of a family member, will provide clues to the cause of the syncope.

---

**QUESTIONS TO ASK**

**Dizziness and Fainting**
*Ask the patient the following questions to help obtain an accurate and impartial history:*
- What do you mean when you say you were dizzy? Felt faint? Did you lose consciousness?
- What were you doing just before you fainted? Did you have any warning that you were going to faint?
- Have you had recurrent fainting spells? If so, how often do you have these attacks?
- What position were you in when you fainted, and did you change positions immediately preceding the event?
- Was the fainting preceded by any other symptom? Nausea? Chest pain? Palpitations? Confusion? Numbness? Hunger? Cough?

---

## SWELLING OF THE ANKLES (DEPENDENT EDEMA)

### Definition

Edema is soft tissue swelling resulting from an abnormal accumulation of fluid. It may be generalized (anasarca), may appear only in dependent body areas (feet and ankles in ambulatory patients or the sacral area in patients on bed rest), or may be limited to a single extremity or organ (such as pulmonary edema). Edema is associated with kidney disease, liver disease, cardiac and pulmonary disease, and obstruction of venous or lymphatic drainage of an extremity.

## Causes

Peripheral (dependent) edema caused by pulmonary diseases occurs when the disease process causes narrowing of the capillaries in the lung, requiring the right ventricle to generate higher and higher pressures to move blood through the lungs. Gradually, the overworked right ventricle becomes enlarged and unable to pump all of its blood through the lungs. This results in a damming effect that causes the venous system to become engorged with blood. Because of the high pressure in the veins, fluid is pushed out into the tissues. At first, the edema is seen only in the lower areas of the body. When the patient has been standing or sitting, the edema is seen in the feet and ankles and is relieved by rest and elevation of the legs. Because patients on bed rest have their legs elevated near the heart level, dependent edema accumulates in the sacral area (back hip area) or at the side of the hip in patients who prefer to lie on their side.

As right-sided heart failure worsens, dependent edema is no longer relieved by rest or changing position and the edema occurs in the abdominal organs, as well as the extremities and dependent areas of the body. As the liver becomes enlarged (hepatomegaly) because of the edema, the patient may also complain of pain just below the ribs on the right side (right upper quadrant pain). Edema of the bowel and ascites (collection of fluid in the abdomen) causes complaints of anorexia, nausea, and sometimes vomiting. Patients may also complain of slowed healing and even skin breakdown in the edematous areas.

Bilateral peripheral, or dependent, edema suggests pulmonary hypertension, heart failure, or venous insufficiency. Unilateral peripheral edema (edema in only one extremity) is most frequently caused by some type of venous obstruction in that extremity, which can occur because of constrictive clothing, jewelry, or wound dressings that surround the extremity and compress venous return. It may also be a danger sign suggesting a deep vein thrombosis (blood clot).

## Descriptions

Patients may report that when they press on their swollen ankles or when they remove their shoes and socks, they notice a depression that remains in place for at least several minutes. When compression of an edematous area with a gloved finger produces a depression that does not fill immediately, pitting edema is present. In the medical history, pitting edema is usually described in general terms such as "the patient denies pitting edema" or "the patient reports pitting edema in both ankles that remains for at least 5 minutes after leg elevation." When the history and physical examination are reported together, pitting edema may be recorded using the scale shown in Table 3.11.

Peripheral edema is both a sign and a symptom. The examiner may find edematous ankles that the patient had not noticed. The presence of edema is such an important factor that the history of the edema should be traced. Precipitating and alleviating factors and associated symptoms should be documented with the history of present illness.

**TABLE 3.11  Pitting Edema Scale**

| Scale | Degree | Refill |
|---|---|---|
| 1+ Trace | Slight | Rapid |
| 2+ Mild | 0-0.6 cm (0-¼ in) | 10-15 sec |
| 3+ Moderate | 0.6-1.3 cm (¼-½ in) | 1-2 min |
| 4+ Severe | >1.3 cm (>½ in) | >2 min |

## FEVER, CHILLS, AND NIGHT SWEATS

Normal body temperature (euthermia) varies between 97.0°F and 99.5°F (36°C and 37.5°C) orally and is 1°F to 2°F (0.5°C to 1°C) higher in the late afternoon than in the early morning. This normal change of temperature during the day is known as the *diurnal variation*. Body temperature is also affected by age (higher in infants and lower in elderly people), exercise (increases to as high as 100°F during exertion and returns to normal within 30 minutes), excitement, sudden changes in environmental temperature, digestion, technique, and route of measurement (about 1°F higher rectally and about 1°F lower axillary), and use of medications containing antipyretics (drugs that decrease temperature).

### Definitions

Fever (hyperthermia or pyrexia) is an elevation of body temperature above the normal range resulting from disease. Fever may be described as sustained (continuously elevated, varying little more than 1°F during a 24-hour period), remittent (continuously elevated with wide, usually diurnal, variations), intermittent (daily elevation with a return to normal or subnormal between spikes), or relapsing (recurring in bouts of several days interspersed with periods of normal temperature). Terms used to describe fever are listed in Table 3.12.

| Fever, Pyrexia | Abnormally High Body Temperature |
|---|---|
| High-grade fever | >101°F (38.2°C) orally |
| Low-grade fever | 99.5°F-101°F (37.5°C-38.2°C) orally |
| Intermittent fever | Daily elevation with a return to normal or subnormal between spikes |
| Remittent fever | Continuously elevated with wide, usually diurnal variations |
| Relapsing fever | Recurring in bouts of several days interspersed with periods of normal temperature |
| Hyperthermia | Elevation of core body temperature above normal |
| Mild hyperthermia | 99°F-102°F (37.2°-38.9°C) |
| Moderate hyperthermia | 102°F-105°F (38.9°C-40.6°C) |
| Critical hyperthermia | >105°F (>40.6°C); medical emergency |
| Malignant hyperthermia | Core body temperature increases 2°F (1°C) every 15 min; occurs in people with an inherited predisposition to the condition |
| Fever of unknown origin (FUO) | Fever >101°F that has occurred several times in the past 3-4 weeks with no known cause |
| Hypothermia | Temperature that is below the normal range |

TABLE 3.12   Terms Used to Describe Fever

Normally, humans increase sweat production about threefold with their diurnal drop in temperature at night. However, when the temperature falls abruptly, as occurs with intermittent fever, sweat production may increase fivefold to eightfold, resulting in diaphoresis. When this profuse sweating occurs at night, soaking the bedclothes, it is clinically significant and is termed night sweats. Night sweats are common in patients with lymphoma, tuberculosis, and some types of pneumonia.

## Causes

Fever is a nonspecific symptom and may be caused by multiple factors, most commonly infection; exposure to a hot environment; dehydration (inadequate fluid volume in the body); reactions to chemical substances, drugs, or protein breakdown; damage to the heat-regulating center in the hypothalamus; malignant neoplasms; connective tissue disease; and a variety of other diseases (Table 3.13). In some patients a cause is never found, in which case the term *fever of unknown origin (FUO)* is used.

Fever is a concern for two important reasons. First, it often signifies that disease is present. The patient with fever should be evaluated for evidence of infection or other causes. Second, fever causes an increase in the metabolic rate of the patient that is proportional to the degree of temperature elevation. This is of little consequence to the patient with a healthy cardiopulmonary system but may represent a major problem to the patient with chronic lung or heart disease. As the body temperature elevates, the demand for oxygen utilization and carbon dioxide removal both increase. As a result, the patient with chronic cardiopulmonary disease is at higher risk for respiratory failure when significant fever is present.

Fever is usually accompanied by many other constitutional symptoms, such as vague aching, malaise (vague discomfort, or uneasiness), irritability, increased heart rate (9 to 10 beats per minute for each 1°F of elevation), and if high enough, confusion, delirium, or convulsions. A rapidly increasing body temperature may be accompanied by chills and shivering or even rigors (bone-shaking, teeth-rattling chills) as peripheral vasoconstriction occurs to conserve heat.

## Fever with Pulmonary Disorders

Because fever is the most common manifestation of infection, it is usually assumed to be caused by an infectious process until proved otherwise. Pulmonary infections, including lung abscess, empyema (infection within the pleural space), tuberculosis, and pneumonia, are accompanied by fever in most patients. Acute bacterial infections are usually accompanied by shaking chills, although the occurrence of a single rigor followed by sustained fever suggests pneumococcal pneumonia. Remittent fever is seen with mycoplasma, pneumonia, Legionnaires' disease, and acute viral respiratory infections.

It cannot be assumed that the patient does not have an infection because there is no fever. Patients vary greatly in the degree of fever accompanying a disease process. Patients taking high doses of steroids and other drugs that can be used as immunosuppressants may have no fever in the presence of a massive infection. In addition, patients with a compromised immune system (e.g., leukemia, acquired immunodeficiency syndrome) may have minimal fever despite the presence of severe infection.

Fever, like swelling and wheezing, can be a sign or a symptom. Once the temperature is taken during the physical examination, it is clearly evident that fever is present. However, many patients report fever or chills but have never taken their temperature. It is important to clarify why patients think they have a fever and whether the temperature was taken to document the route and the patient's technique. The patient should be asked to present any temperature charts that have been made and to describe the pattern of the fever and the accompanying symptoms.

When a cause for fever is not readily apparent, careful attention should also be given to the history of travel, recreation, occupation, and exposure to toxins or carriers of infectious diseases. All drugs used, including over-the-counter medications, vitamins, and illicit drugs, should be listed because many drugs, including antibiotics and blood products, can cause drug-related fever.

## QUESTIONS TO ASK

### Fever, Chills, and Night Sweats

*Ask the patient the following questions to help obtain an accurate and impartial history:*

- How long have you had fever? How did you measure your temperature? What readings did you get?
- Has there been any pattern to the fever? Did it start gradually or suddenly? Did it rise, then disappear, then reappear?
- Have you had other symptoms with the fever such as chills, headache, fatigue, cough, diarrhea, or pain?
- Has your neck felt swollen? Have you had a sore throat or earache?
- Do you have pain when you take a deep breath or cough? Where is the pain?
- Have you had an infection recently? Can you recall a recent exposure to someone who may have had an infection?
- Have you had a recent wound? How did it heal? Is the area still painful?

- Have you traveled to an area where you may have been bitten by a tick? Insect? Spider? Animal?
- Have you been exposed to high temperatures for a prolonged period of time such as playing sports or working out in the heat? How long were you out in the heat? How much water did you drink while you were working or playing?
- Have you had any unusual physical or emotional stress lately? Injury? Anesthetic? Surgery? Blood transfusion?
- Have you taken any new medications in the past few weeks?
- Are you taking thyroid medication? Antidepressants? Amphetamines or diet pills? Medications that keep you from sweating, such as anticholinergics, phenothiazines, monoamine oxidase inhibitors?
- Have you ever been told that you have pneumonia? HIV? Cancer?

## TABLE 3.13   Common Causes and Characteristics of Fever

| Type | Nature of Fever/Patient | Associated Symptoms | Clinical Findings |
|---|---|---|---|
| **Acute** | | | |
| ***Upper Respiratory Infection (URI)*** | | | |
| Viral | Usually <101.5°F orally Any age | Cough, signs of URI, may be systemic symptoms | Oropharynx infected Exposure to URI |
| Bacterial | Often high temperature, >101°F More common in children | Marked signs of URI, few systemic symptoms | Pharyngotonsillar exudates Pulmonary findings Children are restless |
| ***Other Bacterial and Viral Syndromes*** | | | |
| Influenza | Usually mild fever Any age | Muscle aches | Minimal |
| Acute otitis media (middle ear infection) | More common in children, usually >100°F, often follows URI | Ear and face pain, hearing loss | Ear is sensitive to touch, tympanic membrane appears red and bulging |
| Gastroenteritis | Any age | Nausea, vomiting, cramps, diarrhea | Dehydration |
| Urinary tract infection | Often high temperature with chills | Backache | Costovertebral angle tenderness |
| | Adults more common | Usually frequency and urgency | Positive urinalysis |
| Bacterial sepsis | Often high temperature | Chills | |
| Factitious fever | Usually >105°F, can be low grade | No weight loss | Disparity between rectal or oral and urine temperature |
| | Associated with health care | Pulse rate not proportional to fever | May be emotionally disturbed |
| Drug reaction | Often high temperature, acute or chronic | Occasional rash | Taking prescription or OTC medications Fever abates when drug discontinued |
| **Chronic** | | | |
| Infectious mononucleosis | Usually low grade Teenagers, young adults | Fatigue | Enanthema, fever, pharyngitis, splenomegaly, adenopathy (especially postcervical) |
| Tuberculosis | Usually low grade More common in diabetic patients | Cough, fatigue | Chest findings Positive TB test and chest radiograph |
| Hepatitis | Usually low grade More common in intravenous drug users | Fatigue, jaundice, anorexia | Hepatomegaly, jaundice, liver tender to palpation |

*OTC,* Over-the-counter; *TB,* tuberculosis.

## HEADACHE, ALTERED MENTAL STATUS, AND PERSONALITY CHANGES

There are many causes of headaches and psychosocial changes; some are related to pulmonary problems, whereas other causes may be secondary to medications, neurologic dysfunction, or injury. The patient interview and history outlined in Chapter 2 and the physical examination and laboratory studies can provide important clues to the RT or other members of the patient care team about the cause of such symptoms.

It is important to know that many patients with moderate to severe pulmonary disease experience headaches or some form of mood change. In many instances, such problems are related to insufficient oxygen or excessive carbon dioxide in the arterial blood. When patients cannot get adequate oxygen into their blood, as happens with lung disorders, or when the amount of oxygen in the inspired air is low (as at high altitude), the amount of oxygen available to the brain is decreased (cerebral hypoxia), and headache can occur. Likewise, as the carbon dioxide level in the blood increases, the cerebral arterial vessels dilate, causing vascular headaches with throbbing pain over the entire head. Because hypercapnia worsens during sleep in patients with pulmonary disorders, early-morning headaches may be the first indication that the patient is retaining abnormally high amounts of carbon dioxide. If the hypercapnia persists, headaches may be present throughout the day.

As cerebral hypoxia and hypercapnia worsen, progressive changes occur in the patient's mental status. Thought processes and memory deteriorate, the mind wanders, and the patient is easily distracted. Headaches, tremors, uncontrolled movements, hallucinations, and nightmares may occur. If the hypercapnia continues, alertness is affected, progressing to drowsiness, disorientation, stupor, and then coma.

### Personality Changes

Personality changes are not uncommon with advanced pulmonary disorders. The patient may complain of forgetfulness or inability to concentrate. On the other hand, the family may report the patient is depressed, anxious, irritable, demanding, or denying the disease process and refusing to follow the treatment regimen. When chronic lung disease develops from occupational hazards, the patient may be hostile and embittered. Such personality changes may be due to chronic hypoxia or stress or may result from the chronic use of certain medications.

As chronic pulmonary disease progresses, lifestyle options are decreased for the patient and family. Choices of work, play, and even places to live become more limited, and dependency on others increases. Patients must use more of their limited energy to breathe and perform the basic tasks of everyday living. Fears of acute respiratory failure, coughing up blood, another hospitalization, and the possibility of death are always present. As a result, it is not uncommon for patients to deny their illness and refuse to cooperate with treatment, use the illness to demand attention, or channel all of their concerns to the illness and use it as a threat to control others.

However, sudden personality changes or alterations in mental status are indicative of an acute problem. Although such changes are nonspecific and may be seen with neurologic or cardiac disease or intoxication, they also result from hypoxia and hypercapnia. A patient with chronic pulmonary disease who experiences an additional insult, such as trauma, surgery, unusual stress or exertion, pneumothorax, or inhalation of pollutants, may be stressed beyond the ability to adequately oxygenate and remove carbon dioxide from the blood. The patient may have a total change of personality and then deteriorate in a matter of hours. A patient who has been resting quietly and becomes restless deserves the same thorough investigation that would be carried out for the patient who becomes less responsive.

## SNORING AND DAYTIME SOMNOLENCE (SLEEPINESS)

Snoring is often a benign symptom that is reported by the patient's spouse or bed partner. However, it can be a symptom of serious concern when it is accompanied with periods of apnea during sleep, sometimes called sleep disordered breathing. Patients with this combination and accompanying symptoms such as daytime somnolence (sleepiness) must be evaluated for obstructive sleep apnea (OSA) by a polysomnograph (sleep study), as discussed in Chapter 19.

### Incidence and Causes of Snoring

Snoring occurs in about 10% to 12% of children and 10% to 30% of adults. In children snoring occurs equally in boys and girls, but in adults it occurs about twice as often in men. The peak incidence of snoring and OSA occurs at ages 50 to 59 years in men and at ages 60 to 64 years in women.

Snoring is caused by excessive narrowing of the upper airway with breathing during sleep. Some narrowing of the hypopharynx is normal with sleep and is the result of muscle relaxation. Excessive narrowing is common when obesity causes excessive tissue in the airway. For this reason, obesity is one of the most common causes of snoring and OSA. Enlarged tonsils, a large tongue, a short and thick neck, nasal obstruction, a large soft palate, abuse of alcohol or sleeping pills, and anatomic defects of the upper airway are possible precipitating factors in selected patients. In addition, snoring is influenced by sleeping position because gravity influences the position of the tongue and lower jaw. In the supine position, the lower jaw and tongue tend to flop back into the hypopharynx. Thus snoring increases in the supine position and is reduced in the lateral or prone position.

Patients who snore most often have inspiratory snoring. Inspiratory snoring is common because the upper airway tends to narrow naturally during each inspiratory effort as air rushes through. Factors that result in narrowing of the upper airway therefore become more of an issue on inspiration. The addition of sleep to the picture further complicates the problem when the upper airway support muscles relax. In addition, the greater the inspiratory effort, the greater the drop in pressure within the upper airway, and the narrower the airway becomes.

The patient with habitual snoring snores each night and often snores loudly. The occasional snorer most often snores only when he or she is excessively tired, has used alcohol or a sleeping medication, or is sleeping in the supine position.

### Clinical Presentation

Patients who snore and who have OSA or sleep disordered breathing will complain of excessive daytime somnolence (sleepiness) (EDS). If EDS is not present in the patient who snores, the snoring may be relevant only to the spouse or significant other. The EDS associated with OSA is related to the poor quality of sleep that occurs. Upper airway narrowing increases with the effort to breathe and eventually results in total obstruction and apnea. The apnea continues until the patient arouses somewhat (fragmenting the sleep), and the upper airway muscle tone increases in response to the arousal. The patient then is able to breathe until the deeper stage of sleep returns and the pattern cycles again. These cycles may occur hundreds of times each night of sleep. The result is a night of poor-quality sleep in which the deeper stages are not sustained. The patient awakens feeling fatigued and experiences EDS.

EDS often results in serious consequences, such as occupational accidents, motor vehicle crashes, loss of employment, and social dysfunction. In many cases, there is no association made between daytime sleepiness and snoring by the patient, the family, or the patient's family physician. Poor daytime concentration, bedwetting, impotence, high blood pressure, and other complicating factors are seen, especially in more severe cases.

---

### SIMPLY STATED

Patients with loud snoring and excessive daytime sleepiness should be evaluated for obstructive sleep apnea (OSA).

---

## GASTROESOPHAGEAL REFLUX

Gastroesophageal reflux disease (GERD) is defined as symptoms produced by the abnormal reflux of gastric contents into the esophagus. This reflux occurs when the lower esophageal sphincter opens inappropriately. Usually, patients experience heartburn and regurgitation when reflux is present. These symptoms are considered troublesome when they adversely affect the patient's quality of life. In addition to heartburn, patients with reflux may experience a number of extraesophageal symptoms such as laryngitis or hoarseness, asthma, chronic and nocturnal dry cough, chest pain, and dental erosion. Persistent reflux that occurs more than twice a week is often referred to as GERD. People of all ages can have GERD. Obesity, cigarette smoking, and pregnancy are common associated factors. GERD may contribute to the worsening of symptoms in patients with asthma.

---

### ■ KEY POINTS

- Cough is one of the most common symptoms in patients with pulmonary disease. It is the powerful protective reflex arising from stimulation of receptors located in the airways and visceral pleura.
- An acute self-limited cough is usually due to a viral infection involving the upper airway. It usually resolves in a few days. Chronic persistent cough is most commonly caused by postnasal drip syndrome, asthma, COPD, allergic rhinitis, or GERD.
- Sputum is the substance expelled from the tracheobronchial tree, pharynx, mouth, sinuses, and nose by coughing or clearing the throat. The term *phlegm* refers strictly to secretions from the lungs and tracheobronchial tree.

- Excessive sputum production is most often caused by inflammation of the mucous glands that line the airways.
- Hemoptysis, spitting up sputum containing blood, varies in severity from slight streaking to frank bleeding.
- Erosive bronchitis in smokers with chronic bronchitis now accounts for nearly half of the cases of hemoptysis. Bronchogenic carcinoma is the second most frequent cause.
- Dyspnea (*dys,* difficult; *pnea,* breathing) is defined as a subjective experience of breathing discomfort that consists of qualitatively distinct sensations that vary in intensity.
- Dyspnea occurs when the work of breathing is abnormally high for the given level of exertion. This is common with

narrowed airways as in asthma and when the lung is stiff as in pneumonia.

- Orthopnea is present when the patient complains of shortness of breath when lying down.
- Chest pain is the cardinal symptom of heart disease. In its classic presentation, the "viselike" pain of a heart attack is referred down the arms, most often the left, and may radiate into the shoulder, neck, jaw, or back. This type of chest pain is known as *angina* and signals a medical emergency.
- Syncope is a temporary loss of consciousness caused by reduced blood flow and therefore a reduced supply of oxygen and nutrients to the brain.

- Cough (tussive) syncope is the transient loss of consciousness following severe coughing.
- Bilateral peripheral or dependent edema suggests pulmonary hypertension, heart failure, or venous insufficiency.
- Fever (hyperthermia, pyrexia) is an elevation of body temperature above the normal range resulting from disease.
- Patients with snoring and sleep disordered breathing will complain of EDS.

## CASE STUDY

A 66-year-old woman is brought to the emergency department (ED) complaining of rapid onset of SOB, stating, "I cannot catch my breath." She also admits to coughing up a tablespoon of yellowish sputum every 30 minutes to 1 hour, sweating, and feeling warm, although she has not taken her temperature.

### Questions
1. What other key questions should be asked by the interviewer?
2. What pulmonary problems are suggested by the symptoms at this point?
3. Is the fact that the patient complains of sweating significant? If so, why?

### Answers
1. The interviewer should ask the patient if she has chest pain, nausea, dizziness, or blood in her sputum or a history of lung disease, cigarette smoking, or vaping.
2. The pulmonary problems suggested at this point include pneumonia, acute bronchitis, asthma, and acute exacerbation of COPD.
3. The sweating is significant because it is consistent with a fever that may be caused by an infection. If a fever is present, it may be contributing to the patient's SOB because of an increase in oxygen consumption and an increase in the drive to breathe.

## CASE STUDY

A 60-year-old man is brought to the ED complaining of acute chest pain. He was mowing his lawn when he suddenly felt ill. He went indoors to tell his wife, and she called 911. The patient is breathing rapidly while breathing supplemental oxygen through a nasal cannula.

### Questions
1. What questions should the interviewer ask the patient about his chest pain?
2. What other symptoms should the interviewer ask the patient about?
3. What clinical problems may explain the chest pain?

### Answers
1. The interviewer should ask the patient to point to the position of the chest pain on his chest. The patient should also be asked to describe the characteristics of the chest pain; if it radiates to the jaw, shoulder, or back; and if it increases with a deep breath.

2. The patient should be asked about nausea, fever, pedal edema, shortness of breath, cough, and dizziness. The patient's smoking history is important to obtain at some point.
3. If the patient has pain in the center of his chest that radiates to his shoulder or jaw and is accompanied by nausea and/or dizziness, it would be consistent with myocardial ischemia, and the patient may be having a heart attack. If the pain is sharp and located peripherally on the chest, the pain may be related to pleural disease or lung infection.

## CASE STUDY

A 48-year-old morbidly obese construction worker is brought to the ED after crashing his truck into a parked car in the early afternoon. He has sustained a minor head laceration and a bruised forearm. His partner drove him to the ED and says he believes the patient fell asleep while driving. He added that the patient has frequently been making stupid mistakes on the job, cannot do estimates anymore, and has been found snoring loudly during breaks. The patient now seems to be breathing normally while receiving low-flow supplemental oxygen through a nasal cannula.

### Questions

1. What questions should the interviewer ask of the patient about his condition?
2. What clinical problems may explain the daytime sleepiness?
3. What further studies would you recommend?

### Answers

1. The interviewer should ask if the patient believes he fell asleep while driving. Beyond this, and more important, the patient should be asked about alterations in sleeping habits or medications, daytime sleepiness, and other changes, such as difficulty concentrating.
2. Given the predisposing factors of morbid obesity and male gender, as well as the complaints of daytime sleepiness, snoring, and work difficulties, obstructive sleep apnea (OSA) should be strongly suspected.
3. Given the clinical suspicion, the patient should be referred for a polysomnogram (sleep study), as discussed in Chapter 19.

## ASSESSMENT QUESTIONS

1. Which of the following factors may lead to a weak cough?
   a. Reduced lung recoil
   b. Bronchospasm
   c. Weak inspiratory muscles
   d. All of the above

2. A cough described as being persistent for more than 3 weeks would be called which of the following?
   a. Acute
   b. Paroxysmal
   c. Chronic
   d. Nocturnal

3. Which of the following problems is associated with hemoptysis?
   a. Tuberculosis
   b. Lung carcinoma
   c. Pneumonia
   d. All of the above

4. A patient's complaint of breathlessness or air hunger would be defined as which of the following?
   a. Hemoptysis
   b. Wheezing
   c. Dyspnea
   d. Cyanosis

5. What term is used to describe shortness of breath in the upright position?
   a. Orthopnea
   b. Platypnea
   c. Eupnea
   d. Apnea

6. Which of the following is least associated with causing dyspnea?
   a. An increase in the work of breathing
   b. A decrease in the ventilatory capacity
   c. An increase in the drive to breathe
   d. An increase in lung compliance

7. What term is used to describe difficult breathing in the reclining position?
   a. Apnea
   b. Platypnea
   c. Orthopnea
   d. Eupnea

8. Which of the following characteristics is least associated with pleuritic chest pain?
   a. Sharp
   b. Inspiratory
   c. Radiates to the neck
   d. Located laterally

9. Which of the following may cause syncope?
   a. Severe coughing
   b. Pulmonary embolism
   c. Hypovolemia
   d. All of the above

10. Which of the following is (are) true regarding dependent edema caused by lung disease?
    a. It is caused by pulmonary vasodilation
    b. Accompanying hepatomegaly may be present
    c. It is caused by acute systemic hypertension
    d. All of the above

11. Chronic pulmonary hypertension may lead to which of the following clinical findings?
    a. Pedal edema
    b. Inspiratory crackles
    c. Hepatomegaly
    d. a and c

12. Which of the following is associated with night sweats?
    a. Tuberculosis
    b. Congestive heart failure
    c. Asthma
    d. Interstitial pulmonary fibrosis

13. In what decade of life are snoring and obstructive sleep apnea (OSA) most likely to be present in adult males?
    a. 20 to 29 years
    b. 30 to 39 years
    c. 40 to 49 years
    d. 50 to 59 years

14. Which of the following symptoms is least likely to be associated with GERD?
    a. Pedal edema
    b. Hoarseness
    c. Coughing
    d. Wheezing

## BIBLIOGRAPHY

Arikan H, Savci S, Calik-Kutukcu E, Vardar-Yagli N, et al. The relationship between cough-specific quality of life and abdominal muscle endurance, fatigue, and depression in patients with COPD. *Int J Chron Obstruct Pulmon Dis* 2015;**10**:1829.

Bafadhel M, McCormick M, Sahra S, et al. Profiling of sputum inflammatory mediators in asthma and chronic obstructive pulmonary disease. *Respiration* 2011;**22**:88.

Ball J, Dains E, Flynn J, et al. *Seidel's guide to physical examination.* 8th ed. St. Louis: Mosby-Elsevier; 2015.

Benich JJ, Carek PJ. Evaluation of the patient with chronic cough. *Am Fam Physician* 2011;**84**:887.

Bonniaud P, Georges M, Abdulmalak C, et al. Hemoptysis: a frequent diagnostic challenge. *Eur Respir J* 2015;**47**:350.

Eakin EG, Resnikoff PM, Prewitt LM, et al. Validation of a new dyspnea measure: the UCSD shortness of breath questionnaire. *Chest* 1998;**113**:619.

Fordyce CB, Newby DE, Douglas PS. Diagnostic strategies for the evaluation of chest pain: clinical implications from SCOT-HEART and PROMISE. *J Am Coll Cardiol* 2016;**23**:843.

Heuer AJ, Geisler SL, Kamienski M, et al. Introducing medical students to the interdisciplinary health care team: piloting a case-based approach. *J Allied Health* 2010;**39**:76.

Hobbs SB, Walker CM, Carter BW, et al. Progressive dyspnea in a patient with asthma. Insights on computed tomographic imaging of the airway. *Ann Am Thorac Soc* 2016;**13**:292.

Jarvis C. *Physical exam and health assessment.* 7th ed. St. Louis: Mosby-Elsevier; 2016.

Kacmarek RM, Stoller JK, Heuer AJ. *Egan's fundamentals of respiratory care.* 11th ed. St. Louis: Mosby-Elsevier; 2017.

Langridge PJ, Sheehan RL, Denning DW. Microbial yield from physiotherapy assisted sputum production in respiratory outpatients. *BMC Pulm Med* 2016;**16**:23.

Saravi M, Ahmadi Ahangar A, Hojati MM, et al. Etiology of syncope in hospitalized patients. *Caspian J Intern Med* 2015;**6**:233.

Sinz E, Navarro K, Soderberg ES. *Advanced cardiovascular life support provider manual.* Dallas: American Heart Association; 2011.

Tselebis A, Pachi A, Ilias I, et al. Strategies to improve anxiety and depression in patients with COPD: a mental health perspective. *Neuropsychiatr Dis Treat* 2016;**12**:297.

Yorke J, Russell AM, Swigris J, Shuldham C, et al. Assessment of dyspnea in asthma: validation of the dyspnea-12. *J Asthma* 2011;**48**:602.

# 4

# Vital Signs

*Albert J. Heuer*

## LEARNING OBJECTIVES

*After reading this chapter, you will be able to:*

1. Identify the four classic vital signs and the value of monitoring their trends.
2. Recognize the clinical significance of other bedside clinical findings, including abnormal sensorium and level of pain.
3. Describe the normal values of the following vital signs and common causes of deviation from normal in the adult:
   a. Pulse rate
   b. Respiratory rate
   c. Blood pressure
   d. Body temperature
4. Describe the following issues related to body temperature measurement:
   a. Types of devices commonly used
   b. Factors affecting the accuracy of devices
   c. Common sites and temperature ranges of those sites for measurement
5. Describe how fever affects the following:
   a. Oxygen consumption and carbon dioxide production
   b. Respiratory rate
   c. Pulse
6. Define the following terms:
   a. Fever
   b. Tachycardia
   c. Bradycardia
   d. Bradypnea
   e. Pulsus paradoxus
   f. Pulsus alternans
   g. Tachypnea
   h. Systolic blood pressure
   i. Diastolic blood pressure
   j. Hypertension
   k. Hypotension
   l. Pulse pressure
   m. Postural hypotension
7. Describe the technique, common sites for palpation, and characteristics for evaluating the pulse.
8. Describe the techniques for determining respiratory rate and blood pressure.
9. Explain how hypotension affects perfusion and tissue oxygen delivery.
10. Identify the factors that cause erroneously elevated blood pressure measurements.
11. Describe the mechanism by which pulsus paradoxus is produced.

## OUTLINE

## KEY TERMS

| | | |
|---|---|---|
| bradycardia | hypertension | sensorium |
| bradypnea | hypotension | systolic blood pressure |
| diastolic blood pressure | paradoxic pulse | tachycardia |
| fever | postural hypotension | tachypnea |
| Holter monitor | pulse pressure | telemetry |

The previous two chapters focused on subjective data—those that are perceived by the patient. We now turn our attention to more objective data—those that can be measured. Although subjective data are important, objective data are factual information that is generally not influenced by patient opinion or feelings. Therefore they are most often relied on to make important clinical decisions. This chapter focuses mainly on vital signs, the most frequently measured objective data for monitoring vital body functions and often the first and most important indicator that the patient's condition is changing. Given that obtaining vital signs generally requires direct patient interaction, the respiratory therapist (RT) or other member of the patient care team should give proper consideration to the principles relating to preparing for the patient encounter, as outlined in Chapter 1.

Vital signs are used for the following purposes:

- Help determine the relative status of vital organs, including the heart, blood vessels, and lungs, which may be helpful in making many clinical decisions such as when to admit the patient to the hospital
- Establish a baseline (a record of initial measurements against which future recordings are compared)
- Monitor response to therapy, such as surgery and medication administration, as well as selected diagnostic tests
- Observe for trends in the health status of the patient
- Determine the need for further evaluation, diagnostic testing, or intervention

## OBTAINING VITAL SIGNS AND CLINICAL IMPRESSION

The four classic vital sign measurements are temperature, pulse, respirations, and blood pressure. Although they are not always listed as vital signs, the patient's height and weight, level of consciousness and responsiveness (sensorium), level and type of pain, and the general clinical impression are also important observations often included with the vital sign assessment.

Patients who have intravenous or arterial lines and traumatic or surgical wounds have catheter insertion sites, wounds, and extremity checks performed as part of "routine vitals." In addition, pulse oximetry with continuous heart rate and electrocardiogram (ECG) is often monitored along with vital signs of patients in acute care settings.

It should be noted that the vital signs, like other clinical findings, are only as accurate as the clinician or caregiver obtaining them and interpreting the results. Thus it is important to properly obtain and monitor vital signs to help optimize patient care and avoid costly medical errors. In addition, significant inconsistencies among vital signs, clinical impression, and other clinical data can signal an error in measurement or the presence of a potentially serious medical condition despite certain normal findings. For example, a patient who has relatively normal vital signs but whose facial expression and general appearance suggest severe distress may still have an acute medical problem. As a result, it is recommended that RTs "don't treat numbers." Instead, they should rely on the critical analysis of several clinical findings, including but not limited to vital signs, in assessing the patient and making related recommendations.

### SIMPLY STATED

Vital signs are only as accurate as the way in which they are obtained and may be subject to error. Vital signs may also be only minimally affected by serious medical conditions. Therefore they should be considered along with other clinical data to help ensure an accurate diagnosis.

## FREQUENCY OF VITAL SIGNS MEASUREMENT

The frequency of vital signs measurement depends on the condition of the patient; the nature and severity of the disorder; and the procedures, surgery, or treatments being performed. A baseline measurement should be taken on admission and at least at the beginning of each shift.

For acutely ill patients in an intensive care setting, vital signs may be monitored continuously with remote electronic monitoring and alarm interface. For patients with conditions affecting only selected organ systems such as the heart, monitoring can be focused on specific vital signs (including heart rate and rhythm) and can be done continuously through electronic transmitting devices known as telemetry. Similarly, a patient's heart rate and rhythm can be continuously monitored and digitally recorded for review by a physician, outside of the hospital or clinic, using a Holter monitor. However, for more stable patients such as those on medical-surgical floors, "routine vitals" are generally measured and recorded every 4 to 6 hours (at beginning of shift and midshift), unless changes in conditions dictate otherwise.

In addition to acuity, certain procedures may determine the frequency with which vital signs are monitored. For example, patients undergoing a bronchoscopy (see Chapter 17) generally have baseline measurements taken before the procedure, at a maximum of 5-minute intervals during the procedure, and at similar intervals until they recover from moderate sedation and any lingering effects of the procedure. After surgery, vital signs are generally measured frequently to ensure the patient's safety—often every 15 minutes for 2 hours, then every 30 minutes for 1 to 2 hours, then hourly until the patient is stable. The physician's order in the chart is often written as "Vitals q 15 m × 2-4 h, q 30 m × 4 h, q 1 h until stable, then per protocol." Likewise, certain vital signs such as heart rate and respiratory rate should be monitored at a minimum before and after certain standard respiratory treatments such as bronchodilator administration, to evaluate effectiveness of the treatment and for possible side effects.

Of course, vital signs should always be monitored and recorded as often as necessary for the safety of the patient. If the patient's condition worsens unexpectedly, the patient appears to have an adverse reaction to a medical intervention, or the patient suddenly comments about "not feeling well," vital signs should be measured immediately and strong consideration given to activating the Rapid Response Team (also known as the Medical Emergency Team) in the hospital setting or calling 911 in an alternate care setting.

### SIMPLY STATED

Vital signs should be monitored and recorded as often as necessary for the safety of the patient. In general, the frequency with which patients' vital signs are assessed is dictated by the acuity or degree of illness, with those of the more acutely ill patient being assessed more frequently.

## TRENDS IN THE VITAL SIGNS

A single vital sign measurement gives information about the patient at that moment in time. Each measurement may be evaluated to see whether it is high or low compared with the normal value for the patient's age; however, an isolated measurement does not provide much information about what is normal for the individual patient or how the patient is changing or responding to therapy over time. To evaluate whether an individual patient has "normal" vital signs, you must understand what is normal for the patient, given factors such as age, disease, and treatment protocols. Sometimes, chronic disease or treatment modalities cause expected alterations in heart rate, respiratory rate, blood pressure, or body temperature. If you doubt a finding, repeat the measurement, and be sure the patient's position and your technique are correct for the parameter you are measuring. If you still doubt the measurement or if you think the patient may be getting into trouble, get help.

The initial reading is generally referred to as the baseline measurement. A series of vital sign measurements over time establishes a trend and is far more important clinically than any single measurement. Each time vital signs are measured, they should be compared with the baseline values and the most recent measurements. Sometimes, the patient's condition may be changing slowly, and comparison with one or two previous measurements does not indicate the trend, whereas comparison over an entire shift or 24 hours of vital signs may indicate clearly that the patient is slowly deteriorating. Because the trend of vital signs is so important, many physicians insist that vital signs on hospitalized patients be recorded on a multiple-day graph.

Additionally, the patient's vital signs should be viewed in relation to his or her normal level or the values that can typically be obtained for him or her, even when the patient is not necessarily ill. For instance, a heart rate of 96 beats per minute is within normal limits for an adult but may be relatively high and have clinical significance for a patient whose baseline heart rate is generally in the low 60s.

### SIMPLY STATED

To evaluate whether a patient has "normal" vital signs, you must understand what is normal for the patient's age, disease, and environment. A vital sign measurement is only as accurate as the technique used to obtain it.

## COMPARING VITAL SIGNS INFORMATION

Clues to whether a patient's condition may be stable or changing may be obtained by comparing changes in vital signs and other signs and symptoms. For example, patients who are not maintaining adequate blood oxygen levels develop specific changes in general appearance, level of consciousness, heart and respiratory rates, and blood pressure. Table 4.1 lists these common signs of developing acute hypoxemia (partial pressure of arterial oxygen [$Pao_2$] <75 to 80 mm Hg).

In health care, this comparison of multiple signs and symptoms to arrive at the patient's diagnosis is called the *differential diagnosis*. Of course, it takes time for the beginning student

### TABLE 4.1 Signs of Hypoxemia Assessed during Vital Signs Measurement

| Vital Signs Measurement | Sign |
| --- | --- |
| General clinical presentation | Impaired coordination or cooperation |
| | Cool extremities[a] (can be felt while taking the heart rate and blood pressure) |
| | Diaphoresis (profuse sweating) |
| Sensorium (level of consciousness) | Decreased mental function |
| | Impaired judgment, confusion |
| | Loss of consciousness |
| | Decreased pain perception |
| Respiration | Increased rate and depth of breathing |
| | Difficulty breathing, use of accessory muscles |
| Heart rate | Tachycardia |
| | Arrhythmia (irregular heart rate), especially during sleep |
| Blood pressure | Increased blood pressure initially |

[a]Temperature of the extremities, as well as diaphoresis, can be felt at the time the heart rate and blood pressure readings are obtained.

to learn all these relationships, but remember, the difference between the novice and expert clinician is not just knowledge. The distinction is also the ability to assess and compare multiple types of subjective and objective data over time and to identify patterns and relationships in an individual patient. The key to expert assessment of vital signs at the bedside is to be constantly aware and to look for change, as follows:

- Look at the patient: watch facial expressions, body movements, coordination, position, color, skin, anatomic landmarks, and effort to breathe or move.
- Listen to the patient: hear words, tones, sounds, rhythms, patterns, silence, feelings, and fears.
- Touch: feel moisture, temperature, air movement, change in temperature, muscle and skin tone, resistance, and quality of pulses.
- Analyze: collect information in a timely manner; compare it with normal and baseline values. Mentally update this information with each patient encounter. Verify its accuracy. Is the information consistent or inconsistent with the baseline or most recent clinical assessment, or has something changed?
- Trend, trend, trend: what has changed about the patient? How has the patient changed and why? What has not changed? Why? What does it mean? Does the change indicate a need for immediate action?

---

**SIMPLY STATED**

The key to expert assessment of vital signs at the bedside is to be constantly aware: look, listen, touch, question, validate, reassess, analyze, and trend.

---

## HEIGHT AND WEIGHT

Height and weight are routinely measured as part of the physical examination and usually as part of every outpatient appointment. A patient's height is normally taken without shoes or boots, and weight is obtained while the patient is wearing only a hospital gown or indoor clothing. For hospitalized patients, the admitting height and weight are obtained and recorded either when the patient goes to a preadmitting testing service or by the admitting nurse; thereafter, weight is usually measured every day or two. If there is concern about either dehydration or fluid overload, fluid intake and output and weight may be recorded each shift until the patient's fluid balance is stable. Because weight is often used to calculate medication doses and ventilator settings related to ventilator volumes, the weight may be recorded in kilograms (1 kg = 2.2 lb) on the patient's medication record and, if appropriate, the ventilator-patient flow sheet, in addition to the vital signs record. Scales and measurement standards should be selected in sizes and styles appropriate for the age of the patient and should be calibrated regularly to ensure accuracy.

## GENERAL CLINICAL PRESENTATION

General observation begins the moment you first see the patient and continues throughout the examination and care.

The patient's general appearance gives clues to the level of distress and severity of illness, as well as information about the patient's personality, hygiene, culture, and reaction to illness. This first step may dictate the order of care or physical examination. If the patient is in distress, the priority is to evaluate the problem in the most efficient and rapid way possible and to intervene or locate someone who can assist the patient. A more complete examination can be performed when the patient is more stable. Some visual signs of distress include the following:

- Cardiopulmonary distress is suggested by labored, rapid, irregular, or shallow breathing that may be accompanied by coughing, choking, wheezing, dyspnea, chest pain, or a bluish color (cyanosis) of the oral mucosa, lips, and fingers. The patient with cardiopulmonary distress often speaks in short, choppy sentences because of severe dyspnea.
- Anxiety is recognized by restlessness, fidgeting, tense expression, and difficulty communicating normally and may be accompanied by cool hands and sweaty palms.
- Pain is suggested by drawn features, moaning, shallow breathing, guarding (protecting the painful area), and refusal to deep-breathe or cough.
- Bleeding and loss of consciousness are signs of extreme distress that require immediate intervention.

When a patient is not in acute distress, this initial observation provides an opportunity to see the patient as a whole person. Using all your senses—hearing, smelling, seeing, touching, and perception—during this head-to-toe inspection gives information about the patient's apparent age, state of health, body structure, nutritional status, posture, motor activity, physical and sensory limitations, and mental acuity. It helps assess the reliability of the patient as a historian. It also helps identify what type of assistance and teaching the patient may need.

---

**QUESTIONS TO ASK**

**The Clinical Presentation**

*Questions to ask yourself while doing this portion of the examination include the following:*

- What are the general appearance and attitude of the patient?
- Are there inconsistencies between (or among) objective and subjective clinical findings?
- Is the patient in distress and in immediate need of additional care?
- How is the patient responding to the assessment or treatment?
- Are there abnormalities in the patient's face or movements?
- Does the patient have any motor or sensory limitations?
- Will this patient require assistance, safety precautions, or teaching?

---

A written description of these initial observations helps others involved in the patient's care know how to plan care and relate to the patient's needs. Usually, these descriptive statements are written in language everyone can understand (e.g., "J.C. is a cooperative, alert, well-nourished, 43-year-old man who appears younger than his stated age and exhibits no indication of distress. He shows no signs of acute or chronic illness and is admitted for …"). You may occasionally find that more specific terms for body types have been used in the written physical examination report. Box 4.1 lists and defines some of those terms.

A statement is usually made in the documentation of the patient's general appearance regarding the apparent age of the patient relative to his or her stated age. Patients who appear much older than their stated age often suffer from chronic illness, for example, chronic obstructive pulmonary disease patients.

## Pain Level and Type

Pain is referred to by some clinicians as the "fifth vital sign." In the past, the assessment of pain was considered to be mainly a subjective measure. More recently, pain intensity scales have been developed and validated to help accurately quantify a patient's level of pain. One commonly used pain measurement instrument uses a 10-point scale, with 10 being "hurts worst," and corresponding facial expressions and verbal description to assess pain level. In assessing pain it is important to be mindful of certain cultural differences that may affect the patient's accurate reporting of pain or lack thereof. For example, some cultures may deny or understate massive pain because of cultural beliefs and stigmas. With this in mind, when a patient's accurate pain rating score is

coupled with additional information regarding its location and actions that worsen or alleviate it, this information can be quite useful in clinical assessment. For example, chest pain originating from the heart versus an orthopedic injury (e.g., myocardial infarction versus pulled chest muscle) can vary in features such as intensity, location, and duration. In addition, the extent to which a patient's pain has been evaluated and appropriately treated is a focal point for several health care quality programs and initiatives. As a result, rapid assessment of pain and implementing appropriate treatment are essential to providing high-quality patient care.

The use of analgesia (pain-relieving medication) before assessing a patient is somewhat controversial in that the immediate administration of such medications can cause the patient to understate the pain severity, altering the assessment. However, in extreme cases the pain may be so severe that it interferes with the assessment of the patient. In such cases it may be necessary to administer a modest initial dose of analgesic to assess the patient.

---

### QUESTIONS TO ASK

**Pain**

*To ensure a thorough patient examination, the presence and features of pain should be assessed by asking yourself the following questions:*
- Does the patient appear to be in pain?
- Is the patient's subjective response consistent with the presence of pain?
- If the patient is in pain, what are the intensity and location?
- What makes the pain better or worse?
- Was the onset of pain gradual or sudden?
- Is the pain affecting the patient's breathing pattern?
- Did you notify the nurse and the doctor that the patient is in pain?

---

### SIMPLY STATED

Pain is often an important clinical feature and should be quickly evaluated in regard to location, intensity, onset, and what makes it worse or better.

---

## Level of Consciousness (Sensorium)

Evaluation of the patient's level of consciousness is a simple but important task and is discussed in more detail in Chapter 6. Adequate cerebral oxygenation and adequate ventilation to achieve appropriate arterial carbon dioxide levels must be maintained for a patient to be conscious, alert, and oriented. The conscious patient also should be evaluated for orientation to time, place, and person. This is referred to as evaluating the patient's **sensorium** or mental status. The alert patient whose orientation to time, place, and person is accurate is said to be "oriented × 3," and the sensorium is considered normal.

An abnormal sensorium and loss of consciousness may occur when cerebral perfusion is inadequate or when poorly oxygenated blood is delivered to the brain. As cerebral oxygenation deteriorates, the patient initially is restless, confused, and disoriented. If tissue hypoxia continues to deteriorate, the

---

| BOX 4.1 | Terms Used to Describe Body Types |
|---|---|
| Ectomorphic | Slight development, body linear and delicate with sparse muscular development |
| Endomorphic | Soft, roundness throughout the body; large trunk and thighs with tapering extremities |
| Mesomorphic | Preponderance of muscle, bone, and connective tissue, with heavy hard physique of rectangular outline (between endomorphic and ectomorphic) |
| Sthenic | Average height; well-developed musculature, wide shoulders, flat abdomen; oval face |
| Hypersthenic | Short, stocky, may be obese; shorter, broader chest; thicker abdominal wall; rectangular-shaped face |
| Hyposthenic | Tall, willowy, musculature poorly developed; long, flat chest; abdomen may sag; long neck; triangular face |
| Asthenic | Exaggeration of hyposthenic body type |
| Cachectic | Profound and marked malnutrition; wasting; ill health |
| Debilitated | Weak, feeble, lack of strength (with weakness and loss of energy) |
| Failure to thrive | Physical and developmental delay or retardation in infants and children; seen in children with illness but more often in children with psychosocial or maternal deprivation |

patient eventually becomes comatose. An abnormal sensorium also may occur as a side effect of certain medications and in drug overdose cases. Deterioration of the patient's sensorium often indicates the need for mechanical ventilation in the presence of acute respiratory dysfunction.

Evaluation of the patient's sensorium helps determine not only the status of tissue oxygenation but also the ability of the patient to cooperate and participate in treatment. Patients who are alert and oriented can take an active role in their care, whereas those who are disoriented or comatose cannot. The treatment plan is often adjusted according to the evaluation of sensorium.

---

### QUESTIONS TO ASK

**Level of Consciousness**

*Asking yourself questions such as the following while obtaining vital signs will help you assess the patient's sensorium:*

- Is the patient conscious? If the patient is medicated, can he or she be aroused easily?
- Is the patient responding, and is the response appropriate for the stimulus?
- Is the patient alert?
- Is the patient oriented to person, place, and time?
- Can the patient see, hear, and sense touch?
- Is the patient restless, fidgety, or easily distracted?
- Has the patient's responsiveness or behavior changed?

---

### Glasgow Coma Scale

Many systems for evaluating the patient's level of consciousness have been developed. One such assessment tool is the Glasgow Coma Scale, which allows for objective evaluation based on behavioral response in three areas: motor function, verbal function, and eye-opening response. This scale can be quite useful in assessing trends in the neurologic function of patients who have been sedated, have received anesthesia, have suffered head trauma, or are near coma. The Glasgow Coma Scale is described in more detail in Chapter 6.

---

### SIMPLY STATED

An abnormal sensorium may be caused by inadequate oxygenation of the brain resulting from respiratory or cardiac failure.

---

## TEMPERATURE

Normal body temperature for most people is approximately 98.6°F (37°C), with a normal range from 97.0°F to 99.5°F and daily variations of 1°F to 2°F (Table 4.2). The body temperature usually is lowest in the early morning and highest in the late afternoon. Most metabolic functions occur optimally when body temperature is within the normal range. Temperature elevation to between 99°F and 100°F occurs normally during exercise and takes about 15 minutes to return to normal after exercise. In women, normal temperature increases approximately 1°F during ovulation and during the first 4 months of pregnancy.

Body temperature is maintained in the normal range by balancing heat production with heat loss. If the body had no ability to rid itself of the heat generated by metabolism, the body temperature would rise rapidly. The hypothalamus plays an important role in regulating heat loss and can initiate peripheral vasodilation and sweating in an effort to dissipate body heat.

The respiratory system also helps in the removal of excess heat through ventilation. When the inhaled gas is cooler than the body temperature, the airways warm the gas to body temperature. This warming and subsequent exhalation with each breath aid in removing excess body heat. When the inhaled gas is heated to near body temperature before inhalation, this heat loss mechanism is not functional. This most often occurs when the patient is intubated and receiving mechanical ventilation with a heated humidifier in place.

### Fever

An elevation of body temperature above normal (hyperthermia) can result from disease or from normal activities such as exercise. When the temperature is elevated from disease, this elevation is called fever, and the patient is said to be febrile. Terms used to describe fever and its patterns are given in Chapter 3.

Fever most often results from infection somewhere in the body. Infection in the respiratory system can occur in the sinuses, airways, or lungs. However, fever can occur when infection is not present as a side effect of certain medications, with aspiration pneumonia or atelectasis, and after a blood transfusion. Infection is most likely to be the cause of the fever when the body temperature exceeds 102°F.

It is important to remember that not all patients with an infection develop a fever. Some patients are unable to

---

**TABLE 4.2   Normal Temperature Values by Site and Time Requirements for Accuracy When Using a Glass Thermometer**

| Site | NORMAL TEMPERATURE RANGES | | Time Required |
|------|------------|---------|---------------|
| | **Fahrenheit** | **Celsius** | |
| Oral | 97.0°-99.5° | 36.5°-37.5° | 3-5 min[a] |
| Axillary | 96.7°-98.5° | 35.9°-36.9° | 9-11 min |
| Rectal | 98.7°-100.5° | 37.1°-38.1° | 2-4 min |
| Ear | Expected to be very close to rectal if measured correctly | | 2-3 sec |

[a]Wait 15 minutes after eating or drinking.

generate a significant fever despite the presence of major infection. Patients with an inadequate immune system are most prone to this finding. In addition, patients who would otherwise have an elevated body temperature but are taking fever-reducing medication, such as acetaminophen or aspirin, may not be febrile. As a result, a complete assessment of body temperature should address the presence of such medications.

A fever results in an increase in the metabolic rate of the body functions and produces an increase in oxygen consumption and carbon dioxide production by the body tissues. For every 1°C elevation of body temperature, oxygen consumption and carbon dioxide production increase approximately 10%. The demand for an increase in the oxygen supply to the tissues and removal of carbon dioxide must be met by an increase in circulation and ventilation. Examination of the febrile patient often reveals increased heart rate and breathing rate. For the patient with significant cardiac or pulmonary disease, the increased demand on these systems may represent an intolerable stress.

## Hypothermia

When the body temperature is below normal, hypothermia exists. Hypothermia is not common but can occur in persons with severe head injuries that damage the hypothalamus and in persons exposed to cold environmental temperatures. When the body temperature is below normal, the hypothalamus initiates shivering in an effort to generate energy and vasoconstriction to conserve body heat.

Because hypothermia reduces oxygen consumption and carbon dioxide production by the body tissues, the patient with hypothermia usually has slow and shallow breathing and a reduced pulse rate. Mechanical ventilator settings may need significant adjustments in the depth and rate of delivered tidal volumes as the body temperature of the patient varies above and below normal. Likewise, special respiratory interventions, such as heated aerosol, may be helpful in raising the body temperature in hypothermic patients.

## Measurement of Body Temperature

Body temperature is most often measured at one of four sites: the mouth, ear, axilla, or rectum. Rectal temperatures most accurately reflect actual body core temperature but are difficult to obtain in most patients. Tympanic and oral measurement sites are the most commonly used methods for assessing body temperature in children, adolescents, and adults alike.

Temperature is recorded in degrees Fahrenheit (°F) or degrees Celsius (°C), depending on the policies and equipment in each practice setting. Formulas for converting temperature between Fahrenheit and Celsius and an abbreviated conversion table are shown as follows:

$$°F = (°C \times 9/5) + 32$$
$$°C = (°F - 32) \times 5/9$$

Normal temperature ranges vary with the site and method of temperature measurement. When glass thermometers are used, accuracy depends on the length of time the thermometer is allowed to register (see Table 4.2). Electronic thermometers can accurately measure the temperature in approximately 30 seconds or less, provided the probe is positioned correctly and the device is correctly calibrated. To trend temperature over time, the same site and same device should be used for each temperature measurement.

Accurate body temperature measurement is important because variations can be an important clue in properly diagnosing and treating patients. For example, a patient with an elevated body temperature is said to be "febrile," which is often associated with bacterial and viral infections. In addition, variations in body temperature can affect laboratory test results, most notably arterial blood gases (see Chapter 8). Therefore it is often recommended that the patient's body temperature be obtained and recorded just before drawing blood for such purposes.

### Rectal Measurement

Rectal temperatures may be used for patients who are comatose, in intensive care, or confused. The average normal rectal temperature is 99.5°F (37.5°C), which is slightly higher than core temperature. However, despite the relative accuracy of rectal temperatures, the following methods are much more popular alternatives.

### Tympanic (Ear) Measurement

The tympanic method is the most common method for assessing body temperature in children, adolescents, and adults. Tympanic infrared thermometry uses a handheld probe placed in the ear canal to detect infrared emissions from the surfaces of the tympanic membrane and ear canal. No direct contact is made with the tympanic membrane. The temperature is digitized by a computer processor and displayed on a liquid crystal screen in less than 3 seconds. This method has the advantage of being fast, clean, and noninvasive and avoids the embarrassment and time delays associated with the classic forms of temperature measurement. It is commonly used in pediatric outpatient offices and emergency departments around the country. Different companies use different mathematical equations, so ear temperature measurement varies slightly by manufacturer. However, in most cases ear temperature measurements run a few tenths of a degree below core temperature.

### Oral Measurement

Oral temperature measurement remains a common, convenient, and acceptable method for awake adult patients. This method should not be used with infants, comatose patients, or orally intubated patients. Average normal oral temperature in adults is 98.6°F (37°C). Proper placement of the thermometer tip into the posterior sublingual pocket on either side of the mouth is essential, because the temperature in other parts of the mouth may vary as much as 1.7°C. A 10- to 15-minute waiting period is required if a patient has ingested hot or cold liquid or has been smoking.

The oral temperature is not affected significantly by oxygen administration via nasal cannula, simple mask, or air-entrainment mask. Therefore it is not necessary to remove the oxygen or take rectal temperatures in patients receiving oxygen via cannula or mask to obtain accurate oral temperature readings. Heated aerosol or cool mist by facemask may alter oral temperature slightly but probably not enough to alter clinical decisions.

### Axillary Measurement

The axillary method is safe for infants and small children who do not tolerate rectal temperatures. It is the method of choice for neonates because it approximates their core temperature and avoids injury to the rectal tissues. In adults, axillary temperature measurement assesses peripheral or skin temperature rather than core temperature and tends to have a poor correlation to other forms of temperature measurement in febrile adults. Average normal axillary temperature in adults is 97.7°F (36.5°C), approximately 1°F lower than oral temperature and 2°F lower than rectal temperature. It can take up to 11 minutes to obtain an axillary temperature in an adult and approximately 5 minutes in a child. For these reasons, axillary temperature is rarely assessed in the adult.

---

**QUESTIONS TO ASK**

**Temperature**
*To ensure the accuracy of the temperature measurement, ask yourself the following questions:*
- What type of thermometer was used?
- What site was used: oral, axillary, rectal, or tympanic?
- Was an appropriate amount of time used to obtain the temperature for the method of measurement?
- Had the patient just had a treatment, food, liquid, medication (antipyretic), or other event that could alter the accuracy of the measurement?
- Was the patient observed during temperature measurement? Is there any reason to believe that an elevated temperature was "factitious fever," or one artificially created by the patient?
- What is the time of day? Is the temperature highest in the late afternoon and lowest in the early morning, as expected?

---

**SIMPLY STATED**

A body temperature higher than 102°F usually indicates infection.

---

## PULSE

The pulse rate should be evaluated for rate, rhythm, and strength. Normal pulse rate varies with the age and status of the patient. As shown in Table 4.3, the younger the patient, the faster the pulse rate. The normal pulse rate for adults is 60 to 100 beats/min and is regular in rhythm.

A pulse rate exceeding 100 beats/min in an adult is termed tachycardia. Common causes of tachycardia include anxiety, fear, exercise, fever, high ambient temperature, low blood pressure, anemia, reduced arterial blood oxygen levels, and certain medications such as bronchodilators.

**TABLE 4.3 Pulse and Respiratory Rates Referred to Age**

| Age | Resting Pulse (beats/min) | Respiratory Rate (breaths/min) |
|---|---|---|
| Newborn | 90-170 | 35 to 45-70 with excitement |
| 1 year | 80-160 | 25-35 |
| Preschool | 80-120 | 20-25 |
| 10 years | 70-110 | 15-20 |
| Adult | 60-100 | 12-20 |
| Athlete | 40-60 | 12-20 |

A pulse rate lower than 60 beats/min for an adult is termed bradycardia. This is less common but can occur when the heart is diseased, as a side effect of certain medications, or in well-conditioned athletes who typically have resting pulse rates in the 50s. Irregularity of the pulse suggests arrhythmias, which are discussed in Chapter 11.

The amount of oxygen delivered to the tissues depends on the ability of the heart to pump oxygenated blood. The amount of blood pumped through the circulatory system (cardiac output) is a function of pulse rate and stroke volume (volume of blood ejected with each contraction of the left ventricle). When the oxygen content of the arterial blood falls below normal, usually from lung disease, the heart tries to compensate by increasing cardiac output to maintain adequate oxygen delivery to the tissues. An increase in cardiac output is accomplished by an increase in pulse rate in most persons. For this reason, the heart rate is important to monitor in patients with lung disease.

### Measurement of Pulse Rate

The radial artery is the most common site for evaluation of the pulse. The patient's arm and wrist should be relaxed, with the hand at or below heart level. If the patient's wrist is held above the level of the heart, the pulse may be difficult to obtain. The pads of the RT's or other clinician's index and middle fingers are placed lightly over the patient's pulse point and then compressed until the maximal pulsation is felt (Fig. 4.1). The thumb should not be used because pulsations from the artery in the examiner's thumb can be confused with the patient's pulse. The rhythm and strength of pulse are evaluated, the pulse rate is evaluated, and then the pulse rate is counted.

Other common sites available for assessment of the pulse include the brachial, femoral, and carotid arteries. When the blood pressure is abnormally low, the more centrally located pulses, such as the carotid pulse in the neck and femoral pulses in the groin, can be identified more easily than the peripheral pulse.

Ideally, the pulse rate is counted for a full minute to evaluate rate, rhythm, and strength accurately. When the pulse is regular and rhythm and strength are normal, the pulse rate may be counted for 15 seconds and multiplied by 4 or counted for 30 seconds and multiplied by 2. However, if any irregularity is felt, the pulse is counted for a full minute. The pulse

**FIG. 4.1** Technique for assessment of radial pulse.

rate, or heart rate as it is called on some vital signs records, is always recorded as beats per minute.

## Pulse Rhythm and Pattern

The rhythm of the pulse is the relative equality of the intervals between beats. The rhythm can be described as regular, regularly irregular, or irregularly irregular. A regularly irregular rhythm is a pulse with an irregularity that occurs in a continuous pattern (e.g., beat, beat, pause, beat, beat, pause). Bigeminy is a rhythm coupled in pairs. Trigeminy is a rhythm grouped as three beats and a pause. An irregularly irregular pulse has no pattern and is generally an unfavorable clinical finding.

When the rhythm is very irregular, it may be necessary to count the heart rate using a stethoscope placed over the heart (auscultation). During very irregular heart rhythms, some heartbeats cannot generate a strong enough pulse wave to be felt in the peripheral pulse. The difference between the number of auscultated beats and peripheral pulse beats is termed the *pulse deficit*. Irregular pulse rhythms are best evaluated by an ECG and may indicate the need for continuous ECG monitoring (see Chapter 11).

The strength of the pulse is assessed by how the artery feels as the blood flows through it with each beat. The strength of the pulse can be described as bounding, full, normal, weak, thready, or absent. A normal pulse is easy to feel, does not fade in and out, and is not easily obliterated by finger pressure. A bounding pulse is a full pulse that is difficult to depress with the fingertips. A weak, thready, or feeble pulse is not strong and can be compressed easily. An absent pulse cannot be felt.

There are slight variations in numeric systems used to describe pulses; some scales are 0 to 3, others are 0 to 4, and some rating systems add plus signs (+). Because of this variation, it is important to clarify which scale is used in each health care facility. Two commonly accepted grading systems for pulse strength are shown later. If the preferred grading system is not indicated on the charting forms, it is better to use the descriptive terms for pulse strength.

The fullness of the pulse can be reduced for many reasons, including an arterial blood clot, atherosclerosis, diabetes mellitus, dehydration, or any other condition that would cause the blood flow through the artery to decrease.

Spontaneous ventilation may influence the strength of the pulse. When the patient's pulse strength notably decreases with spontaneous inhalation, it is referred to as pulsus paradoxus. Pulsus alternans is an alternating succession of strong and weak pulses and usually is not related to respiratory disease. These concepts are described in more detail in the discussion of blood pressure later in this chapter.

---

### QUESTIONS TO ASK

**Pulse**
*To ensure the accuracy of the pulse rate, ask yourself the following questions:*
- What is the pulse rate? Rhythm? Quality?
- Has the patient been doing something that might raise the pulse temporarily? Is the patient usually anxious at this time?
- Should I take the pulse again later when the patient is resting?
- If the pulse is irregular, did I count it for a full minute?
- Does the pulse vary with respirations?
- How does the current measurement compare with previous measurements?

---

### SIMPLY STATED

An irregular pulse should be counted for a full minute to determine heart rate accurately.

---

## RESPIRATORY RATE AND PATTERN

Respiratory rates vary by age and condition of the patient. Table 4.3 gives reference ranges for patients of various ages. A respiratory rate of 40 breaths/min is unusual for an adult, and greater than 60 breaths/min is abnormal at any age. If carefully measured, respiratory rate is a sensitive and reasonably specific marker of acute respiratory distress. Likewise, the respiratory pattern relates to the regularity and depth of the breaths, which can vary in the presence of certain diseases.

Tachypnea is the term used to describe respiratory rates above normal. Rapid respiratory rates may occur as the result of certain respiratory disorders such as atelectasis, reduced arterial blood oxygen content, and increased arterial carbon dioxide. Tachypnea in the postoperative patient is common when significant fever develops or when the lungs partially collapse (atelectasis) as a side effect of the surgery. Atelectasis causes the lung volumes to decrease below normal, and the patient adopts a breathing pattern that is made up of rapid and shallow breaths as a compensatory mechanism. The degree of atelectasis determines the degree of tachypnea in such cases.

Alternatively, tachypnea can stem from nonrespiratory conditions such as anxiety, pain, and exertion. In addition, various forms of metabolic acidosis place extra stress on the respiratory system as a compensatory response and can cause an increase in rate and depth of breathing. In the case of ketoacidosis resulting from uncontrolled diabetes, a fast and deep breathing pattern known as Kussmaul's breathing is often evident. Evaluation of abnormal respiratory patterns is described in Chapter 5. In any event, a thorough history and interview, as well as an appropriate bedside patient assessment, will often help distinguish the root cause of tachypnea and thus facilitate appropriate treatment.

A slow respiratory rate, referred to as bradypnea, is uncommon but may occur in patients with head injuries or hypothermia, as a side effect of certain medications such as narcotics, and in patients with drug overdose.

Other medical terms used to describe respiratory rate and depth are listed in Table 4.4. Intermittent breathing, flaring nostrils, external sounds (e.g., wheezing or stridor), intercostal and sternal retractions, and use of accessory muscles when breathing are all indications that the patient is in acute distress and requires immediate intervention (see Chapter 5).

## Measurement of Respiratory Rate and Pattern

The respiratory rate is counted by watching the abdomen or chest wall move in and out with breathing. With practice, even the subtle breathing movements of the healthy person at rest can be identified easily. In some patients, the RT or other clinician may need to place his or her hand on the patient's abdomen to identify the breathing rate.

Never ask the patient to "breathe normally" while you are assessing the rate of respiration. When individuals think about their breathing, they often voluntarily change their breathing rate and pattern. A better technique is to observe the patient's chest as you finish counting the radial pulse and evaluate the respirations while still holding the wrist. The patient will not be aware that you stopped counting the pulse, so voluntary changes in breathing usually do not occur. When the respiratory rate is regular, counting the number of respirations in 30 seconds and multiplying the number by 2 provides an accurate respiratory rate. The depth and pattern of breathing should also be assessed and recorded with the respiratory rate. Assessment of breathing pattern is discussed in Chapter 5.

### TABLE 4.4   Terms Commonly Used to Describe Breathing Patterns

| Medical Term | Definition |
| --- | --- |
| Apnea | Absence of spontaneous ventilation |
| Eupnea | Normal rate and depth of breathing |
| Bradypnea | Less than normal rate of breathing |
| Tachypnea | Rapid rate of breathing |
| Hypopnea | Decreased depth of breathing |
| Hyperpnea | Increased depth of breathing with or without an increased rate |
| Sighing respiration | Normal rate and depth of breathing with periodic deep and audible breaths |
| Intermittent breathing | Irregular breathing with periods of apnea |

### QUESTIONS TO ASK

**Respiratory Rate**

*To ensure the accuracy of the respiratory rate, ask yourself the following questions:*

- What is the respiratory rate? Regularity? Pattern?
- What is the depth of respiration?
- Are accessory muscles used for respiration?
- Did the patient's awareness that respirations were being counted alter the rate or pattern of respiration?
- Did I count the rate for a full minute if the rate was unusually fast, slow, or irregular?
- How does this current respiratory rate compare with previous measurements?
- Does the change in respiratory rate originate from nonrespiratory causes such as pain, anxiety, or a metabolic problem?

### SIMPLY STATED

The respiratory rate should be assessed without the patient being aware of the assessment.

### SIMPLY STATED

An abnormal respiratory rate and pattern may indicate respiratory distress but can also be caused by other problems such as pain, anxiety, or metabolic problems.

## BLOOD PRESSURE

Arterial blood pressure is the force exerted against the walls of the arteries as the blood moves through the arterial vessels. Arterial systolic blood pressure is the peak force exerted during contraction of the left ventricle. Diastolic blood pressure is the force occurring when the heart is relaxed. Blood pressure is recorded with the systolic pressure listed over diastolic pressure: 120/80 mm Hg.

Pulse pressure is the difference between systolic and diastolic pressures. Normal pulse pressure is 35 to 40 mm Hg. When pulse pressure is less than 30 mm Hg, the peripheral pulse is difficult to detect. Patients with heart failure and inadequate stroke volume usually have a reduced pulse pressure.

Arterial blood pressure is determined by the force of left ventricular contraction, the peripheral vascular resistance, and the blood volume. The normal values for blood pressure change with age, as shown in Table 4.5. Blood pressure lower than 120/80 mm Hg is considered normal for an adult and is associated with a favorable cardiovascular risk.

A blood pressure persistently higher than 140/90 mm Hg is termed hypertension. Persistent pressures above this level are associated with an escalating risk for development of heart, vascular, and renal diseases. Risk increases progressively: the higher the blood pressure and number of concurrent risk factors, the more advanced the degree of target organ damage.

Although hypertension is one of the major modifiable risk factors for stroke, coronary heart disease, congestive heart failure, and peripheral vascular disease, it is estimated that approximately half of those affected are not aware of their hypertension. Table 4.6 lists adult blood pressure and hypertension classifications.

Although hypertension is a common problem in the United States and around the world, the exact cause in most cases is not known. Hypertension most often occurs when either the contractility of the heart or the peripheral vascular resistance is abnormally increased. In most cases of hypertension, the cause is complex and involves many factors, including genetics, environment, diet, smoking history, and stress level. In addition, the presence of select disorders, such as obstructive sleep apnea, may cause chronic hypertension.

It is now recognized that a systolic blood pressure of 150 mm Hg or more and/or a diastolic pressure of 90 mm Hg or more are a major cause of morbidity and mortality, especially on those 60 years old or older. As a result, if an assessment reveals a blood pressure of 150/90 mm Hg or more, pharmacologic treatment is generally recommended as part of the management plan, especially in individuals older than 59. Lower blood pressure thresholds are now used to consider initiating pharmacologic therapy for those with certain comorbidities, including a threshold of 140/90 for those 18 years old or older with chronic kidney disease.

Hypotension is defined as an arterial blood pressure that is less than 90/60 mm Hg in adults. Low blood pressure is relative and may be clinically significant if it drops suddenly, is unusually low, or is associated with symptoms such as dizziness or fainting. Hypotension may occur as the result of peripheral vasodilation, left ventricular failure, or low blood volume. Perfusion of vital body organs may be significantly reduced with hypotension. Without adequate circulation, oxygen delivery to the tissues is impaired, and tissue hypoxia occurs. Adequate pressure and perfusion must be reestablished to prevent organ failure. In cases of hypotension caused by dehydration, this can often be accomplished by the administration of intravenous fluids. However, in other cases, severe hypotension may need to be managed with medication.

Changes in posture may produce abrupt changes in the arterial blood pressure, especially in the hypovolemic patient. Normally, when the patient moves from the supine to the sitting position, blood pressure changes very little, but when hypovolemia or vasodilation is present, blood pressure may fall significantly when the patient sits up; this is referred to as postural (or orthostatic) hypotension.

## Measurement of Blood Pressure

The most common technique for measuring arterial blood pressure uses a sphygmomanometer (an occluding cuff, stethoscope, and manometer). This technique measures blood pressure indirectly by determining the pressure required to collapse the artery in an arm or leg (Fig. 4.2). The cuff is applied to the extremity, usually the upper arm, and inflated. When the pressure in the cuff exceeds the systolic blood pressure, blood flow through the artery is occluded and the pulse can no longer be felt. When the cuff is gradually deflated, blood flow in the artery resumes and the pulsations can be felt, heard with a stethoscope, or sensed by a flow probe or sensor. The cuff pressure at the time the blood flow resumes is used as the systolic arterial pressure.

The blood pressure cuff consists of an inflatable rubber bladder encased in a nondistensible cuff. Blood pressure cuffs are made in many different sizes to accommodate various sizes and ages of patients. Some of the most commonly used sizes are listed in Table 4.7. The bladder inside the cuff can be removed for cleaning or repair, so it is important to ensure that the correct size bladder is inside the cuff. Selection of the proper size cuff and bladder is essential to obtain an

### TABLE 4.5  Median Blood Pressure by Age and Sex

| Age | MEDIAN BLOOD PRESSURE (MM HG) | |
| | Male | Female |
| --- | --- | --- |
| 1 year | 85/37 | 86/40 |
| 5 years | 95/53 | 93/54 |
| 10 years | 102/61 | 102/60 |
| 13 years | 108/62 | 107/63 |
| 17 years | 118/67 | 111/66 |
| 20+ years | 120/80 | 120/80 |

Data from The fourth report on the diagnosis, evaluation, and treatment of high blood pressure in children and adolescents, *Am Fam Physician* 71:1014, 2005.

### TABLE 4.6  Classification of Blood Pressure and Hypertension for Adults (18+ Years)

| Category | Systolic Blood Pressure (mm Hg) | Diastolic Blood Pressure (mm Hg) | Potential Management and Treatment Recommendations |
| --- | --- | --- | --- |
| Normal | <120 | <80 | |
| Prehypertensive | 120-139 | 80-89 | Lifestyle modification with possible drug therapy |
| **Hypertension** | | | |
| Stage 1 (mild) | 140-159 | 90-99 | Lifestyle modification, drug therapy, frequent monitoring |
| Stage 2 (moderate) | >159 | >99 | Lifestyle modification, drug therapy, possibly with multiple drugs, frequent monitoring |

Data from The seventh report of the Joint National Committee on Prevention, Detection, Evaluation, and Treatment of High Blood Pressure, *JAMA* 289:2560-2571, 2004.

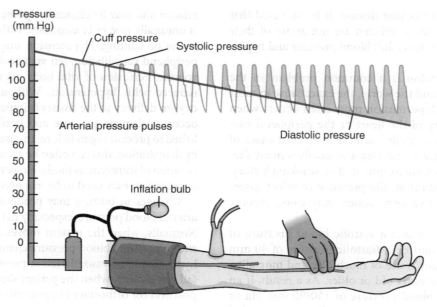

**FIG. 4.2** When the pressure within the sphygmomanometer cuff is increased above arterial blood pressure, the arteries under the cuff are occluded, and no pulse can be palpated at the wrist. As the cuff pressure is gradually released, the systolic peaks of pressure finally exceed cuff pressure, and blood spurts into the arteries below the cuff, producing palpable pulses at the wrist. The sudden acceleration of blood below the cuff produces vibrations that are audible through a stethoscope. The pressure displayed in the manometer at the time the pulse is heard or felt indicates systolic pressure. As cuff pressure is diminished, the sounds increase in intensity and then rather suddenly become muffled at the level of diastolic pressure where the arteries remain open throughout the entire pulse wave. At still lower pressures, the sounds disappear completely when laminar flow is reestablished. (Modified from Rushmer RF: *Cardiovascular dynamics,* ed 3, Philadelphia, 1970, WB Saunders.)

### TABLE 4.7   Acceptable Bladder Dimensions for Arms of Different Sizes

| Cuff | Bladder Width (cm) | Bladder Length (cm) | (Maximum) Arm Circumference[a] (cm) |
|---|---|---|---|
| Newborn | 4 | 8 | 10 |
| Infant | 6 | 12 | 15 |
| Child | 9 | 18 | 22 |
| Small adult | 10 | 24 | 26 |
| Adult | 13 | 30 | 34 |
| Large adult | 16 | 38 | 44 |
| Adult thigh | 20 | 42 | 52 |

[a]Calculated so that the largest arm would still allow the bladder to encircle the arm by at least 80%.
Data from the National High Blood Pressure Education Program Working on High Blood Pressure in Children and Adolescents: The fourth report on the diagnosis, evaluation, and treatment of high blood pressure in children and adolescents, *Am Fam Physician* 71:1014, 2005.

accurate pressure reading. The length of the bladder should be long enough to cover 80% of the distance around the arm in an adult and 100% of the arm circumference of a child. Overlapping the end of the bladder in children does not produce an error in the measurement. Using too wide a bladder produces a pressure that is lower than actual pressure. Using a bladder that is too narrow or too short results in overestimation of the blood pressure. The error of overestimation is greater, so if the correct size cuff is not available, a larger cuff should be selected.

### Auscultatory Blood Pressure Measurement

The auscultatory method of pressure measurement uses the stethoscope to listen for the sounds produced by the arterial pulse waves (Korotkoff sounds) when blood flow in the artery resumes. As the pressure is reduced during deflation of the occluding cuff, the Korotkoff sounds change in quality and intensity. The five phases of this change are characterized in Table 4.8.

The pressure at which the first sound is heard corresponds to the systolic pressure. There has been debate over whether to use the muffling or disappearance of the sounds as the diastolic pressure. There is now general consensus that phase V, disappearance of sounds, should be used as the diastolic pressure for most children, adolescents, and adults. In situations where sounds can be heard at levels far below those at which muffling occurs, such as that which may occur in pregnant women and patients with aortic insufficiency, phase IV may be used as the diastolic pressure. When there is a large discrepancy between muffling and disappearance of sounds, both pressures should be recorded (e.g., 110/60/30 mm Hg).

## TABLE 4.8 Korotkoff Sounds and Characteristics

| Korotkoff Sounds | Characteristic | Pressure Measured |
|---|---|---|
| Phase I | First appearance of clear, repetitive tapping sounds; coincides approximately with the reappearance of a palpable pulse | Systolic pressure |
| Phase II | Sounds are softer and longer, with the quality of an intermittent murmur | Auscultatory gap may occur |
| Phase III | Sounds become crisper and louder | Auscultatory gap may occur |
| Phase IV | Sounds are muffled, less distinct, and softer | Diastolic pressure in pregnant women, patients with high cardiac outputs or peripheral vasodilation, and some small children |
| Phase V | Sounds disappear completely | Diastolic pressure in adults and children |

## BOX 4.2 Technique for Measurement of Blood Pressure by Sphygmomanometry and Auscultation

The intent and purpose of the measurement should be explained to the patient in a reassuring manner, and every effort should be made to put the patient at ease and properly prepare for the patient encounter as described in Chapter 1.

The sequential steps for measuring the blood pressure in the upper extremity should include the following:

1. Prepare for the actual patient encounter (see Chapter 1), including scanning the medical record, gathering all necessary equipment, and ensuring there is a means to record the blood pressure readings immediately after being obtained.
2. Identify the patient, and explain the procedure to the patient.
3. Have the patient sit up, if possible, and minimize noise and other potential distractions, which can artificially alter measurements or interfere with the measurement process.
4. Position the patients with their bare arm resting so that the middle portion of the upper arm is approximately at the level of the heart.
5. Estimate the circumference of the bare upper arm at the midpoint between the shoulder and elbow, and select an appropriately sized cuff. The bladder inside the cuff should encircle about 80% of the arm in adults and about 100% of the arm in children younger than 13 years. If in doubt, use a larger cuff.
6. Palpate the brachial artery, and apply the cuff so that the midline of the bladder is over the arterial pulsation, then wrap and secure the cuff snugly around the patient's bare upper arm. Avoid rolling up the sleeve too tightly to prevent constricting blood flow. Loose application of the cuff results in overestimation of the pressure. The lower edge of the cuff should be 1 inch or about 2 cm above the inside bend (antecubital fossa).
7. Place the pressure manometer so that the center of it is easily visible at about eye level and the tubing from the cuff is unobstructed.
8. First inflate the cuff rapidly to 70 mm Hg, and then increase it in 10–mm Hg increments while palpating the radial pulse. Note the level of pressure at which the pulse disappears. Then gradually deflate the cuff, and note the pressure at which the pulse subsequently reappears during deflation. This procedure, called the *palpatory method,* provides a necessary preliminary approximation of the systolic blood pressure to ensure an adequate level of inflation when the actual auscultatory measurement is made. It may be useful to avoid underinflation of the cuff in patients with an auscultatory gap and overinflation in those with very low blood pressure.
9. Place the stethoscope ready to auscultate, and ensure that the stethoscope head is in the low-frequency position (bell).
10. Place the head of the stethoscope over the brachial artery pulsation, just above and medial to the inside of the elbow (antecubital fossa) but below the lower edge of the cuff, and hold it firmly in place, making sure that the head makes contact with the skin around its entire circumference.
11. Inflate the bladder rapidly to a pressure 20 to 30 mm Hg above the level previously determined by palpation, then partially unscrew (open) the valve and gradually deflate the bladder at 2 mm/s while listening for the appearance of the Korotkoff sounds.
12. As the cuff pressure declines, note the level of the pressure on the manometer at the first appearance of repetitive sounds (phase I), at the muffling of these sounds (phase IV), and when they disappear (phase V). While the Korotkoff sounds are audible, the rate of deflation should be no more than 2 mm per pulse beat, thereby compensating for both rapid and slow heart rates.
13. After the last Korotkoff sound is heard, deflate the cuff slowly for at least another 10 mm Hg, to ensure that no further sounds are audible, and then rapidly deflate it.
14. Both systolic (phase I) and diastolic (phase V) pressures should be promptly recorded, rounded off (upward) to the nearest 2 mm Hg. All values should be recorded in the medical record with the date and time of the measurement, the arm on which the measurement was made, the patient's position, and the cuff size (when a nonstandard size is used).
15. The procedure should be repeated after at least about 1 minute and the two readings averaged.

Occasionally, the Korotkoff sounds disappear during phases II or III and reappear as the cuff pressure decreases. The period of silence is called the *auscultatory gap* and is most common in older patients with high blood pressure. The auscultatory gap can generally be eliminated by elevating the arm overhead for 30 seconds before inflating the cuff then bringing the arm to the usual position to continue measurement.

The technique for obtaining an auscultatory blood pressure as specified by the American Heart Association is included in Box 4.2. The student is encouraged to obtain a copy of the recommendations and to check periodically for updates.

| A | B | C |
|---|---|---|
| **Cuff applied properly** | **Narrow cuff** | **Cuff applied loosely** |
| Tissue pressure = cuff pressure | Tissue pressure ≠ cuff pressure | Tissue pressure ≠ cuff pressure |

**FIG. 4.3 A,** When a sphygmomanometer cuff of sufficient width in relation to the diameter of the arm is properly applied, the tissue pressure around deep arteries under the cuff equals cuff pressure. However, pressure under the edge of the cuff does not penetrate as deeply as that under the center of the cuff. **B,** A cuff that is too narrow in relation to the diameter of the limb does not transmit its pressure to the center of the limb. Under these conditions, the cuff pressure must greatly exceed arterial pressure to produce complete occlusion of the artery, and erroneously high systolic and diastolic pressures are read from the pressure manometer or digital read-out. **C,** If a cuff of sufficient width is applied too loosely, it becomes rounded before exerting pressure on the tissues and produces the same sort of error as a narrow cuff produces.

## Errors in Blood Pressure Measurement

Causes of arterial blood congestion above the cuff that result in erroneously high cuff pressure measurements include the following (Fig. 4.3):

- Too narrow a cuff
- Cuff applied too tightly
- Cuff applied too loosely (when the loose bladder is inflated, the edges rise, so the portion pressing on the artery has a tourniquet effect)
- Excessive pressure placed in the cuff during measurement
- Inflation pressure held in the cuff
- Incomplete deflation of cuff between measurements

A low pressure reading is obtained if the cuff is too wide; however, this produces errors in the range of 3 to 5 mm Hg rather than the 40–mm Hg error often obtained when using too narrow a cuff.

Erroneous diastolic pressures occur when pressure is maintained on the artery so that laminar flow is not reestablished. Because turbulent flow can be heard, muffling or disappearance of sound may not occur. Causes include applying the cuff too tightly and pressing the stethoscope too tightly over the artery. Static electricity, ventilators, extraneous room sounds, and the presence of an auscultatory gap may also cause erroneous cuff measurements.

## Effects of the Respiratory Cycle on Blood Pressure and Pulse Intensity

Systolic blood pressure usually decreases slightly (by 2 to 4 mm Hg) with normal inhalation. This decrease in systolic blood pressure is more significant during a forced maximal inhalation. When the systolic pressure drops more than 10 mm Hg during inhalation at rest, a definite abnormality exists; this is termed paradoxical pulse. Paradoxic pulse, also called *pulsus paradoxus,* occurs in various circulatory and respiratory conditions such as asthma and cardiac tamponade. The most probable mechanism responsible for this fluctuation in blood pressure centers around the negative intrathoracic pressure created by the respiratory muscles during inhalation. The negative intrathoracic pressure encourages venous blood to return to the right ventricle and discourages arterial blood flow out of the left ventricle. The increased venous return to the right ventricle during inspiration increases the right ventricular filling pressures, which causes the interventricular septum to distend toward the left ventricle. This results in reduced left ventricular filling, reduced stroke volume, and decreased systolic blood pressure simultaneous with inhalation. It should be noted that the pulsus paradoxus should not be confused with abdominal paradox (see Chapter 5), which is the inward movement of the abdomen on inhalation and is associated with diaphragmatic fatigue.

The fluctuation in systolic blood pressure with breathing can be identified most accurately with a sphygmomanometer; however, if the pulse can be felt to wane with inspiration in several accessible arteries, paradoxic pulse is probably present. To confirm and quantify the presence of paradoxic pulse, a blood pressure cuff is used. The cuff is inflated until no sounds are heard with the stethoscope bell over the brachial artery, and then it is gradually deflated until sounds are heard on exhalation only. The cuff pressure then is reduced slowly until sounds are heard throughout the respiratory cycle. The difference between the systolic pressure heard only during expiration and systolic pressure heard throughout the respiratory cycle indicates the degree of paradoxic pulse. A reading in excess of 10 mm Hg is significant.

Pulsus paradoxus is commonly seen in patients with restrictions around their heart such as cardiac tamponade, constrictive pericarditis, or restrictive cardiomyopathy. It may also occur in patients with severe pulmonary disease such as acute asthma.

---

**QUESTIONS TO ASK**

**Blood Pressure**
*To ensure the accuracy of the blood pressure reading, ask yourself the following questions:*
- Is the correct cuff size being used? Is the cuff applied correctly?
- Is the arm in the standard position when the blood pressure is measured?
- Is the same arm used as was used in previous measurements? Which arm has higher blood pressure?
- Is the pressure manometer at eye level?
- Has the patient been in the same position long enough to obtain a stable reading?
- Does the blood pressure change when the patient changes position from supine or sitting to standing?
- Does the patient complain of symptoms such as dizziness when changing position?
- Are things occurring in the environment that would artificially alter the patient's blood pressure?
- If the blood pressure is high, does it decrease if measured again in a few minutes?

---

**SIMPLY STATED**

Hypotension occurs when the left ventricle is weak, the blood volume is reduced, or vasodilation is excessive. These problems can occur as a side effect of certain medications (e.g., β-blockers, diuretics).

---

## KEY POINTS

- The respiratory therapist (RT) who accurately measures vital signs, properly trends these data, and views such information collectively with other clinical findings can be a valuable asset in diagnosing and treating patients with respiratory dysfunction.
- Vital signs are only as accurate as the way in which they are obtained. Therefore vital signs should be analyzed along with other clinical data to help ensure an accurate diagnosis.
- The four classic vital signs are temperature, pulse, respirations, and blood pressure.
- Other clinical indicators available to RTs include general clinical impression, height and weight, sensorium, and pain.
- The frequency for obtaining vital signs depends on the patient's condition and the procedures being performed, but vital signs should be obtained at least every 4 to 6 hours and as often as every 15 minutes or even continuously for acutely ill patients.
- The RT should trend vital signs to monitor a patient's status over time.
- The normal body temperature is 98.6°F (37.0°C) with daily variations of 1°F to 2°F. A patient with a temperature above that is febrile and below that range is hypothermic.
- For every 1°C elevation of body temperature, oxygen consumption and carbon dioxide production increase approximately 10%.
- For an adult, the normal pulse rate is 60 to 100 beats per minute. A pulse rate above that is termed *tachycardia* and below that is *bradycardia.*
- The normal respiratory rate for an adult is 12 to 20 breaths per minute. *Tachypnea* is a respiratory rate higher than 20, and *bradypnea* is when the respiratory rate is below 12.
- In addition to assessing pulse and respiratory rate, the RT should also assess the pattern and intensity of a patient's pulse and respirations.
- Pulsus paradoxus (or paradoxic pulse) is a decrease in systolic blood pressure, and pulse intensity during inhalation should not be confused with abdominal paradox, which is the inward movement of the abdomen on inhalation and is associated with diaphragmatic fatigue.
- A blood pressure slightly below 120/80 mm Hg is considered normal for an adult. Hypertension is a blood pressure above 140/90 mm Hg, and hypotension is below 90/60 mm Hg.
- There are several errors that can occur when measuring blood pressure. For example, using a cuff that is too narrow or tight can result in falsely high readings.
- A paradoxic pulse occurs when systolic pressure drops more than 10 mm Hg during inhalation and may occur during a severe asthma attack or during cardiac tamponade.

---

## ASSESSMENT QUESTIONS

1. All of the following are included in the measurement of vital signs *except:*
   a. Pulse
   b. Respiratory rate
   c. Urinary output
   d. Blood pressure
2. Which of the following changes is consistent with a fever?
   a. Decreased respiratory rate
   b. Increased pulse rate

c. Decreased oxygen consumption

d. Decreased blood pressure

3. Which of the following methods of temperature measurement are most common for adults?

a. Oral and rectal

b. Axillary and tympanic

c. Rectal and axillary

d. Tympanic and oral

4. What is the normal value of the resting pulse rate in the adult?

a. 30 to 60 beats/min

b. 60 to 100 beats/min

c. 80 to 120 beats/min

d. 100 to 150 beats/min

5. What is the normal range of the respiratory rate for adults?

a. 6 to 10 breaths/min

b. 8 to 12 breaths/min

c. 12 to 20 breaths/min

d. 15 to 25 breaths/min

6. Which of the following causes tachycardia in the adult?

a. Hypothermia

b. Hypoxemia

c. Hypertension

d. Polycythemia

7. Which of the following arterial sites is the most common for evaluating the pulse in the adult patient?

a. Pedal

b. Temporal

c. Radial

d. Femoral

8. Which of the following causes tachypnea in the adult?

a. Hypothermia

b. Narcotic overdose

c. Metabolic acidosis

d. Hyperoxia

9. Which of the following causes an erroneously low blood pressure measurement?

a. Inflation pressure held in the cuff between measurements

b. Use of blood pressure cuff that is too narrow

c. Not enough pressure used in the cuff during measurement

d. Tachycardia

10. Hypotension may often be associated with all of the following *except:*

a. Reduced perfusion

b. Less oxygen delivery to the tissues

c. Excessive salt intake

d. Dehydration

11. The peak pressure in the arteries is known as which of the following?

a. Pulse pressure

b. Diastolic pressure

c. Systolic pressure

d. Pulse pressure

12. A decrease in the intensity of the palpated pulse during inhalation is a definition of which of the following?

a. Abdominal paradox

b. Pulse pressure

c. Pulsus paradoxus

d. Pulsus alternans

13. What is the normal range for pulse pressure?

a. 10 to 20 mm Hg

b. 20 to 25 mm Hg

c. 30 to 50 mm Hg

d. 35 to 40 mm Hg

14. If a patient experiences syncope when moving from the supine to the upright position, what is the likely cause?

a. Left ventricular failure

b. Postural hypotension

c. Excessive vasoconstriction

d. Pulsus paradoxus

## BIBLIOGRAPHY

Ball J, Dains J, Flynn JA, et al. *Mosby's guide to physical examination.* 8th ed. St. Louis: Mosby-Elsevier; 2015.

Blumenthal D, McGinnis JM. Measuring vital signs: an IOM report on core metrics for health and health care progress. *JAMA* 2015;**313**:1901.

Curatolo M. Regional anesthesia in pain management. *Curr Opin Anaesthesiol* 2016;**120**:198.

DesJardins T, Burton GG. *Clinical manifestations and assessment of respiratory disease.* 7th ed. Maryland Heights, MO: Mosby-Elsevier; 2016.

Halbach SM, Hamman R, Yonekawa K, Hanevold C. Utility of ambulatory blood pressure monitoring in the evaluation of elevated clinic blood pressures in children. *J Am Soc Hypertens* 2016;**10**:406.

Hingorani P, Karnad DR, Rohekar P, et al. Arrhythmias seen in baseline 24-hour holter ECG recordings in healthy normal volunteers during phase I clinical trials. *J Clin Pharmacol* 2015;**10**:103.

Jarvis C. *Physical examination and health assessment.* 7th ed. St. Louis: Mosby-Elsevier; 2016.

Kacmarek RM, Stoller JK, Heuer AJ. *Egan's fundamentals of respiratory care.* 11th ed. St. Louis: Mosby-Elsevier; 2017.

Riley M, Bluhm B. High blood pressure in children and adolescents. *Am Fam Physician* 2012;**85**:693.

Salota V, Slovakova Z, Panes C, et al. Is postoperative tympanic membrane temperature measurement effective? *Br J Nurs* 2016;**12**:490.

# 5

# Fundamentals of Physical Examination

*Albert J. Heuer and Kathleen Smith-Wenning*

## LEARNING OBJECTIVES

*After reading this chapter, you will be able to:*

1. Describe the four components of the physical examination.
2. Explain the importance of reviewing the history of present illness before performing a physical examination.
3. Describe the significance of the following during examination of the head and neck:
   a. Nasal flaring
   b. Cyanosis
   c. Pursed-lip breathing
   d. Diaphoresis
   e. Changes in pupillary size in response to light
   f. Deviated tracheal position
   g. Jugular venous distention
4. Identify the correct method for measuring jugular venous pressure and expected normal findings.
5. Locate the topographic position of the following:
   a. Thoracic cage landmarks (suprasternal notch, sternal angle [angle of Louis], vertebral spinous processes [C7 and T1])
   b. Lung fissures (oblique [major] and horizontal [minor])
   c. Tracheal bifurcation anteriorly and posteriorly
   d. Right and left diaphragm anteriorly and posteriorly
   e. Lung borders
6. Define the following terms used to classify thoracic configuration during inspection of the chest:
   a. Pectus carinatum
   b. Pectus excavatum
   c. Kyphosis
   d. Scoliosis
   e. Kyphoscoliosis
   f. Barrel chest
   g. Flail chest
7. Define the following terms used to describe breathing pattern during inspection of the chest:
   a. Apnea
   b. Biot breathing
   c. Cheyne-Stokes breathing
   d. Kussmaul breathing
   e. Apneustic
   f. Paradoxic breathing

8. Describe the breathing patterns associated with restrictive and obstructive lung disease.
9. Identify the muscles of inspiration.
10. Describe the clinical significance of accessory muscle use and retractions and bulging.
11. Define the following terms and state their significance:
    a. Abdominal paradox
    b. Respiratory alternans
    c. Peripheral cyanosis
    d. Central cyanosis
    e. Hoover sign
12. Describe the clinical significance of peripheral versus central cyanosis.
13. List causes of increased and decreased tactile fremitus.
14. List causes of decreased thoracic expansion as assessed during chest palpation.
15. Describe subcutaneous emphysema and its clinical significance.
16. List causes of increased and decreased resonance during percussion of the lung.
17. Identify the four basic parts of a stethoscope and their uses.
18. Describe the proper technique for auscultation of the lungs.
19. Identify the four characteristics of breath sounds that should be evaluated during auscultation.
20. Define the following terms used to describe lung sounds and the mechanisms responsible for producing the sounds:
    a. Adventitious
    b. Tracheal
    c. Bronchovesicular
    d. Vesicular (normal)
    e. Diminished/absent
    f. Harsh/bronchial
21. Define the following terms used to describe abnormal lung sounds and the mechanisms responsible for producing the sounds:
    a. Crackles
    b. Rhonchi
    c. Wheezes
    d. Stridor
    e. Pleural friction rub

22. Use qualifying adjectives to describe lung sounds, and explain the importance of using these qualifying adjectives.
23. Describe the significance of the following auscultatory findings:
    a. Early inspiratory crackles
    b. Late inspiratory crackles
    c. Monophonic wheezes
    d. Polyphonic wheezes
    e. Stridor
    f. Late inspiratory crackles
    g. Inspiratory and expiratory crackles
    h. Pleural friction rub
24. Define bronchophony and its cause.
25. Identify the topographic location of the apex and base of the heart during examination of the precordium.
26. Identify the point of maximal impulse, its normal location, and the factors that may cause it to shift to the right or left.
27. Describe the best location for auscultating sounds produced by the aortic, pulmonic, mitral, and tricuspid valves.

28. Describe what produces the first ($S_1$) and second ($S_2$) heart sounds, which are normal, as well as the third ($S_3$) and fourth ($S_4$) heart sounds, which are typically not normal.
29. Describe what is meant by a gallop rhythm and what it signifies.
30. List the factors that increase or decrease the intensity of the heart sounds.
31. Describe the clinical significance of a loud $P_2$ heard during auscultation of the heart.
32. Describe the factors that cause systolic and diastolic heart murmurs.
33. Define the term *hepatomegaly* and its significance in the cardiopulmonary patient.
34. Define the following terms and their significance during examination of the extremities:
    a. Digital clubbing
    b. Cyanosis
    c. Pedal edema
    d. Capillary refill
    e. Peripheral skin temperature and turgor

## OUTLINE

## KEY TERMS

abdominal paradox
accessory muscles
acrocyanosis
adventitious
angle of Louis
ascites
attenuation
auscultation
barrel chest
bronchial breath sounds
bronchophony
bulging
central cyanosis
clubbing

crackles
cyanosis
diaphoresis
diplopia
early inspiratory crackles
flail chest
gallop rhythm
harsh breath sounds
heave
hepatomegaly
Hoover sign
hyperresonant
intercostal
kyphoscoliosis

kyphosis
late inspiratory crackles
loud $P_2$
lymphadenopathy
miosis
mydriasis
nystagmus
palpation
pectus carinatum
pectus excavatum
pedal edema
percussion
peripheral cyanosis
pleural friction rub

## KEY TERMS—cont'd

| | | |
|---|---|---|
| pleurisy | rhonchi | tactile fremitus |
| point of maximal impulse (PMI) | scalene | tracheal breath sound |
| precordium | scoliosis | vesicular breath sound |
| ptosis | sternocleidomastoid | vocal fremitus |
| respiratory alternans | stridor | wheeze |
| retractions | subcutaneous emphysema | |

Physical examination is the process of examining the patient for the physical signs of disease. It is an efficient way to obtain immediate and pertinent information about the patient's health status. The four basic components of the physical examination are inspection, palpation, percussion, and auscultation.

The patient initially is examined to help the physician and other members of the patient care team determine the correct diagnosis and to establish the patient's baseline clinical status. Once a tentative diagnosis is made, subsequent examinations are valuable in monitoring the patient's treatment plan and evaluating the patient's response to it. Each examination should be modified according to the patient's history, the patient's physical limitations, and the purpose of the assessment. If possible, the examination should be performed in a quiet, well-lighted private setting. In addition, the respiratory therapist (RT) or other clinician should avoid exposing the patient to unnecessary physical or emotional discomfort and should respect privacy, as well as cultural and religious preferences.

This chapter emphasizes the techniques of examination used in assessment of the patient with cardiopulmonary disease. Because cardiopulmonary disease may indirectly alter other body systems, examination of the whole patient is important. The techniques used in examination of the thorax and other body systems for the abnormalities often associated with respiratory disease are reviewed. The typical order in which the initial physical examination is performed and recorded is presented in Box 5.1. See Chapter 4 for a complete discussion of the initial impression and assessment of the vital signs.

A review of the patient's history of present illness and past medical history before examination is quite important. This review gives the patient care team insight into the anticipated physical examination findings and suggests the techniques to emphasize.

## EXAMINATION OF THE HEAD AND NECK

### Head and Face

An examination of the head should first identify the patient's facial expression. This may help determine whether the patient is in acute distress or is experiencing physical pain. The facial expression can also help evaluate alertness, mood, general character, and mental capacity. Nasal flaring

---

**BOX 5.1   Typical Format for Recording the Physical Examination**

**Initial Impression**
Age, height, weight, general appearance, and gender

**Vital Signs**
Pulse rate, respiratory rate, temperature, and blood pressure

**Heent (Head, Ears, Eyes, Nose, and Throat)**
Inspection findings

**Neck**
Inspection and palpation findings

**Thorax**
Lungs: inspection, palpation, percussion, and auscultation findings
Heart: inspection, palpation, and auscultation findings

**Abdomen**
Inspection, palpation, percussion, and auscultation findings

**Extremities**
Inspection and palpation findings

---

is identified by observing the external nares flare outward during inhalation. This may occur in patients of any age but is most often seen in neonates and young children with respiratory distress. It suggests that an increase in the work of breathing is present. It may be seen in a large variety of clinical conditions, including upper airway obstruction (e.g., croup), bronchiolitis, pneumonia, and respiratory distress syndrome.

Cyanosis may be detected, especially around the lips and oral mucosa, when respiratory disease results in reduced oxygenation of the arterial blood. Cyanosis is a bluish cast to the skin that clinically may be difficult to detect, especially in a poorly lighted room, in patients with dark-pigmented skin, and in those with moderate to severe anemia. The presence of cyanosis is strong evidence that tissue oxygenation may be less than optimum; further investigation (e.g., arterial blood gas analysis) is indicated. The absence of cyanosis does not indicate that tissue oxygenation is adequate because a sufficient hemoglobin concentration must exist before cyanosis can be identified (see Inspection for Central Cyanosis).

Patients with chronic obstructive pulmonary disease (COPD) may use pursed-lip breathing during exhalation. This technique often is taught to patients and may even be used by patients who have not had instruction on its benefits. Some patients naturally begin to pucker their lips during exhalation to provide a slight resistance to the exhaled breath. This resistance provides a modest backpressure in the airways during exhalation and prevents their premature collapse. This exhalation technique alters the inspiratory-to-expiratory (I:E) ratio, extending expiratory time and thus allowing a more complete exhalation.

Excessive sweating by the patient is known as diaphoresis. It usually occurs at many sites in the body at the same time but is often first appreciated during inspection of the patient's face. It is a common finding in patients in acute respiratory distress and in those having severe pain. It also may be seen with exercise, eating spicy foods, fever, menopause, and other scenarios. Diaphoresis is also common in patients experiencing a myocardial infarction. For this reason, diaphoresis should always be taken seriously, especially in the patient at risk for heart disease.

## Eyes

The pupillary reflexes are evaluated as part of the neurologic examination. Cranial nerves II and III must be intact for normal pupillary reflexes to be present. If the pupils are equal in size, round, and reactive to light and accommodation, the physician may simply write PERRLA (*p*upils *e*qual, *r*ound, *r*eactive to *l*ight and *a*ccommodation) in the patient's chart. Head trauma, tumors, central nervous system disease, and certain medications can cause abnormal findings. Brain death, catecholamines, and atropine can cause the pupils to become dilated and fixed (mydriasis). Atropine is a common medication used during cardiopulmonary resuscitation, and its administration minimizes the use of assessing pupillary reflexes as a measure of the patient's neurologic status. Parasympathetic stimulants and opiates can cause pinpoint pupils (miosis). Examination of the pupillary reflexes is also discussed in Chapter 6.

Examination of the eyelids is useful when the RT or other clinician suspects disease of the cranial nerves. Drooping of the upper lid (ptosis) may be an early sign of disease involving the third cranial nerve. Congenital defects, cranial tumors, and neuromuscular diseases, such as myasthenia gravis, may cause ptosis. Ptosis may be an early warning sign of respiratory failure when a descending neuromuscular disease, such as myasthenia gravis, is occurring. Neuromuscular diseases affecting the cranial nerves also may result in blurred or double vision (diplopia) and involuntary, cyclic movement of the eyeballs known as nystagmus.

## Neck

Inspection and palpation of the neck are of value in determining the tracheal position, estimating the jugular venous pressure (JVP), and identifying whether the patient's accessory muscles are in use. Normally, the trachea is located centrally in the neck when the patient is facing forward. The midline of the neck can be identified by palpation of the suprasternal notch at the base of the anterior neck. The midline of the trachea should be directly below the center of the suprasternal notch.

The trachea may be shifted from midline with atelectasis, pneumothorax, pleural effusion, or lung tumors. In instances of atelectasis or lung resection (removal of one part of a lung), the trachea shifts toward the affected side as it moves toward the side with reduced lung volumes. Conversely, the trachea often shifts (deviates) away from a tension pneumothorax, pleural effusion, or lung tumor because of the effect that excessive air, fluid, or tissue outside of the lung has on pushing the trachea away from the affected side toward the unaffected side. It should also be noted that abnormalities in the lower lung fields may not shift the trachea unless the defect is severe.

The JVP is estimated by examining the level of the column of blood in the jugular veins. JVP reflects the volume and pressure of the venous blood in the right side of the heart. Both the internal and external jugular veins can be assessed, although the internal jugular is most reliable. Persons with an obese or muscular neck may not have visible neck veins, even with distention.

In the supine position, the neck veins of a healthy person are full. When the head of the bed is elevated gradually to a 45-degree angle from horizontal, the level of the column of blood descends to a point no more than a few centimeters above the clavicle with normal venous pressure. With elevated venous pressure, the neck veins may be distended as high as the angle of the jaw, even when the patient is sitting upright (Fig. 5.1). The degree of venous distention can be estimated by measuring the distance the veins are distended above the sternal angle. The sternal angle has been chosen universally because its distance above the right atrium remains nearly constant (approximately 5 cm) in all positions. With the head of the bed elevated to a 45-degree angle, venous distention greater than 3 to 4 cm above the sternal angle is abnormal (Fig. 5.2).

Exact quantification of the jugular pressure in terms of centimeters above the sternal angle is difficult and probably exceeds the accuracy needed for most observers. A simple grading scale of normal, increased, and markedly increased is acceptable.

The level of jugular venous distention may vary with breathing. During inhalation, the level of the column of blood may descend toward the thorax and return to the previous position with exhalation. For this reason, JVP should always be estimated at the end of exhalation.

The most common cause of jugular venous distention is right-sided heart failure. Right-sided heart failure may occur secondary to left-sided heart failure or chronic hypoxemia. Hypoxemia initiates pulmonary vasoconstriction and increases the resistance to blood flow through the pulmonary vasculature, increasing the workload of the right ventricle. Persistent lung disease with hypoxemia may result in right-sided heart failure and jugular venous distention. Jugular venous distention also may occur with hypervolemia and when the venous return to the right atrium is obstructed by tumors in the mediastinum.

## SIMPLY STATED

Jugular venous distention most often is the result of right-sided heart failure. It occurs because of the backup of blood to the jugular veins, which are in close proximity to the failing right side of the heart. Right-sided heart failure occurs for many reasons, including as a result of chronic left-sided heart failure or when chronic hypoxemic lung disease is present.

**FIG. 5.1** Photograph of jugular venous distention. (From Daily EK, Schroeder JP: *Techniques in bedside hemodynamic monitoring*, ed 5. St. Louis, 2000, Mosby.)

**FIG. 5.2** Estimation of jugular venous pressure. (Modified from Malasanos L, Barkauskas V, Stoltenberg-Allen K: *Health assessment*, ed 4. St. Louis, 1990, Mosby.)

Contraction of the sternocleidomastoid muscle in the neck is an indication that the patient's work of breathing is increased. It is a common finding in patients with airway obstruction and is discussed in the section on chest inspection.

The attending physician often examines the patient's neck for enlarged lymph nodes (lymphadenopathy) during the initial examination. Lymphadenopathy is a common finding in patients with respiratory infections, and the lymph nodes are usually enlarged and tender to palpation in this situation. Nontender lymphadenopathy may be caused by malignancy or human immunodeficiency virus.

The carotid pulse in the neck is palpated to evaluate the strength of the left ventricular contraction and the condition of the aortic valve. Heart disease that results in poor left ventricular contraction causes the carotid pulse to become weak. Stenosis of the aortic valve also causes a weak carotid pulse along with a systolic murmur (see Examination of the Precordium). An incompetent aortic valve that causes regurgitation of blood back into the left ventricle results in a pulse that rises and descends sharply. This is called a water-hammer pulse. The left and right carotid pulses must not be palpated simultaneously because this may significantly reduce blood flow to the brain.

The strength of the pulse at any location is described on a scale of 0 to 4, as follows:

0 = Absent, not palpable
1 = Diminished, barely palpable
2 = Expected normal amplitude
3 = Full and stronger than expected
4 = Bounding

## LUNG TOPOGRAPHY

Understanding how the lungs are situated within the chest is vital when preparing to perform an accurate physical assessment of the respiratory system. Topographic (surface) landmarks of the chest are helpful in identifying the location of underlying structures and describing the location of abnormalities.

### Imaginary Lines

On the anterior chest, the midsternal line divides the chest into two equal halves. The left and right midclavicular lines parallel the midsternal line and are drawn through the midpoints of the left and right clavicles, respectively (Fig. 5.3).

The midaxillary line divides the lateral chest into two equal halves. The anterior axillary line parallels the midaxillary line and is situated along the anterolateral chest. The posterior axillary line is also parallel to the midaxillary line and is located in the posterolateral chest (Fig. 5.4).

Three imaginary vertical lines are drawn on the posterior chest. The midspinal line divides the posterior chest into two equal halves. The left and right midscapular lines parallel the midspinal line and pass through the inferior angles of the scapulae in the relaxed upright patient (Fig. 5.5).

## Thoracic Cage Landmarks

On the anterior chest, the suprasternal notch is located at the top of the manubrium and can be located by palpation of the depression at the base of the neck. Directly below this notch is the sternal angle, which is also called the angle of Louis. The sternal angle can be identified by palpating down from the suprasternal notch until the ridge between the gladiolus and the manubrium is identified. This important landmark is visible in most persons. The second rib articulates with the top of the gladiolus at this point (Fig. 5.6). Rib identification on the anterior chest can now be accomplished with this as a reference point. It is recommended that ribs be counted to the side of the sternum because individual costal cartilages that attach the ribs to the sternum are not identified as easily near the sternum.

On the posterior chest, the spinous processes of the vertebrae are useful landmarks (Fig. 5.7). The spinous process of the seventh cervical vertebra (C7) usually can be identified by having the patient extend the head and neck forward

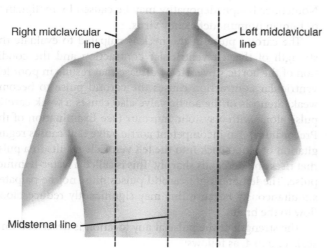

**FIG. 5.3** Imaginary lines on anterior chest wall. (From Kacmarek RM, Stoller JK, Heuer AJ: *Egan's fundamentals of respiratory care,* ed 11. St. Louis, 2017, Mosby-Elsevier.)

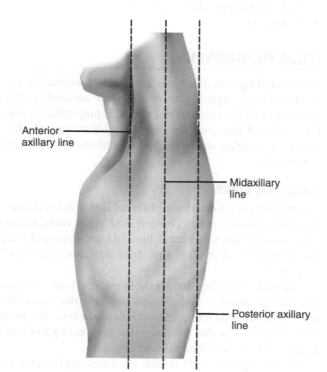

**FIG. 5.4** Imaginary lines on lateral chest wall. (From Kacmarek RM, Stoller JK, Heuer AJ: *Egan's fundamentals of respiratory care,* ed 11. St. Louis, 2017, Mosby-Elsevier.)

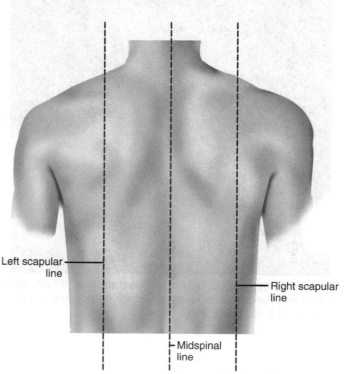

**FIG. 5.5** Imaginary lines on posterior chest wall. (From Kacmarek RM, Stoller JK, Heuer AJ: *Egan's fundamentals of respiratory care,* ed 11. St. Louis, 2017, Mosby-Elsevier.)

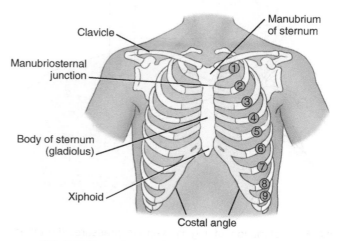

**FIG. 5.6** Thoracic cage landmarks on anterior chest.

and slightly down. At the base of the neck, the most prominent spinous process that can be visualized and palpated is C7. The spinous process just below C7 belongs to the first thoracic vertebra (T1). The scapular borders also can be useful landmarks on the posterior chest. With the patient's arms raised above the head, the inferior border of the scapula lies almost directly over the oblique fissure that separates the upper from the lower lobes on the posterior chest.

## Lung Fissures

Between the lobes of the lungs are the interlobar fissures. Both lungs have an oblique fissure that begins on the anterior chest at approximately the sixth rib at the midclavicular line. This fissure extends laterally and upward until it crosses the fifth rib on the lateral chest in the midaxillary line and continues on the posterior chest to approximately T3 (Figs. 5.8 and 5.9).

The right lung also has a horizontal fissure that separates the right upper lobe from the right middle lobe. The horizontal fissure extends from the fourth rib at the sternal border around to the fifth rib at the midaxillary line. The left lung rarely has a horizontal fissure.

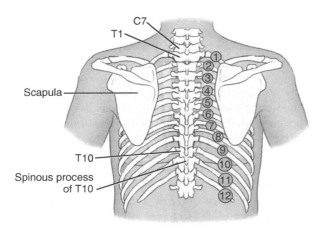

**FIG. 5.7** Thoracic cage landmarks on posterior chest.

**FIG. 5.8** Topographic position of lung fissures on anterior chest.

## Tracheal Bifurcation

On the anterior chest, the carina (tracheal bifurcation) is located approximately beneath the sternal angle (angle of Louis) and on the posterior chest at approximately T4.

## Diaphragm

The diaphragm is a dome-shaped muscle that lies between the thoracic and abdominal cavities and moves up and down during normal ventilation. At the end of a tidal expiration, the right dome of the diaphragm is located at the level of T9 posteriorly and the fifth rib anteriorly. On the left, the diaphragm comes to rest at the end of expiration at T10 posteriorly and the sixth rib anteriorly. The right hemidiaphragm is usually a little higher anatomically than the left hemidiaphragm because of the placement of the liver.

## Lung Borders

Superiorly on the anterior chest, the lungs extend 2 to 4 cm above the medial third of the clavicles. The inferior borders on the anterior chest extend to approximately the sixth rib at the midclavicular line and to the eighth rib on the lateral chest wall. On the posterior chest, the superior border extends to T1, and the inferior border varies with ventilation between approximately T9 and T12 (see Fig. 5.9).

# EXAMINATION OF THE THORAX

## Inspection

Visual examination of the chest is of value in assessing the thoracic configuration and the pattern and effort of breathing. For inspection to be adequate, the room must be well lighted, and the patient should be sitting upright. If the patient is too ill to sit up, the clinician must roll the patient carefully onto one side to examine the posterior chest. Male patients should be stripped to the waist. Female patients should be given some type of drape to prevent possible embarrassment from exposure of their breasts.

### Thoracic Configuration

The normal adult thorax has an anteroposterior diameter less than the transverse (side-to-side) diameter. The anteroposterior diameter normally increases gradually with age and prematurely increases in patients with COPD. This abnormal increase in anteroposterior diameter is called a barrel chest and is commonly seen in patients with emphysema due to hypertrophy of the accessory muscles of breathing and chronic hyperinflation of the lungs. When the anteroposterior diameter increases, the ribs lose their normal 45-degree angle of slope in relation to the spine and become horizontal (Fig. 5.10). Other abnormalities of the thoracic configuration include the following:

Pectus carinatum: outward sternal protrusion anteriorly

Pectus excavatum: depression of part or all of the sternum

Kyphosis: spinal deformity in which the spine has an abnormal anteroposterior curvature (Fig. 5.11)

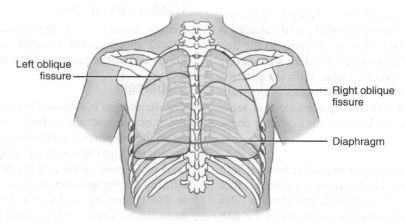

Left oblique fissure

Right oblique fissure

Diaphragm

**FIG. 5.9** Topographic position of lung fissures on posterior chest.

A                    B

**FIG. 5.10 A,** Patient with normal thoracic configuration. **B,** Patient with increased anteroposterior diameter. Note contrasts in angle or slope of ribs and development of accessory muscles.

**Scoliosis:** spinal deformity in which the spine has a lateral curvature (see Fig. 5.11)

**Kyphoscoliosis:** combination of kyphosis and scoliosis (see Fig. 5.11)

It should be noted that several of these abnormalities, depending on their severity, can result in a restrictive lung defect. In particular, the abnormalities of pectus excavatum and kyphoscoliosis may produce such a restriction. Severe trauma to the chest cage can result in fractures of the ribs and sternum. Abnormal configuration of the thoracic cage may result, especially if multiple ribs are broken. A section of the rib cage may move paradoxically with breathing when

multiple ribs are fractured at more than one site. The paradoxic motion is seen as a sinking inward of the affected region with each spontaneous inspiratory effort and an outward movement with subsequent exhalation. This paradoxical motion of the affected rib cage is called **flail chest.**

## Breathing Pattern and Effort

The healthy adult at rest has a consistent rate and rhythm of ventilation. The diaphragm and the intercostal muscles are the primary muscles of ventilation, actively working to increase the thoracic cavity dimension during normal inspiratory effort. During normal breathing at rest, the diaphragm performs the majority of the work of breathing. The effort of breathing is minimum on inhalation and passive on exhalation. Men typically breathe with the diaphragm, causing the stomach to move slightly outward during inhalation. Women tend to use a combination of intercostal muscles and the diaphragm, producing more chest wall movement than men. Table 5.1 describes the abnormal patterns of breathing. See Chapter 4, Table 4.4, for further descriptions of terms commonly used to describe breathing rates associated with patterns of breathing.

Additional muscles of ventilation, called **accessory muscles,** are also slightly active during normal, resting breathing. When ventilatory demands increase, these accessory muscles become more active in assisting the primary muscles of ventilation in the work of breathing. The predominant accessory muscles include the intercostal, scalene, sternocleidomastoid, pectoral, trapezius, and abdominal wall muscles. The accessory muscles of inspiration specifically include the external intercostals, scalene, sternocleidomastoids, trapezius, pectoralis minor, and pectoralis major. Changes in the patient's breathing pattern can provide important clues to the type of respiratory problem present. Patients with restrictive lung disease (reduced lung volumes) typically breathe with a rapid (tachypnea) and shallow (hypopnea) pattern. (See Chapter 4, Table 4.4, for further discussion of breathing rate and pattern terminology.) The more lung volume lost, the greater increase in the respiratory rate. Acute obstruction of intrathoracic airways, as occurs with asthma, results in a prolonged exhalation time. The approximate I:E ratio can be determined by timing the two phases of breathing. Normal I:E ratio is approximately 1:2.

**FIG. 5.11** Examples of chest cage abnormalities. **A,** Scoliosis. **B,** Kyphosis. **C,** Kyphoscoliosis.

| TABLE 5.1 | **Abnormal Breathing Patterns** | |
|---|---|---|
| **Pattern** | **Characteristics** | **Causes** |
| Tachypnea | Rapid rate of breathing | Loss of lung volume, arterial hypoxemia, metabolic acidosis |
| Apnea | No breathing | Cardiac arrest |
| Biot | Irregular breathing with long periods of apnea | Increased intracranial pressure |
| Cheyne-Stokes | Irregular type of breathing; breaths increase and decrease in depth and rate with periods of apnea | Diseases of central nervous system, congestive heart failure |
| Kussmaul | Deep and fast | Metabolic acidosis |
| Apneustic | Prolonged inhalation | Brain damage |
| Paradoxic | Injured portion of chest wall area moves in the opposite direction to the rest of the chest | Chest trauma |
| Abdominal paradox | Contraction of accessory muscles to aid inspiratory effort; diaphragm is pulled upward and abdomen sinks inward during inspiration | Fatigue of diaphragm, paralysis |

With more severe cases of airway obstruction, the I:E ratio may be 1:3, 1:4, or even longer at 1:5 or greater. Acute upper airway obstruction, as occurs with croup or epiglottitis, often results in a prolonged inspiratory time.

### SIMPLY STATED

The patient's breathing pattern often provides strong clues to the underlying pathologic condition. Rapid and shallow breathing suggests a loss of lung volume, a prolonged expiratory time indicates intrathoracic airway obstruction, and a prolonged inspiratory time indicates upper airway obstruction.

Any respiratory abnormalities that increase the work of breathing may cause the accessory muscles of breathing (most visibly the scalenes and sternocleidomastoids) to become active during breathing at rest. This is common in acute and chronic diffuse airway obstruction, acute upper airway obstruction, and disorders that reduce lung compliance such as pneumonia or acute respiratory distress syndrome.

Significant increases in the effort of breathing cause large swings in pleural pressure. As a result, the skin overlying the chest cage may sink inward between the ribs during inspiration and bulge outward during exhalation, when the work of breathing is increased. Inward depression of the skin during inspiration is known as retractions. Retractions may be seen between ribs (intercostal), below the ribs (subcostal), or above the clavicles (supraclavicular).

The opposite movement of the skin during exhalation is known as bulging. Obesity and muscular chest walls prevent retractions and bulging from occurring unless the abnormality is severe.

The diaphragm may be nonfunctional in patients with spinal injuries or neuromuscular disease and severely limited in patients with COPD. When this occurs, the accessory muscles of breathing become active, even at rest. The respiratory accessory muscles may also become active during acute airway obstruction. However, its absence does not rule out the possibility that severe airway obstruction is present.

In patients with emphysema, the lungs lose their elastic recoil and become hyperinflated. This results in the diaphragm assuming a lower, less functional position. The accessory muscles must assist ventilation by raising the anterior chest in an effort to increase thoracic volume. Significant use of the accessory muscles of breathing at rest is a sign of more severe chronic obstructive lung disease.

Normally, the abdomen moves gently outward with inspiration and inward with exhalation. When the diaphragm becomes fatigued, the accessory muscles of breathing attempt to maintain ventilation by becoming more active. As the accessory muscles contract in an effort to cause gas to flow into the lung, negative intrathoracic pressure causes the diaphragm to be pulled upward and the abdomen to sink inward during inspiration. This is known as abdominal paradox, which is an important finding that occurs with paralysis or fatigue of the diaphragm. Diaphragm fatigue is common in patients with COPD, especially during weaning from mechanical ventilation. It should be noted that abdominal paradox should not be confused with the term *paradoxic pulse* (also known as *pulsus paradoxus*), which is when the systolic blood pressure drops by more than 10 mm Hg during inspiration, described in more detail in Chapter 4.

Abdominal paradox may be accompanied by respiratory alternans. Respiratory alternans consists of periods of breathing using only the chest wall muscles alternating with periods of breathing entirely by the diaphragm. It is not as common as abdominal paradox but also is an indication that the diaphragm is fatigued. Not all patients with diaphragm dysfunction develop abdominal paradox or respiratory alternans, but when these clinical signs are present, they indicate significant inspiratory muscle fatigue.

COPD patients with severe hyperinflation have a low, flat diaphragm with limited mobility. Contraction of the flattened diaphragm pulls the lateral margins of the chest wall inward during each inspiratory effort. This abnormal movement of the lateral chest wall during breathing in COPD patients with severe hyperinflation is known as Hoover sign.

Patients with brain injury may have an abnormal pattern of breathing. The pattern of breathing often proves useful in determining the degree of brainstem function, which is discussed in Chapter 6.

### Inspection for Central Cyanosis

Central cyanosis is present when the patient's trunk or oral mucosa is cyanotic. This occurs when the lungs are not oxygenating the blood adequately or when congenital heart disease causes venous blood to be shunted into the arterial system without passing through the lungs. Central cyanosis is an indication that tissue oxygenation may not be adequate and that further investigation is needed (e.g., arterial blood gas analysis). Cyanosis is apparent only when a significant amount of reduced (deoxygenated) hemoglobin is present. In patients with severe anemia (hemoglobin of 4 to 5 grams or less per deciliter of blood), cyanosis is generally not detected until advanced oxygenation problems are present.

---

**SIMPLY STATED**

Central cyanosis generally indicates hypoxemia or cyanotic heart disease. Further investigation is needed.

---

## Palpation

Palpation is the act of touching the chest wall in an effort to evaluate underlying lung structure and function. Palpation is performed to evaluate vocal fremitus, estimate thoracic expansion, and assess the skin and subcutaneous tissues of the chest. Palpation is used in selected patients to confirm or rule out suspected problems suggested by the history and initial physical examination.

### Vocal Fremitus

The term vocal fremitus refers to the vibrations created by the vocal cords during phonation. These vibrations are transmitted down the tracheobronchial tree and through the alveoli to the chest wall. When these vibrations are felt on the chest wall, they are called tactile fremitus.

During the assessment of tactile fremitus, the patient is directed to repeat the word "ninety-nine" while the clinician systematically palpates the thorax. The clinician can use the palmar aspect of the fingers or the ulnar aspect of the hand as illustrated in Fig. 5.12. If one hand is used, it should be moved from one side of the chest to the corresponding area on the other side. The anterior, lateral, and posterior chest wall should be evaluated.

The vibrations of tactile fremitus may be increased, decreased, or absent. Increased fremitus results from the transmission of the vibration through a more solid medium. The normal lung structure is a combination of solid and air-filled tissue. Any condition that tends to increase the density of the lung, such as the consolidation of pneumonia, atelectasis, lung tumors, or masses, results in an increased intensity of fremitus. If the area of consolidation or atelectasis is not in connection with a patent bronchus, for instance, due to mucous obstruction of a bronchus, fremitus will be absent or decreased.

A reduced tactile fremitus is often present in patients who are obese or overly muscular. In addition, when there is a bronchial obstruction such as a mucous plug or foreign object, or when the pleural space lining the lung becomes filled with air (pneumothorax) or fluid (pleural effusion), the vocal fremitus is reduced significantly or is absent.

The lungs become hyperinflated, with a significant reduction in the density of lung tissue, in patients with emphysema. In this situation, the vocal vibrations from the larynx transmit poorly through the lung tissue, resulting in a bilateral reduction in tactile fremitus. The bilateral reduction in tactile fremitus is more difficult to detect than the unilateral increase in fremitus associated with lobar consolidation. The causes of abnormal tactile fremitus are summarized as follows:

*Increased.*
- Pneumonia
- Lung tumor or mass
- Atelectasis (with patent bronchiole)

**FIG. 5.12** Palpation for assessment of vocal fremitus. **A,** Use of palmar surface of fingertips. **B,** Use of ulnar aspect of hand. (From Cuppett M, Walsh K: *General medical conditions in the athlete,* ed 2. St. Louis, 2012, Mosby.)

***Decreased.***
- Unilateral
  - Bronchial obstruction with mucous plug or foreign object
  - Pneumothorax
  - Pleural effusion
- Diffuse
  - COPD with hyperinflation
  - Muscular or obese chest wall

The passage of air through airways contaminated with thick secretions may produce palpable vibrations called *rhonchial fremitus*. Rhonchial fremitus often is identified during inhalation and exhalation and may clear if the patient produces an effective cough. It often is associated with a coarse, low-pitched sound that is audible without a stethoscope.

### Thoracic Expansion

The normal chest wall expands symmetrically during deep inhalation. This expansion can be evaluated on the anterior and posterior chest. Anteriorly, the RT's or other clinician's hands are placed over the anterolateral chest with the thumbs extended along the costal margin toward the xiphoid process. On the posterior chest, the hands are positioned over the posterolateral chest with the thumbs meeting at approximately T8 (Fig. 5.13). The patient is instructed to exhale slowly and completely while the clinician's hands are positioned as described. When the patient has exhaled maximally, the clinician gently secures the tips of his or her fingers against the sides of the chest and extends the thumbs toward the midline

until the tip of each thumb meets at the midline. The patient is then instructed to take a full, deep breath. The clinician should make note of the distance each thumb moves from the midline. Normally, each thumb moves an equal distance of approximately 3 to 5 cm.

Diseases that affect expansion of both lungs cause a bilateral reduction in chest expansion. This is seen commonly with neuromuscular diseases and COPD. A unilateral (one-sided) reduction in chest expansion occurs with respiratory diseases that reduce the expansion of one lung or a major part of one lung. This may occur with lobar consolidation, atelectasis, pleural effusion, and pneumothorax.

### Skin and Subcutaneous Tissues

The chest wall can be palpated to determine the general temperature and condition of the skin. When air leaks from the lung into subcutaneous tissues, fine beads of air produce a crackling sound and sensation when the chest wall is palpated. This is called subcutaneous emphysema.

### Percussion of the Chest to Assess Resonance

Percussion is the act of tapping on a surface in an effort to evaluate the underlying structure. Percussion of the chest wall produces a sound and a vibration useful in the evaluation of the underlying lung tissue. The vibration created by percussion penetrates and thus evaluates the lung to a depth of 5 to 7 cm below the chest wall.

The technique most often used in percussion of the chest wall is called mediate or indirect percussion. The RT or other

**FIG. 5.13** Estimation of thoracic expansion. **A,** Exhalation. **B,** Maximal inhalation. (From Kacmarek RM, Stoller JK, Heuer AJ: *Egan's fundamentals of respiratory care,* ed 11. St. Louis, 2017, Mosby-Elsevier.)

clinician places the middle finger of the left hand (if the clinician is right-handed) firmly against the chest wall parallel to the ribs with the palm and other fingers held off the chest. The tip of the middle finger on the right hand or the lateral aspect of the right thumb strikes the finger against the chest near the base of the terminal phalanx with a quick, sharp blow. Movement of the hand striking the chest should be generated at the wrist and not the elbow or shoulder (Fig. 5.14).

The percussion note is clearest if the clinician remembers to keep the finger on the chest firmly against the chest wall and to strike this finger and immediately withdraw. The two fingers should be in contact for only an instant.

### Percussion over Lung Fields

Percussion of the lung fields should be performed systematically, testing comparable areas on both sides of the chest consecutively. Percussion over the bony structures and breasts of the female patient is not of value and should be avoided. The RT or other clinician can ask the patient to raise his or her arms above the shoulders, which helps move the scapulae laterally and minimizes interference with percussion on the posterior chest wall.

The sounds generated during percussion of the chest are evaluated for intensity (loudness) and pitch. Percussion over normal lung fields produces a moderately low-pitched sound that can be heard easily. This sound is best described as normal resonance. When the percussion note is louder and lower in pitch than normal, the resonance is said to be increased. A hollow-sounding pitch during percussion is said to be hyperresonant. Percussion may produce a sound with

**FIG. 5.14** Technique for indirect chest percussion.

characteristics just the opposite of resonance, referred to as dull or flat. This sound is high pitched, short in duration, and not loud. It is simply described as decreased resonance.

*Clinical Implications.* By itself, percussion of the chest is of little value in making a diagnosis. When the percussion note is considered along with the history and other physical findings, it may contribute significantly. Any abnormality that tends to increase the density of the lung tissue, such as the consolidation of pneumonia, lung tumors, or alveolar collapse (atelectasis), results in a loss of resonance and a dull percussion note over the affected area. Percussion over pleural spaces filled with fluid, such as blood or water, also results in decreased resonance.

An increase in resonance is detected in patients with hyperinflated lungs. Hyperinflation can occur as a result of acute bronchial obstruction (asthma) and chronic bronchial obstruction (emphysema). When the pleural space contains large amounts of air (pneumothorax), the percussion note increases in resonance over the affected side.

### SIMPLY STATED

Increased resonance to percussion indicates excessive air trapped in the pleural space or lung; decreased resonance to percussion indicates fluid in the pleural space or consolidation of the lung.

Unilateral abnormalities are easier to detect than are bilateral abnormalities because the normal side provides an immediate comparison. The decreased resonance heard from percussion over consolidation is a distinct sound that is easier to detect than the subtle increase in resonance associated with hyperinflation or pneumothorax.

Percussion of the chest has limitations that are often clinically important. Abnormalities of the lungs are difficult to detect if the patient's chest wall is obese or overly muscular. Abnormalities that are small or more than 5 cm below the surface are not likely to be detected during percussion of the chest. Percussion to assess lung resonance is not performed routinely on most patients. However, it is useful in selected situations such as in the acutely ill patient suspected of having tension pneumothorax.

### Diaphragmatic Excursion

The range of diaphragm movement may be estimated by percussion and is assessed best on the posterior chest wall (Fig. 5.15). For the clinician to estimate diaphragm movement, the patient first is instructed to take a deep, full inspiration and to hold it. The clinician then determines the lowest margin of resonance by percussing over the lower lung field and moving downward in small increments until a definite change in the percussion note is detected. The patient then is instructed to exhale maximally, holding this position while the percussion procedure is repeated. The clinician should work rapidly to prevent the patient from becoming short of breath. The normal diaphragmatic excursion during a deep breath is approximately 5 to 7 cm. The range of diaphragm movement is less than normal in certain neuromuscular diseases and in patients with severe pulmonary hyperinflation (e.g., emphysema).

The exact range of movement and position of the diaphragm are difficult to determine by percussion. This probably is because the diaphragm is a dome-shaped muscle, with the center of the dome 15 cm beneath the surface of the posterior chest. Percussion can only approximate the position and degree of movement of the diaphragm.

### Auscultation of the Lungs

Auscultation is the process of listening for sounds produced in the body. Auscultation over the thorax is performed to

**FIG. 5.15** Assessment of diaphragmatic excursion by percussion. *Horizontal lines* indicate position of diaphragm at maximal inhalation *(dashed line)* and exhalation *(solid line).*

**FIG. 5.16** Acoustic stethoscope. (From Kacmarek RM, Stoller JK, Heuer AJ: *Egan's fundamentals of respiratory care,* ed 11. St. Louis, 2017, Mosby-Elsevier.)

identify normal or abnormal lung sounds. Careful assessment of the patient's lung sounds is useful in making the initial diagnosis and evaluating the effects of treatment. A stethoscope is used during auscultation for better transmission of sounds to the clinician. The room must be as quiet as possible whenever auscultation is performed.

### Stethoscope

The stethoscope includes four basic parts: a bell, a diaphragm, tubing, and earpieces (Fig. 5.16). The bell detects a broad spectrum of sounds and is of particular value in listening to low-pitched heart sounds. It is also valuable in auscultation of the lungs in certain situations such as in the emaciated patient whose rib protrusion restricts placement of the diaphragm flat against the chest. The bell piece should be pressed lightly against the chest when the clinician is attempting to auscultate low-frequency sounds. If the bell is pressed too firmly against the chest wall, the skin will be stretched under the bell and may act as a diaphragm, filtering out certain low-frequency sounds.

The diaphragm piece is used most often in auscultation of the lungs because most lung sounds are high frequency. It is also useful in listening to high-frequency heart sounds. The diaphragm piece should be pressed firmly against the chest so that external sounds are not heard.

The ideal tubing should be thick enough to exclude external noises and should be approximately 19 inches in length, with the total length of the stethoscope from the binaurals to the diaphragm being a standard 27 inches. Longer tubing may compromise transmission of lung sounds, and shorter tubing often is inconvenient in reaching the patient's chest.

The stethoscope should be examined regularly for cracks in the diaphragm, wax or dirt in the earpieces, and other defects that may interfere with the transmission of sound. It should be wiped with isopropyl alcohol regularly to prevent a buildup of microorganisms.

### Technique

The patient should be sitting upright in a relaxed position when possible. The patient is instructed to breathe a little deeper than normal with the mouth open. Inhalation should be an active process and exhalation passive. The bell or diaphragm is placed directly against the chest wall to eliminate clothing as a factor in most cases. However, a thin gown or shirt/blouse probably offers little interference and may make the female patient more comfortable during the procedure. The tubing should not be allowed to rub against any objects because this may produce extraneous sounds. Auscultation of the lungs should be systematic, including all lobes on the anterior, lateral, and posterior chest. It is recommended that clinicians begin at the bases, compare side with side, and work toward the lung apices. The examination begins at the lung bases because certain abnormal lung sounds (described later) that occur primarily in the dependent lung zones may be altered by several deep breaths (Fig. 5.17). The clinician should listen to at least one full ventilatory cycle at each position on the chest wall. Auscultation over the neck is useful whenever upper airway narrowing may be present.

Four characteristics of breath sounds are to be identified. First, the pitch, either high or low pitch (vibration frequency), is identified. Second, the amplitude or intensity (loudness) is noted. Third, the clinician listens for the distinctive characteristics. Fourth, the duration of inspiratory

**FIG. 5.17** The normal sequencing for auscultation of the posterior (**A**); anterior (**B**); left lateral (**C**); and right lateral chest wall (**D**). Note that the clinician compares the breath sounds from side to side using the corresponding location on each side of the chest.

sound is compared with that of expiration. The acoustic characteristics of breath sounds can be illustrated in breath sound diagrams (Fig. 5.18). RTs and other members of the patient care team must have a clear understanding of the characteristics of the normal breath sounds described in Table 5.2 to identify subtle changes that may signify respiratory disease.

### Terminology

In healthy persons, the sound heard over the trachea has a loud, tubular quality called a tracheal breath sound. Tracheal breath sounds are high-pitched sounds with an expiratory component equal to or slightly longer than the inspiratory component.

A slight variation to the tracheal breath sound is heard around the upper half of the sternum on the anterior chest and between the scapulae on the posterior chest (Fig. 5.19). This is not as loud as the tracheal breath sound, is slightly lower in pitch, and has equal inspiratory and expiratory components. It is called a bronchovesicular breath sound. It is not evaluated in most clinical situations.

Auscultating over the lung parenchyma of a healthy person yields a soft, muffled sound. This is called a vesicular breath sound, or normal breath sound, and is lower in pitch and intensity (loudness) than the tracheal breath sound. The vesicular sound is somewhat difficult to hear and is heard primarily during inhalation with only a minimal exhalation component (see Table 5.2).

Respiratory disease may alter the intensity of normal breath sounds heard over the lung fields. A slight variation in intensity is difficult to detect even for experienced clinicians. Breath sounds are described as diminished when the intensity decreases and absent in extreme cases. Breath sounds are described as harsh when the intensity increases. Harsh breath sounds may have an expiratory component equal to the inspiratory component and are described as bronchial breath sounds in such cases.

Abnormal lung sounds produced by the movement of air in the lungs are called adventitious sounds. The term adventitious refers to sounds that are added sounds or extra sounds produced within a normal sound or heard in a place within the lung where that particular sound is not normally heard, such as tracheal or bronchial breath sounds heard over lung parenchyma. Clinicians may also use the term adventitious as a synonym to mean abnormal lung sounds. Most adventitious lung sounds can be classified as either continuous or discontinuous sounds. Continuous lung sounds are defined as those having a duration longer than 25 ms. (This definition is derived from recording and spectral analysis of lung sounds. Clinicians are not expected to time the lung sounds.) Discontinuous lung sounds are characteristically intermittent, crackling, or bubbling sounds of short duration (Fig. 5.20).

### SIMPLY STATED

Lung sounds are classified in two basic categories: normal breath sounds and adventitious lung sounds. The normal breath sounds are the expected sounds of breathing heard when auscultating each area of the lung, and the adventitious lung sounds are the abnormal sounds superimposed on the normal breath sounds or sounds not normally heard in the particular area of auscultation.

**FIG. 5.18** Diagrammatic representation of normal breath sound. Upstroke represents inhalation, downstroke represents exhalation, length of upstroke represents duration, thickness of stroke represents intensity, and angle between upstroke and horizontal line represents pitch. The example in this figure illustrates a normal vesicular breath sound. (Modified from Kacmarek RM, Stoller JK, Heuer AJ: *Egan's fundamentals of respiratory care*, ed 11. St. Louis, 2017, Mosby-Elsevier.)

Experts have debated for many years about the terms to use in the description of abnormal lung sounds. *Rales* is an outdated term that had a long, evolving history and in the past was used to describe discontinuous abnormal lung sounds. Like the term *rales*, the term *rhonchi* has a confusing history and has been applied to more than one type of abnormal lung sound by various health care professionals. However, the American Thoracic Society (ATS) and the American College of Chest Physicians (ACCP) Joint Committee on Pulmonary Nomenclature have suggested that the term crackles be used to describe discontinuous, abnormal lung sounds and the term rhonchi be used to describe low-pitched, continuous, abnormal lung sounds. Crackles may be heard when air moves through excessive fluid or secretions in the airways, when collapsed airways pop open during inspiration.

| Breath Sound | Pitch | Intensity | Location | Diagram of Sound |
|---|---|---|---|---|
| Vesicular or normal | Low | Soft | Peripheral lung areas | |
| Bronchovesicular | Moderate | Moderate | Around upper part of sternum, between scapulae | |
| Tracheal | High | Loud | Over trachea | |

**TABLE 5.2  Characteristics of Normal Breath Sounds**

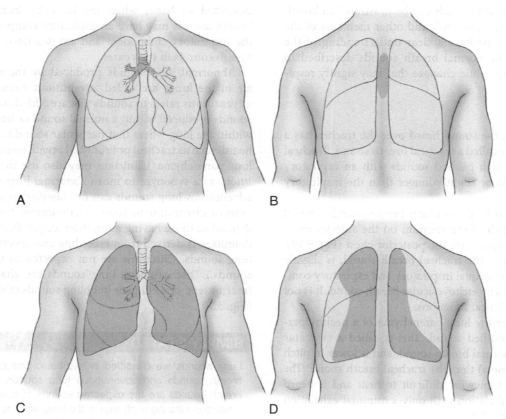

**FIG. 5.19** Location on chest wall where normal bronchovesicular and vesicular breath sounds are heard. **A,** Anterior bronchovesicular. **B,** Posterior bronchovesicular. **C,** Anterior vesicular. **D,** Posterior vesicular.

**FIG. 5.20** Time-expanded waveforms demonstrating inspiratory crackles **(A)** and expiratory polyphonic wheezes **(B).** (Modified from Wilkins RL et al: Lung sound terminology used by respiratory care practitioners, *Respir Care* 34:36, 1989.)

Low-pitched "coarse" crackles (a crackling sound) that are continuous are often referred to as rhonchi.

The term **wheeze** is used to describe the musical sounds heard from the chest of the patient with intrathoracic airway obstruction (e.g., asthma). Wheezes are classified as continuous sounds and are easily recognized in most cases.

**SIMPLY STATED**

The term *crackles* should be used for discontinuous abnormal lung sounds. Both the terms *wheeze* and *rhonchi* are classified as continuous adventitious lung sounds. Wheeze is an abnormal musical sound, and rhonchi describes low-pitched, continuous, abnormal lung sounds.

Another continuous type of adventitious lung sound, heard primarily over the larynx and trachea during inhalation when upper airway obstruction is present, is known as **stridor.** This is a loud, high-pitched sound that often may be heard without the aid of a stethoscope. Stridor is readily recognized by most clinicians.

Because there is a lack of standardization of lung sound terminology among clinicians, authors of other publications may use different terms to describe abnormal lung sounds. Table 5.3 provides a list of alternative terms that may be used by others.

When abnormal lung sounds are identified, their location and specific characteristics should be noted. Abnormal lung sounds may be high or low pitched, loud or faint, scanty or profuse, and inspiratory or expiratory (or both). The timing during the respiratory cycle should also be noted (e.g., late inspiratory). The RT or other clinician must pay close

## TABLE 5.3   Recommended Terminology for Lung Sounds and Other Terms Used

| Recommended Term | Classification | Other Terms Used |
|---|---|---|
| Crackles | Discontinuous | Rales<br>Crepitations |
| Rhonchi | Low-pitched, continuous | Coarse crackles |
| Wheezes | High-pitched, continuous | Sibilant rales<br>Musical rales<br>Sibilant rhonchus |

attention to these characteristics of abnormal lung sounds because they help determine the functional status of the lungs. The importance of using appropriate qualifying adjectives to describe abnormal lung sounds is further emphasized in the next paragraphs.

### Mechanisms and Significance of Lung Sounds

The exact mechanisms responsible for the production of normal and abnormal lung sounds are not understood in detail. However, there is enough agreement among investigators to allow a general description. This knowledge should provide a better understanding of the lung sounds often heard through a stethoscope.

*Normal Breath Sounds.* Lung sounds heard over the chest of the healthy person are generated primarily by turbulent flow in the larger airways. Turbulent flow creates audible vibrations in the airways, producing sounds that are transmitted through the lung and the chest wall. As the sound travels to the lung periphery and the chest wall, it is altered by the normal lung. Normal lung tissue acts as a low-pass filter, which means it preferentially passes low-frequency sounds. This filtering effect can be demonstrated easily by listening over the periphery of the lung while a subject speaks. The muffled voice sounds are difficult to understand because of the filtering properties of the normal lung. The alteration of sounds that travel through the lung is known as attenuation. Attenuation accounts for the characteristic differences between tracheal and bronchovesicular breath sounds heard directly over larger airways and vesicular sounds heard over the periphery of the lung.

Normal vesicular lung sounds are at least partly produced locally in the underlying lobe being auscultated.

### SIMPLY STATED

All normal breath sounds are produced primarily by turbulent flow in the airways.

The stability of normal breath sounds over time has been studied. Results indicate that normal vesicular breath sounds remain very stable from one day to the next in healthy persons with regard to pitch and amplitude. This suggests that significant changes in the pitch or loudness of breath sounds in the patient breathing with a similar pattern over time are not normal, and further investigation is indicated.

Auscultation for normal breath sounds following intubation is common practice. This is performed in an attempt to confirm that the endotracheal tube is placed properly in the trachea and not in the esophagus or one of the main stem bronchi. The finding of bilateral vesicular breath sounds is strong evidence that the tube is in the trachea. Confirmation by a chest film is recommended because the breath sounds may be difficult to hear in some patients, and air entering the esophagus may be misinterpreted as breath sounds.

*Abnormal Bronchial Breath Sounds.* Bronchial breath sounds may replace the normal vesicular sound when the lung increases in density, as occurs in pneumonia and certain types of atelectasis. When the normal air-filled lung becomes consolidated, the attenuation of sound is reduced, and similar sounds are heard over large upper airways and the consolidated lung (Fig. 5.21).

*Diminished Breath Sounds.* Diminished breath sounds occur when the sound intensity at the site of generation (larger airways) is reduced or when the sound transmission properties of the lung or chest wall are reduced. The intensity of sound created by turbulent flow through the bronchi is reduced with shallow or slow breathing patterns (e.g., major sedation). Obstructed airways (e.g., mucous plugs) and hyperinflated lung tissue (e.g., emphysema) increase attenuation of breath sounds through the lungs. Air (pneumothorax) or fluid (e.g., pleural effusion) in the pleural space and obesity reduce the transmission of breath sounds through the chest wall.

### SIMPLY STATED

Diminished breath sounds are produced by shallow breathing or when the turbulent flow sounds of the larger airways are not transmitted through the lung or chest wall. This attenuation of breath sounds is increased with mucous plugging or pleural effusion that absorbs or reflects sound.

*Wheezes.* Wheezes are generated by the vibration of the wall of a narrowed or compressed airway as air passes through at high velocity (Fig. 5.22). The diameter of an airway may be reduced by bronchospasm, mucosal edema, increased mucus production, or foreign object obstruction. The pitch of the wheeze is independent of the length of the airway but is related directly to the degree of airway compression—the tighter the compression, the higher the pitch. Low-pitched continuous sounds often are associated with the presence of excessive sputum in the airways. A sputum flap vibrating in the airstream may produce low-pitched wheezes that clear after the patient coughs.

When wheezes are identified, certain characteristics should be noted. RTs and other clinicians should identify the pitch and intensity and the portion of the respiratory cycle occupied by the wheezing. Improvement in the patient's airway caliber with bronchodilator therapy often results in a decrease in pitch and intensity of the wheezing and in a reduction in the portion of the respiratory cycle occupied

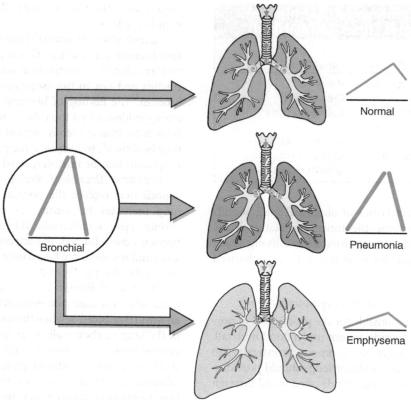

FIG. 5.21 Examples of how the normal bronchial breath sound is altered as it passes through normal (top), consolidated (middle), and emphysematous (bottom) lung tissue.

FIG. 5.22 Proposed mechanism for wheezing. **A,** Normal airway, where internal and external airway wall pressures are equal. **B,** Slight narrowing of the airway, which causes an increase in the velocity of airflow and a decrease in the lateral wall pressure inside the airway relative to the outside. **C,** Greater narrowing of the airway to the point that forward flow is inhibited and lateral wall pressure increases relative to outside pressure. **D,** Fluttering of the airway walls between position of **B** and **C**.

by wheezing. For example, before treatment, the patient may have loud, high-pitched wheezing that is heard during inspiration and expiration. After bronchodilator therapy, the wheezing may decrease in pitch and intensity and be heard only during the latter part of exhalation. Because the intensity of wheezing is related to the flow, loud wheezing indicates that air movement is occurring, whereas soft wheezing may occur with fatigue and the onset of respiratory failure. The clinician must never rely solely on changes in the intensity (loudness) of wheezing in assessing the patient's response to therapy.

Wheezing may be polyphonic (having several different musical notes) or monophonic (having a single note). Polyphonic wheezing is limited to exhalation, and its many different musical notes begin and end simultaneously, indicating that multiple airways are constricted, as in asthma. Monophonic wheezes may occur in one or more than one bronchus, with each one indicating obstruction of a bronchus. When multiple monophonic wheezes are present, the multiple notes often begin and end at different times; therefore these single-note wheeze sounds may overlap. The illusion of widespread airway obstruction results from a few loud notes transmitting to most areas of the chest wall. A single monophonic wheeze indicates obstruction of a single airway. This may be present in the patient with an airway tumor that is partially obstructing a major airway or with aspiration of a foreign object. The clinician who hears a monophonic wheeze over the patient's chest should also auscultate over the patient's neck. If the wheeze is heard loudest over the neck, the upper airway is the source of the sound.

*Stridor.* Stridor is produced by mechanisms similar to those of wheezing. Rapid airflow through a narrow site of the upper airway causes the lateral walls to vibrate and produce a high-pitched sound often heard without a stethoscope. The diameter of the upper airway is most often narrowed because of infection, as in croup or epiglottitis, or with inflammation after extubation. Stridor is most often heard during inhalation because the upper airway tends to narrow with significant inspiratory efforts. It may also be heard during inhalation and exhalation when the upper airway obstruction is severe and fixed (airway opening does not vary with breathing). This is seen in patients with laryngeal tumor.

Stridor can be a life-threatening sign that indicates ventilation may be compromised. The patient with stridor should be monitored closely, and equipment and personnel needed to perform emergency intubation, cricothyroidotomy, or tracheostomy should be nearby. The simultaneous presentation of stridor and cyanosis is a particularly ominous sign because the cyanosis probably is the result of hypoxemia caused by hypoventilation. Like wheezing, stridor can occur only when significant airflow is present through the site of obstruction. As a result the lack of stridor should never be interpreted as a sign of a healthy upper airway in the patient with a history of, or other clinical findings consistent with, upper airway abnormalities.

*Crackles.* Crackles often are produced by the movement of excessive secretions or fluid in the airways as air passes through. In this situation, crackles usually are coarse and heard during inspiration and expiration. They often clear if the patient coughs, and they may be associated with rhonchial fremitus.

Airway closure may occur in peripheral bronchioles or in more proximal bronchi. Crackles also occur in patients without excess secretions when collapsed airways pop open during inspiration. The crackling sound in this situation is caused by the explosive equalization of pressure between the collapsed airways and the patent airways above. The source of the crackles in this situation may be suggested by certain characteristics described in the next paragraphs.

Larger, more proximal bronchi may close during expiration when there is an abnormal increase in bronchial compliance, such as in the case of severe emphysema. In this situation, crackles usually occur early in the inspiratory phase and are called early inspiratory crackles. Early inspiratory crackles are usually few in number but may be loud or faint. They often are transmitted to the mouth and are not silenced by a cough or change in position. They occur most often in patients with COPD, as in chronic bronchitis, and emphysema, and may indicate that a more severe airway obstruction is present.

Peripheral alveoli and airways may close during exhalation when the surrounding intrathoracic pressure increases. Crackles produced by the sudden opening of peripheral airways usually occur late in the inspiratory phase and are called late inspiratory crackles (Fig. 5.23). They are more

**FIG. 5.23** Proposed mechanism for late inspiratory crackles. Peripheral airways pop open when inspiratory effort is sufficient to overcome the forces causing the atelectasis.

common in the dependent regions of the lungs, where the gravitational stress predisposes the peripheral airways to collapse during exhalation. They are often identified in several consecutive respiratory cycles, producing a recurrent rhythm. They may clear with changes in posture or if the patient performs several deep inspiratory maneuvers. Coughing or maximal exhalation by the patient may produce the reappearance of late inspiratory crackles. Patients with respiratory disorders, such as atelectasis, pneumonia, pulmonary edema, and fibrosis, that reduce lung volume (restrictive disorders) are most likely to have the late inspiratory type of crackles (Table 5.4).

### SIMPLY STATED

Wheezing indicates intrathoracic airway obstruction, whereas late inspiratory crackles suggest atelectasis or other conditions of the lung that cause a loss of lung volume. Fine crackles indicate the sudden opening of airways. Rhonchi or coarse crackles indicate excess airway mucus moving with airflow into and out of the lung.

*Pleural Friction Rub.* A pleural friction rub is a creaking or grating type of sound that occurs when the inflamed pleural membranes (pleurisy) rub together. It may be heard only during inhalation but often is identified during both phases of breathing, with the intensity of sound increasing during deep breaths. Pleural rubs are rarely encountered in the clinical setting and for this reason often are not identified correctly when present. Pleural rubs may be heard in patients with pneumonia, pulmonary fibrosis, or pulmonary embolism, or after thoracic surgery.

*Voice Sounds.* If inspection, palpation, percussion, or auscultation of the patient's chest suggests any respiratory abnormality, vocal resonance may be useful. Vocal resonance is produced by the same mechanism as vocal fremitus, described earlier. The vibrations created by the vocal cords during

**TABLE 5.4    Application of Adventitious Lung Sounds**

| Lung Sounds | Possible Mechanism | Characteristics | Causes |
|---|---|---|---|
| Rhonchi | Airflow through mucus | Discontinuous, coarse | Pneumonia, bronchitis, bronchiectasis, cystic fibrosis, other lung infections |
| Wheezes | Rapid airflow through obstructed airways caused by bronchospasm, mucosal edema | High pitched; most often occur during exhalation | Asthma, congestive heart failure, bronchitis |
| Stridor | Rapid airflow through obstructed upper airway caused by inflammation or fixed obstruction | High pitched; often occurs during inhalation | Croup, epiglottitis, postextubation airway edema, laryngeal tumor |
| Crackles | | | |
|   Inspiratory and expiratory | Excess airway secretions moving with airflow | Coarse and often clears with cough | Bronchitis, respiratory infections |
|   Early inspiratory | Sudden opening of proximal bronchi | Scanty, transmitted to mouth; not affected by cough | Bronchitis, emphysema, congestive heart failure |
|   Late inspiratory | Sudden opening of peripheral airways | Diffuse, fine; occur initially in the dependent regions | Atelectasis, pneumonia, pulmonary edema, fibrosis |

phonation travel down the tracheobronchial tree and through the peripheral lung units to the chest wall. The patient is instructed to repeat the words "one, two, three" or "ninety-nine" while the clinician listens over the chest wall with the aid of a stethoscope, comparing side with side. The normal, air-filled lung tissue filters the voice sounds, resulting in a significant reduction in intensity and clarity. Pathologic abnormalities in lung tissue alter the transmission of voice sounds, resulting in either increased or decreased vocal resonance.

An increase in intensity and clarity of vocal resonance is called bronchophony. Bronchophony occurs as a result of an increase in lung tissue density, as in the consolidation of pneumonia, and is the result of the better transmission of vocal vibrations through consolidation. Bronchophony is easier to detect when it is unilateral and is often associated with bronchial breath sounds, dull percussion note, and increased vocal fremitus.

Egophony is when the spoken voice sounds increase in intensity through the chest wall and the quality sounds nasal or bleating. This is assessed by the clinician when the patient is asked to say "e-e-e" but the sound is heard as "a-a-a" through the stethoscope. The area where it is heard may indicate a compressed lung above a pleural effusion. Whispering pectoriloquy is a technique to assess a patient for lung consolidation. Whispering of the words "one, two, three" by the patient creates high-frequency vibrations that are selectively filtered by normal lung tissue. Normally, whispers are heard as muffled, low-pitched sounds through the stethoscope. If the clinician hears high-pitched sounds, this suggests that lung consolidation is present.

Vocal resonance is reduced in similar lung abnormalities that result in reduced breath sounds and decreased tactile fremitus. Hyperinflation of lung parenchyma, pneumothorax, bronchial obstruction, and pleural effusion reduce the transmission of vocal vibrations through the lung or chest wall, producing decreased vocal resonance.

# EXAMINATION OF THE PRECORDIUM

As mentioned previously, chronic diseases of the lungs may and often do cause abnormalities in other body systems. Recognition of these abnormalities is helpful in identifying respiratory disease and in quantifying its severity. Because of the close working relationship between the heart and lungs, the heart is especially at risk for developing problems secondary to lung disease. The techniques for physical examination of the chest wall overlying the heart (precordium) include inspection, palpation, and auscultation. Percussion is of little or no value in the examination and is omitted. For the sake of convenience, most clinicians perform the examination of the precordium simultaneously with the examination of the lungs.

## Review of Heart Topography

The heart lies between the lungs within the mediastinum and is situated so that the right ventricle is more anterior than the left ventricle. The upper portion of the heart consists of both atria and commonly is called the *base of the heart*. The base lies directly beneath the upper-middle portion of the gladiolus (sternum). The lower portion of the heart, which consists of the ventricles, is called the *apex*. The apex points downward and to the left, extending to a point near the midclavicular line, and usually lies directly beneath the lower left portion of the gladiolus and near the costal cartilage of the fifth rib (Fig. 5.24).

## Inspection and Palpation

The purpose of inspecting and palpating the precordium is to identify any normal or abnormal pulsations. Pulsations on the precordium are affected by the thickness of the chest wall and the quality of the tissue through which the vibrations must travel. The normal apical impulse is produced by the thrust of the contracting left ventricle and usually is identified near the

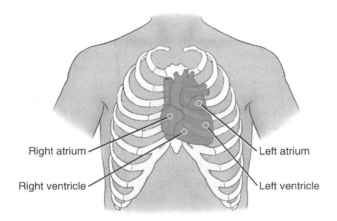

**FIG. 5.24** Topographic position of the heart.

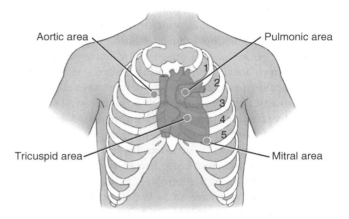

**FIG. 5.25** Position on the chest where each heart valve is best auscultated. Note that the stethoscope chestpiece is placed between the ribs to better hear the underlying heart sounds and to avoid interference by bony structures.

midclavicular line in the fifth intercostal space. This systolic thrust may be felt and visualized in many healthy persons; it may be called the **point of maximal impulse (PMI)**.

Right ventricular hypertrophy, a common manifestation of chronic lung disease, often produces a systolic thrust (**heave**) that is felt and may be visualized near the lower left sternal border. The palmar aspect of the clinician's right hand is placed over the lower left sternal border for identification. Right ventricular hypertrophy may be the result of chronic hypoxemia, pulmonary valve disease, or pulmonary hypertension.

In patients with chronic pulmonary hyperinflation (emphysema), identification of the apical impulse is more difficult. The increase in anteroposterior diameter and the alteration in lung tissue contribute to poor transmission of the vibrations of systole to the surface of the chest. Therefore in patients with pulmonary emphysema, the intensity of the PMI often is reduced or not identifiable.

The PMI may shift to the left or right with shifts in the mediastinum. Pneumothorax or lobar collapse often shifts the mediastinum, resulting in a shift of the PMI toward the lobar collapse but usually away from the pneumothorax. Patients with emphysema and low, flat diaphragms may have the PMI located in the epigastric area.

The second left intercostal space near the sternal border is called the *pulmonic area* and is palpated in an effort to identify accentuated pulmonary valve closure. Strong vibrations may be felt in this area with pulmonary hypertension (Fig. 5.25).

## Auscultation of Heart Sounds

Normal heart sounds are created primarily by the closure of the heart valves. The first normal heart sound is $S_1$, produced by the sudden closure of the mitral and tricuspid valves (often called the *atrioventricular [AV] valves*), which happens virtually simultaneously during contraction of the ventricles (systole). The second normal heart sound is $S_2$. When systole ends, the ventricles relax and the pulmonic and aortic (semilunar) valves close, which signals the onset of diastole and creates the second heart sound ($S_2$). Because the left side of the heart has a significantly higher pressure created during

systole, closure of the mitral valve is louder and contributes more to the $S_1$ sound than the closure of the tricuspid valve in the healthy person. For the same reason, closure of the aortic valve usually contributes more to the production of $S_2$. Both $S_1$ and $S_2$ heart sounds are normally heard in all populations. The $S_3$ and $S_4$ heart sounds are only normal in small children and may indicate a murmur in adults.

A split in the $S_1$ sound is heard when the tricuspid valve closure is delayed, and the sounds of the mitral and tricuspid valve are heard separately. This significant splitting of $S_1$ usually indicates heart disease. Defects in the electrical conduction system of the heart, such as bundle branch block, cause the two ventricles to lack synchrony during systole, causing a splitting of $S_1$.

Splitting of $S_2$ occurs when the semilunar valves (pulmonic and aortic) do not close simultaneously. A physiologically normal, narrow splitting of $S_2$ is due to the effects of spontaneous breathing on blood flow into the heart. During inhalation, there is a decrease in intrathoracic pressure, increasing venous return to the right side of the heart, which further delays pulmonic valve closure. The splitting of $S_2$ decreases or disappears on exhalation. Wide splitting of the second heart sound (significantly delayed closure of the pulmonic valve after the aortic valve) is usually a sign of disease and is seen with pulmonary hypertension, right bundle branch block, pulmonary embolism, and right-sided heart failure.

A third heart sound ($S_3$) may be identified early in diastole. $S_3$ is thought to be produced by rapid ventricular filling immediately after systole. The rapid distention of the ventricles causes the walls of the ventricles to vibrate briefly and produce a sound of low intensity and pitch. It is best heard over the apex with the bell of the stethoscope. It is normal in young healthy children and is called physiologic $S_3$ in this situation. However, in patients older than 40 years of age and especially in those with a history of heart disease, an $S_3$ is usually a sign of disease. $S_3$ usually indicates a ventricular abnormality (e.g., myocardial infarction) or some condition in which ventricular filling in volume or pressure is increased, such as an enlarged, failing ventricle. A fourth heart sound ($S_4$) also may be identified during diastole. $S_4$ occurs late in diastole just before $S_1$. $S_4$ is produced by active filling of the ventricles from atrial contraction just before systole. It may occur in healthy persons but most often is considered a sign of heart disease. The presence of an $S_4$ heart sound suggests decreased ventricular compliance with increased resistance to filling (increased end-diastolic pressure) as occurs with systemic hypertension, ventricular hypertrophy with outflow obstruction, ischemic heart disease, aortic stenosis, and acute mitral valve regurgitation. Most patients with an acute myocardial infarction have an $S_4$ if a sinus rhythm is present as seen on the electrocardiogram (see Chapter 11). The patient with an $S_4$ is often incorrectly thought to have a split $S_1$ because the timing of $S_4$ is normally very close to the first heart sound (Fig. 5.26).

A gallop rhythm is an abnormal condition in which a third ($S_3$) or fourth ($S_4$) heart sound is present. The spacing of the heart sounds results in a unique sequence of sounds that resembles the gallop of a horse. A gallop rhythm suggests that the left or right ventricle is being overdistended during diastole. When an $S_3$ or $S_4$ is present and originates in the right ventricle, it is best heard at the left sternal border near the apex. When the $S_3$ or $S_4$ originates in the left ventricle, it is best heard at the midclavicular line over the apex of the heart.

Auscultation of the heart sounds may identify alterations in the loudness of $S_1$ or $S_2$. A reduction in the intensity of the heart sounds may be the result of cardiac or extracardiac abnormalities. Extracardiac factors include alteration in the tissue between the heart and the surface of the chest. Pulmonary hyperinflation, pneumothorax, and obesity make identification of both $S_1$ and $S_2$ difficult. $S_1$ and $S_2$ intensity may also be reduced when the force of ventricular contraction is poor, as in heart failure, or when valvular abnormalities exist.

Pulmonary hypertension increases intensity of $S_2$ as a result of more forceful closure of the pulmonic valve; this is called an increased or loud $P_2$. A loud $P_2$ is a common finding in patients with pulmonary hypertension, cor pulmonale, and pulmonary embolism because high pulmonary artery pressures cause the pulmonic valve to close with more force. An increased $P_2$ is identified best over the pulmonic area of the chest (see Fig. 5.25). A loud aortic valve component (loud $A_2$) is commonly heard in patients with systemic hypertension. The best location to auscultate each heart valve is presented in Fig. 5.25.

> **SIMPLY STATED**
>
> A gallop rhythm is an abnormal condition in which a third ($S_3$) or fourth ($S_4$) heart sound is present in the adult. A loud pulmonic valve component to the second heart sound is called a *loud $P_2$* and suggests pulmonary hypertension, cor pulmonale, and/or pulmonary embolism. A loud aortic valve component (*loud $A_2$*) is commonly heard in patients with systemic hypertension.

Cardiac murmurs are identified whenever the heart valves are incompetent (incomplete closure) or stenotic (narrowed). Murmurs usually are classified as either systolic or diastolic. Systolic murmurs occur during systole and are heard following $S_1$. These murmurs are produced by an incompetent AV valve as in mitral valve regurgitation or a stenotic semilunar valve as in aortic valve stenosis. An incompetent mitral valve allows a backflow of blood into the left atrium, usually producing a high-pitched whooshing noise simultaneously with $S_1$. A stenotic aortic valve produces a similar sound because a narrowed valve creates an obstruction of blood flow out of the ventricle during systole.

Diastolic murmurs occur during diastole and are heard following $S_2$. These murmurs are created by either an incompetent semilunar valve, as in aortic regurgitation, or a stenotic AV valve, as in mitral stenosis. In aortic regurgitation, an incompetent aortic valve allows a backflow (reflux) of blood from the aorta into the left ventricle simultaneously with or immediately after $S_2$. A stenotic mitral valve obstructs blood flow from the left atrium into the left ventricle creating a turbulent murmur sound.

A murmur may also be created by rapid blood flow across normal valves. In summary, murmurs are created by a backflow of blood through an incompetent valve, forward flow through a stenotic valve, and rapid flow through a normal valve.

When indicated, auscultation of heart sounds is usually performed at the same time as auscultation of lung sounds. The diaphragm of the stethoscope is most useful for higher-frequency sounds such as $S_1$, $S_2$, and systolic murmurs. The bell side of the stethoscope is best used for low-frequency sounds such as gallops ($S_3$ and $S_4$) and diastolic murmurs. The heart sounds may be easier to identify if the patient leans forward or lies on the left side because anatomically this moves the heart closer to the chest wall. When the peripheral pulses are difficult to identify, auscultation over the precordium may be an easier method of assessing the heart rate.

## EXAMINATION OF THE ABDOMEN

An in-depth discussion of the abdominal examination is beyond the scope of this text; however, the abnormalities associated with respiratory disease are reviewed here.

The abdomen should be inspected and palpated for evidence of distention and tenderness. Abdominal distention

**FIG. 5.26** Timing of the first, second, third, and fourth heart sounds.

may cause impairment of excursion of the diaphragm and contribute to respiratory failure. Distention may also inhibit the patient from coughing and deep breathing, both of which are extremely important in preventing respiratory complications in the postoperative patient.

Palpation and percussion are used on the right upper quadrant (Fig. 5.27) of the abdomen in an effort to estimate the size of the liver. An enlarged liver may be found when chronic right-sided heart failure has occurred as a consequence of chronic respiratory disease. Any respiratory disease that results in a reduction of the oxygen level in the blood causes pulmonary vasoconstriction. If this occurs over a period of months or years, the right ventricle becomes enlarged and fails to pump blood effectively. The venous blood flow returning to the right ventricle is reduced, and engorgement of major veins and organs may occur. The hepatic vein that empties into the inferior vena cava may become engorged in this situation, and the liver may increase in size. This is called hepatomegaly.

To identify hepatomegaly, the clinician locates the superior and inferior borders of the liver by percussion. Normally, the liver spans approximately 10 cm at the right midclavicular line. If the liver extends more than 10 cm, it is considered enlarged.

Hepatomegaly may be accompanied by the collection of serous fluid in the peritoneal cavity known as ascites. Ascites most often results from interference with venous return to the right side of the heart, as occurs in heart failure. Cirrhosis of the liver, depletion of plasma proteins, and sodium retention

are common contributing factors. Severe ascites may restrict diaphragm movement, as mentioned earlier, and contribute to the onset of respiratory failure.

Obesity causes the abdomen to enlarge as a result of the collection of fatty tissue in the abdominal wall. This will restrict movement of the diaphragm especially during exertion when larger tidal volumes are needed. For this reason, obese patients often complain of shortness of breath during minimal exercise.

## EXAMINATION OF THE EXTREMITIES

Respiratory disease may result in numerous abnormalities, identified during inspection of the extremities. These abnormalities include digital clubbing, cyanosis, and pedal edema, and each is discussed briefly.

### Clubbing

Clubbing of the digits is a significant manifestation of cardiopulmonary disease. The mechanism responsible for clubbing is not known, but it is often associated with a chronic cardiopulmonary disease. It is identified most commonly in patients with cyanotic congenital heart disease, bronchogenic carcinoma, COPD, cystic fibrosis, and bronchiectasis.

Clubbing is characterized by a painless bulbous enlargement of the terminal phalanges of the fingers and toes, developing over many years. The angle of the fingernail to the nail base advances past 180 degrees, and the base of the nail feels spongy. The profile view of the digits allows easier recognition of clubbing (Fig. 5.28).

> **SIMPLY STATED**
>
> Clubbing of the digits is most commonly seen in patients with cyanotic congenital heart disease, bronchogenic carcinoma, COPD, cystic fibrosis, and bronchiectasis.

### Cyanosis

Examination of the fingertips and toes indicates the presence or absence of cyanosis, a blue, gray, or purplish

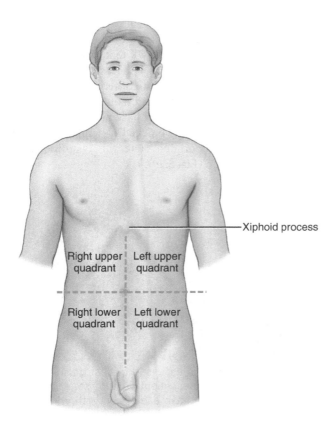

FIG. 5.27 Division of the abdomen into quadrants.

FIG. 5.28 Lateral view of digital clubbing of the index finger. (Courtesy Lawrence Cox. From Seidel HM, Ball J, Dains J, et al: *Mosby's guide to physical examination*, ed 7. St. Louis, 2011, Mosby-Elsevier.)

appearance of the skin, common in patients with severe cardiopulmonary disease. The ability to observe cyanosis depends on the patient's skin pigmentation and lighting in the room and may be masked by severe anemia. The presence of cyanosis in the digits of a pediatric or adult (peripheral cyanosis or acrocyanosis) indicates that the blood flow contains a reduction in oxygen-saturated hemoglobin. The patient with peripheral cyanosis resulting from poor perfusion also has extremities that are cool to the touch because vasoconstriction may occur due to cold ambient temperature. Tissue oxygenation may be compromised in such situations. However, it should be noted that acrocyanosis in a newborn (blue color of hands and feet alone) is usually a normal finding at birth and is not a reliable indicator of hypoxemia.

### SIMPLY STATED

The ability to see peripheral or acrocyanosis depends on the lighting in the room, the patient's skin pigmentation, and the patient's hemoglobin level. This is different from the condition of central cyanosis. If a patient is anemic, central and peripheral cyanosis will be masked and unapparent on visual examination.

## Pedal Edema

Pedal edema may be a manifestation of chronic lung disease. Because hypoxemia produces pulmonary vasoconstriction, the right ventricle must work harder than normal whenever significant hypoxemia exists. This chronic workload on the right ventricle may result in right ventricular hypertrophy and poor venous blood flow return to the heart. When the venous return to the right side of the heart is reduced, the peripheral blood vessels engorge, resulting in an accumulation of fluid in the subcutaneous tissues of the ankles, called pedal edema. The ankles most often are affected because they naturally are maintained in a gravity-dependent position throughout the day. The edematous tissues pit (indent) when pressed firmly with the fingertips. The severity of edema usually is characterized by the examining physician using a scale of 1+ to 4+, with 1+ indicating slight edema and 4+ indicating severe edema. Pitting edema, or that which leaves an indentation on the patient's leg after the clinician's gloved finger releases moderate pressure, should be evaluated for the level of occurrence above the ankle in an effort to quantify the degree of right-sided heart failure. For example, pitting edema occurring at a level well above the knee is much more significant than pitting edema around the ankles only.

### SIMPLY STATED

Pedal edema may occur in patients with chronic lung disease that has resulted in cor pulmonale or chronic right-sided heart failure.

## Capillary Refill

Capillary refill is assessed by pressing firmly for a brief period on the fingernail and identifying the speed at which the blood flow returns. When cardiac output is reduced and digital perfusion is poor, capillary refill is slow, taking several seconds to appear. In normal persons with good cardiac output and digital perfusion, capillary refill should take less than 3 seconds.

## Peripheral Skin Temperature

When the heart does not circulate the blood at a sufficient rate, compensatory vasoconstriction occurs in the extremities to shunt blood toward the vital organs. The reduction in peripheral perfusion results in a loss of warmth in the extremities. Palpation of the patient's feet and hands may provide general information about perfusion. Cool extremities usually indicate inadequate perfusion.

Actual extremity temperature can be compared with room temperature. The extremity should be at least 2°C warmer than room temperature (unless room temperature is equal to or greater than body temperature). When there is less than 2° C difference, perfusion is reduced; a 0.5°C difference indicates that the patient has serious perfusion problems.

## Assessment of Hydration: Skin Turgor

Physical assessment also includes assessing the skin for clues as to the hydration status of the patient. Skin turgor is the normal tension or resiliency of the skin attributable to the outward pressure of cells and interstitial fluid. It is assessed by pulling up on the skin on the back of the patient's hand or wrist in a gentle pinching motion with the thumb and pointer finger. The skin of the patient will tent upward as the clinician pinches it. When the skin is released, it should immediately return to its original state of tension on the hand or wrist, indicating adequate hydration of the patient. When the skin does not immediately snap back and return to its original state, but remains in a pinched or tented position with a slower return to its original state, this is an indication of possible dehydration (Fig. 5.29).

FIG. 5.29 Skin turgor is assessed by first grasping a fold of skin on the back of the patient's hand, sternum, forearm, or abdomen. Note the ease and speed with which the skin returns to place. (From Jarvis C: *Physical examination and health assessment*, ed 5, Philadelphia, 2008, Saunders.)

## KEY POINTS

- Physical examination of the patient with cardiopulmonary disease is performed to determine the cause and severity of the patient's problem and the effects of treatment. A review of the patient's history of present illness and past medical history before examination gives the clinician insight into the expected physical examination findings and suggests the techniques to emphasize.

- Diaphoresis is a sign of severe stress in the patient with cardiopulmonary disease. In patients prone to heart disease, it is consistent with myocardial infarction.

- Distention of the neck veins is consistent with right-sided heart failure and cor pulmonale.

- Lymphadenopathy in the neck is often palpated when respiratory infection is present.

- The degree of venous distention can be estimated by measuring the distance the veins are distended above the sternal angle. With the head of the bed elevated to a 45-degree angle, venous distention greater than 3 to 4 cm above the sternal angle is abnormal.

- In unilateral lung disease, the trachea tends to shift toward large-scale atelectasis and away from the side with a pneumothorax, pleural effusion, or lung mass.

- On the anterior chest, directly below the suprasternal notch is the sternal angle (the angle of Louis). The carina (tracheal bifurcation) is located approximately beneath the angle of Louis.

- A barrel chest is seen as an abnormal enlargement in the anteroposterior diameter of the chest due to accessory muscle hypertrophy and lung hyperinflation. It is a common finding in patients with COPD.

- The diaphragm and the intercostal muscles are the primary muscles of ventilation, actively working to increase the thoracic cavity dimension during normal inspiratory effort.

- When ventilatory demands increase, these accessory breathing muscles become more active in assisting the primary muscles of ventilation in the work of breathing.

- Abdominal paradox is a sign of diaphragm fatigue and impending respiratory failure and should not be confused with a paradoxic pulse, which is characterized by a drop in systolic blood pressure during inspiration.

- Patients with restrictive lung disease breathe with a rapid and shallow breathing pattern.

- Patients with obstructive lung disease breathe with a prolonged expiratory time.

- Retractions are a sign of significant respiratory distress.

- Any respiratory abnormalities that increase the work of breathing may cause the accessory muscles of breathing to become active during breathing at rest.

- Increased tactile fremitus results from the transmission of the vibration through a more solid medium such as the consolidation of pneumonia, atelectasis, lung tumors, or masses.

- A reduced tactile fremitus is often found in patients with obesity, overly muscular body type, hyperinflation (COPD), a bronchial obstruction such as a mucous plug or foreign object, or pleural space lining the lung that becomes filled with air (pneumothorax) or fluid (pleural effusion).

- A unilateral decrease in chest expansion is always abnormal and is consistent with pneumonia, pneumothorax, or atelectasis.

- Subcutaneous emphysema is when air leaks from the lung into subcutaneous tissues and fine beads of air produce a crackling sound and sensation when the chest wall is palpated. It may be caused by barotrauma to the alveoli due to positive-pressure ventilation.

- An increase in resonance during percussion of the chest indicates hyperinflation of the lungs as in emphysema or an accumulation of air in the pleura as in pneumothorax.

- A decrease in resonance during percussion of the chest is consistent with an abnormality that causes consolidation of the lungs such as pneumonia, atelectasis, or pleural effusion.

- The four characteristics of breath sounds to be identified during auscultation are the pitch (vibration frequency), the amplitude or intensity (loudness), distinctive characteristics, and the duration of inspiratory sound compared with expiratory sound.

- All normal breath sounds are created by turbulent flow in the airways. Listening directly over the trachea allows direct auscultation of this sound. Listening over the lung provides an attenuated, softer version of the turbulent flow sounds in the larger airways.

- Diminished breath sounds occur with shallow breathing or when attenuation of the breath sounds is increased due to hyperinflation of the lung (e.g., emphysema).

- Adventitious bronchial breath sounds are heard when the lung attenuation ability is reduced due to consolidation of the lung (e.g., pneumonia).

- Wheezes are consistent with diseases of airway obstruction such as asthma and bronchitis.

- Coarse crackles are heard when air moves through excessive airways secretions, whereas fine crackles are most commonly heard with the sudden opening of collapsed peripheral airways during deep breathing in the patient with restrictive lung disease or with fluid-filled alveoli.

- Stridor is a high-pitched sound and an ominous sign that indicates the patency of the upper airway is compromised.

- The normal point of maximal impulse (PMI) is created by contraction of the ventricles. Normal location is near the fifth intercostal space at the left midclavicular line. A shift to the left or right of the mediastinum, as occurs in lower lobe atelectasis, will cause the PMI to shift to one side.

- The normal heart sounds are created by closure of the atrioventricular valves during systole ($S_1$) and closure of the semilunar valves during diastole ($S_2$).

- $S_3$ is thought to be produced by rapid ventricular filling immediately after systole. $S_4$ is produced by active filling of the ventricles from atrial contraction just before systole.

- A gallop rhythm is present when $S_3$ and $S_4$ are present. A gallop rhythm is consistent with cardiac disease, including a recent myocardial infarction.

- Pulmonary hypertension increases intensity of $S_2$ as a result of more forceful closure of the pulmonic valve. A loud $P_2$ is also consistent with cor pulmonale and pulmonary embolism.
- A loud aortic valve component (loud $A_2$) is considered an increase in the intensity of a heart sound and is commonly heard in patients with systemic hypertension.
- Cardiac murmurs are identified whenever the heart valves are incompetent (incomplete closure) or stenotic (narrowed).

- An enlarged liver (hepatomegaly) is frequently seen in patients with right-sided heart failure caused by chronic lung disease (cor pulmonale).
- Cyanosis of the oral mucosa provides evidence that the lungs are not oxygenating the blood at normal levels.
- Pedal edema is a sign of heart failure. Edema that extends above the ankles suggests a more severe case of heart failure.
- Skin turgor is the normal tension or resiliency of the skin attributable to the outward pressure of cells and interstitial fluid and can indicate the hydration status of the patient.

## ASSESSMENT QUESTIONS

1. Which of the following is not a typical component of the physical examination?
   a. Inspection
   b. Palpation
   c. Auscultation
   d. Interviewing
2. Pursed-lip breathing is most often seen in patients with which of the following diseases?
   a. Pulmonary fibrosis
   b. COPD
   c. Pneumonia
   d. Congestive heart failure
3. Which of the following is an unlikely cause of diaphoresis?
   a. Myocardial infarction
   b. Fever
   c. Pulmonary fibrosis
   d. Exercise
4. In which of the following conditions is lymphadenopathy of the neck seen?
   a. Infection of the upper airway
   b. Asthma
   c. Cystic fibrosis
   d. Atelectasis
5. Which of the following may cause an increased jugular venous distention?
   1. Chronic hypoxemia
   2. Right-sided heart failure secondary to left-sided heart failure
   3. Right-sided heart failure alone
   a. 1 and 2 only
   b. 2 and 3 only
   c. 1, 2, and 3
   d. 3 only
6. What spinous process is most prominent with the patient sitting and with the head bent forward?
   a. T1
   b. C1
   c. C7
   d. S3
7. At which of the following topographic locations is the bifurcation of the trachea located on the anterior chest?
   a. Over the upper part of the manubrium
   b. Beneath the sternal angle

   c. The fourth rib at the sternum
   d. Under the xiphoid process
8. The minor (horizontal) fissure begins at which of the following locations on the anterior chest?
   a. Second rib at the sternal border
   b. Fourth rib at the sternal border
   c. Sixth rib at the sternal border
   d. Seventh rib at the sternal border
9. "An inward depression of the sternum" describes which of the following thoracic configurations?
   a. Kyphosis
   b. Pectus excavatum
   c. Flail chest
   d. Barrel chest
10. What type of lung problem is associated with severe kyphoscoliosis?
    a. COPD
    b. Restrictive lung disease
    c. Pneumothorax
    d. Pulmonary fibrosis
11. Which of the following best describes an apneustic breathing pattern?
    a. Prolonged exhalation
    b. Prolonged inhalation
    c. Deep and fast
    d. Absence of breathing
12. What is indicated by the presence of retractions?
    a. Heart failure
    b. An increase in the work of breathing
    c. Pneumothorax
    d. Restrictive lung disease
13. Which of the following I:E ratios is consistent with a severe asthma attack?
    a. 3:1
    b. 2:1
    c. 1:1
    d. 1:3
14. Which of the following breathing patterns is associated with narrowing of intrathoracic airways?
    a. Prolonged inspiratory time
    b. Prolonged expiratory time
    c. Rapid and shallow
    d. Rapid and deep

15. Which of the following indicate diaphragmatic fatigue?
    1. Paradoxic pulse
    2. Abdominal paradox
    3. Respiratory alternans
    4. Biot breathing pattern
       a. 1 and 2 only
       b. 2 and 3 only
       c. 3 and 4 only
       d. 1 and 4 only
16. Which of the following causes an increased tactile fremitus?
    a. Air movement through retained secretions
    b. Pleural effusion
    c. Emphysema
    d. Obesity
17. Which of the following causes a bilateral decrease in chest expansion?
    a. Lung tumor
    b. Pneumothorax
    c. COPD
    d. Pleural effusion
18. Which of the following causes an increased resonance to percussion of the chest?
    a. Lobar consolidation
    b. Pneumothorax
    c. Pleural effusion
    d. Atelectasis
19. What clinical condition would cause the range of diaphragm movement to be reduced bilaterally?
    a. Severe emphysema
    b. Left lower lobe atelectasis
    c. Congestive heart failure
    d. Pneumonia
20. Normal tracheal breath sounds are produced by which of the following mechanisms?
    a. Turbulent airflow through large airways
    b. Filtered sounds through lung tissue
    c. Passage of air through secretions
    d. Passage of air through narrowed airways
21. Which of the following terms is used to describe discontinuous adventitious lung sounds?
    a. Wheeze
    b. Crackles
    c. Rhonchi
    d. Stridor
22. The finding of late inspiratory crackles on auscultation of a patient might indicate which of the following?
    1. Atelectasis
    2. Pulmonary fibrosis
    3. Bronchospasm
    4. Pneumonia
       a. 1 only
       b. 1 and 3 only
       c. 1, 2, and 3 only
       d. 1, 2, and 4 only

23. What clinical condition is most closely associated with polyphonic wheezing?
    a. Pneumonia
    b. Pneumothorax
    c. Asthma
    d. Pulmonary fibrosis
24. Which of the following lung sounds is commonly heard in the patient with partial upper airway obstruction?
    a. Polyphonic wheeze
    b. Fine inspiratory crackles
    c. Coarse inspiratory and expiratory crackles
    d. Inspiratory stridor
25. Which of the following is the normal topographic location of the PMI?
    a. Third intercostal space at the anterior axillary line
    b. Fourth intercostal space at the anterior axillary line
    c. Fifth intercostal space at the midclavicular line
    d. Sixth intercostal space at the midsternal line
26. Which of the following locations is best for auscultating the mitral valve?
    a. Third intercostal space at the anterior axillary line
    b. Fourth intercostal space at the anterior axillary line
    c. Fifth intercostal space at the midclavicular line
    d. Sixth intercostal space at the midsternal line
27. What produces the sounds associated with the first heart sound?
    a. Closure of the atrioventricular (AV) valves
    b. Closure of the semilunar valves
    c. Left ventricular muscle movement
    d. Blood flow through normal valves
28. What clinical condition is most closely associated with a gallop heart rhythm?
    a. Pneumonia
    b. Pericarditis
    c. Congestive heart failure
    d. Aortic stenosis
29. Which of the following may cause an increased $P_2$ component of the second heart sound?
    1. Pulmonary hypertension
    2. Pulmonary embolism
    3. Cor pulmonale
    4. Systemic hypertension
       a. 1 and 3 only
       b. 2 and 3 only
       c. 1, 2, and 3 only
       d. 1, 2, 3, and 4
30. Which of the following is/are associated with right-sided heart failure?
    1. Jugular venous distention
    2. Hepatomegaly
    3. Pedal edema
    4. Systemic hypertension
       a. 1 only
       b. 1 and 2 only
       c. 1 and 3 only
       d. 1, 2, and 3

## BIBLIOGRAPHY

Ball J, Dains J, Flynn JA, et al. *Mosby's guide to physical examination.* ed 8. St. Louis: Mosby-Elsevier; 2015.

Bickley LS. *Bates' guide to physical examination and history taking.* ed 11. Philadelphia: Wolters Kluwer Health/Lippincott Williams & Wilkins; 2013.

DesJardins T, Burton GG. *Clinical manifestations and assessment of respiratory disease.* ed 7. Maryland Heights, MO: Mosby-Elsevier; 2016.

Jarvis C. *Physical examination and health assessment.* ed 7. St. Louis: Mosby-Elsevier; 2016.

Kacmarek RM, Stoller JK, Heuer AJ. *Egan's fundamentals of respiratory care.* ed 11. St. Louis: Mosby-Elsevier; 2017.

Kattwinkel J, Niermeyer S, Nadkarni V, et al. Advisory statement from the Pediatric Working Group of the International Liaison Committee on Resuscitation. *Pediatrics.* April 1999;103(4). Available at http://www.pediatrics.org/cgi/content/full/103/4/e56 Date retrieved: 6/2/2017.

LeBlond RF, Brown DD, DeGowin RL. *DeGowin's diagnostic examination.* ed 9. New York: McGraw-Hill; 2009.

Seidel HM, Ball J, Dains J, et al. *Mosby's guide to physical examination.* ed 9. St. Louis: Mosby-Elsevier; 2015.

Shumway NM, Wilson RL, Howard RS, et al. Presence and treatment of air hunger in severely ill patients. *Respir Med.* 2008;102:27.

Talley NJ, O'Connor S. *Clinical examination: a systematic guide to physical diagnosis.* Chatswood, Australia: Elsevier; 2014.

# 6

# Neurologic Assessment

*Ruben D. Restrepo*

## LEARNING OBJECTIVES

*After reading this chapter, you will be able to:*

1. Define key terms related to neurologic assessment.
2. Describe the functional anatomy of the nervous system.
3. Explain the cortical function of the different lobes of the brain.
4. Describe the functions of the brainstem, the cerebellum, and the 12 pairs of cranial nerves.
5. Describe common techniques used to assess the mental status.
6. Obtain and interpret Glasgow Coma Scale assessment.
7. Describe the importance of assessing level and content of consciousness in intensive care unit patients.
8. Distinguish among common techniques used to assess the cranial nerves, the sensory system, the motor system, coordination, and gait.
9. Describe common techniques used to assess deep, superficial, and brainstem reflexes.
10. Explain the control of the breathing and circulation by the central nervous system.
11. Briefly describe ancillary tests used in neurologic assessment.
12. Identify the importance of intracranial pressure monitoring and the value of assessing cerebral perfusion pressure.
13. Give an overview of brain death declaration.

## OUTLINE

## KEY TERMS

afferent
anisocoria
ataxia
ataxic breathing
Babinski sign
Biot breathing
brain death
central nervous system (CNS)
cerebral perfusion pressure (CPP)
Cheyne-Stokes respiration
content of consciousness

corneal reflex
Cushing triad
decerebrate posture
decorticate posture
deep tendon reflexes
delirium
doll's eyes reflex
efferent
electroencephalogram (EEG)
gag reflex
gait

Glasgow Coma Scale (GCS)
intracranial pressure (ICP)
level of consciousness
lower motor neuron (LMN)
lumbar puncture (LP)
Mini-Mental State Examination (MMSE)
miosis
mydriasis
nystagmus
oculocephalic reflex

Neurologic assessment is a comprehensive evaluation of the patient's mental status, cranial nerve function, motor system, coordination, sensory system, and various reflexes. Injuries that involve the nervous system often affect the patient's respiratory system and the ability of the patient to cooperate with respiratory care procedures. As a result, the respiratory therapist (RT) should become familiar with the key components of the neurologic assessment. The neurologic examination of an intubated, restrained, and frequently sedated patient in the intensive care unit (ICU) presents its own set of challenges. This chapter reviews the clinical neurologic assessment with special emphasis on patients with respiratory illness and the terminology related to such assessment.

### SIMPLY STATED

Injuries that involve the nervous system often affect a patient's respiratory system and the ability to cooperate with respiratory care procedures. Thus the RT should become familiar with the key components of the neurologic assessment, especially when managing critically ill patients.

Although obtaining a thorough history from the patient or family members can help the clinician characterize the dysfunction, the neurologic examination can assist in localizing and quantifying its severity. The initial interaction (e.g., how patient responds appropriately to verbal stimuli) often provides information that might affect the patient's adherence to respiratory care and performance of complex tasks that require coordination of multiple sensorimotor systems (e.g., the use of a pressurized metered-dose inhaler). The initial examination establishes baseline data, and subsequent examinations gauge the patient's response to the clinician's interventions. The frequency of these assessments will depend on the patient's diagnosis, acuity of the condition, and how rapidly changes are occurring or expected to occur.

### SIMPLY STATED

The frequency and depth of neurologic assessments depend on the patient's diagnosis, acuity of the condition, and how rapidly changes are occurring or expected to occur.

## FUNCTIONAL NEUROANATOMY

The neurologic system is made up of two major parts: the central and peripheral nervous systems. The central nervous system (CNS) contains the brain and spinal cord (Fig. 6.1), and the peripheral nervous system is composed of the 12 cranial nerves and the 31 spinal nerves. The brain consists of three parts: the cerebrum, the brainstem, and the cerebellum.

The peripheral nervous system is organized according to its function into sensory and motor divisions. This functional organization allows the clinician to understand how signals are transmitted to and from the CNS (Fig. 6.2).

The cerebrum is the largest part of the brain and is made up of two hemispheres and areas that control specific intellectual or motor functions (Fig. 6.3). Lesions in the cerebrum can lead to abnormalities in functions such as movement, level of consciousness, ability to speak and write, emotions, and memory.

The brainstem is the lower part of the brain where it connects to the spinal cord. It consists of the midbrain, pons, and medulla oblongata (Fig. 6.4). Most of the cranial nerves originate in the brainstem. Many neurologic functions of particular importance to the RT, such as regulation of heart rate, blood pressure, and breathing, are located in the brainstem. In addition, the brainstem contains reflex centers for certain cranial nerve functions such as the pupillary reflex, which is discussed later in this chapter. Lesions in the brainstem can cause a wide range of breathing problems from hyperventilation to apnea.

### SIMPLY STATED

Many neurologic functions of particular importance to the RT, such as regulation of heart rate, blood pressure, and breathing, are located in the brainstem.

The cerebellum is located in the posterior part of the brain and is responsible for controlling equilibrium, muscle tone, and coordination of muscle movements. Lesions in the cerebellum cause characteristic symptoms such as loss of muscle coordination (ataxia), tremors, and disturbances in gait and balance.

The spinal cord connects the brain to the various parts of the body for motor and sensory function. It spans a distance of approximately 45 cm in the average adult and extends from the base of the brain down to the level of the first lumbar (L1) vertebra (see Fig. 6.1). The rest of the space between the vertebral bodies is a collection of nerve roots termed the *cauda equina* (Latin for horse's tail).

Two sets of nerve fibers called *spinal nerves* project from both sides of the spinal column at 31 locations along the spine. There are 8 cervical (C1 to C8), 12 thoracic

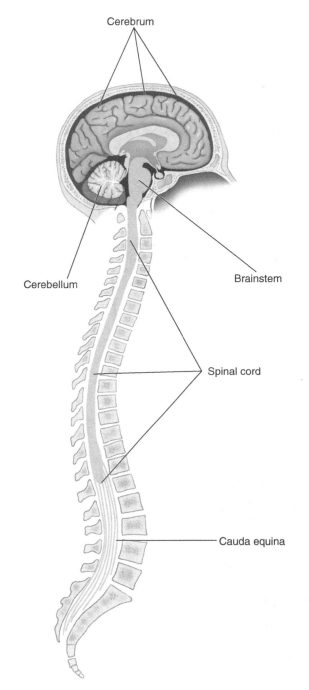

**FIG. 6.1** The central nervous system: cerebrum, brainstem, cerebellum, and spinal cord.

(T1 to T12), 5 lumbar (L1 to L5), 5 sacral (S1 to S5), and 1 coccygeal pair of spinal nerves. Sensory (dorsal) and motor (ventral) nerve roots separate as they exit the spinal cord until their fibers combine at the level of the dorsal root ganglion. Each nerve root has the ability to provide sensory input to the brain (e.g., feel pain) and the ability to cause muscle movement (e.g., extend the arm on command) (Fig. 6.5).

A herniated vertebral disk is the most common nerve root pathology that results in compression on the nerve roots. This

usually results in pain with radiation into the affected area of skin (dermatome) supplied with afferent nerve fibers by a single posterior spinal root (Fig. 6.6).

### SIMPLY STATED

A herniated vertebral disk is the most common nerve root pathology, and it causes pain with radiation into the affected area of skin (dermatome) supplied with afferent nerve fibers by a single posterior spinal root.

Two spinal nerves important for respiratory function are the right and left phrenic nerves that innervate the diaphragm to control breathing. The phrenic nerves arise from the cervical spine roots of C3 to C5. Damage to this portion of the spinal cord (or above) can result in complete paralysis of the diaphragm and the intercostal muscles and make the patient dependent on a ventilator for life. The additional muscles of respiration, such as intercostal muscles, are innervated by the spinal nerves that originate in the thoracic portion of the spinal cord. These nerves, although normal, will be cut off from the efferent impulses originating above the injury (C3 to C5 level or above) and will be rendered ineffective. Figs. 6.6 and 6.7 illustrate the typical outcome after spinal cord or root injury.

### SIMPLY STATED

The phrenic nerves arise from the cervical spine roots of C3 to C5. Damage to this portion of the spinal cord can result in complete paralysis of the respiratory muscles and ventilator dependency.

## ASSESSMENT OF CONSCIOUSNESS

The cerebral hemispheres (or lobes) represent the highest and most complex level of neurologic function. Although a great deal of the mental status reflects integration of cortical function, it can still be divided into functional areas that correspond to anatomic regions of the cerebral hemispheres (Fig. 6.8). Table 6.1 gives a brief overview of areas of cortical function that can be assessed by components of the mental status examination.

### Assessing Consciousness

Assessment of the level of consciousness (wakefulness and alertness) and the content of consciousness (awareness and thinking) begins when you first encounter the patient. Different levels of consciousness from full alertness to coma have been defined (Box 6.1). The assessment of the content of consciousness starts with orientation. A fully oriented patient will be expected to answer those questions in detail—for example, first and last name, month, day and year, and the ward and name of the hospital. Such patients can be described as *alert and oriented times three* (one score for each name, date, and location).

FIG. 6.2 Functional organization of the central nervous system.

**FIG. 6.3** Left lateral view of the cerebrum showing the four cerebral lobes (frontal, parietal, temporal, and occipital) and its anatomic relationship with the cerebellum and the brainstem.

The two common conditions often present in hospitalized patients are coma and delirium. Although coma is characterized by the absence of arousal and awareness, a patient with **delirium** has alternating levels of consciousness and marked deficits in attention and organized thinking (confusion). Several studies have shown that delirium occurs in 60% to 80% of mechanically ventilated patients and that it is independently associated with longer hospital stay, higher mortality rate, and poor long-term

cognitive function. The causes of delirium are frequently multifactorial, including one or more of the following: hypoxia, electrolyte or acid-base imbalance, concomitant medical illness, sleep deprivation, use (previous or current) of sedation, unfamiliarity with surroundings, and side effects of medications. A patient with preexisting dementia may present similarly to a patient with delirium, and it may be difficult to tell them apart without knowledge of the patient's medical history (see Chapter 2).

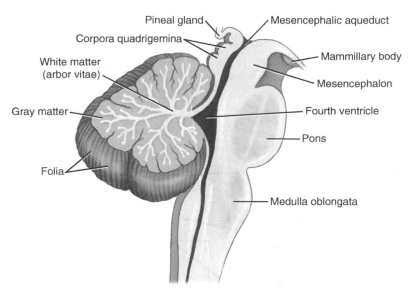

**FIG. 6.4** Left lateral view of the cerebellum showing its anatomic relationship with the brainstem.

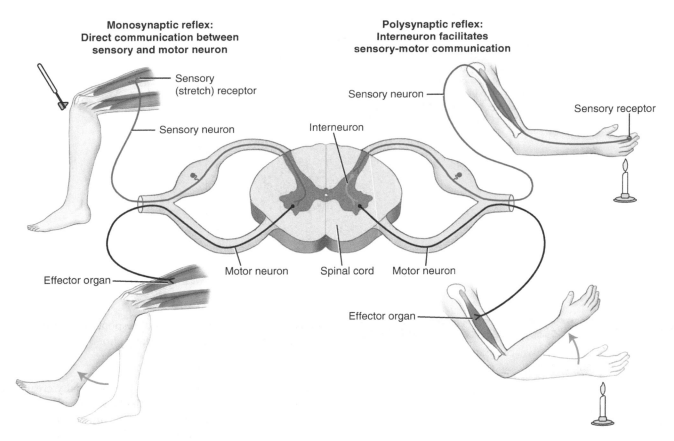

**FIG. 6.5** Caudal view of the spinal cord. The diagram shows the motor neuron (anterior) and the sensory neuron (posterior) before they come together as a spinal nerve. The sensory neuron provides sensory input to the brain to elicit a motor response.

Patients with high cervical cord lesions seldom survive without immediate ventilatory support.

Patients who survive a lesion above C7 usually remain dependent on others for daily care.

Sparing of the C7 segment retains elbow and wrist extension and enables transfer from wheelchair to bed, providing a degree of independence.

Patients with thoracolumbar injuries usually regain full independence.

A mixed cord and lumbar root lesion may occur at this level. Fortunately roots are more resistant to injury—"root escape"—and the outlook is more favorable.

C1

C4

C7
T1

T9

T10

L1

Spinal cord damage

Root damage

**FIG. 6.6** Outcome after spinal cord or root injury.

---

### SIMPLY STATED

Coma and delirium are two common dysfunctions of the level and content of consciousness, respectively, that are often present in hospitalized patients, especially in the ICU. Delirium occurs in 60% to 80% of mechanically ventilated patients and is associated with longer hospital stay, higher mortality rate, and poor long-term cognitive function.

Some patients who partially recover from their initial severe neurologic injury will remain in a persistent vegetative state. Although these patients' eyes may be open, they are not aware of their surroundings, do not respond to verbal stimuli or commands in a meaningful way, do not track objects or individuals, and do not respond to environmental changes. Overall prognosis is usually poor.

### Glasgow Coma Scale

The Glasgow Coma Scale (GCS) was originally created to assess the neurologic status of patients with head injury and has become the most widely used instrument for quantifying neurologic impairment. It tests the best motor response, best verbal response, and eye opening. The simplicity of the scale makes it widely useful for nearly every member of the health care team. However, it is poorly suited to patients who have impaired verbal responses caused by aphasia, hearing loss, or tracheal intubation or more subtle alterations of consciousness, such as delirium. A scale that goes from 3

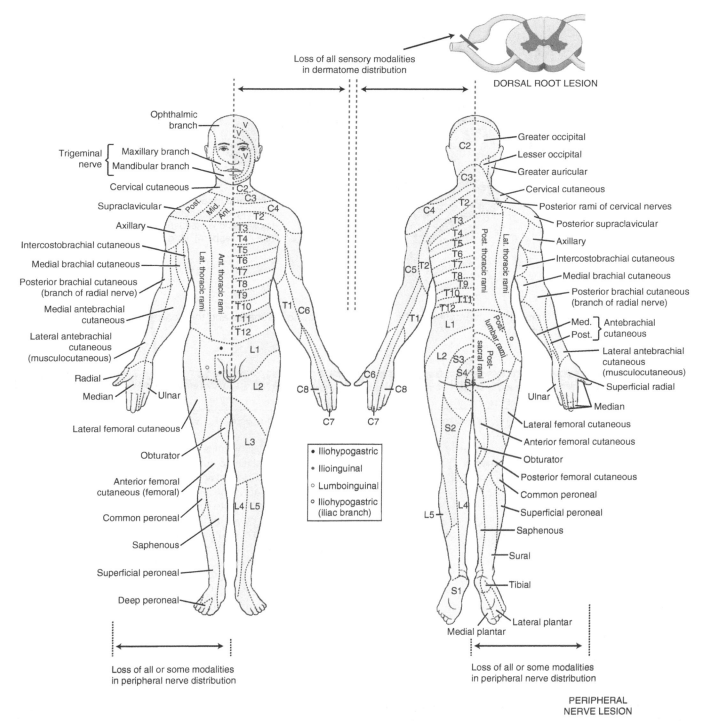

**FIG. 6.7** Schematic representation of dermatomes.

(deep coma or death) to 15 (fully awake) is useful for rapid triage (Table 6.2). Endotracheal intubation makes it impossible to test the patient's verbal response, so the letter "T" is often attached to the GCS score to indicate the presence of the tube (e.g., GCS 5T).

Patients with GCS scores of 12 to 15 often do not require ICU admission. Scores of 9 to 12 indicate a significant insult with a moderate coma, and patients with GCS scores lower than 8 or 9 have a severe coma and typically require endotracheal intubation for airway protection and ventilatory assistance ("less than eight, intubate"). For example, patients with head trauma and low GCS score may need to be intubated because they will have a prolonged recovery period, but patients with more transient neurologic deficit (such as drug or alcohol overdose) may not benefit from intubation based solely on their GCS score.

**Parietal lobe**
Recognition of right/left
differentiation, sensation,
recognition of body parts

**Frontal lobe**
Judgment, humor, social mores,
affect, personality, motor movement,
expressive speech (Broca, left
hemisphere), spatial and perceptual
information (right hemisphere)

**Occipital lobe**
Interpretation of written
language (left hemisphere).
Visual interpretation

**Temporal lobe**
Hearing, comprehension of
spoken and written language
(left hemisphere), long-term memory

**FIG. 6.8** Graphic representation of the cerebral lobes or hemispheres and their corresponding cortical function.

| TABLE 6.1 | Assessment of Cerebral Cortical Function | |
|---|---|---|
| **Cerebral Lobe** | **Cortical Function** | **Assessment** |
| Frontal | Attention: working memory | Digit span, spelling backward, and naming months of the year backward |
| | Judgment: abstract reasoning | Problem solving, verbal similarities, and proverbs |
| | Set generation | Verbal fluency and the ability to generate a set of items |
| Temporal | Orientation, memory | Questions about month, date, day of week, and place |
| | | Three-word recall (recent memory) |
| | | Naming U.S. presidents (remote memory) |
| Frontal-temporal | Receptive language | Following commands (spoken and written language) |
| | Expressive language | Fluency and correctness of content and grammar |
| | | Reading comprehension |
| Parietal (dominant) | Gnosis | Identifying objects placed in the hand and numbers written on the hand with eyes closed |
| | Constructional | Attending to the contralateral side of the body |
| | | Drawing a face, clock, or geometric figures |
| | | Right-left orientation, naming fingers, and calculations |
| Parietal (nondominant) | Praxis | Performing skilled motor tasks without any nonverbal prompting |
| Occipitotemporal | Visual recognition | Recognition of colors and faces |

**SIMPLY STATED**

The GCS is the most widely used instrument for quantifying neurologic impairment. Patients with GCS scores of less than 8 typically require endotracheal intubation.

## Mini-Mental State Examination

The Mini-Mental State Examination (MMSE), or Folstein test, is a brief questionnaire used to assess cognition and classify dementia. It can be used to screen for cognitive impairment, to estimate the severity of cognitive impairment at a given point in time, to follow the course of cognitive changes

in an individual over time, and to document an individual's response to treatment.

## Assessment of Consciousness in the Intensive Care Unit

The Richmond Agitation Sedation Scale (RASS) helps to measure the sedation and agitation of patients in the ICU and is often considered when titrating sedation medications (Table 6.3). The RASS assigns a 0 (zero) for an alert and calm patient and goes as high as +4 for a combative and violent patient, to a low of −5 for a patient who cannot be aroused.

## BOX 6.1　Levels of Consciousness

*Full consciousness:* The patient is alert and attentive, follows commands, responds promptly to external stimulation if asleep, and once awake, remains attentive.

*Lethargy:* The patient is drowsy but partially awakens to stimulation; the patient will answer questions and follow commands but will do so slowly and inattentively.

*Obtundation:* The patient is difficult to arouse and needs constant stimulation to follow a simple command. Although there may be verbal response with one or two words, the patient will drift back to sleep between stimuli.

*Stupor:* The patient arouses to vigorous and continuous stimulation; typically, a painful stimulus is required. The only response may be an attempt to withdraw from or remove the painful stimulus.

*Coma:* The patient does not respond to continuous or painful stimulation. There are no verbal sounds and no movement, except possibly by reflex.

## TABLE 6.2　Glasgow Coma Scale

| Action | Response | Score |
|---|---|---|
| Eyes open | Spontaneously | 4 |
| | To speech | 3 |
| | To pain | 2 |
| | None | 1 |
| Best verbal response | Oriented | 5 |
| | Confused | 4 |
| | Inappropriate words | 3 |
| | Incomprehensive sounds | 2 |
| Best motor response | Obeys commands | 6 |
| | Localized pain | 5 |
| | Flexion withdrawal | 4 |
| | Abnormal flexion | 3 |
| | Abnormal extension | 2 |
| | Flaccid | 1 |
| **Total** | | **15** |

Delirium is frequently evaluated with the Confusion Assessment Method for the ICU (CAM-ICU). Delirium is an acute change or fluctuation in mental status plus inattention and either disorganized thinking or an altered state of consciousness at the time of assessment. Delirium occurs in many mechanically ventilated patients and has been associated with longer hospital stays and poor clinical outcomes. Because many aspects of delirium in the ICU may be preventable or treatable, it is recommended that RTs become familiar with these assessment tools.

## CRANIAL NERVE EXAMINATION

There are 12 cranial nerves (CNs) connected to the brain (Fig. 6.9). Assessment of the CNs allows the clinician to examine the entire brainstem, which is divided into three levels: the midbrain, the pons, and the medulla. Because CNs never cross, except for CN IV, clinical findings are always on the same side as the CN involved (Table 6.4).

## TABLE 6.3　Richmond Agitation Sedation Scale (RASS)

| Target RASS | RASS Description |
|---|---|
| +4 | Combative, violent, danger to staff |
| +3 | Pulls or removes tube(s) or catheter(s); aggressive |
| +2 | Frequent nonpurposeful movement, fights ventilator |
| +1 | Anxious, apprehensive, but not aggressive |
| 0 | Alert and calm |
| −1 | Awakens to voice (eye opening/contact) >10 s |
| −2 | Light sedation, briefly awakens to voice (eye opening/contact) <10 s |
| −3 | Moderate sedation, movement, or eye opening; no eye contact |
| −4 | Deep sedation, no response to voice, but movement or eye opening to physical stimulation |
| −5 | Unarousable, no response to voice or physical stimulation |

Some functions are controlled by several CNs. The pupillary response (CNs II and III), the corneal reflex (CNs V and VII), and the gag reflex (CNs IX and X) depend on more than one CN. Although a stroke is the most common cause of CN dysfunction, other abnormalities should be considered (Table 6.5). Many of the nerves cannot be tested without the patient's cooperation, so the CN assessment of a comatose patient may not be viewed as complete.

### SIMPLY STATED

The gag reflex (CNs IX and X), the pupillary reflex (CNs II and III), and the corneal reflex (CNs V and VII) depend on more than one CN.

## SENSORY EXAMINATION

Sensory evaluation is performed by having the patient respond to stimuli at a specific location. The principal sensory modalities are pain and temperature. Others include vibratory sense, position sense, and discriminatory or integrative sensations. Comparing one side with the other is valuable in localizing the specific site of abnormality.

## MOTOR EXAMINATION

A bedside neurologic assessment almost always includes an evaluation of motor function. The clinician assesses the patient's ability to move on command; therefore the patient must be awake, willing to cooperate, and able to understand what the examiner is asking.

Motor strength is assessed bilaterally, and each extremity is graded using a motor scale from 0 (no movement) to +5 (full range of motion with full strength). In an unconscious patient, the assessment of motor response is performed by applying

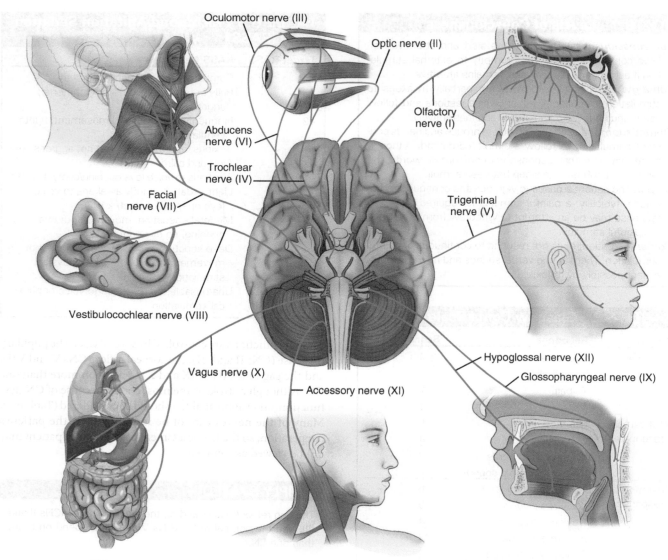

**FIG. 6.9** The cranial nerves. Ventral surface of the brain showing attachment to the cranial nerves.

| TABLE 6.4 | **Assessment of the Cranial Nerves** | | |
|-----------|------------------|----------------|------------|
| **Cranial Nerve** | **Classification** | **Major Functions** | **Assessment** |
| I: Olfactory | Sensory | Smell | Have patient identify a familiar scent with eyes closed (usually deferred). |
| II: Optic | Sensory | Vision (acuity and field of vision) | Have patient read from a card, one eye at a time. Test visual fields by having patient cover one eye, focus on your nose, and identify the number of fingers you are holding up in each of four visual quadrants. |
| | | Pupil reactivity to light and accommodation (afferent impulse) | |
| III: Oculomotor | Motor | Eyelid elevation | Check pupillary responses by shining a bright light on one pupil; both pupils should constrict (consensual reflex). Do the same for the other eye. To check for accommodation, move your finger toward the patient's nose; the pupils should constrict and converge. Check EOMs by having patient look up, down, laterally, and diagonally. |
| | | Pupil size and reactivity (efferent impulse) | |
| | | Most EOMs | |
| IV: Trochlear | Motor | EOM (turns eye downward and laterally) | Have patient look down and in. |

## TABLE 6.4   Assessment of the Cranial Nerves—cont'd

| Cranial Nerve | Classification | Major Functions | Assessment |
|---|---|---|---|
| V: Trigeminal | Both | Chewing | Ask patient to hold the mouth open while you try to close it and to move the jaw laterally against your hand. With patient's eyes closed, touch her face with cotton and have her identify the area touched. In comatose patients, brush the cornea with a wisp of cotton; the patient should blink. |
| | | Facial and mouth sensation | Facial and mouth sensation |
| | | Corneal reflex (sensory) | Corneal reflex (sensory) |
| VI: Abducens | Motor | EOM (turns eye laterally) | Have patient move the eyes from side to side. |
| VII: Facial | Both | Facial expression | Ask patient to smile, raise eyebrows, and keep eyes and lips closed while you try to open them. |
| | | Taste | Have patient identify salt or sugar placed on the tongue. |
| | | Corneal reflex (motor) | |
| | | Eyelid and lip closure | |
| VIII: Acoustic | Sensory | Hearing | To test hearing, use tuning fork, rub your fingers, or whisper near each ear. |
| | | Equilibrium | |
| IX: Glossopharyn-geal | Both | Gagging and swallowing (sensory) | Touch back of throat with sterile tongue depressor or cotton-tipped applicator. Have patient swallow. |
| | | Taste | |
| X: Vagus | Both | Gagging and swallowing (motor) | Assess gag and swallowing with CN IX. |
| | | Speech (phonation) | Assess vocal quality. |
| XI: Spinal accessory | Motor | Shoulder movement | Have patient shrug shoulders and turn head from side to side. |
| | | Head rotation | |
| XII: Hypoglossal | Motor | Tongue movement | Have patient stick out tongue and move it internally from cheek to cheek. |
| | | Speech (articulation) | Assess articulation. |

*CN*, Cranial nerve; *EOM*, extraocular movement.

## TABLE 6.5   Etiology of Cranial Nerve Malfunction

| Cranial Nerve | Cause of Impairment |
|---|---|
| I | Trauma to the cribriform plate, frontal lobe mass or stroke, and nasal problems (e.g., allergic or viral) |
| II | Eye disease or injury, diabetic retinopathy and glaucoma major causes, occipital lobe mass or stroke |
| III, IV, and VI | Brainstem injury or compression (e.g., tumor, stroke, intracranial bleeding, diabetic neuropathy [can cause temporary palsies]) |
| V | Stroke in the contralateral sensory cortex |
| VII | Stroke induced (central palsy) |
| VIII | Sensorineural hearing loss as a result of age or noise exposure, tumors at cerebellopontine angle, acoustic neuroma, earwax, or middle ear disease can cause temporary hearing loss. |
| IX and X | Stroke |
| XI | Neck injury |
| XII | Stroke |

a noxious stimulus and observing the patient's response to it. Central stimulation, such as sternal pressure, produces an overall body response and is more reliable than peripheral stimulation. In an unconscious patient, peripheral stimulation, such as nail bed pressure, can elicit a reflex response, which is not a true indicator of motor activity. If central stimulation is necessary, it should be performed judiciously because deep sternal pressure can easily bruise the soft tissue above the sternum. A less traumatic alternative to sternal pressure is to squeeze the trapezius muscle. Supraorbital pressure should not be used for central stimulation in patients with facial fractures or vagal nerve sensitivity. The response to pain varies depending on the level of neurologic function. Normally, pain causes the patient to attempt to remove the source of the pain or to withdraw from the painful stimulation. If the cerebral cortex is functioning, there is withdrawal from painful stimuli in a predictable and reflexive manner. The symmetry and pattern of the motor response to noxious stimuli, as well as associated neurologic symptoms, should be documented for all patients suspected of having a neurologic disease.

The motor system is usually divided into the direct corticospinal tract or upper motor neuron (UMN) and lower motor neuron (LMN). The corticospinal tract has its main influence on the motor neurons that innervate the muscles of the distal extremities such as the hand and the foot. The clinical findings from a UMN lesion include loss of distal extremity strength, dexterity, and a Babinski sign (see the next section) plus increased tone, hyperreflexia, and the clasp-knife phenomenon (from loss of control of the indirect brainstem centers). A UMN lesion above the level of the red nucleus (a collection of neurons in the anterior part of the midbrain) will result in decorticate posture (thumb tucked under flexed fingers in fisted position, pronation of forearm, and flexion at elbow with the lower extremity in extension with foot inversion), whereas a lesion

Decorticate posture

Decerebrate posture

**FIG. 6.10** Decorticate posture is indicated by flexed wrist and arm and extended legs and feet. Decerebrate posture is indicated by arm and leg extension. (Modified from McCance K, Heuther S: *Pathophysiology,* ed 6. St. Louis, 2009, Mosby-Elsevier.)

below the level of the red nucleus will result in **decerebrate posture,** in which the upper extremity is in pronation and extension and the lower extremity is in extension (Fig. 6.10). If there is a lesion in the medulla the patient would be acutely flaccid.

### SIMPLY STATED

A UMN lesion above the level of the red nucleus will result in decorticate posture (thumb tucked under flexed fingers in fisted position, pronation of forearm, and flexion at elbow with the lower extremity in extension and foot inversion), whereas a lesion below the level of the red nucleus will result in decerebrate posture (upper extremity in pronation and extension and the lower extremity in extension).

Lesions of the LMN result in loss of strength, tone, and reflexes, with muscle showing wasting and fasciculations. Table 6.6 summarizes some of the clinical findings of UMN and LMN lesions.

## DEEP TENDON, SUPERFICIAL, AND BRAINSTEM REFLEXES

Reflex assessment encompasses deep tendon, superficial, and brainstem reflexes.

### Deep Tendon Reflexes

**Deep tendon reflexes,** such as the **patellar reflex** or *knee jerk,* evaluate spinal nerves. They should be tested in any patient

**TABLE 6.6    Clinical Signs of Upper Motor Neuron (UMN) and Lower Motor Neuron (LMN) Lesions**

| Clinical Sign | UMN Lesion | LMN Lesion |
|---|---|---|
| Weakness | + | + |
| Atrophy | − | + |
| Fasciculation | − | + |
| Reflexes | ↑ | ↓ |
| Tone | ↑ | ↓ |
| Babinski | + | − |

with a spinal cord injury or symptoms consistent with a neurologic problem (Fig. 6.11). The reflexes are graded on a scale from 0 to 5, with 0 being no reflex, 2 being normal, and 5 being hyperreflexia with clonus (repeated rhythmic contractions). Abnormal or absent deep tendon reflexes indicate abnormalities in anatomic components required for the reflex arc to occur. These structures include the muscle, the nerve fibers going from the tendon to the spinal cord, and the nerve fibers returning from the spinal cord to the muscle. Table 6.7 illustrates the spinal nerve level assessed with each reflex. Absent deep tendon reflexes may be a sign that the patient is at risk for respiratory failure.

### Superficial Reflexes

The **plantar reflex** is the only superficial reflex that is commonly assessed and should be tested in comatose

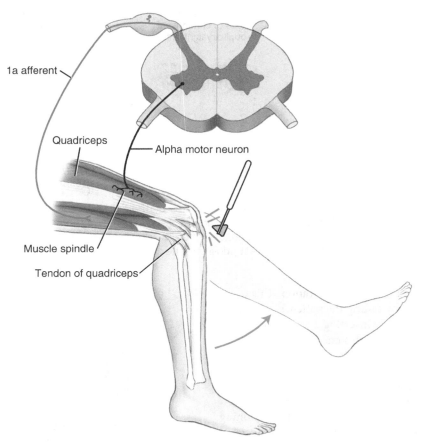

**FIG. 6.11** Patellar reflex arc. Forward knee jerk is elicited by tapping of the tendon of the quadriceps.

| TABLE 6.7 | **Deep Tendon Reflex** |
|---|---|
| **Reflex** | **Spinal Nerve** |
| Biceps | C5-C6 |
| Triceps | C7-C8 |
| Patellar | L2-L4 |
| Achilles | L5-S1 |

patients and in those with suspected injury to the L4 to L5 or S1 to S2 areas of the spinal cord. Striking the lateral plantar aspect of the foot elicits a plantar flexion (curling under) of the toes. Dorsiflexion of the great toe with fanning of remaining toes (**Babinski sign**) is abnormal, except in children up to 12 to 18 months of age (Fig. 6.12). The presence of Babinski sign could indicate a lesion of the UMN or brain disease caused by damage to the corticospinal tract.

**FIG. 6.12** Babinski sign. Dorsiflexion of the great toe with fanning of remaining toes after stroking the outer aspect of the sole in the direction of the *arrow*.

## Brainstem Reflexes

Brainstem reflexes are evaluated in stuporous or comatose patients to determine whether the brainstem is intact. Protective reflexes, such as coughing, gagging, and the corneal response, are usually evaluated as part of the assessment of the CNS.

### Gag Reflex

CNs IX and X are especially important to the RT because they control a variety of functions. CN IX controls the muscles of

---

**SIMPLY STATED**

The presence of Babinski sign (dorsiflexion of the great toe with fanning of remaining toes) while testing the plantar reflex could indicate a lesion of the UMN or brain disease.

**Normal—**
both pupils constrict

**CN III lesion—**
loss of consensual
pupillary light reflex

**CN II lesion—**
loss of direct
pupillary light reflex

A                    B                    C

**FIG. 6.13** Pupillary reflex. **A,** Shining of a light source on the right may cause a constriction of both pupils in normal individuals. **B,** Constriction of the pupil only on the right eye in patients with lesions of CN III and loss of consensual reflex. **C,** Pupillary constriction of the opposite eye in lesions of CN II and loss of direct pupillary reflex.

swallowing that are needed to prevent aspiration. This function of CN IX is evaluated by testing the patient's gag reflex. This test is performed by gently inserting a tongue depressor into the back of the throat. Although some healthy individuals have a minimal or absent gag reflex, its absence may increase the risk for aspiration, and endotracheal intubation may be necessary to protect the lungs. CN IX also has a branch that extends to the carotid sinus and plays a major role in the control of blood pressure. The ability to cough with suctioning can be tested in an intubated patient and implies an intact CN X. This test should not be attempted in nonintubated patients in the ICU because of the risk for aspiration. Stimulation of CN X while suctioning the airway may result in bradycardia caused by vagal stimulation. Excessively aggressive suctioning may also cause airway injury from the mechanical trauma. To decrease the vagal stimulation, as well as airway injury, it is recommended that suctioning time (catheter in the airway) be limited to 10 to 15 seconds and that an appropriate pressure setting be used during suctioning.

---

**SIMPLY STATED**

Although some healthy individuals have a minimal or absent gag reflex (CNs IX and X), its absence may increase the risk for aspiration, and endotracheal intubation may be necessary to protect the airway and lungs. The ability to cough with suctioning can be tested in an intubated patient and implies an intact CN X.

---

### Pupillary Reflex

Pupillary light reflexes provide information regarding the status of the brain and the sympathetic and parasympathetic nervous systems. Pupillary reflex is determined by briefly passing a bright light in front of both open eyes while carefully watching the iris in both eyes for movement. Pupil size, congruency, and response to light and accommodation should be described. The acronym PERRLA is commonly used to refer to normal pupils that are equal, round, and reactive to light and accommodation (movement) (see Chapter 5). Any

CORNEAL REFLEX

Wisp of cotton

No orbicularis oculi contraction in
response to corneal stimulation

**FIG. 6.14** Corneal reflex. Lightly touching the cornea with a wisp of cotton should be followed by blinking of both eyes.

visible change in the pupils' size is noted. Anisocoria is a neurologic term indicating that one pupil is larger than the other. Mydriasis, or pupillary dilation, may be caused by serious brain injury or inadvertent exposure of the eyes to inhaled anticholinergics. Miosis, or small "pinpoint" pupils, usually results from pontine hemorrhage or from ingestion of narcotics or organophosphates. Pupillary responses almost always remain intact in metabolic causes of coma. Midposition and fixed pupils often indicate severe cerebral damage (Fig. 6.13).

---

**SIMPLY STATED**

The acronym PERRLA refers to normal *p*upils that are *e*qual, *r*ound, and *r*eactive to *l*ight and *a*ccommodation. Pupillary function is controlled by the midbrain and evaluates CNs II and III.

---

### Corneal Reflex

The corneal reflex is used to test the afferent CN V and the efferent CN VII. The test is performed by lightly touching the cornea with a cotton swab. The normal response is that the patient blinks both eyes. Most clinicians omit the corneal reflex test unless there is sensory loss on the face as per history or examination or cranial nerve palsies are present at the pontine level (Fig. 6.14).

### Oculocephalic and Oculovestibular Reflexes

Abnormalities of extraocular movement (CNs II, III, IV, and VI) have prognostic importance in the ICU. Normal movement of the eyes requires an intact midbrain connection. The resting position of the gaze, the presence of nystagmus, and the response to head movements and cold tympanic membrane stimulation should be identified. To test the oculocephalic reflex, or doll's eyes reflex, turn the patient's head briskly from side to side; the eyes should turn to the left while the head is turned to the right, and vice versa. If this reflex is absent, there will be no eye movement when the patient's head is moved side to side. To test the oculovestibular reflex, also known as the *ice caloric* or *cold caloric reflex,* a physician instills at least 20 mL of ice water into the ear of a comatose patient. In patients with an intact brainstem, the eyes will move laterally toward the affected ear. In patients with severe brainstem injury, the gaze will remain at midline.

## COORDINATION, BALANCE, AND GAIT EXAMINATION

The principal area of the brain that is examined by the coordination, balance, and gait examination is the cerebellum. Although the cortex initiates the volitional movements, the cerebellum ensures its coordination, precision, and timing. Therefore cerebellar dysfunction results in disintegration of movements and undershooting and overshooting of goal-directed movements (dysmetria). Disintegration of movement and dysmetria are the main elements of ataxia.

---

**SIMPLY STATED**

Cerebellar dysfunction results in breakdown of coordinated movements and leads to undershooting and overshooting of goal-directed movements (dysmetria).

---

## VITAL ORGAN FUNCTION AND THE NEUROLOGIC SYSTEM

### Control of Breathing

The nervous system is intricately connected to the mechanics of respiration. Automatic breathing is regulated primarily by lower brainstem nuclei (Fig. 6.15). A healthy awake individual has rhythmic and regular respiratory cycles, occasionally interrupted by the cortical commands (e.g., hyperventilation during anxiety or irregular breathing during speaking). The breathing is even more regular during sleep, when the responses to the exogenous stimuli are minimal. It is debated whether a true "pacemaker" exists that works at a subconscious level and results in rhythmic contraction and relaxation of the respiratory muscles. Alternatively, it is argued that the respiratory centers in the brainstem receive impulses from multiple receptors and the rhythmic breathing is the result of integration of these various excitatory or inhibitory stimuli. The major receptors that influence the breathing are central and peripheral chemoreceptors. Central chemoreceptors are

located in the brainstem and respond to changes in $Paco_2$ indirectly (Fig. 6.16). The cellular membrane of these receptor cells is impermeable to the hydrogen ions ($H^+$) but freely permeable to $CO_2$ (see Fig. 6.16). As $CO_2$ travels across the membrane, it combines with water and forms $H^+$ and $HCO_3^-$. It is the hydrogen ion that forms from this reaction, not the $CO_2$ itself that the central chemoreceptors respond to. Peripheral chemoreceptors are located in the aortic and carotid bodies and are further subdivided into receptors that sense pH and $Pao_2$. Unlike the central receptors, peripheral chemoreceptors directly respond to the hydrogen ion concentration. The response to the fluctuation in any one of these individual variables (pH, $Paco_2$, and $Pao_2$) depends on the status of the other variables. For example, the response to $Paco_2$ elevation is exaggerated during relative hypoxia or acidosis and blunted during relative hyperoxia (Fig. 6.17). A good example of hyperventilation caused by severe acidosis is Kussmaul breathing (Fig. 6.18B). Other types of breathing dysrhythmias from various of brainstem lesions are also depicted in Fig. 6.19.

In a normal awake individual, the brain is very sensitive to even minor fluctuations in $Paco_2$ causing great increase in minute ventilation. This type of response keeps $Pao_2$ in the 90- to 100-mm Hg range, which does not change the activity of the oxygen-sensing chemoreceptors. For this reason, it is stated that normal individuals have *hypercapnic drive* to breathe. In patients with chronic respiratory acidosis (advanced chronic obstructive pulmonary disease [COPD] or other alveolar hypoventilation syndromes), $Pco_2$ is often consistently elevated, and the respiratory system's response to $Paco_2$ fluctuations is blunted. In such situations the patient becomes more dependent on the peripheral chemoreceptors (especially the ones that sense $Pao_2$). Such patients are said to have *hypoxic drive* to breathe. This mechanism becomes very important when patients with chronic hypercarbia are given supplemental oxygen. Many myths and misconceptions exist regarding the situation when a patient with chronic compensated respiratory acidosis and hypoxia is given oxygen. Some of these patients develop worsening hypercarbia, probably due to various factors, the important ones being ventilation/perfusion ratio (V/Q) mismatch and the abolition of hypoxic drive. Although conceptually easy to understand, the abolition of hypoxic drive has been difficult to prove during experimental research, leading many clinicians to explain the worsening hypercarbia on the basis of V/Q mismatch. During the periods of hypoxia, there is vasoconstriction of the pulmonary vessels, which is reversed once supplemental oxygen is given. This reversal leads to perfusion of the lung areas that are not well ventilated—creation of additional lung units with poor ventilation but good perfusion, an equivalent of alveolar dead space—causing worsening hypercarbia. This leads to a dilemma of either leaving the patient hypoxic or giving supplemental oxygen at the risk for hypercarbia and the potential need for ventilatory support, with neither option being optimal. In reality, many of these patients may be well managed with low levels of supplemental oxygen (keeping $Spo_2$ in the 90% to 92% range) with careful monitoring of their clinical status and gas exchange.

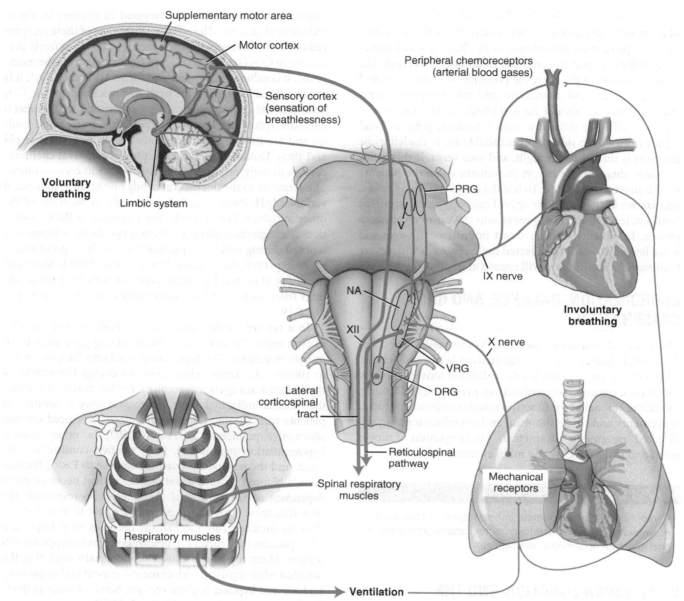

**FIG. 6.15** Schematic representation of the neural control of breathing. Central chemoreceptors; *DRG*, dorsal respiratory group; *NA*, nucleus ambiguus; *PRG*, pontine respiratory group; *V*, sensory nucleus of V; *VRG*, ventral respiratory group.

Other peripheral receptors are less important in minute-to-minute control of breathing but still have significant effects on the system. They include receptors that are located in the bronchial tree that sense temperature (bronchospasm and coughing when breathing cold air); stretch receptors located in the lung (after a period of inactivity and relatively low minute ventilation, we all sigh to take a deep breath and "stretch" the lungs—an event mostly dictated by the stretch receptors); and musculoskeletal receptors that sense the movement of the muscles and joints and increase the minute ventilation even when no extra work is done by the muscles.

Higher brain centers have some control of the lower centers located in the midbrain. For example, we can all hyperventilate or hold our breath on command. However, at some

point, the influence of these higher centers seizes, and the midbrain takes over. Breath holding is usually terminated by the combination of hypoxia and hypercarbia that results from it. Similarly, hyperventilation will lead to syncope, leading to relative hypoventilation until $Pao_2$ and $Paco_2$ levels are corrected. Another illustrative example of integrated responses to breathing is high-altitude physiology. When a person dwelling at sea level arrives at high altitude (usually altitudes higher than 3000 m or 10,000 feet), he or she will start to hyperventilate because of relative hypoxia from low inspired $Po_2$. Although this hyperventilation will only modestly increase the $Pao_2$, it will cause significant changes in $Paco_2$ and pH, causing severe respiratory alkalosis and limiting further increases in minute ventilation. Within the next 24 to 48

**FIG. 6.16** How carbon dioxide affects respiratory drive. *CSF,* Cerebrospinal fluid. (From Beachey W: *Respiratory care anatomy and physiology,* ed 3. St. Louis, 2013, Mosby-Elsevier.)

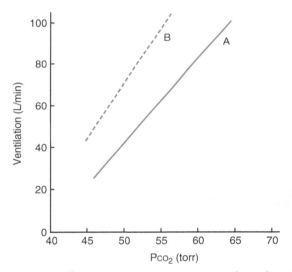

**FIG. 6.17** Ventilatory response to progressive elevation of $P_{CO_2}$ in normal individual. **A,** *Solid line* shows response when simultaneous $P_{O_2}$ is high (hyperoxic conditions). **B,** *Dashed line* shows heightened response when simultaneous $P_{O_2}$ is low (hypoxic conditions). (From Weinberger S, Cockrill B, Mandel J: *Principles of pulmonary medicine.* 2013, ed 6. Saunders.)

hours, other compensatory mechanisms (usually bicarbonate wasting by the kidneys) will correct the alkalosis and allow further increases in minute ventilation and $Pa_{O_2}$. For this reason, it is imperative that individuals climbing high altitudes regularly stay at base camps to acclimate before climbing. Use of alcohol and other CNS depressants while at high altitudes is also incrementally dangerous because it adds undue stress to the already strained respiratory drive.

As described earlier, the normal breathing pattern is rhythmic and regular. Lesions at various levels from the brain to the upper cervical cord cause abnormal changes of the breathing pattern (see Fig. 6.18). The most common abnormal respiratory pattern seen in patients with neurologic disorders is Cheyne-Stokes respiration, which consists of phases of hyperpnea that regularly alternate with episodes of apnea. Fig. 6.19 was obtained from a patient with a stroke and shows tidal volume waxing in a smooth crescendo and, once a peak is reached, waning in an equally smooth decrescendo. Cheyne-Stokes respiration usually has an intracranial cause, although it can be caused by hypoxemia and cardiac failure. Ataxic breathing (also called Biot breathing) is a marker of severe brainstem dysfunction seen as an irregular and unpredictable breathing pattern that indicates that all brain function above the medulla is absent.

---

### SIMPLY STATED

The most common abnormal respiratory pattern seen in patients with neurologic disorders is Cheyne-Stokes respiration, which consists of phases of hyperpnea that regularly alternate with episodes of apnea.

---

### Control of the Cardiovascular System

Because the brainstem and vagus nerve play an important role in vasomotor tone, conditions affecting these areas can cause vital signs to change. However, a change in vital signs is not a very sensitive indicator of neurologic deterioration because the change often happens too late to prevent irreversible brain damage. Increased intracranial pressure (ICP), such as in brainstem herniation syndromes, produces a specific set of changes known as Cushing triad (see more details on ICP monitoring in later sections of the chapter). Cushing triad consists of increasing systolic blood pressure with a widening pulse pressure, bradycardia, and bradypnea. Cushing triad is, however, a late sign of increased ICP. Once this pattern of vital signs occurs, brainstem herniation is already in progress, and it may be too late to reverse it.

## ANCILLARY TESTING OF THE NEUROLOGIC SYSTEM

### Imaging of the Neurologic System

Computed tomography (CT) scanning and magnetic resonance imaging (MRI) are two commonly used imaging studies to assess structural integrity of the neurologic system (also see Chapter 10). Although CT is quick and easy to perform, MRI provides higher-quality images. Both studies can be enhanced with contrast material, which is often used for the better visualization of the vasculature. When it comes to brain imaging, CT scan is frequently done in the emergency department or in other urgent scenarios for a rapid evaluation, whereas MRI is reserved for more stable patients, in whom detailed information about structural anatomy of the

**FIG. 6.18** Correlation of intraaxial brainstem lesions at different levels and the associated type of respiratory dysrhythmia. **A,** Cheyne-Stokes respiration. **B,** Central neurogenic hyperventilation (Kussmaul breathing). **C,** Apneustic breathing. **D,** Cluster breathing. **E,** Ataxic breathing (Biot breathing).

**FIG. 6.19** Cheyne-Stokes respiration showing the typical tidal volume waxing in a smooth crescendo and decrescendo pattern. $V_T$, Tidal volume.

nervous system is necessary. In the evaluation of the spinal cord, MRI is far superior to CT (even with contrast enhancement), so it is often the test of choice. See Chapter 10 for the safety issues and precautions associated with CT and MRI scanning. Special types of imaging (angiography or radionuclide testing) may be performed to confirm brain death (see Declaration of Brain Death).

## Electroencephalography

An electroencephalogram (EEG) is a recording of the brain's electrical activity, just as an electrocardiogram is a recording of the heart's electrical activity. A major role of the EEG is to evaluate a patient with seizures. It is commonly used to distinguish true seizures from false seizures (malingering, conversion disorder, or involuntary movements that resemble seizures). Other common indications include assessment of patients with altered consciousness or as a confirmatory test during determination of brain death. Multiple electrodes are placed on the patient's skull to record the electrical activity. The tracings are acquired digitally and interpreted by a physician, typically a neurologist. In most situations, an approximately 1-hour-long recording is enough to make a diagnosis. In complicated or equivocal cases, 24-hour EEG monitoring (to extend the observation period) or video EEG monitoring

**TABLE 6.8  Sequence of Loss of Brainstem Function**

| Highest Level of Brainstem Function | Breathing | Oculocephalic Reflex | Pupils | Pain Response |
|---|---|---|---|---|
| High midbrain | Normal | Normal | Normal | Withdrawal |
| Mid-midbrain | Cheyne-Stokes | Present | Small but reactive | Decorticate |
| Pons | Hyperventilation | Minimal | Mid-fixed | Decerebrate |
| Medulla | Ataxic | None | Mid-fixed | None |

(to correlate the patient's symptoms and movements with waveform tracings) may be necessary. A simplified version of EEG is also performed during an overnight sleep study (poly-somnogram), which is discussed in detail in Chapter 19.

## Lumbar Puncture

The brain and the spinal cord are surrounded by the cerebro-spinal fluid (CSF) and are often described to be floating in it. CSF is a clear, colorless fluid that insulates the brain from mechanical injury, provides a favorable biochemical environment, and decreases the weight of the brain within the skull. Lumbar puncture (LP) is done to obtain a sample of CSF. The major utility of CSF analysis is in patients with suspected infection. In other cases, it is done to determine the presence of elevated protein levels (Guillain-Barré syndrome) or to look for inflammatory or malignant conditions. The fluid is typically sent for cell count and differential, smears and culture, and biochemical analysis. Cytology and serologic studies are ordered to diagnose malignancy and other inflammatory conditions. LP involves inserting a long 20-gauge catheter into the space between the lower lumbar vertebrae.

## Intracranial Pressure Monitoring

The main purpose of ICP monitoring is to assess cerebral perfusion. As the blood flows across the pressure gradient, the cerebral perfusion will be proportional to the difference between the mean arterial pressure (MAP) and the ICP. This pressure difference is often called cerebral perfusion pressure (CPP). Assuming CPP = MAP – ICP, the cerebral perfusion worsens as ICP increases. Mean ICP of a supine patient is normally 10 to 15 mm Hg. Although small fluctuations are normal during the cardiac cycle, variability greater than 10 mm Hg is suggestive of serious neurologic compromise. Elevations in ICP to 15 to 20 mm Hg compress the capillary bed and compromise microcirculation. At ICP levels of 30 to 35 mm Hg, edema develops, even in normal tissue. Cerebral perfusion cannot be maintained if ICP increases to within 40 to 50 mm Hg of the MAP. When ICP approximates MAP, perfusion stops, which causes severe ischemic brain injury and even brain death.

ICP monitoring is commonly done in patients with increased risk for brainstem herniation, such as with stroke or anoxic brain injury. As the brain swells, the pressure rises within the confined space of the skull, and CPP decreases. During incremental elevation of the ICP, brainstem functions are lost in a predictable sequence (Table 6.8). In cases of significant swelling, parts of the brain (commonly the brainstem) are displaced (herniated) from their original location and thus become injured. Hyperventilation (goal $Paco_2 \sim 30$) is sometimes used to decrease the intracranial blood volume and lower ICP, especially because it is one of the fastest ways to decrease the ICP. However, it is extremely important to remember that hypoventilation also affects the overall blood flow to the brain, and its final effect on the CPP (a measure of brain perfusion) may be misjudged by only examining the effects of hyperventilation on ICP. The overall effect of the hyperventilation on CPP is complex and not completely understood. These effects are also short lived, limiting the usefulness of hyperventilation to the initial 24 hours or so. Owing to the complexity of the situation, the decision of whether to hyperventilate the patient for the purposes of ICP lowering is often made in consultation with various subspecialty physicians.

### SIMPLY STATED

Although hyperventilation is associated with lower ICP values, CPP is the most critical element to monitor.

## DECLARATION OF BRAIN DEATH

Brain death is an irreversible condition that occurs when all perceptible brain activity has ceased. It usually follows a devastating brain injury, commonly caused by a prolonged cardiac arrest or a massive stroke. In most situations, the determination of brain death will be the grounds to pronounce the patient dead (even if the heart is still beating) and remove the mechanical ventilator and other support devices. Because of the nuances of various protocols and exceptions from this general rule, the reader is encouraged to become familiar with the local laws and regulations regarding brain death; only a general overview of the topic is given here.

Typically a clinical examination by a physician and a confirmatory test (EEG or an imaging study) are performed. The absence of pupillary, corneal, gag, and oculovestibular reflexes, as well as the absence of respirations during an apnea test, provides confirmation of lack of brain activity. Other important clinical features that need to be documented by the physician before the declaration of brain death are the absence of reversible conditions, such as the following:

- Hypothermia
- Effects of sedative medications

- Effects of neuromuscular blockade
- Major metabolic disturbances
- Shock

A physician and RT routinely administer an apnea test. Many patients with brain injury may have been hyperventilated for various reasons, and respiratory alkalosis will suppress the drive to breathe. For this reason, the arterial blood gases are normalized before the apnea test. After documentation of normal or near-normal $PaO_2$ and $PaCO_2$, the patient is disconnected from the ventilator, and 100% oxygen is administered through an endotracheal tube. Some protocols require administration of oxygen through a transtracheal catheter, but this technique may lead to increased intrathoracic pressures and barotrauma and should be done very carefully. The patient is closely monitored during the apnea test, with the emphasis on spontaneous breathing, oxygenation, and cardiovascular status. Many patients, already terminally ill, will deteriorate during the apnea test, leading to termination of

the test by the attending physician. In the absence of spontaneous breathing movement and the evidence of clinical deterioration, the patient is monitored for 8 to 10 minutes, arterial blood gases are redrawn, and the patient is placed back on the ventilator. An increase of $PaCO_2$ to 60 mm Hg or 20 mm Hg above the baseline in the absence of spontaneous respirations is indicative of a positive apnea test (i.e., the patient was apneic) and suggestive of brain death.

It must be remembered that although designed to measure spontaneous respiratory drive, the apnea test truly measures the respiratory effort. For example, the patient may have a preserved drive but weak effort due to comorbidities (neuromuscular disease), leading to shallow and ineffective respirations that do not make the chest rise or affect $PaCO_2$ levels. Proper and timely administration of brain death protocol are of paramount importance to the patient and the family, as well as to ensuring maintenance of other organ functions (e.g., kidney, liver, heart) if organ donation is a consideration.

## KEY POINTS

- Injuries that involve the nervous system often affect the patient's respiratory system and the ability of the patient to cooperate with respiratory care procedures.
- Many neurologic functions of particular importance to the RT, such as regulation of heart rate, blood pressure, and breathing, are located in the brainstem.
- Damage to cervical spine roots of C3 to C5 may result in complete paralysis of the diaphragm.
- The GCS is the most widely used instrument for quantifying neurologic impairment.
- Delirium in ventilated patients is associated with longer stays in the hospital and poor clinical outcomes.
- An absent gag reflex (CNs IX and X) may increase the risk for aspiration.

- The ability to cough with suctioning implies an intact CN X.
- The most common abnormal respiratory pattern seen in patients with neurologic disorders is Cheyne-Stokes respiration.
- CPP is the most critical element to monitor in patients with head injury when monitoring ICP.
- Brain death is an irreversible condition when all perceptible brain activity has seized. Absence of brainstem reflexes and spontaneous respiratory drive is a critical feature of brain death.
- There several ancillary tests, including ICP and EEG monitoring, as well LP, that can be done to help clinicians assess the patient's neurologic status.

## ASSESSMENT QUESTIONS

1. The knowledge of neurologic function and its assessment is important in the daily practice of the respiratory therapist (RT) because:
   a. The RT is often the first health care professional to encounter a patient with stroke
   b. The RT is an important member of neurology clinic staff
   c. Many respiratory conditions also affect the central nervous system
   d. Many central nervous system conditions also affect the respiratory system
2. Anatomically, the brain is divided into the:
   a. Cerebrum, cerebellum, and brainstem
   b. Cerebrum, cerebellum, brainstem, and cranial nerves
   c. Cerebrum, cerebellum, brainstem, and spinal cord
   d. Cerebrum, cerebellum, brainstem, spinal cord, cranial nerves, and spinal nerves

3. The centers that regulate autonomous respiratory function are located in the:
   a. Brain cortex
   b. Brainstem
   c. Cerebellum
   d. Spinal cord
4. Which of the following is the most common cause of nerve root pathology caused by compression?
   a. Herniated vertebral disk
   b. Spinal tumor
   c. Spinal cord injury
   d. Infection
5. A patient with C3-level spinal cord injury is likely to demonstrate:
   a. Ventilatory insufficiency
   b. Babinski sign
   c. Normal patellar reflex
   d. Altered content of consciousness

6. Injury to the cervical spine roots C2 to C4 is associated with which of the following abnormalities?
   a. Absence of deep tendon reflexes
   b. Babinski sign
   c. Paralysis of the diaphragm
   d. Doll's eyes reflex

7. A patient in stupor will have a major deficit during this part of the neurologic assessment:
   a. Sensory examination
   b. Motor examination
   c. Level of consciousness
   d. Deep tendon reflexes

8. What is the most widely used instrument to quantify neurologic impairment?
   a. Merck Gait Evaluation
   b. Glasgow Coma Scale
   c. APACHE III score
   d. Apnea test

9. A Glasgow Coma Scale score below this number is typically an indication for endotracheal intubation:
   a. 8
   b. 10
   c. 12
   d. 14

10. Which of the following cranial nerves are evaluated with the gag reflex?
    a. II and III
    b. V and VII
    c. I and II
    d. IX and X

11. Dislodgment of the endotracheal tube is most likely to occur during:
    a. Lumbar puncture
    b. ICP monitoring
    c. CAM-ICU assessment
    d. EEG lead placement

12. The presence of dorsiflexion of the great toe with fanning of remaining toes while testing the plantar reflex is known as which of the following?
    a. Babinski sign
    b. Jerk reflex
    c. Patellar reflex
    d. Quadriceps reflex

13. Which of the following is the most useful test in assessing delirium?
    a. Glasgow Coma Scale
    b. Richmond Agitation Sedation Scale
    c. CAM-ICU assessment
    d. Cranial nerve examination

14. PERRLA is used to describe findings while examining which of the following?
    a. Pupils
    b. Gag reflex
    c. Deep tendon reflexes
    d. Level of consciousness

15. A patient with Kussmaul breathing is likely to have:
    a. Severe acidosis
    b. Hypoxic drive to breathe
    c. Brain death
    d. Normal minute ventilation

16. Which of the following respiratory patterns consists of phases of hyperpnea that regularly alternate with episodes of apnea?
    a. Biot
    b. Kussmaul
    c. Apnea
    d. Cheyne-Stokes

17. Which of the following is the most critical parameter to keep in mind when managing a patient with intracranial hypertension?
    a. Mean arterial pressure
    b. Cerebral perfusion pressure
    c. Intracranial pressure
    d. Pulse pressure

## BIBLIOGRAPHY

Abdo WF, Heunks L. Oxygen-induced hypercapnia in COPD. *Crit Care*. 2012;16(5):323–328.

Caruana-Montaldo B, Gleeson K, Zwillich CW. Control of breathing in clinical practice. *Chest*. 2000;117:205.

DeMyer WE. *Technique of the neurologic examination*. ed 5. New York: McGraw-Hill; 2014.

Ely EW: Confusion assessment method for the ICU (CAM-ICU): complete training manual. Retrieved August 31, 2016, from http://www.mc.vanderbilt.edu/icudelirium/docs/CAM_ICU_training.pdf. Last revised October 2010.

Kacmarek RM, Stoller JK, Heuer AJ. *Egan's fundamentals of respiratory care*. ed 11. St. Louis: Mosby-Elsevier; 2017.

Kutchak FM, Debesaitys AM, Rieder Mde M, et al. Reflex cough PEF as a predictor of successful extubation in neurological patients. *J Bras Pneumol*. 2015;41(4):358–364.

Singh B, Mielke MM, Parsaik AK, et al. A prospective study of chronic obstructive pulmonary disease and the risk for mild cognitive impairment. *JAMA Neurol*. 2014;71(5):581–588.

Teasdale G, Jennett BJ. Assessment of coma and impaired consciousness. A practical scale. *Lancet*. 1974;2(7872):81–84.

Teasdale G, Maas A, Lecky F, et al. The Glasgow Coma Scale at 40 years: standing the test of time. *Lancet Neurol*. 2014;13(8):844–854.

# 7

# Clinical Laboratory Studies

*Nadine A. Fydryszewski and Elaine M. Keohane*

## LEARNING OBJECTIVES

*After reading this chapter, you will be able to:*

1. Explain the three phases of laboratory testing.
2. Describe the composition of blood.
3. Explain the importance of specimen integrity and effects on laboratory test results.
4. Define laboratory test sensitivity, specificity, and positive and negative predictive value.
5. Discuss the meaning of the term *reference interval.*
6. Describe the clinical applications and general clinical significance of increases and decreases for each component of the complete blood count, the reticulocyte count, and erythrocyte sedimentation rate.
7. Define leukocytosis, leukopenia, relative and absolute count, neutrophilia, neutropenia, lymphocytosis, lymphopenia, monocytosis, eosinophilia, basophilia, leukemia, anemia, and hemostasis.
8. Describe the body's response to anemia and the potential effects of uncompensated anemia.
9. Differentiate primary, secondary, and relative polycythemia, and describe the adverse effects of polycythemia.
10. Describe the clinical applications of the activated partial thromboplastin time, prothrombin time, and platelet count in assessing hemostasis.
11. Explain the clinical application and significance of the quantitative D-dimer assay.
12. Describe the clinical applications and general clinical significance of increases and decreases in electrolyte concentrations, glucose levels, blood urea nitrogen, and creatinine.
13. Discuss the importance of renal and hepatic panel tests as related to the management of patients with respiratory disorders.
14. Relate lipid panel measures to the risk for atherosclerosis and heart disease.
15. Identify the current cardiac biomarkers used to help identify acute coronary syndrome and congestive heart failure.
16. Describe the preanalytical testing phase in clinical microbiology.
17. Discuss the common examination methods of microbiology specimens (e.g., Gram stain, acid-fast stains).
18. Explain the purpose of microbiology culture and antimicrobial sensitivity tests.
19. Describe collection and transport protocols for pulmonary secretions.
20. Discuss the importance of macroscopic and microscopic examination of sputum.
21. List the microscopic criteria used to assess the quality of a sputum sample.
22. Explain the significance of sputum eosinophilia.
23. Describe the indications for and method of performing a bronchoalveolar lavage.
24. Describe the macroscopic, microscopic, and chemical significance of pleural fluid examination.
25. Explain the purpose of histologic and cytologic examinations.
26. List the malignant tumors responsible for producing most primary lung cancers.
27. List the types of pulmonary samples that can be examined cytologically.
28. Discuss the general concept of skin testing and two methods to screen for tuberculosis.
29. Given a variety of patient presentations, identify the common laboratory tests helpful in assessing the problem.

## OUTLINE

## KEY TERMS

| | | |
|---|---|---|
| analyte | hypochloremia | neutrophilia |
| anemia | hypochromic | normoblasts |
| anergy | hypoglycemia | normochromic |
| basophilia | hypokalemia | normocytic |
| blasts | hyponatremia | polycythemia |
| cytology | left shift | polycythemia vera |
| eosinophilia | leukocytosis | pseudoneutropenia |
| glycosuria | leukopenia | pseudoneutrophilia |
| granulocytes | lymphocytopenia | reticulocyte |
| hemostasis | lymphocytosis | sensitivity |
| hyperchloremia | macrocytic | serum |
| hyperglycemia | macrophage | specificity |
| hyperkalemia | microcytic | spurious |
| hypernatremia | monocytosis | thrombocytopenia |
| hypoalbuminemia | neutropenia | thrombocytosis |

## CLINICAL LABORATORY OVERVIEW

The practice of medicine would be impossible without the diagnostic tests performed by medical laboratory scientists in the clinical laboratory. Clinical laboratory tests are used to diagnose, treat, monitor, and prevent disease. Laboratory scientists analyze body fluids and other medical specimens, providing laboratory data and vital information to other members of the health care team.

The clinical laboratory includes several specialized disciplines: microbiology, hematology, immunology, transfusion medicine, clinical chemistry, and molecular diagnostics. Most hospitalized patients with respiratory disease undergo many laboratory tests, and it is important for respiratory therapists (RTs) to have a basic understanding of the commonly ordered tests. This chapter provides key information related to the preanalytical, analytical, and postanalytical phases of laboratory testing. Although the emphasis is on laboratory tests and data related to patients with respiratory disease, most of the concepts described are applicable to any patient.

### Phases of Laboratory Testing

Laboratory testing involves preanalytical, analytical, and postanalytical phases. The preanalytical phase is related to selection of the appropriate assays for the patient's condition, patient identification and preparation, and specimen selection, collection, and transport. The RT may be involved in this phase, particularly in collection of arterial blood samples and pulmonary secretions for laboratory testing. The analytical phase is the actual testing performed by laboratory scientists. The postanalytical phase involves reporting and interpretation of results.

Most laboratory tests are performed using blood collected from peripheral veins, arteries, or capillaries. For most tests, the site of blood collection has no effect on the analysis or the results. Exceptions include blood gases and lactic acid, which may vary significantly by collection site. Therefore it is important that appropriate selection, collection, and transport be used. Blood collection tubes with color-coded caps, with and without additives, must be matched to the analytes being tested. Other specimens submitted for laboratory tests include body fluids, secretions such as sputum, pleural fluid, cerebrospinal fluid, urine, feces, biopsy material, and sweat.

### Composition of Blood

Blood consists of two major components: cells (45%) and the plasma (55%). There are three types of cells: white blood cells (leukocytes), red blood cells (erythrocytes), and platelets (thrombocytes). Blood cells are derived from hematopoietic stem cells (the precursor of all blood and immune cells) and develop in the bone marrow or lymphoid tissue (lymph nodes, spleen, thymus). The plasma consists of water and soluble substances including electrolytes, clotting factors, immunologic factors, proteins, lipids, and hormones. Almost every substance the cells use must be transported by the plasma. Serum is the fluid remaining when the blood is allowed to clot. It closely resembles plasma but lacks some coagulation factors.

## Specimen Integrity and Effect on Test Results

Specimen integrity is critical to quality and accurate laboratory testing. Test results can be affected by hemolysis, storage times and temperature, method of transport, interfering conditions of the blood (icterus, lipemia, turbidity), inadequate blood volume when using tubes with additives, and using the wrong collection tube. For example, a specimen that is hemolyzed can yield falsely elevated results for several analytes, such as potassium, magnesium, calcium, and iron. Maintenance of specimen integrity for microbiologic samples commonly gathered by RTs is discussed later in this chapter. Specimen integrity for arterial blood gas samples is covered in Chapter 8.

## Laboratory Test Parameters

A quality test result is accurate and precise but also must provide useful information to clinicians for making a diagnosis or monitoring disease. The usefulness of a test is evaluated in terms of its predictive value, which includes measurements of clinical (diagnostic) sensitivity, clinical (diagnostic) specificity, positive predictive value, and negative predictive value. If a test is positive in a patient with disease, it is considered a true positive (TP). If the test is negative in a patient with disease, it represents a false negative (FN). A negative test in a disease-free patient is considered a true negative (TN). On the other hand, if a positive test occurs in a disease-free patient, the result would be considered a false positive (FP). TP, FN, TN, and FP can be grouped into statistical parameters describing the accuracy of the test results in relation to a particular disease.

- Sensitivity: frequency of positive test results in patients with disease. *Example:* A sensitivity of 98% means that 98% of the patients with the disease will be detected by the test (TP), and 2% of the patients with the disease will be negative with the test (FN). Another way to express sensitivity is, "If the patient has the disease, the test will be positive." If the result of a test with high sensitivity is negative, one can confidently rule out the disorder in question.
- Specificity: frequency of negative test results in patients without disease. *Example:* A specificity of 98% means that 98% of the patients without the disease will be negative for the test (TN), and 2% of the patients without the disease will be positive for the test (FP). Another way to express specificity is, "If the patient does *not* have the disease, the test will be negative." If the result of a test with high specificity is positive, one can confidently rule in the disorder in question.

Laboratory test results are often interpreted based on comparison to a reference interval or range. Reference intervals depend on many factors, including patient age, gender,

sample population, and test method. The laboratory report will contain specific reference intervals that have been established for that facility or population. Reference intervals are calculated to include 95% of a healthy population (2 standard deviations). The reference intervals mentioned in this chapter represent those typical of many laboratories. Clinicians should abandon using the terms "normal value" and "normals" because they are misleading. A test result falling outside a reference interval does not necessarily mean that the patient has the abnormal condition or disease. Trends in results, comparison with related test results, and clinical findings must be taken into consideration. Correlation of clinical findings with laboratory test results leads to appropriate diagnosis and treatment.

## HEMATOLOGY

Clinical laboratory tests in hematology can be divided into two main categories: (1) general hematology tests for evaluating normal and abnormal blood cells and (2) coagulation studies for evaluating blood clotting. General hematology tests covered here include the complete blood count (CBC), including the white blood cell differential count and reticulocyte count and erythrocyte sedimentation rate. Routine coagulation tests discussed in this section include the prothrombin time (PT)/ international normalized ratio (INR) and the activated partial thromboplastin time (APTT). Routine hematology and coagulation tests are important for assessing wellness and health status, detecting and initial investigation of various disease states, and monitoring certain therapies.

## Complete Blood Count

The CBC is an overall assessment of the quantity and morphology (appearance) of the white blood cells (WBCs), red blood cells (RBCs), and platelets. The CBC includes a total WBC count, a count of the different types of WBCs (called a *differential count*), the RBC count, hemoglobin (Hb) level, hematocrit (Hct), the RBC indices, a platelet count, and a reticulocyte count. Table 7.1 contains sample adult reference intervals for the CBC components in both common units and standard international (SI) units.

The following discussion focuses first on WBCs and the differential count and then shifts to RBCs and platelets. Coagulation studies are discussed last.

### White Blood Cells

WBCs function as part of the immune system in protecting the body from various pathogenic microorganisms and foreign antigens. WBCs develop in the bone marrow or lymphoid tissue through the influence of growth factors and are released into the peripheral blood when mature. The WBCs that are present in the peripheral blood of healthy individuals include segmented neutrophils, eosinophils, basophils, lymphocytes, and monocytes.

*White Blood Cell Differential Count.* CBC analyzers determine the total number of WBCs per microliter or liter of blood and perform an automated differential count in which

### TABLE 7.1 Sample Reference Intervals for the Complete Blood Count (CBC) in Adults

| CBC Component Conventional Units (SI units) | Reference Intervals |
|---|---|
| WBC count × 10³/µL (× 10⁹/L) | 4.0-11.0 |
| RBC count × 10⁶/µL (× 10¹²/L) | M: 4.20-6.00 |
| | F: 3.80-5.20 |
| Hemoglobin g/dL (g/L) | M: 13.5-18.0 (135-180) |
| | F: 12.0-15.0 (120-150) |
| Hematocrit % (L/L) | M: 40-54 (0.40-0.54) |
| | F: 35-49 (0.35-0.49) |
| **Erythrocyte Indices** | |
| Mean cell volume (MCV) (fL) | 80-100 |
| Mean cell hemoglobin (pg) | 26-34 |
| Mean cell hemoglobin concentration (MCHC) (g/dL) | 32-36 |
| Platelet count × 10³/µL (× 10⁹/L) | 150-450 |
| Reticulocytes % | 0.5-2.5 |
| Reticulocytes × 10³/µL (× 10⁹/L) | 20-115 |

*F*, Female; *M*, male; *RBC*, red blood cell; *SI*, standard international; *WBC*, white blood cell.

### TABLE 7.2 Sample Reference Intervals for the Differential White Blood Cell Count in Adults

| Cell Type | Relative(%) | Absolute[a] |
|---|---|---|
| Segmented neutrophils | 50-70 | 1.5-7.5 |
| Eosinophils | 1-3 | 0-0.4 |
| Basophils | 0-1 | 0-0.1 |
| Lymphocytes | 20-45 | 1.0-4.0 |
| Monocytes | 2-11 | 0.1-1.3 |

[a]× 10³/µL (× 10⁹/L).

The primary function of neutrophils is to destroy invading microorganisms, foreign material, and dead cells. They accomplish this by phagocytosis, a process in which the neutrophil engulfs and destroys the particles through release of various enzymes and reactive molecules.

### SIMPLY STATED

There are five different types of WBCs, the most common of which is the segmented neutrophil. It is the first line of defense against bacterial infections.

the percentage and absolute number of each type of WBC are determined. If the instrument count is abnormal, or a sample is flagged for suspected abnormal or immature cells, a manual slide review and differential count are performed by a laboratory scientist. In addition, the morphology of all the cells is assessed, and the presence of immature and abnormal cells is noted.

The relative count is the percentage of a particular cell among all the WBCs counted. The absolute count for that cell type is determined by the CBC analyzer by multiplying its percentage or relative count by the total WBC count. Table 7.2 provides sample reference intervals for the relative and absolute counts of each type of WBC.

Because the relative count is influenced by increases or decreases of the other WBC types, the absolute count provides a more useful assessment. In a simplified example, if an adult patient had a total WBC count of $20 \times 10^9$/L with a relative count of 85% neutrophils and 15% lymphocytes, the absolute counts are $17 \times 10^9$/L for neutrophils and $3 \times 10^9$/L for lymphocytes. Comparing these results to the reference intervals in Table 7.2, there is both a relative and an absolute increase in neutrophils. On the other hand, although the relative count for the lymphocytes is decreased, the absolute count is within the reference interval.

*White Blood Cell Functions.* Neutrophils, eosinophils, and basophils are included in a general category of cells called granulocytes because of their prominent granules. However, they have different functions.

Segmented neutrophils (previously called polymorphonuclear leukocytes) are the most numerous cell type in the peripheral blood, constituting 50% to 70% of circulating WBCs. A band is a slightly less mature neutrophil in which the nucleus has not yet segmented. Bands represent less than 5% of the circulating WBCs in healthy individuals. Circulating bands are included in the segmented neutrophil count.

Neutrophils are produced and stored in the bone marrow, a process that takes 10 to 12 days. However, if the demand for neutrophils increases—as may occur in an acute bacterial infection—their time in the bone marrow may be shortened to a few days. In these cases, some immature neutrophils may be released. Once released into the peripheral blood, neutrophils have a very short half-life of approximately 6 to 8 hours.

In the peripheral blood, neutrophils are continuously exchanged between two intravascular pools, with about half the cells in the circulating pool and half in the marginated pool. The circulating neutrophils are those counted in the CBC. Marginated neutrophils adhere to the walls of the blood vessels and are not counted. Neutrophils are able to rapidly shift from one pool to the other based on physiologic conditions (discussed subsequently).

Eosinophils constitute 1% to 3% of WBCs, whereas basophils are even more rare at 0% to 1%. Both cell types are involved in immune system regulation, control of parasitic infections, and allergic reactions. Eosinophils also accumulate at the site of allergic reactions.

Lymphocytes constitute 20% to 45% of circulating WBCs in adults; in healthy children, the relative and absolute lymphocyte counts are higher. Lymphocytes are particularly important in the body's defense against foreign microorganisms and cells. There are three major types of lymphocytes: T cells, B cells, and natural killer (NK) cells. T and B cells participate in the body's adaptive or specific immune response by recognizing foreign antigens and tagging them for destruction. T cells are involved in cell-mediated immunity, which is particularly important in eliminating viruses and other intracellular organisms. B cells are involved in humoral immunity and develop into antibody-producing cells. NK cells are able to destroy certain virally infected cells and tumor cells.

Enumeration of the different types of lymphocytes is not done routinely but can be accomplished using specialized instruments and monoclonal antibodies. Approximately 50% to 85% of circulating lymphocytes are T cells, with B cells and NK cells comprising approximately 5% to 20% each. T lymphocytes also can be separated into subcategories. For example, knowledge of the $CD4^+$ T-lymphocyte cell count provides important information about the severity and prognosis of patients with acquired immunodeficiency syndrome (AIDS; see later discussion of lymphocytopenia).

Monocytes constitute 2% to 11% of circulating WBCs. In tissues, the monocyte is known as a macrophage. The primary functions of the monocyte are phagocytosis (engulfment) of organisms and other foreign material invading the body and initiation and regulation of the specific immune response with T lymphocytes. In the lung, alveolar macrophages play a key role in clearing inhaled particulate matter.

*Nonmalignant White Blood Cell Abnormalities.* Leukocytosis is an increase in the WBC count above the reference interval, whereas leukopenia is a decrease in the WBC count below the reference interval. Abnormalities in the WBC count can be defined more specifically by referring to the specific cell type that is increased or decreased using similar terminology. For example, an increase in neutrophils is called neutrophilia, and a decrease is called neutropenia. Increases in the cell counts may be primary (a result of uncontrolled proliferation of cells in the bone marrow) or secondary (a result of stimulation of the bone marrow secondary to other diseases or disorders). Similarly, decreases in cell counts may be caused by either primary bone marrow failure or increased destruction of the cells peripherally. Bone marrow failure can occur as a side effect of various drugs and disorders (secondary) or as a result of unknown causes (primary or idiopathic).

Neutrophilia is a common response to acute bacterial infections, such as bacterial pneumonia (Box 7.1). Neutrophilia also may occur in response to fungal, parasitic, or early viral infections. In addition, neutrophilia also occurs in inflammation due to autoimmune disorders or tissue damage that occurs after surgery, burns, myocardial infarction, or traumatic injury. Acute hemorrhage or hemolysis, metabolic disorders (such as acidosis or uremia), and certain drugs, toxins, and chemicals also cause neutrophilia. When the bone marrow is stimulated to release neutrophils at a rate faster than it can produce them, it releases them at increasingly more immature stages. This is called a left shift. The degree of the left shift and the severity of the neutrophilia usually correlate with the severity of the infection. A left shift is reported as the presence of immature granulocytes on some CBC instruments.

## SIMPLY STATED

The typical response to an acute bacterial infection is a neutrophilia with a left shift (increase in bands and presence of immature granulocytes in the peripheral blood).

---

### BOX 7.1  Common Causes of Nonmalignant or Reactive Neutrophilia

**Pathologic**
Acute bacterial infections
Other infections (fungal, parasitic, early stages of viral infections)
Inflammatory responses
Tissue damage (burns, surgery, traumatic injury, myocardial infarction)
Autoimmune disorders
Acute hemorrhage or hemolysis
Metabolic disorders (acidosis, uremia)
Certain drugs, chemicals, or toxins

**Physiologic (Pseudoneutrophilia)**
Physical or emotional stress
Strenuous exercise
Exposure to temperature extremes
Epinephrine administration
Anesthesia

---

### BOX 7.2  Causes of Neutropenia

**Decreased Neutrophil Production**
Drugs, chemicals, physical agents (e.g., chemotherapy, benzene, radiation)
Disorders of stem cells, acquired and inherited
Cancers infiltrating the bone marrow
Vitamin $B_{12}$ or folate deficiency (megaloblastic anemia)

**Increase in Neutrophil Destruction**
Overwhelming bacterial infection
Immune disorders (antibody production against neutrophils)

**Pseudoneutropenia**
Some antipsychotic drugs

---

Pseudoneutrophilia, also called physiologic neutrophilia, occurs when marginated neutrophils are shifted to the circulating pool and are counted in the CBC. Shock, stress, strenuous exercise, labor, trauma, or epinephrine administration can cause pseudoneutrophilia. This type of neutrophilia is immediate and typically transient, lasting less than an hour. Because the marginated cells are mature neutrophils, there is no left shift as seen in pathologic neutrophilia.

Neutropenia may occur as a result of decreased bone marrow production or increased destruction of circulating neutrophils (Box 7.2). Many drugs, some chemicals, and radiation therapy can cause neutropenia by destroying the blood cell precursors in the bone marrow, thus decreasing bone marrow production. One of the most common causes of neutropenia is cancer chemotherapy. Because of their short half-life, the neutrophils are the first blood cell type to decrease with chemotherapy. The absolute neutrophil count is closely monitored during chemotherapy, and adjustments in therapy are made if it drops too low. Other causes of decreased production include acquired and hereditary defects in stem cells, hematologic malignancies, infiltration of cancer cells into the bone marrow, immune disorders, and deficiencies of vitamin $B_{12}$ or folate. Neutrophils can also be quickly depleted by overwhelming infections or be destroyed as a result of the production of antibodies against them. Pseudoneutropenia is a transient shift of the neutrophils from the circulating pool to the marginated pool. Morning pseudoneutropenia has been reported in some patients taking antipsychotic drugs.

Neutrophils are the first-line defense against microorganisms, so patients with neutropenia have a high risk for developing life-threatening bacterial or fungal infections. The lower the absolute neutrophil count and the longer the duration of the neutropenia, the greater the risk for serious infection.

### SIMPLY STATED

Neutropenia is often a sign of a serious health problem and usually occurs as a result of decreased bone marrow production or increased destruction of neutrophils in the peripheral blood.

Eosinophilia (increase in eosinophils) is often seen in parasitic infestations and allergic states (such as hay fever, dermatitis, and drug reactions). Patients with extrinsic or atopic asthma often have eosinophilia. Basophilia (increase in basophils) is usually associated with myeloproliferative neoplasms (discussed later in the chapter).

Lymphocytosis (increase in lymphocytes) is typically seen in viral infections and certain bacterial (pertussis) and parasitic (toxoplasmosis) infections. In some viral infections, especially infectious mononucleosis, many of the lymphocytes are enlarged and have a characteristic appearance, being labeled as reactive lymphocytes. Interpretation of lymphocytosis should take into account the patient's age because children normally have higher counts than adults. Lymphocytopenia (decrease in lymphocytes) is seen in acquired and congenital immune deficiency states and in various conditions such as acute inflammation, malnutrition, and after treatment with chemotherapy, radiation, or corticosteroids. Lymphocytopenia is an important feature of human immunodeficiency virus (HIV) infection, the virus that causes AIDS. The virus infects and destroys the CD4+ helper T lymphocytes, resulting in their depletion. As the CD4+ cells decline, the immune system becomes more compromised, leading to increased risk for certain cancers and infections. Peripheral blood CD4+ counts, along with the HIV viral load, are used to monitor the progression of the disease.

Monocytosis (increase in monocytes) is characteristic of certain infections, including tuberculosis, syphilis, typhoid fever, and subacute bacterial endocarditis. A monocytosis often signals the recovery stage of an acute infection. Monocytosis also may occur in inflammatory conditions and autoimmune states.

*Malignant White Blood Cell Abnormalities.* Hematologic malignancies or neoplasms occur due to mutations in a stem cell or blood precursor cell that disrupt the normal blood development process. Those that involve the bone marrow and peripheral blood are generally called leukemias, whereas those confined mainly to the lymphoid tissue are called lymphomas.

In acute leukemia, mutations cause a maturation arrest in a blood cell precursor at an early stage of development. Typically, blasts, which are the most immature stage of a cell type, accumulate in the bone marrow and peripheral blood. These blasts quickly replace all other cells in the bone marrow and, if left untreated, will cause a rapid death of the patient. WBC counts are variable, but the key feature in the WBC differential is the presence of blasts. The normal WBCs, along with RBCs and platelets, are decreased. Acute lymphoblastic leukemia usually occurs in young children, whereas acute myeloid leukemia most often occurs in older adults. Acute leukemias are classified by the World Health Organization according to the presence of recurrent genetic abnormalities in the leukemia cells.

Chronic leukemias result from a slower growth and accumulation of more mature cells in the peripheral blood and bone marrow. Chronic lymphocytic leukemia is the most common type of adult leukemia and occurs predominantly in elderly people. The WBC count is increased, and the differential count shows a preponderance of mature lymphocytes. Chronic myelogenous leukemia (CML) occurs predominantly in middle-aged adults. It is caused by a mutation in a stem cell that results in uncontrolled proliferation of granulocytes. The WBC count is increased, and the bone marrow and peripheral blood contain markedly increased numbers of neutrophils including all stages of maturation, as well as eosinophils and basophils. Platelets are also increased, and there is progressive anemia. Without treatment, CML terminates in acute leukemia, known as *blast transformation.*

Polycythemia vera is a neoplasm characterized by a proliferation of erythrocytic, granulocytic, and platelet precursors in the bone marrow. Patients typically present with very high RBC counts and hemoglobin concentration, in addition to an increase in WBCs and platelets. Myelodysplastic syndromes result from stem cell mutations that cause ineffective blood cell production in the bone marrow and a progressive decrease in WBCs, RBCs, and platelets in the peripheral blood. They occur predominantly in the elderly. Lymphomas can initiate in all types of lymphoid cells. Lymphoma cells can sometimes circulate in the peripheral blood, but they are usually confined to lymphoid tissues and detected by lymph node biopsy.

### Red Blood Cells

RBCs are produced in the bone marrow by maturation of nucleated erythrocytic precursor cells known as normoblasts. Under normal circumstances, as the normoblasts mature, the cytoplasm acquires a pink color as a result of the development of hemoglobin. Before the RBC is released from the bone marrow to circulate in the peripheral blood, the nucleus is removed. RBCs have a life span of approximately 120 days.

Normal RBCs assume the shape of a biconcave disk to facilitate their primary function of carrying oxygen and to provide maximal deformability to bend as they pass through

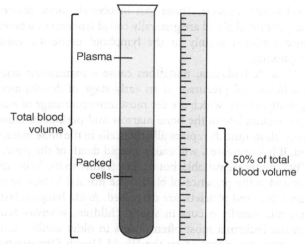

Plasma

Total blood volume

Packed cells

50% of total blood volume

**FIG. 7.1** Determination of hematocrit (Hct) from centrifuging blood sample. Packed cell volume is half the total blood volume; therefore the Hct is 50% in this example.

small capillaries. The major component of mature RBCs (erythrocytes) is hemoglobin, which imparts to blood its normal red color when carrying oxygen. The RBC count is reported in number of cells per microliter or liter of blood (see Table 7.1 for reference intervals). An adequate number of RBCs with an adequate concentration of hemoglobin and a functionally normal hemoglobin molecule are needed for transport of sufficient oxygen from the lungs to the tissues.

### SIMPLY STATED

RBCs act as carriers of hemoglobin, which is needed to transport oxygen throughout the body.

*Hematocrit (Packed Cell Volume).* The hematocrit is the ratio of the packed RBC volume to the volume of whole blood. A manual hematocrit is performed by centrifuging whole blood to pack the blood cells to the bottom of a small capillary tube and then measuring the percentage or fraction of the total blood volume occupied by the RBCs (Fig. 7.1). CBC analyzers determine the hematocrit using various automated technologies. Because it measures the volume of the hemoglobin-containing RBCs, one can estimate the hematocrit by multiplying the hemoglobin content times a factor of 3.

*Hemoglobin.* Hemoglobin is the protein that carries oxygen to the tissues; it is the major component of RBCs. Hemoglobin also is important in maintaining acid-base balance by acting as a buffer and by carrying carbon dioxide ($CO_2$) from the tissues to the lungs. The hemoglobin molecule consists of four heme groups, each with an iron molecule capable of binding oxygen, and four globin chains.

Hemoglobin is reported in grams per deciliter or liter of blood. The reference intervals for the RBC count, hematocrit, and hemoglobin vary by gender, with men having higher levels than women because of the positive influence of testosterone on RBC production (see Table 7.1). Age also affects hemoglobin levels, with higher values in newborns and slightly lower values in elderly people.

*Red Blood Cell Indices.* Three RBC indices are the mean cell volume (MCV), mean cell hemoglobin (MCH), and mean cell hemoglobin concentration (MCHC). They are calculated from the RBC count, hemoglobin, and hematocrit. The MCV is the average volume of the patient's RBCs. A decrease in the MCV indicates the RBCs are smaller, or microcytic, whereas an increase in the MCV indicates the RBCs are larger, or macrocytic. A normal MCV indicates the RBCs are normal in volume, or normocytic, although the presence of an equal number of smaller and larger RBCs could produce a normal MCV. The MCH is the average weight of hemoglobin in the patient's RBCs. The interpretation of the MCH correlates with that of the MCV. The MCHC is the concentration of hemoglobin in the patient's RBCs. A decrease in the MCHC indicates the RBCs have less hemoglobin, called hypochromic, whereas a normal MCHC indicates the RBCs have a normal complement of hemoglobin, called normochromic.

*Red Blood Cell Abnormalities.* Anemia is a decrease in the RBC mass of the body that results in a decrease in the oxygen-carrying capacity of the blood. It can be due to a decrease in hemoglobin concentration or a defect in hemoglobin function. Anemia is clinically defined by a decrease in the hemoglobin concentration below the reference interval for an individual's gender and age.

One of the body's responses to hypoxia is an increase in secretion of erythropoietin by the kidneys, which accelerates the maturation and release of new RBCs into the circulation. The circulatory system also responds to severe or sudden anemia by increasing the heart rate, respiration rate, and cardiac output to deliver oxygen more quickly to the tissues and by redirecting blood flow from the skin to the heart, brain, and muscles.

General symptoms of anemia include pallor, fatigue, and dyspnea, but various other symptoms may also occur depending on the cause of the anemia. In severe anemia, tachycardia and hypotension also occur, which if untreated can lead to cardiac failure. The severity of the symptoms depends on the degree of hemoglobin reduction, the state of the patient's cardiovascular system, and the rate of development and duration of the anemia.

Anemias may be classified by pathophysiology into those caused by a decrease in RBC production and those caused by an increase in RBC destruction or loss. However, a more practical approach is to use the MCV to classify anemias into microcytic, macrocytic, or normocytic types.

The most common type of anemia worldwide is the result of iron deficiency. Iron deficiency anemia occurs when there is a dietary deficiency of iron, increased need for iron that is not met (pregnancy, infancy, adolescent growth spurts), malabsorption of iron, or chronic blood loss. In chronic blood loss, the iron contained in the RBCs slowly leaves the body instead of being recycled. Iron is required for hemoglobin synthesis, and with sustained, low iron levels, the bone marrow begins to produce smaller RBCs with a decreased amount of hemoglobin, and the RBC indices become microcytic and hypochromic.

Anemia also can result from chronic inflammation that causes an impairment of iron regulation and RBC production in the bone marrow. The resulting anemia is often normocytic, but it can be microcytic in diseases of long duration. Macrocytic anemia is most often caused by either folate or vitamin $B_{12}$ deficiency. Low folate or vitamin $B_{12}$ levels impair DNA synthesis in the nucleus and result in ineffective blood cell production and macrocytic RBCs.

The hemolytic anemias constitute a large group of disorders in which excessive destruction of RBCs in the circulation exceeds the capacity of the bone marrow to replace the cells that are lost. Hemolytic anemia may be due to intrinsic defects in the RBCs (such as sickle cell anemia) or abnormalities extrinsic to the RBCs (such as hemolysis caused by antibodies, malaria, or drugs). A dilutional anemia can result from administration of excessive fluids that disproportionally increase the plasma volume compared to the RBC mass. There is a relative (spurious) but not absolute decrease in the hemoglobin, hematocrit, and RBC count because of the hemodilution.

Hemoglobin may be converted to an inactive form through oxidation, denaturation, or other chemical reaction. The most common forms of inactive hemoglobin are carboxyhemoglobin (COHb) and methemoglobin (metHb). The measurement of these abnormal hemoglobin combinations and their impact on oxygen transport are discussed in detail in Chapter 8.

### SIMPLY STATED

Patients with anemia have a decreased oxygen-carrying capacity of the blood. The response to severe and chronic anemia is increased erythropoietin secretion by the kidneys to stimulate more RBC production and increased heart rate and cardiac output to deliver more oxygen to the tissues. The latter can result in high-output cardiac failure.

Polycythemia is an increase in the RBC count, hemoglobin, and hematocrit and may be primary, secondary, or relative (spurious). Primary polycythemia vera is an uncommon neoplasm caused by mutations in myeloid precursor cells resulting in an uncontrolled growth and accumulation of RBCs, WBCs, and platelets in the bone marrow and peripheral blood (polycythemia vera, previously discussed).

Secondary polycythemia is more common and is seen in patients who have chronic stimulation of the bone marrow to produce more RBCs secondary to some other disorder or condition. Examples include patients with chronic hypoxemia due to disease (e.g., chronic obstructive pulmonary disease [COPD]), obstructive sleep apnea, pulmonary fibrosis, chronic heart failure) or as compensation for the low oxygen pressures breathed by those living at high altitude. In these cases, chronic hypoxemia stimulates erythropoietin production by the kidneys, causing the bone marrow to produce and release additional RBCs to compensate for the oxygen deficit.

Heavy smokers also may exhibit secondary polycythemia. The carbon monoxide associated with cigarette smoke binds tightly with the hemoglobin and reduces oxygen transport. This results in a functional anemia to which the bone marrow responds by increasing RBC production.

In the presence of significant hypoxia due to severe anemia, the maturation time of RBCs in the bone marrow is decreased, resulting in the release of immature nucleated RBCs (NRBCs), which are not normally seen in the blood of adults. As a result of the hypoxic conditions in utero, NRBCs are normally present in fetal blood and newborns but disappear 3 to 4 days after birth. NRBCs may also occur in patients who have infiltration of the bone marrow with benign or malignant cells.

Both primary and secondary polycythemias involve an absolute increase in the total RBC mass. Sometimes, relative polycythemia occurs because of a decrease in the plasma volume. This is seen in patients who are dehydrated. Relative polycythemia does not represent a true increase in the number of circulating RBCs.

Although polycythemia is helpful in increasing the oxygen-carrying capacity of the blood, it can be detrimental to the heart and circulatory system. Polycythemia increases the viscosity of the blood, causing both an increased cardiac workload and a greater risk for clot formation and thrombosis. Treatment focuses on management of the underlying cause and in some patients may include restoring a normal hematocrit by controlled removal of whole blood through phlebotomy.

### SIMPLY STATED

Patients with chronic hypoxemia may develop a secondary polycythemia to compensate for the reduction in blood oxygen levels; polycythemia can increase cardiac workload and the incidence of thrombosis.

*Reticulocyte Count.* The reticulocyte is the final erythrocyte development stage before the RBC is fully mature. These slightly immature RBCs lack a nucleus and differ from mature RBCs in that they are slightly larger and have not yet assumed a biconcave shape. A reticulocyte count is performed by obtaining the percentage of reticulocytes among the RBCs. Normally about 1% of the circulating RBCs are reticulocytes, with slightly higher values in newborns. The reticulocyte count is also reported as an absolute count by multiplying the reticulocyte percentage by the RBC count. Reference intervals are provided in Table 7.1.

The reticulocyte count helps to assess the bone marrow response to an anemia. If the absolute reticulocyte count is high in a patient with anemia, it indicates that the bone marrow is responding to the anemia by increasing production of RBCs. In this case the cause of the anemia is likely due to excessive peripheral blood loss or destruction. However, if the reticulocyte count is low, the anemia is likely the result of decreased bone marrow production.

### Platelet Count

Platelets are the smallest cells in the peripheral blood. After injury to a blood vessel, they participate in clot formation at the site of the injury to stop the bleeding. The platelet count routinely is provided as part of the CBC. Table 7.1 provides the reference interval for the platelet count. Like other blood cells, platelets may be decreased as a result of increased destruction in the peripheral blood or decreased production in the bone marrow. A reduction in the platelet count below the reference interval is called thrombocytopenia.

Thrombocytopenia usually manifests as small skin hemorrhages (petechiae, purpura, and ecchymoses) and bleeding from mucosal surfaces (such as epistaxis or menorrhagia). When the platelet count is decreased significantly (<20 × $10^3/\mu L$), patients are more likely to have bleeding problems, especially with trauma such as surgery or arterial punctures. However, when the platelet count becomes extremely low (<10 × $10^3/\mu L$), the patient is at risk for serious spontaneous bleeding, including intracranial hemorrhage. There are many disorders that cause thrombocytopenia, including side effects of drugs such as chemotherapy or heparin, bone marrow diseases, and immune thrombocytopenic purpura, an autoimmune disorder in which autoantibodies are produced against the platelets, marking them for destruction in the spleen.

An increase in platelets (thrombocytosis) may be due to a reactive (secondary) process after hemorrhage, surgery, splenectomy, stress, or inflammation or by a malignant process associated with one of the myeloid neoplasms. A markedly increased platelet count increases the risk for thrombosis.

## Erythrocyte Sedimentation Rate

Although not part of the CBC, the erythrocyte sedimentation rate (ESR) is a commonly ordered test to monitor inflammatory diseases. If whole blood is placed in a vertical tube, the RBCs tend to fall to the bottom. The ESR measures the distance (in millimeters) that the RBCs fall in a vertical tube in 1 hour. The ESR is a nonspecific test that is increased in many disorders, especially inflammatory processes. This is largely because of an increase in various plasma proteins (such as globulins and fibrinogen) that reduce the negative charge on the surface of the RBCs, causing them to aggregate or stack on each other and fall at an increased rate. Anemia falsely increases the ESR because the RBCs fall faster in a whole blood specimen with a lower concentration of RBCs per microliter.

## Coagulation Screening Tests

Hemostasis (ability to prevent hemorrhage, form a blood clot, keep blood flowing in circulation) involves a complex system of clot-forming and anticoagulant forces that are in balance to promote localized clot formation and to prevent unintended clotting under other circumstances.

Hemostasis testing is complex and is done to evaluate patients who are bleeding, as well as those who have excessive clotting. In the clinical laboratory, however, the ability to form a clot is assessed in a plasma-based system (without platelets and vascular cells) and is divided into intrinsic, extrinsic, and common pathways that use different groups of clotting factors. Three basic screening tests are generally used for the initial assessment of bleeding: the platelet count (already discussed), the APTT, and the PT/INR.

The APTT assesses the clotting factors in the intrinsic and common pathways by measuring the length of time required for plasma to form a fibrin clot once the intrinsic pathway is activated. The reference interval varies by laboratory but is usually about 25 to 35 seconds. The PT assesses the clotting factors in the extrinsic and common pathways and is performed similarly, using activation of the extrinsic system as an initiation point. The reference interval for the PT generally falls between 12 and 15 seconds. An INR is calculated from the PT result using a formula that takes into account the specific reagents and instrument used for the test. Because there are many different reagent-instrument combinations that can affect the PT result, the INR allows for a comparison of results between different laboratories.

Prolongation of the APTT or PT/INR indicates a reduction in blood-clotting ability. These tests are abnormal if one or more of the involved clotting factors are decreased significantly. Further studies are then required to delineate the specific factors implicated. Factor deficiencies may be either congenital (e.g., hemophilia A, which is a congenital decrease or absence of factor VIII) or acquired (e.g., liver disease with a decrease in multiple clotting factors). The APTT is one of the tests used for monitoring intravenous unfractionated heparin therapy, whereas PT/INR is used for monitoring warfarin (Coumadin) therapy. The INR should be between 2.0 and 3.0 in patients taking warfarin who have atrial fibrillation or a history of pulmonary emboli and generally between 2.5 and 3.5 in patients with a mechanical heart valve. Patients on warfarin with an INR lower than 2 are below the therapeutic range and are at risk for thrombosis. Patients with an INR greater than 4.0 have an increased the risk for hemorrhage, and patients with an elevated INR and anatomic bleeding should be treated as a medical emergency.

---

### SIMPLY STATED

Respiratory therapists should review the patient's platelet count, PT/INR, and APTT before performing an arterial puncture; if results indicate a decrease in blood-clotting ability, extra precautions should be taken to ensure hemostasis.

---

Tests used for the assessment of excessive thrombosis are complex, but one important assay to consider is D-dimer. D-dimer is produced as a result of the breakdown of fibrin clots that form in the vasculature. The upper reference interval for D-dimer in the plasma is about 240 ng/mL, but the value varies depending on each laboratory's methods. An increase in D-dimer is nonspecific and can be observed in many conditions with excessive clotting, as well as in inflammation, renal disease, and even pregnancy. However, because the D-dimer test has high sensitivity, a level below the upper limit of the reference interval can help rule out both systemic thrombosis, such as disseminated intravascular coagulation, and local thrombosis, such as pulmonary embolism and deep vein thrombosis.

# CHEMISTRY

The clinical chemistry laboratory provides key information to clinicians to assess the health status of the body or disease processes. This is accomplished by measurements of specific biochemical compounds, both those normally present in the body (endogenous chemicals) and external or exogenous substances that are administered or ingested, such as drugs, alcohol, and poisons. It is beyond the scope of this chapter to discuss the hundreds of laboratory tests available. This section will focus on the commonly ordered tests used to assess patient status and those directly related to the needs of the RT for patient management.

It is important to emphasize again that laboratory reference values depend on many factors, including patient age, gender, sample population, and test method. The reference intervals used in this section are based on general averages. However, test interpretation should always be based on the values established within one's institution.

Chemistry tests typically are ordered by clinicians in groupings called *panels.* The common chemistry panels discussed here and the reference intervals for their constituent tests are provided in Table 7.3.

## Basic Metabolic Panel

The basic metabolic panel is the most commonly ordered group of chemistry tests. It includes the four major electrolytes, the fasting glucose level, and two renal-function tests, blood urea nitrogen (BUN) and creatinine.

### Electrolytes

Normal cell function depends on proper concentrations of electrolytes, and the body must maintain electrolytes in a balanced state. Monitoring electrolyte concentrations is extremely important in patients whose body fluids are being endogenously or exogenously manipulated (e.g., intravenous therapy, renal disease, or diarrhea). Electrolytes are measured in the blood using either a plasma or serum sample. The four primary electrolytes are sodium ($Na^+$), potassium ($K^+$), chloride ($Cl^-$), and total $CO_2$.

Sodium is the major cation in extracellular fluid. The kidney, influenced by hormones secreted by the adrenal gland (aldosterone) and hypothalamus (antidiuretic hormone [ADH]), closely regulates the concentration of $Na^+$ in the blood. Sodium is mainly responsible for the osmotic pressure of the extracellular fluid. Increased serum $Na^+$ (hypernatremia) is seen when the body loses water without salt (e.g., profuse sweating, diarrhea, renal diseases, or prolonged hyperpnea), when water intake is insufficient, or when certain hormonal abnormalities are present. Patients with hypernatremia typically complain of excessive thirst and a dry, sticky mouth.

Decreased $Na^+$ concentration (hyponatremia) is caused by either excess water intake/retention or excess sodium loss. Theoretically, healthy people could become hyponatremic by drinking too much water, but water retention is most commonly associated with excessive secretion of ADH.

**TABLE 7.3 Common Chemistry Panels with Sample Test Reference Intervals**

| Panel and Analytes Measured | Common Reference Intervals |
|---|---|
| **Basic Metabolic Panel** | |
| Sodium ($Na^+$) | 135-145 mmol/L |
| Potassium ($K^+$) | 3.5-5.0 mmol/L |
| Chloride ($Cl^-$) | 98-107 mmol/L |
| Total $CO_2$ | 22-30 mmol/L |
| Glucose (fasting) | 70-99 mg/dL |
| Blood urea nitrogen (BUN) | 7-20 mg/dL |
| Creatinine | 0.7-1.3 mg/dL |
| **Renal Panel** | |
| Blood urea nitrogen (BUN) | See basic metabolic panel |
| Creatinine | See basic metabolic panel |
| Glomerular filtration rate (GFR) | 90-120 mL/min/1.73 m² |
| Urinalysis | Multiple tests—see discussion |
| **Hepatic Panel** | |
| Albumin | 3.5-5.0 g/dL |
| Total protein | 6.3-8.0 g/dL |
| Alkaline phosphatase (ALP) | 38-126 U/L |
| Alanine aminotransferase (ALT) | 10-40 U/L |
| Aspartate aminotransferase (AST) | 5-30 U/L |
| Bilirubin (total) | 0.3-1.9 mg/dL |
| **Lipid Profile** | |
| Total cholesterol | <200 mg/dL |
| High-density lipoprotein cholesterol (HDL-C) | >39 mg/dL |
| Low-density lipoprotein cholesterol (LDL-C) | <100 mg/dL |
| Triglycerides | 30-149 mg/dL |
| **Cardiac Biomarkers** | |
| Total creatine kinase (CK) | 50-200 U/L |
| Creatine kinase isoenzyme (CK-MB) | <5 % total CK |
| Troponin I (cTnI) | <0.01 ng/ML |
| Myoglobin | 19-92 µg/L |
| B-type natriuretic peptide (BNP) | <20 pg/L |

Excessive ADH secretion can occur with many illnesses, most commonly neurologic, pulmonary, or malignant. Patients with these conditions may become severely hyponatremic despite normal total body salt stores. Hyponatremia caused by actual loss of $Na^+$ is most often seen in patients receiving diuretics but can also be caused by diarrhea, severe sweating, or Addison disease (impaired production of aldosterone). Patients with severe hyponatremia (<115 mmol/L) may show confusion, abnormal sensorium, muscle twitching, and sometimes seizures.

Potassium is the major cation within cells. Extracellular concentration normally is low, with serum concentrations

---

**BOX 7.3** **Causes of Hypokalemia**

**Decreased Potassium Intake**
Low-potassium diet
Alcoholism

**Increased Loss of Potassium**
Gastrointestinal loss
Renal disease
Diuretics

**Extracellular-to-Intracellular Shift of Potassium**
Alkalosis
Increased plasma insulin
Diuretic use

---

**BOX 7.4** **Causes of Hyperkalemia**

**Increased Potassium Intake**
High-potassium diet
Oral potassium supplement
Transfusion of old blood

**Decreased Potassium Excretion**
Renal failure
Hypoaldosteronism

**Intracellular-to-Extracellular Shift of Potassium**
Acidosis
Crush injuries
Tissue hypoxia

**Pseudohyperkalemia**
Hemolysis
Leukocytosis

---

typically in the 3.5 to 5.0 mmol/L range. Hypokalemia occurs when there is increased loss of potassium or decreased intake or when $K^+$ ions shift from the extracellular to intracellular space (Box 7.3). Increased loss of potassium occurs when $K^+$-containing fluid is lost (e.g., vomiting, nasogastric suctioning), with some kidney diseases, and with the use of some diuretics. Decreased intake of potassium is often a dietary problem. Total body potassium depletion is present in such cases.

Metabolic alkalosis causes a shift of $K^+$ from the extracellular to the intracellular space, decreasing its serum concentration. This shift occurs in exchange for $H^+$ and is necessary to maintain electrolytic neutrality between these two spaces (see Chapter 8). This type of hypokalemia is not associated with true depletion of body potassium stores.

Hypokalemia is important to detect because it can be associated with cardiac, skeletal muscle, and gastrointestinal dysfunction. Weaning from mechanical ventilation may be difficult if hypokalemia is present. Patients with hypokalemia often have nausea, vomiting, abdominal distention, muscle cramps, lethargy, confusion, muscle weakness, and dysrhythmias. Electrocardiogram (ECG) abnormalities and dysrhythmias include flattened or inverted T waves, ST-segment depression, premature atrial contractions, and atrial or ventricular fibrillation (see Chapter 11).

Hyperkalemia can occur with increased intake, with decreased output, or when $K^+$ shifts from the intracellular to extracellular space (Box 7.4). Pseudohyperkalemia may occur when $K^+$ leaks out of RBCs or WBCs. This can be caused by improper collection technique causing hemolysis, delay in processing the specimen, or specimens from patients with abnormally high numbers of platelets, WBCs, or RBCs. As with hypokalemia, hyperkalemia can have major effects on the heart, causing telltale ECG abnormalities such as peaked T waves, shortened QT intervals, increases in the PR interval, and widening of the QRS complex (see Chapter 11). Untreated high serum potassium levels can lead to ventricular fibrillation and asystole.

Hyperkalemia caused by increased intake is often the result of dietary supplementation. Decreased output of $K^+$ is seen in some kidney disorders and with use of certain diuretics. Metabolic acidosis causes an increased level of $H^+$ in the extracellular fluid. In an effort to buffer this acidosis, intracellular $K^+$ ions exchange with extracellular $H^+$. This helps maintain a more neutral extracellular pH but leads to increased extracellular levels of $K^+$. Correcting the acidosis usually corrects the hyperkalemia.

Chloride is the chief anion in the extracellular fluid. Hypochloremia occurs when there is prolonged vomiting (loss of HCl), chronic respiratory acidosis (which elevates $HCO_3^-$ levels), addisonian crisis, and certain kidney diseases. Hyperchloremia is seen with prolonged diarrhea (loss of $HCO_3^-$), certain kidney diseases, and sometimes hyperparathyroidism.

Total $CO_2$ is technically not an electrolyte because the measure includes both physically dissolved $CO_2$ and that dissociated into $HCO_3^-$. Because about 95% of the total $CO_2$ consists of $HCO_3^-$, the two measures are often used interchangeably. As the second most plentiful anion in the serum and the key element in the carbonic acid buffer system, $HCO_3^-$ plays a major role in acid-base balance (see Chapter 8). Increased serum $HCO_3^-$ and $CO_2$ levels are observed in metabolic alkalosis or as compensation for respiratory acidosis. On the other hand, $HCO_3^-$ and $CO_2$ levels decrease in metabolic acidosis or as compensation for respiratory alkalosis.

Other electrolyte concentrations that are often measured include calcium ($Ca^{2+}$), phosphorus ($PO_4^-$), and magnesium ($Mg^{2+}$). $Ca^{2+}$ levels are controlled by parathyroid hormone (PTH). Patients with increased PTH have hypercalcemia. Because bone contains a large amount of calcium, certain bone diseases or metastasis of cancer to bone may result in hypercalcemia. Hypocalcemia occurs in vitamin D deficiency (rickets) and in various other hormonal aberrations. $PO_4^-$ metabolism is closely linked to that of $Ca^{2+}$. Abnormalities of $Mg^{2+}$ concentrations are common in the intensive care unit. Hypomagnesemia and hypocalcemia have been associated with respiratory muscle weakness, which makes ventilator weaning difficult.

## SIMPLY STATED

Normal electrolyte concentrations are essential for proper physiologic function of the body. Assessment of a patient's electrolytes can help identify causes of abnormalities such as irregular heart rhythms or respiratory muscle weakness.

Electrolyte values can be used to approximate the anion gap between the measured anions and cations and those that are not measured. Calculating the anion gap helps classify the acid balance status and define the cause of a metabolic acidosis. Chapter 8 provides details on the measurement and interpretation of the anion gap.

Analysis of the electrolyte concentration of sweat can assist in diagnosis of cystic fibrosis. The test is called a *sweat chloride test, sweat electrolytes,* or *iontophoretic sweat test.* The sweat glands of patients with cystic fibrosis have a diminished ability to reabsorb $Na^+$ and $Cl^-$. As a result, a high concentration of $Na^+$ and $Cl^-$ (>60 mmol/L) is present in the sweat.

### Glucose

Glucose is the major carbohydrate found in the blood. It is produced through digestion of dietary carbohydrates and used as a primary energy source by most body tissues, as well as by various blood cells. A common reference interval for fasting plasma glucose level (blood drawn after an overnight fast) is 70 to 99 mg/dL. After ingestion of carbohydrates, the glucose level normally rises in the first 60 to 90 minutes and then returns to the normal fasting level within 2 hours.

Glucose metabolism is regulated primarily by insulin, a hormone produced by the pancreas that decreases blood glucose levels. The most common glucose imbalance is **hyperglycemia**, most frequently caused by type 1 or type 2 diabetes. Patients with type 1 diabetes have decreased blood insulin levels as a result of failure of the pancreas to produce this hormone. Type 1 diabetes accounts for about 10% of cases in the United States. Patients with type 1 diabetes require daily doses of insulin for the rest of their life. Type 2 diabetes accounts for 90% of diabetes cases. Type 2 diabetes occurs when insulin made by the body is ineffective because of a problem in structure, function, or release.

Patients with diabetes are at greater risk for stroke, cardiovascular disease, serious infection, and renal failure. For this reason, patients with diabetes must regularly check their blood sugar levels and adjust their medication accordingly. Inadequate insulin dosing can result in impaired glucose metabolism, which forces the body to turn to fats and proteins as an energy source. The result is an abnormal accumulation of ketoacids. This buildup of organic acids causes a form of metabolic acidosis called ketoacidosis, which can represent a medical emergency often manifested by Kussmaul respirations (see Chapter 8). On the other hand, administration of too much insulin can cause hypoglycemia (discussed later).

Medications such as steroids, diuretics, antihypertensive drugs, birth control pills, and some immunosuppressive drugs also can cause hyperglycemia. Other conditions associated with hyperglycemia are acute stress (e.g., trauma, heart

### TABLE 7.4  Interpretation of Tests for Assessing Glucose Imbalances

|  | Fasting Blood Glucose | 2 hr Oral Glucose Tolerance Test | Glycosylated Hemoglobin |
|---|---|---|---|
| Non-diabetic | <100 mg/dL | <140 mg/dL | <5.7% |
| Prediabetes | 100-125 mg/dL | 140-199 mg/dL | 5.7%-6.4% |
| Diabetes | >125 mg/dL | ≥200 mg/dL | ≥6.5% |

attack, stroke), chronic renal failure, excessive food intake, hyperthyroidism, pancreatic cancer, and pancreatitis.

**Hypoglycemia** is a relatively uncommon problem caused by either pancreatic overproduction or excessive administration of insulin. Excessive production may occur in response to a rapid rise in blood sugar or as a result of insulin-producing pancreatic tumors. Both overproduction and excessive administration have the same effect, that is, a rapid fall in blood glucose. Hypoglycemia causes sweating, shaking, weakness, headaches, lethargy, and in severe cases, coma. Other conditions associated with hypoglycemia are excessive alcohol intake, severe liver disease, hypothyroidism, and starvation.

In 2016 the American Diabetes Association issued new diagnosis guidelines emphasizing that no one test is preferred over another for diagnosis of diabetes. The testing recommendations are as follows: (1) fasting plasma glucose (FPG), (2) the oral glucose tolerance test (OGTT), (3) the glycosylated Hb (HbA1c) test, and (4) a random plasma glucose in a patient with classic symptoms of hyperglycemia. The FPG is performed after an overnight fast. For the OGTT, an initial FPG test is performed. Then patients drink a standard amount of glucose solution. Two hours after this "challenge" to their system, a repeat plasma glucose test is performed. The HbA1c test measures the percentage of hemoglobin that is bound with glucose. In contrast to the FPG and OGTT tests, which provide "snapshots" of diabetic control, the HbA1c indicates average blood glucose control for the prior 2 to 3 months. However, it does not eliminate the need for patients' daily self-testing of their blood glucose levels. Several variables must be taken into consideration when using the A1c for diagnosis. These include age, race/ethnicity, and anemia/hemoglobinopathies. Table 7.4 summarizes the interpretation of these tests for glucose imbalances.

### Blood Urea Nitrogen and Creatinine

BUN and creatinine are common screening tests used to assess renal function and as such are included in both the basic metabolic and renal panels (see Table 7.3). Urea is a waste product of protein metabolism and is synthesized in the liver from amino groups and ammonia generated during protein catabolism. Therefore urea is constantly being formed and is excreted by the kidneys. BUN levels depend on renal function, diet, and liver function.

Many kidney diseases result in decreased filtration and thereby increased retention of urea, leading to an elevated BUN level. Other conditions that are associated with elevated BUN include increased metabolism (e.g., fever and stress), malignancy, congestive heart failure, ketoacidosis and dehydration in diabetes, gastrointestinal bleeding, sepsis, high-protein diet, some antibiotics, and burns. Conditions causing a decreased BUN include pregnancy, decreased dietary protein, and some antibiotics.

Creatinine is a waste product of creatine metabolism and produced in muscle. It enters the blood and is filtered out by the kidneys. Diet (e.g., protein intake), water intake, exercise, and urine output do not effect creatinine levels; thus increased creatinine levels are directly associated with renal function impairment. Creatinine serum levels usually remain nearly constant, reflecting the balance between its production and its filtration by the renal glomerulus. Creatinine can be elevated in shock, hypotension, congestive heart failure, dehydration, muscle atrophy, urinary obstruction caused by kidney stones, prostatic cancer, and anabolic steroid administration. Decreased creatinine levels are seen in muscle wasting conditions. Neither the BUN nor the creatinine level is sensitive to early renal disease.

When the BUN and creatinine are elevated as a result of renal failure, metabolic acidosis may be present (see Chapter 8). To compensate for metabolic acidosis, the respiratory system normally tries to restore the pH by increasing ventilation and reducing $Paco_2$ levels. Therefore patients with renal failure may have increased respiratory rates and may appear to be short of breath. However, if the patient with metabolic acidosis also has a concurrent respiratory disorder, respiratory compensation may not be possible, and the pH may remain dangerously low.

## Renal Panel

The renal panel includes BUN and creatinine and two non-blood analyses, the glomerular filtration rate (GFR) and urinalysis.

The ratio of BUN to creatinine can help determine the cause of increases in these analytes. The reference interval is usually between 10:1 and 20:1. An increased BUN-to-creatinine ratio can be observed in conditions causing decreased renal blood flow (e.g., congestive heart failure, dehydration). A decreased ratio may be observed with liver disease and malnutrition.

### Glomerular Filtration Rate

The GFR is used to measure kidney function and assess the stage of kidney disease. This is not a laboratory test per se but rather a calculation based on the serum creatinine level and the patient's age, gender, height, weight, and race. All else being equal, as the serum creatinine increases, the GFR decreases. The common reference interval is 90 to 120 mL per minute per 1.73 $m^2$. Older people will have lower normal GFR levels because GFR decreases with age. Levels below 60 mL per minute per 1.73 $m^2$ for 3 or more months are a sign of chronic kidney disease. A GFR below 15 mL per minute per 1.73 $m^2$ indicates renal failure and the need for immediate medical attention.

### Urinalysis

Routine urinalysis includes assessment of appearance, specific gravity, pH, protein, glucose, ketones, blood, bilirubin, urobilinogen, and other chemical compounds. A microscopic examination of the urine sediment may be performed if abnormalities are detected in the chemical analysis.

The appearance simply denotes the color and whether the urine appears clear or cloudy. The specific gravity indicates the concentration of the urine. More concentrated urine (specific gravity > 1.03) is seen in dehydration, whereas more dilute urine (specific gravity < 1.002) occurs with high fluid intake and when the kidneys are unable to concentrate urine normally. The pH of the urine reflects the acid-base status of the patient, typically ranging between 5 and 7. Lower urine pH levels indicate increased acid production.

Normally little to no protein appears in the urine. The presence of protein (proteinuria) usually indicates renal disease. Glucose in the urine (**glycosuria**) appears most commonly in diabetes but sometimes is caused by renal disease. Ketones occur with starvation and in diabetes mellitus. Hematuria, or RBCs in the urine, is a nonspecific finding caused by a variety of problems and some drugs. Bilirubin is present in urine in the conjugated form and is seen in liver disease and bile duct obstruction. Urobilinogen is normally present in the urine in small amounts but increases in some liver diseases and hemolytic states. A high urine WBC count suggests inflammation, most commonly associated with a urinary tract infection.

In addition to its analysis in the blood, urine creatinine also may be measured. By comparing creatinine concentrations in the blood and urine, the creatinine clearance test can help clinicians evaluate the efficiency of renal filtration. The average creatinine clearance is 90 to 125 mL per minute for males and 80 to 115 mL per minute for females. Clearance decreases approximately 1 mL per minute per year after age 50 years. Levels below the reference intervals indicate impaired kidney function or decreased renal blood flow.

## Hepatic Panel

The hepatic panel includes tests for blood proteins, liver-associated enzymes, and bilirubin. These tests are used primarily to help assess liver function.

### Proteins

There are two primary classes of proteins found in the blood, albumin and globulin. Albumin is produced by liver cells and makes up a large percentage of the total serum protein. There are more than 500 proteins classified as globulins, including enzymes and antibodies.

Albumin functions as a transport and storage vehicle for many hormones, drugs, and electrolytes. Albumin is also important in maintaining the oncotic pressure of blood, which helps keep water within the vascular space. In addition, albumin plays a primary role in lipid metabolism. Decreased albumin levels (hypoalbuminemia) are seen in various forms of protein malnutrition and in severe liver disease. Significant hypoalbuminemia leads to loss of fluid from the vascular space and can cause edema throughout the body, including in the lungs (pulmonary edema).

Total protein represents the sum of the albumin and globulins in the blood. Total protein analysis provides information on nutritional status and possible disease conditions. A decrease in total protein occurs in severe liver disease (many proteins are produced by the liver), in nephrotic syndrome (albumin lost through kidneys), and in severe malnutrition. Increased total protein is seen in inflammatory disorders and infections such as hepatitis and HIV or in certain bone marrow disorders such as multiple myeloma.

The total protein level has many limitations, in part because it does not reveal which of the many serum proteins may be abnormal. That information requires serum protein electrophoresis. For example, in multiple myeloma, a characteristic narrow band or spike pattern appears on electrophoresis, indicating a high concentration of a specific immunoglobulin.

### Liver-Associated Enzymes

There are three liver-associated enzymes in the hepatic panel: alkaline phosphatase, alanine aminotransferase, and aspartate aminotransferase. Abnormalities in these enzymes can indicate liver dysfunction or failure, which can lead to pulmonary complications such as hydrothorax, pulmonary hypertension, and hepatopulmonary syndrome.

Alkaline phosphatase (ALP) is an enzyme produced in the bile ducts that increases in response to obstruction of the duct, such as occurs in cholelithiasis. ALP also is present in bone, placenta, spleen, kidney, and intestine, where isoenzyme (different forms of the enzyme based on where it is produced) evaluation can often identify the source. For example, elevated bone ALP indicates increased new bone formation, as occurs in growing children.

Alanine aminotransferase (ALT) is found in high concentrations primarily in liver cells (hepatocytes). For this reason, ALT levels increase dramatically in acute liver damage, such as viral hepatitis.

Like ALT, aspartate aminotransferase (AST) is present in liver cells, but it also occurs in substantial concentrations in cardiac and skeletal muscle. As with ALT, very high AST levels occur with acute liver damage but may also indicate muscle trauma. High levels of AST in the presence of normal levels of ALT suggest extrahepatic injury. At one time, AST also was used as a biomarker for acute myocardial infarction (AMI). However, this test has been replaced by more sensitive and specific indicators of myocardial damage.

### Bilirubin

Bilirubin is a byproduct of the spleen's normal breakdown of hemoglobin. This unconjugated form of bilirubin is bound to albumin and cleared from the blood by the liver. Hepatocytes process the bilirubin into a water-soluble form called *conjugated bilirubin* that is excreted into the bile and eliminated through stool in the lower gastrointestinal tract. An increase in total blood levels of bilirubin (hyperbilirubinemia) can be due to (1) increased production (e.g., hemolytic anemia), (2) liver damage (e.g., cirrhosis, hepatitis), or (3) impaired excretion (e.g., bile duct obstruction). If the total bilirubin is increased, knowledge of the conjugated portion can help reveal the cause of the hyperbilirubinemia. An increased total bilirubin with a normal proportion of conjugated bilirubin indicates either an increase in RBC hemolysis or failure of the liver to process the bilirubin load (previously cited causes 1 and 2). On the other hand, if the total bilirubin and conjugated portion are both elevated, the likely cause is bile duct obstruction.

### Lipid Panel

Lipids are organic compounds used throughout the body as a fuel source, as building blocks for cell structure, and in many other important biologic functions. The lipid panel includes measurement of cholesterol, lipoproteins, and triglycerides.

Cholesterol is a steroid that is essential for the function of cells, tissues, and organs and is used to make hormones and bile. The body produces cholesterol, but it is also found in certain food sources, particularly those with high saturated fat content such as eggs and fatty meats. Unlike tests intended to diagnose disease states, cholesterol testing is used to estimate the risk for atherosclerosis and heart disease. As such, this test is an important component of preventive health care management.

Lipoproteins are complex combinations of both proteins and lipids. There are four major groups of lipoproteins, of which two are routinely tested: high-density lipoprotein cholesterol (HDL-C) and low-density lipoprotein cholesterol (LDL-C). HDL is referred to as the "good cholesterol" because it removes excess cholesterol from the circulation. LDL is referred to as the "bad cholesterol" because it deposits cholesterol on blood vessel walls, which can then lead to atherosclerosis.

Triglycerides are the main storage form of fat in humans, and fatty tissue is primarily made up of these substances. Accurate results require that patients follow a stable diet 2 weeks before the testing, avoid drinking alcohol for several days, and fast 9-12 hours before blood collection. Although very high levels are associated with a risk for pancreatitis, triglycerides are best assessed in combination with cholesterol and lipoproteins. Table 7.5 outlines the interpretation of these lipid panel measures by their common reference intervals.

### Cardiac Biomarkers

Cardiac biomarkers are chemicals that appear in the blood as a result of either ischemic myocardial damage or stress. They are helpful in diagnosing and monitoring patients with either acute coronary syndrome or congestive heart failure. Biomarkers of ischemic myocardial damage include total creatine kinase (CK) and its heart-specific isoenzyme CK-MB, myoglobin, and troponin. The current biomarker used to help diagnose congestive heart failure is B-type natriuretic peptide (BNP).

CK is primarily contained in skeletal muscle, myocardium, and brain tissue. Total CK values are elevated in AMI and various skeletal muscle diseases. Because high total CK levels are not very specific, testing for the more heart-specific CK-MB isoenzyme is needed to distinguish myocardial from general muscle damage. In AMI, CK-MB is elevated 4 to 6 hours after onset of symptoms, peaks at 24 hours, and returns to normal in 2 to 3 days (Fig. 7.2).

## TABLE 7.5   Lipid Profile Interpretation

| Test Result | Interpretation |
| --- | --- |
| **Total Cholesterol** | |
| <200 mg/dL | Desirable; low risk for heart disease |
| 200-239 mg/dL | Borderline; moderate risk for heart disease |
| >240 mg/dL | High; high risk for heart disease |
| **Low-Density Lipoprotein Cholesterol (LDL-C)** | |
| <100 mg/dL | Optimal |
| 100-129 mg/dL | Near optimal/above optimal |
| 130-159 mg/dL | Borderline high |
| 160-189 mg/dL | High |
| >190 mg/dL | Very high |
| **High-Density Lipoprotein Cholesterol (HDH-C)** | |
| <40 mg/dL (men); <50 mg/dL (women) | Low—increased risk |
| 40-50 mg/dL (men); 50-59 mg/dL (women) | Average level |
| >60 mg/dL (men and women) | Optimal |
| **Triglycerides (fasting)** | |
| <150 mg/dL—desired | |
| 150-199 mg/dL—borderline | |
| 200-299 mg/dL—high | |
| >500 mg/dL—very high | |

FIG. 7.2 Cardiac biomarkers plotted showing the multiples of the cutoff for acute myocardial infarction (AMI) over time. The *dashed horizontal line* shows the upper limit of normal, defined as the 99th percentile from a normal healthy reference population. (Reprinted with permission from Anderson JL, Adams CD, Antman EM, et al: ACC/AHA 2007 guidelines for the management of patients with unstable angina/non-ST-elevation myocardial infarction: a report of the American College of Cardiology/American Heart Association Task Force on Practice Guidelines. *J Am Coll Cardiol* 50:e1-e157, 2007.)

Myoglobin is a heme protein present in cardiac and skeletal muscle. Whenever there is significant muscle damage, myoglobin is elevated and can be measured. Although it is not specific for AMI, it is useful as an early biomarker because it is released from damaged myocardium or skeletal muscle within 2 to 4 hours after onset of infarction, peaks at 6 to 12 hours, and returns to normal within 24 to 36 hours (see Fig. 7.2).

Troponin is a complex of three proteins (troponin T, troponin I, troponin C) that helps regulate muscle contraction and normally is present in very small quantities in the blood. Only troponins I and T are found in the heart. Troponin I is considered the more specific of the two for the diagnosis of AMI and is considered the single best marker for acute coronary syndrome. Troponin I can be detected in the serum 3 to 6 hours after an AMI, peaks in about 12 hours, and can persists for 7 days or more (see Fig. 7.2). Troponin T is useful in patients who do not seek immediate medical attention for their symptoms because it peaks later (2 days) and remains elevated longer (7 to 10 days) than troponin I. High-sensitivity cardiac troponin (hs-cTn) appears to have better diagnostic accuracy but has not yet been approved by the Food and Drug Administration (FDA) for use in the United States.

BNP is a cardiac neurohormone secreted from membrane granules in the cardiac ventricles as a response to ventricular volume expansion and pressure overload. BNP levels lower than 100 pg/mL have a 90% negative predictive value and are thus useful in ruling out congestive heart failure (CHF).

A comparable positive predictive value for ruling in the diagnosis of CHF occurs with BNP levels greater than 500 pg/mL. Intermediate values are less helpful and may occur in conditions with similar symptoms, including renal insufficiency, cor pulmonale, and acute pulmonary embolism. As with all laboratory tests, BNP is not recommended as a stand-alone test, and clinical presentation and other laboratory test results should be considered in the patient assessment.

### SIMPLY STATED

Troponin I is the single best marker for diagnosis of acute coronary syndrome. As with all laboratory tests, the clinical presentation and other test results (e.g., ECG) should be considered in patient assessment.

## MICROBIOLOGY

Clinical microbiology includes routine bacteriology and the subspecialties of mycology, parasitology, virology, and mycobacteriology. Laboratory scientists specializing in microbiology isolate and identify microorganisms from body tissues and fluids and perform antimicrobial susceptibility testing on pathogens to determine which antibiotics will be most effective. Although bacteria are the most common organisms isolated, most microbiology laboratories can identify fungi, parasites, mycobacteria (tuberculosis [TB]), rickettsia, and viruses. If the microbiology laboratory does not have the ability to isolate and/or identify these rarer organisms, specimens are sent to a referral laboratory.

## Preanalytical Phase: Specimen Selection, Collection, and Transport

The preanalytical phase of analysis, specimen selection, collection, and transport is critical to producing quality results. All specimens for microbiologic analysis should be collected as soon as possible on onset of symptoms and before administration of antimicrobial therapy. Specimens should be transported in appropriate transport devices, containers, or special media to preserve the integrity and viability of organisms. After specimen collection, timely transport to the laboratory for processing and testing is also critical.

Specific guidelines have been established for collection and transport of specimens for health care providers who obtain microbiologic samples. Specimen selection is determined by the site of infection and suspected organism causing the infection or disease. Patient history and clinical information are vital in directing the appropriate management of microbiologic specimens.

Many body sites are normally sterile, and the isolation of any organisms from these sites may be significant. Normally, blood, pleural fluid, ascitic fluid, spinal fluid, urine, and tissue samples do not contain microorganisms and, if collected in a sterile manner, will not grow organisms when cultured. Other samples, such as stool and sputum, contain normal flora. Normal flora refers to microorganisms that under normal circumstances colonize or are present in a body site and do not cause disease. These organisms may contaminate a specimen during the collection process. Precautions should be taken during specimen collection to minimize the amount of normal flora. Another important consideration is antibiotic therapy. In general, specimens for microbiology analysis should be collected *before* use of antibiotics. If a patient has been receiving antibiotics, the organism causing the infection may not grow in culture, causing an invalid test result.

### Microscopic Examination of Specimens

Initial screening of a specimen is accomplished using a direct smear. Various stains are used, and the laboratory scientist selects the staining methods based on the type of organism suspected.

The most common stain is the Gram stain, which separates bacteria into gram-positive (purple) or gram-negative (red) groupings. The basic morphologic form of the organisms can be determined from the smear and be identified as predominantly spherical (cocci) or rod shaped (bacilli). For example, *Streptococcus pneumoniae* (the most common cause of bacterial pneumonia) appears as encapsulated, lancet-shaped, gram-positive diplococci (pairs). *Staphylococcus aureus* appears as gram-positive cocci in clusters. *Klebsiella pneumoniae* appears as short, fat, encapsulated gram-negative rods and *Haemophilus influenzae* as very short gram-negative rods often described as coccobacilli. For pulmonary specimens, and other specimens where mycobacteria (e.g., TB) are suspected, an acid-fast stain may be performed.

In combination with relevant clinical information, the Gram stain report provides the clinician with preliminary information helpful in making a proper diagnosis.

In addition, antibiotic treatment may be initiated based on this preliminary information.

### Culture and Sensitivity

Most specimens sent to the microbiology laboratory are for culture and sensitivity. Specimens are inoculated onto nutrient, selective, and differential agar or media that support the growth of various organisms. Although most organisms grow in 24 to 48 hours, some (e.g., mycobacteria, fungi) may require up to 6 weeks. The laboratory scientist observes the morphology of organisms growing on the media and determines whether potential pathogens are present. Definitive organism identification is accomplished through biochemical and enzymatic reactions or molecular diagnostic tests. Traditional biochemical tests may require an additional 24 to 48 hours for full identification. Along with the culture, a sensitivity test often is performed. The bacteria are grown in the presence of various antibiotics, thereby determining whether an organism is sensitive to a particular drug. This information is clinically important in selecting the proper antibiotic therapy.

Molecular diagnostic methods, such as polymerase-chain reaction (PCR), for bacteria, viruses, mycobacteria, fungi, and some antibiotic-resistance genes, are replacing many of the standard culture and biochemical identification assays. Results are reported in 30 minutes to 2 hours based on the method.

### Examination of Pulmonary Secretions

Three types of pulmonary specimens are acceptable for assessment of lower respiratory infections: (1) bronchoalveolar specimens (includes lavage fluid, brush sample, washing, and endotracheal aspirates); (2) expectorated sputum; and (3) induced sputum. Table 7.6 provides general guidelines for collection, transport, and storage of respiratory specimens.

#### Sputum Collection

Expectorated sputum is the preferred specimen for diagnosis of pneumonia. The goal of sputum collection is to obtain fresh, uncontaminated secretions from the tracheobronchial tree. This goal is readily achieved when the alert patient is carefully instructed by a trained health care provider, such as an RT, on the proper collection procedure (see Table 7.6). If tuberculosis is suspected, three sputum specimens are recommended to ensure recovery of mycobacteria. An early-morning specimen is optimum and will have the highest yield of mycobacteria (AFB bacilli). The minimum quantity is 3 to 5 mL.

Occasionally, sputum induction is needed to obtain an adequate sample. Sputum induction is accomplished by having the patient breathe a slightly irritating mist, usually hypertonic saline. The mist increases flow of bronchial secretions (bronchorrhea) and stimulates a cough, which usually results in a specimen of adequate volume. Patient preparation for and transport of induced sputum samples are the same as for expectorated sputum.

If a culture is required but the patient is unwilling or unable to produce a sputum specimen (such as a young child or unconscious adult), either tracheobronchial suctioning or bronchoscopic lavage may be needed. Bronchoscopic lavage is performed by a physician during a bronchoscopy, usually with the assistance of an RT (see Chapter 17).

### Sputum Examination

*Macroscopic Examination.* Gross examination of the sample should be conducted at the bedside to determine its origin. Appropriate sputum samples from the tracheobronchial tree typically are more viscous and purulent than saliva. A specimen obviously containing mostly saliva usually is discarded. Macroscopic examination of the sputum also identifies such characteristics as color, presence of blood, general viscosity, and odor, which can provide a presumptive diagnosis (see Chapter 3).

*Microscopic Examination.* On receipt of the sputum specimen in the microbiology laboratory, the laboratory scientist performs a Gram stain. This examination assesses specimen quality and provides information about microorganisms present in the sample. A good specimen will have few squamous epithelial cells and numerous polymorphonuclear leukocytes. A high number of epithelial cells suggests oral contamination. Depending on the laboratory protocol, this type of specimen may be rejected, and no further testing will be performed.

If the specimen is deemed acceptable, the microscopic examination will also provide a preliminary report of the microbial composition of the sputum along with quantitation. For example, the report may indicate numerous gram-positive cocci in pairs (diplococcic) suggestive of pneumococci or numerous gram-negative diplococci suggestive of *H. influenzae*. This preliminary screening information provides a quick presumptive organism identification that will aid in diagnosis and early initiation of antibiotic treatment.

The specimen is then set up for culture on agar plates. The purposes of specimen culturing are to (1) determine whether a pathogen actually is present, (2) definitively identify it, and (3) assess its susceptibility to antimicrobial agents. Typically, culture results are provided within 24 to 48 hours.

After a patient has been on a regimen of antimicrobial therapy, the Gram stain and culture results can change. If the antibiotic is effective against the pathogen causing the infection, the Gram stain and culture will no longer demonstrate the pathogen but instead will reveal organisms consistent with normal flora. If, on the other hand, the antibiotic is not effective against the organism responsible for the patient's infection, the Gram stain and culture will continue to demonstrate the pathogen.

---

**SIMPLY STATED**

Sputum Gram stain, culture, and antimicrobial sensitivity can be useful in determining the organism responsible for the respiratory infection and the appropriate antimicrobial therapy to treat the infection; use of antibiotics by the patient before collecting the specimen can influence results of the Gram stain, culture, and antimicrobial susceptibility results.

---

Additional microscopic examination of sputum may be performed using others stains, such as the Wright stain or Giemsa stain. These stains can be used to determine sputum eosinophil counts. If the leukocytes observed in a sputum stain are predominantly eosinophils, exposure to an allergen is likely. Sputum eosinophil counts are useful in differentiating among asthma phenotypes and monitoring the condition once therapy is discontinued. Besides asthma, eosinophilia has been associated with certain microbial infections, particularly some parasitic infections.

### Bronchoalveolar Lavage

Bronchoalveolar lavage (BAL) is performed during bronchoscopy by injecting a large volume of sterile fluid into the patient's lung (see Chapter 17). This fluid mixes with the respiratory secretions within the airways and alveoli and is subsequently withdrawn for analysis in the laboratory. BAL has two main functions: (1) to evaluate the need for therapy in patients with interstitial lung disease (diseases that often cause pulmonary fibrosis) by analysis of the cells obtained in the lavage solution and (2) to collect a quality specimen that can be analyzed for the presence of microorganisms that cause pneumonia. BAL is contraindicated in patients with severely reduced pulmonary function, hypoxemia, severe cardiovascular disease, or serious electrolyte disturbances.

---

| TABLE 7.6 | Respiratory Specimen Collection, Transport, and Storage Guidelines | |
|---|---|---|
| **Specimen Type** | **Collection Procedure** | **Transport/Storage** |
| Sputum | No food for 1-2 h before collection | Sterile container, >1 mL |
| Expectorated or induced | Brush teeth, gums, tongue Rinse/gargle with water Deep cough Collect in sterile container Minimize contamination with saliva | Room temperature if transported to laboratory within 2 h Refrigerate if delay in transport to laboratory up to 24 h |
| Bronchoalveolar (BAL) Bronchial brushings/washings, Tracheal aspirates | Collect liquids in sterile sputum trap Place brush in sterile container with 1 mL sterile saline | Sterile container, >1 mL Room temperature, if transported to laboratory within 2 h Refrigerate if delay in transport to laboratory up to 24 h |

After the lavage solution is recovered from the patient, the sample is sent to the laboratory for microscopic analysis. Lavage solution obtained from healthy nonsmokers is 91% to 95% macrophages, 6% to 8% lymphocytes, and 1% granulocytes (neutrophils and eosinophils). The cellular composition of this fluid shows characteristic alterations in diseases such as pulmonary sarcoidosis and hypersensitivity pneumonitis.

## Pleural Fluid Examination

Normal pleural fluid is clear and pale yellow. Usually, only small amounts of fluid (3 to 20 mL) are present in the pleura. Pleural fluid (effusion, transudate, thoracentesis, empyema) is collected by percutaneous needle aspiration or surgery. A volume of at least 1 mL is required for microbiology workup; however, as much fluid as possible should be sent to the laboratory for analysis, particularly if additional testing is required. Fluid is immediately transported to the laboratory in a sterile screw-cap tube or anaerobic transport system at room temperature, and the specimen should *not* be refrigerated.

It is important to differentiate between the types of pleural fluid to aid in diagnosis of the disease or condition. A set of pleural fluid-to-serum ratios, known as *Light's criteria,* are used to distinguish between transudates and exudates. According to these criteria, the presence of any one of the following defines the fluid as an exudate:

- The ratio of pleural fluid protein to serum protein is greater than 0.5.
- The ratio of pleural fluid lactic dehydrogenase (LDH) to serum LDH is greater than 0.6.
- Pleural fluid LDH is greater than 0.6 times the normal upper limit for serum.

Additional criteria used by some laboratories to distinguish between transudates and exudates are summarized in Table 7.7.

After the type of fluid is determined, additional tests may be performed to confirm the diagnosis. Transudates usually require no further testing and are often caused by cirrhosis, CHF, and chronic renal failure. Exudates are associated with several conditions and diseases and usually require additional testing. Exudates may be caused by infections such as bacterial pneumonia or TB, pulmonary abscess, pulmonary infarction, fungal or viral infection, trauma, various cancers, and pancreatitis. Additional tests include glucose (decreased in infection and inflammation), lactate level (increased in infection and inflammation), amylase (increased in pancreatitis), triglycerides (extremely elevated in thoracic duct leakage), pH, and biomarkers for certain tumors.

Normal pleural fluid may have a few WBCs but no RBCs or microorganisms present. Pleural fluid associated with bacterial infection will be cloudy and have increased WBCs (neutrophils), and Gram or other stains will demonstrate microorganisms. A culture and sensitivity test will provide definitive identification of the pathogen and data on appropriate antibiotics to treat the patient. Pleural fluid associated with pulmonary infarction will demonstrate an increase in the RBC count.

## HISTOLOGY AND CYTOLOGY

Biopsy of lung tissue may be done either through a bronchoscope or by means of thoracotomy or thoracoscopy. Biopsy specimens are sent to the histology or surgical pathology laboratory. The tissue is processed, cut very thin, placed on a glass slide, and stained. The pathologist examines the cells with a microscope. This can yield valuable information about infectious processes, chronic lung diseases, and benign and malignant tumors. An acid-fast (Ziehl-Neelsen) stain can be done on tissue to identify mycobacteria (TB or TB-like organisms). Gomori methenamine silver (GMS) and periodic acid–Schiff (PAS) stains may be used to identify fungal organisms. GMS stain can also demonstrate *Pneumocystis* organisms, a cause of pneumonia in immunosuppressed patients, such as those with AIDS. Tissue Gram stains may also be performed.

Surgical removal of lung cancer requires close cooperation between the surgeon and surgical pathologist. The surgical pathologist must provide immediate reports to the surgeon regarding the presence of cancer in the resected lung, the type of cancer present, whether the surgical margins are clear, and whether there are metastases in local or regional lymph nodes. Because of the need for prompt feedback during surgery, specimens cannot be processed in the usual way. Instead the tissue is frozen so that it can be immediately sectioned and reviewed under the microscope. The frozen sections are thicker and more difficult to evaluate than standard sections but are usually adequate for surgical guidance. Final histology reports are issued after surgery, when standard processing and stains have been completed.

Tumors of the lung may be benign or malignant. A classification of malignant lung tumors is shown in Box 7.5. Benign lung tumors are less common than malignant tumors, with hamartoma (a benign proliferation of elements normally occurring in the lung) being seen most often. The non–small

### TABLE 7.7 Criteria for Pleural Fluid Differentiation

| Test | Transudate | Exudate |
|---|---|---|
| Physical characteristics | Clear | Cloudy |
| Protein | <25 g/L | >35 g/L |
| Fluid-to-serum protein ratio | <0.5 | >0.5 |
| Fluid-to-serum LDH ratio | <0.67 | >0.67 |
| Fluid cholesterol | <60 mg/dL | >60 mg/dL |
| Fluid-to-serum cholesterol ratio | <0.3 | >0.3 |
| Fluid-to-bilirubin ratio | <0.6 | >0.6 |

### BOX 7.5 Histologic Classification of Malignant Lung Tumors

1. Non–small cell lung cancer (NSCLC)
   a. Adenocarcinoma
   b. Squamous cell carcinoma
   c. Large cell carcinoma
2. Small cell lung cancer (SCLC)

cell lung cancers (squamous cell carcinoma, adenocarcinoma, and large cell carcinoma) represent approximately 80% to 85% of the primary lung tumors, whereas small cell lung cancer represents about 10% to 15%. These tumors collectively are called *bronchogenic carcinoma*. They are usually related to smoking (with the possible exception of adenocarcinoma) and are highly malignant. Tumors consisting of a mixture of cell types and other rare types of tumors may occur. Secondary or metastatic tumors to the lung are also common. Metastases to the lung arise from squamous carcinomas originating from the gastrointestinal tract or adenocarcinomas from breast, colon, and kidney, as well as hematopoietic malignancies.

Cytology is the study of fluids, secretions, or other body samples that contain cellular material but not actual fragments of intact tissue. The cells are spread on a glass slide, stained with the Papanicolaou stain, and examined by a cyto-technologist and pathologist. Often, the presence of malignancy and even the type of malignancy can be determined in this manner. Pulmonary samples that can be examined cytologically include sputum, bronchial washings, bronchial brushings, pleural fluid, and fine-needle aspiration (FNA) of lung tissue or lung masses. In FNA, a small needle is inserted into a mass, and some of the cellular material is aspirated and spread onto a slide. The slide is stained and examined, often yielding accurate information about the nature of the mass. FNA of lung masses is performed under radiologic guidance. For many years, this procedure has been widely used to evaluate lung masses and has proved to be a safe, simple, and effective way to diagnose malignant tumors and other processes without requiring major surgery.

## SKIN TESTING

Historically, skin testing was used to help diagnose selected infections (such as TB and coccidioidomycosis) and allergic disorders. The procedure involves injecting a small amount of the protein essence of the organism or allergen into the subcutaneous layer of the skin. The development of an inflammatory nodule at the location of the injection indicates an immune response to the foreign material. Unfortunately, many people develop immune unresponsiveness to foreign material, a condition called anergy. For this reason, many skin tests used to assess for infections and allergens have been replaced by serologic testing of the patient's immune responses.

The exception is the Mantoux tuberculin skin test for TB, also referred to as the *PPD test*. The test is performed by administering 0.1 mL of tuberculin purified protein derivative (PPD) by injection into the subcutaneous layer of skin, and the site is evaluated in 48 to 72 hours. The test is positive if an intradermal or subdermal nodule develops at the site of injection. This is a cellular reaction and indicates that the patient has been infected by TB or a TB-like organism. TB causes the strongest reaction, but other nontuberculous mycobacteria can produce weakly positive reactions. Because of this cross-reactivity, there is a set of criteria for interpreting a positive PPD. A normal healthy person without risk for exposure to TB is classified as PPD skin test positive only if the skin reaction produced a 15-mm diameter welt, whereas an HIV-positive or other immunocompromised patient is classified as positive with a 5-mm diameter skin nodule.

Older patients may have had a positive skin test in the past that eventually reverts to negative. A two-step skin test with the second test performed 3 weeks after the first test often shows a true positive when the first test produced a negative result. Multiple skin tests performed on a patient who has never been exposed to TB do not cause a positive result. Bacille Calmette-Guérin (BCG) vaccination, which is common in countries with a high prevalence of TB, causes a positive PPD skin test up to 10 years after vaccination; therefore positive PPD skin tests more than 10 years after BCG vaccination usually suggest a true TB infection.

An alternative to the TB skin test (PPD) is the interferon-γ release assay (IGRA). This is a blood test that measures how the immune system reacts to the bacteria that cause TB. This test only requires one visit to have blood drawn, unlike the two-step PPD skin test. The blood test results are available in 24 to 48 hours. Another advantage is that prior BCG vaccination does not cause a false-positive test result. There are two IGRA tests FDA approved for use in the United States: QuantiFERON-TB Gold In-Tube test (QFT-GIT) and T-SPOT TB Test (T-Spot).

Neither the TB skin test nor the TB blood test confirms a diagnosis of TB. A positive test result only indicates that a person has been infected with TB bacteria. Neither test is able to indicate whether a person has latent TB infection or active TB disease. Additional tests such as a chest radiograph and sputum AFB stain and culture are required to confirm a diagnosis of TB.

---

**SIMPLY STATED**

The PPD skin test and the IGRA blood tests for TB must be interpreted in light of the patient's medical history, and additional tests such as x-ray and sputum AFB stain and culture are required to confirm TB disease.

---

## RECOMMENDED LABORATORY TESTS

Assessment of lung disease and pulmonary function is covered in detail in various chapters of this book. The clinical laboratory provides testing associated with care of patients with respiratory disorders, including analysis of arterial blood gases (see Chapter 8), CBC, various chemistry panels, pulmonary specimen culture, special stains (TB), and cytologic examination. Table 7.8 provides a brief overview of the common recommended laboratory tests based on patient presentation. Results from these tests may suggest additional diagnostic tests. The need for additional testing depends on each individual presentation, the clinician's practice protocols, and test algorithms and protocols established by each facility. Consultation with a clinical laboratory scientist is recommended if additional advanced testing is indicated.

TABLE 7.8    **Common Laboratory Tests Related to Respiratory Care**

| Patient Presentation | Recommended Tests |
| --- | --- |
| Evidence of tissue hypoxia but with normal $Pao_2$, $Spo_2$ (e.g., fatigue, cognitive disturbances) | CBC, reticulocyte count, lactic acid, CO-oximetry (see Chapter 8) |
| Postoperative patient with low-grade fever—possible pneumonia | CBC with differential, blood culture, sputum culture |
| Fluid balance disturbances | CBC, electrolytes, urinalysis |
| Decreased or absent urine output | Electrolytes, BUN, creatinine, GFR urinalysis |
| Chest pain, suspected MI or ischemia | Electrolytes, cardiac biomarkers |
| Hepatic disease (e.g., suspected hepatitis, history of alcohol or drug abuse) | Electrolytes, hepatic panel, acute viral hepatitis serology |
| Acid-base disturbances | ABGs (see Chapter 8), electrolytes, BUN, creatinine, GFR, urinalysis |
| PVCs or cardiac dysrhythmias without history of cardiac disease | Electrolytes, lipid panel |
| Uncontrolled bleeding or monitoring anticoagulation therapy | CBC and WBC differential, platelet count, PT/INR, APTT |

*ABGs,* Arterial blood gases; *APTT,* activated partial thromboplastin time; *BUN,* blood urea nitrogen; *CBC,* complete blood count; *GFR,* glomerular filtration rate; *MI,* myocardial infarction; *PT/INR,* prothrombin time/international normalized ratio; *PVCs,* premature ventricular contractions; *WBC,* white blood cell.

## KEY POINTS

- Blood consists of two major components: plasma and blood cells (WBCs, RBCs, and platelets).
- Tests that evaluate the cellular elements of the blood include the CBC, platelet count, and reticulocyte count.
- WBCs that can be seen in the peripheral blood of healthy individuals are neutrophils, eosinophils, basophils, lymphocytes, and monocytes.
- Neutrophils usually constitute 50% to 70% of the blood's WBCs and are the body's first line of defense against microbial infections.
- Lymphocytes are particularly important in the body's defense against viral, TB, and intracellular organisms. Lymphocytes normally comprise 20% to 45% of circulating WBCs.
- Leukocytosis is an increase in the WBC count above the reference interval. A decrease in the WBC count is called leukopenia.
- Neutrophilia is a common response to inflammation and infection.
- Lymphocytosis (increase in lymphocytes) typically is seen in viral infections, especially infectious mononucleosis.
- Monocytosis (increase in monocytes) is characteristic of chronic infections, including TB, syphilis, typhoid fever, and subacute bacterial endocarditis.
- RBCs are produced in the bone marrow by maturation of nucleated cells known as normoblasts; RBCs have a life span of approximately 120 days.
- Anemia is a decrease in the oxygen-carrying capacity of the blood and is clinically defined by a decrease in the hemoglobin level below the reference interval for the gender and age of the patient.
- Polycythemia is an increase in the RBC count, hemoglobin, and hematocrit and may be primary, secondary, or relative.
- Platelets are the smallest cells in the peripheral blood and play a vital role in hemostasis and clot formation at the site of an injury to a blood vessel.
- A decrease in the platelet count is called thrombocytopenia.
- The four electrolytes measured in the basic metabolic panel are $Na^+$, $K^+$, $Cl^-$, and total $CO_2$.

- Increased serum $Na^+$ concentration (hypernatremia) is seen when the body loses water without salt (e.g., profuse sweating, diarrhea, renal diseases, or prolonged hyperpnea) and if there is lack of sufficient water intake.
- Decreased $Na^+$ concentration (hyponatremia) is caused by either excess free water intake and retention or excess sodium loss.
- Hypokalemia (decreased serum $K^+$) occurs when there is increased loss of potassium or decreased intake or when $K^+$ ions shift from extracellular to intracellular water space.
- Hyperkalemia (elevated serum $K^+$) can occur with increased intake, with decreased output, or when $K^+$ ions shift from intracellular to extracellular water space.
- The anion gap is the difference between the measured and unmeasured anions and cations which can help classify the cause of metabolic acidosis.
- Elevated blood glucose level is called hyperglycemia. It occurs for a variety of reasons but is most often related to diabetes.
- The most common screening tests in assessing renal function are the BUN and creatinine.
- High levels of AST occur with acute hepatitis. ALP is useful in evaluating liver disease and bone disease.
- Troponin I is the most specific current biomarker for identifying ischemic myocardial damage.
- Proper specimen selection, collection, and transport are prerequisites to obtaining quality microbiology test results.
- Microscopic examination of sputum will assess specimen quality; a high epithelial cell count indicates oral contamination and that the specimen is not useful for diagnostic purposes.
- Results of the sputum Gram stain and culture normally are affected by antibiotic therapy.
- The most commonly used skin test is the Mantoux tuberculin skin test for TB (PPD test).
- An alternative to the TB skin test is the interferon-$\gamma$ release assay, or IGRA, which measures how the immune system reacts to the presence of mycobacteria.

## CASE STUDY 7.1

A 22-year-old woman was brought to the emergency department by her mother with chief complaints of cough, fever, and chills for the past 3 days. The patient has a history of Down syndrome and lives at home with her parents. Initial examination reveals tachycardia, tachypnea, fever, and normal blood pressure. Chest auscultation identifies bronchial breath sounds and inspiratory and expiratory crackles over the right lower lobe. The admitting physician orders a sputum Gram stain and culture, CBC, and chest film. The initial laboratory results are as follows:

| CBC | Result | Reference Interval |
|---|---|---|
| WBC ($\times 10^3/\mu$L) | 19.5 | 4.0-11.0 |
| RBC ($\times 10^6/\mu$L) | 4.53 | 4.00-5.40 |
| Hb (g/dL) | 10.6 | 12.0-16.0 |
| Hct (%) | 34.9 | 35-49 |
| MCV (fL) | 77.0 | 80.0-100.0 |
| MCHC (g/dL) | 30.4 | 32-36 |

**White Blood Cell Differential (%)**

| | | |
|---|---|---|
| Segmented neutrophils | 90 | 50-70 |
| Lymphocytes | 8 | 20-45 |
| Monocytes | 2 | 2-11 |
| Eosinophils | 0 | 1-3 |
| Basophils | 0 | 0-1 |
| Left shift/immature granulocytes present | | |

Sputum: Gram stain: 2+ gram-positive cocci in chains, pairs tetrads, and groups; 1+ WBCs with many epithelial cells

**Interpretation**

Leukocytosis is present and is the result of an increase in the neutrophils consistent with a bacterial infection (probably pneumonia). The left shift indicates the presence of immature granulocytes (bands or younger neutrophils) due to the stress on the bone marrow to release more neutrophils to fight the infection. The relative decrease in the percentage of lymphocytes is caused by the absolute increase in the number of neutrophils and is not an abnormality.

The RBC count is within the reference interval; however, the decreases in hemoglobin, hematocrit, MCV, and MCHC are consistent with a mild microcytic, hypochromic anemia. Further investigation is needed to identify the cause, but iron deficiency anemia is a common reason.

The Gram stain of the sputum revealed many epithelial cells indicating contamination with saliva. The sample should be discarded and another sputum sample obtained.

## CASE STUDY 7.2

A 65-year-old woman was brought to the emergency department by her husband. The patient is complaining of severe shortness of breath, weakness, and cough. She has a long history of COPD and a 90 pack-year smoking history, currently admitting to smoking 1 pack/day. In the emergency department, she appears acutely and chronically ill and is found to be using her accessory muscles to breathe. She is cyanotic and has decreased breath sounds bilaterally. The patient is started on oxygen by nasal cannula, and the attending physician orders a CBC, electrolyte determination, and other tests. The results are as follows:

| Test | Result | Reference Interval |
|---|---|---|
| WBC ($\times 10^3/\mu$L) | 19.9 | 4.0-11.0 |
| RBC ($\times 10^6/\mu$L) | 5.1 | 4.00-5.40 |
| Hb (g/dL) | 15.8 | 12.0-16.0 |
| Hct (%) | 48.5 | 35-49 |
| MCV (fL) | 95.1 | 80.0-100 |
| MCHC (g/dL) | 32.6 | 32-36 |

**White Blood Cell Differential (%)**

| | | |
|---|---|---|
| Segmented neutrophils | 78 | 50-70 |
| Lymphocytes | 12 | 20-45 |
| Monocytes | 7 | 2-11 |
| Eosinophils | 3 | 1-3 |
| Basophils | 0 | 0-1 |

**Electrolytes (mmol/L)**

| | | |
|---|---|---|
| Na$^+$ | 137 | 135-145 |
| K$^+$ | 4.8 | 3.5-5.0 |
| Cl$^-$ | 87 | 98-107 |
| Total CO$_2$ | 41 | 22-30 |

**Interpretation**

The increase in WBCs indicates leukocytosis and is the result of an increase in the number of circulating neutrophils. This may be in response to a bacterial infection or acute stress. The RBC count, hemoglobin, and hematocrit are in the upper reference interval. These findings are consistent with secondary polycythemia typical for patients with a chronic lung disease in which the arterial blood oxygen levels are persistently low.

The electrolyte values reveal a decreased serum Cl$^-$ and an increased serum CO$_2$. This probably is related to the patient's long-term history of COPD. Some patients with COPD chronically retain CO$_2$ because of poor pulmonary function. To compensate for the elevated CO$_2$, the kidneys retain increased levels of serum HCO$_3^-$ in an effort to maintain a near-normal serum pH. The resulting metabolic buildup of serum HCO$_3^-$ is reflected as an increased total CO$_2$ in the venous blood sample. The increase in serum CO$_2$ (HCO$_3^-$) causes the kidneys to excrete more than the usual amount of Cl$^-$ in an effort to maintain electrical neutrality. As a result, serum Cl$^-$ levels typically are reduced in patients with chronically elevated serum CO$_2$.

## CASE STUDY 7.3

A 27-year-old man has a CD4 count of 120 (reference interval, 550 to 1600/μL). He is concerned about his chronic cough and sputum production. The sputum has been negative for WBCs and bacteria. A PPD skin test was placed on his right forearm 2 days ago, and a 3-cm reddened area and a 5-mm nodule have appeared at the skin test site. Initial laboratory data results are as follows:

| CBC | Result | Reference Interval |
|---|---|---|
| WBC ($\times10^3$/μL) | 5.0 | 4.0-11.0 |
| Hb (g/dL) | 14 | 14.0-18.0 |
| Hct (%) | 42 | 40-54 |
| MCV (fL) | 92 | 80-100 |

| White Blood Cell Differential (%) | | |
|---|---|---|
| Segmented neutro-phils | 70 | 50-70 |
| Lymphocytes | 20 | 20-45 |
| Monocytes | 6 | 2-11 |
| Eosinophils | 4 | 0-3 |
| Basophils | 0 | 0-1 |
| Sedimentation rate (mm/hr) | 40 (elevated) | 0-15 |

### Interpretation

The low CD4 count suggests that the patient is moderately immunocompromised, possibly caused by HIV. The elevated sedimentation rate suggests inflammation, which could be caused by TB or other infection. The large area of redness around the skin test site is not significant. The 5-mm nodule in this immunocompromised patient indicates TB infection. It is anticipated that sputum cultures will be positive in 6 weeks. A PCR test for TB bacilli in the patient's sputum is likely to be positive. This patient's normal CBC is expected despite his chronic infection because TB does not usually cause an elevated WBC count.

## CASE STUDY 7.4

A 20-year-old man was brought to the emergency department by ambulance following a motor vehicle crash. He was driving in a local canyon when a deer ran out in front of his car and caused him to lose control. The vehicle left the road and rolled over in the canyon. He complains of a stiff neck and left leg pain. Although very upset and scared, he is conscious and able to move all extremities. Vital signs are normal except for a heart rate of 110 beats per minute. His initial CBC reveals the following:

| Test | Result | Reference Interval |
|---|---|---|
| WBC ($\times10^9$/L) | 14.9 | 4.0-11.0 |
| RBC ($\times10^{12}$/L) | 5.1 | 4.60-6.00 |
| Hb (g/dL) | 15.0 | 14.0-18.0 |
| Hct (%) | 45.5 | 40-54 |
| MCV (fL) | 89.2 | 80.0-100.0 |
| MCHC (g/dL) | 33.0 | 32-36 |

| White Blood Cell Differential (%) | | |
|---|---|---|
| Segmented neutro-phils | 77 | 50-70 |
| Lymphocytes | 13 | 20-45 |
| Monocytes | 5 | 2-11 |
| Eosinophils | 4 | 1-3 |
| Basophils | 1 | 0-1 |

No WBC abnormalities noted.

### Interpretation

The RBC count, hemoglobin, hematocrit, and indices are all within their reference intervals. The elevated WBC count suggests possible infection; however, the lack of fever and absence of a left shift or immature granulocytes on the WBC differential suggest otherwise. This is most likely a case of pseudoneutrophilia, in which marginated neutrophils are released into circulation as a result of sudden stress (the accident). This type of neutrophilia is usually transient and resolves spontaneously in a matter of hours.

## ASSESSMENT QUESTIONS

1. Which of the following is not a component of the cellular elements of the blood?
   a. RBCs
   b. Lipids
   c. WBCs
   d. Platelets
2. What is the medical name for platelets?
   a. Leukocytes
   b. Thrombocytes
   c. Reticulocytes
   d. Erythrocytes
3. What is the primary role of white blood cells?
   a. Carry oxygen
   b. Promote blood clotting
   c. Fight infection
   d. Boost metabolism

4. What is the reference interval for WBCs?
   a. 1000 to 3000/μL
   b. 3000 to 5000/μL
   c. 4000 to 11,000/μL
   d. 600 to 14,000/μL
5. Which of the following white cell types normally represents the largest percent in the WBC differential?
   a. Neutrophils
   b. Eosinophils
   c. Basophils
   d. Lymphocytes
6. A left-shifted white cell differential is evidenced by which of the following findings?
   a. An increase in the number of eosinophils
   b. A decrease in the number of segmented neutrophils
   c. An increase in the number of bands (immature neutrophils)
   d. A decrease in the number of lymphocytes

7. Which of the following is a common finding in patients with bacterial pneumonia?
   a. Neutrophilia
   b. Leukopenia
   c. Lymphocytopenia
   d. Eosinophilia

8. Which of the following is a common finding in a patient with an allergic reaction?
   a. Neutropenia
   b. Leukopenia
   c. Eosinophilia
   d. Monocytosis

9. Viral infections typically produce which of the following abnormalities?
   a. Lymphocytosis
   b. Eosinophilia
   c. Basophilia
   d. Monocytosis

10. Your patient has AIDS. The most useful test to identify the prognosis of AIDS is:
    a. Leukocyte count
    b. CD4 count
    c. Monocyte count
    d. Hemoglobin A1c

11. Chemotherapy used to treat cancer can cause a suppression of blood counts for which of the following cells?
    a. Neutrophils
    b. Erythrocytes
    c. Thrombocytes
    d. All of the above

12. Your patient may have active TB. What laboratory finding is most consistent with this suspicion?
    a. Lymphocytosis
    b. Anemia
    c. Monocytosis
    d. Eosinophilia

13. Which of the following statements is (are) true regarding hemoglobin?
    a. It functions in oxygen transport
    b. It is the main component of RBCs
    c. It functions in $CO_2$ transport
    d. All of the above

14. Which of the following is the most common cause of anemia?
    a. Drug-induced RBC lysis
    b. Acute blood loss
    c. Iron deficiency
    d. None of the above

15. Which of the following is not true regarding polycythemia?
    a. It can be caused by chronic hypoxemia
    b. It is defined as an increase in RBCs, Hb, and Hct
    c. It increases the oxygen-carrying capacity of the blood
    d. It decreases the workload on the heart

16. Which of the following tests is used to assess the patient's blood-clotting ability?
    a. RBC count
    b. Hemoglobin
    c. Hematocrit
    d. Prothrombin time

17. Which of the following electrolytes closely affects muscle function?
    a. Sodium
    b. Potassium
    c. Chloride
    d. Phosphorus

18. Which of the following electrolytes is mainly responsible for extracellular water balance?
    a. Calcium
    b. Sodium
    c. Magnesium
    d. Potassium

19. Anion gap is useful in assessing the cause of:
    a. Metabolic alkalosis
    b. Metabolic acidosis
    c. Respiratory acidosis
    d. Respiratory alkalosis

20. An increase in the sweat electrolyte concentration is seen in:
    a. Cystic fibrosis
    b. Patent ductus arteriosus
    c. Bronchiectasis
    d. Epiglottitis

21. Which of the following tests is (are) a measure of kidney function?
    a. BUN
    b. Creatine kinase
    c. Creatinine
    d. a and c

22. The recommend test for early detection of myocardial infarction is:
    a. AST
    b. LDH
    c. CPK
    d. Troponin

23. Which of the following bacteriologic tests is used to determine the effectiveness of antibiotics on a particular organism?
    a. Gram stain
    b. Culture
    c. Sensitivity
    d. Acid-fast stain

24. A Ziehl-Neelsen stain is used to identify which of the following organisms?
    a. *Staphylococcus aureus*
    b. *Pseudomonas aeruginosa*
    c. *Streptococcus pneumoniae*
    d. *Mycobacterium tuberculosis*

25. Which of the following items are evaluated during a macroscopic (gross) sputum examination?
    a. Color
    b. Consistency
    c. Volume
    d. All of the above
26. Which of the following is the most common cause of bacterial pneumonia?
    a. *Streptococcus pneumoniae*
    b. *Pseudomonas aeruginosa*
    c. *Haemophilus influenzae*
    d. *Klebsiella pneumoniae*
27. Which of the following findings is (are) consistent with pleural infection?
    a. Bloody pleural fluid
    b. Low pleural fluid protein levels
    c. Opaque or turbid pleural fluid
    d. All of the above
28. Which of the following tests performed during urinalysis could be helpful in diagnosing diabetes mellitus?
    a. Glucose
    b. pH
    c. Ketones
    d. All of the above
29. Proteinuria usually is indicative of which of the following?
    a. COPD
    b. Kidney disease
    c. Cardiovascular disease
    d. Spinal meningitis
30. Which of the following may cause a patient to have a negative reaction to a skin test?
    a. He or she does not have the disease
    b. He or she is anergic
    c. The disease has progressed to a point beyond treatment
    d. a and b
31. Which of the following is true regarding a PPD?
    a. It is positive with coccidioidomycosis infection
    b. It is often positive if the patient has previously had a BCG vaccination
    c. It is negative if the induration produced is 12 mm in diameter
    d. None of the above

# BIBLIOGRAPHY

Amodio G, Antonelli G, Di Serio F. Cardiac biomarkers in acute coronary syndromes: a review. *Curr Vasc Pharmacol* 2010;8:388–93.

Anoop SVS, et al. High-sensitivity cardiac troponin I at presentation in patients with suspected acute coronary syndrome: a cohort study. *Lancet* 2016;386(10012):2481–8.

Apple F, Sandoval Y. Implementing high sensitivity cardiac troponin assays. *Clinical Laboratory News*. EJIFCC. 2016;27(3):217–23.

Arneson W, Brickell J. *Clinical chemistry: a laboratory perspective*. Philadelphia: FA Davis; 2007.

Bishop ML, Fody EP, Schoeff LE. *Clinical chemistry techniques, principles, correlations*. 6th ed. Philadelphia: Lippincott Williams & Wilkins; 2010.

Caliendo AM, Gilbert DN, Ginocchio CC, et al. Better tests, better care: improved diagnostics for infectious diseases. *Clin Infect Dis* 2013;57(Suppl. 3):S139–70.

Cefalue W, editor-in-chief. American diabetes association standards of medical care in diabetes. *Diabetes Care* 2016;39(Suppl. 1).

Chabot-Richards DS, George T. Leukocytosis. *Int J Lab Hematol* 2014;36:279–88.

Chung KF. Inflammatory biomarkers in severe asthma. *Curr Opin Pulm Med* 2012;18:35–41.

Farrell PM, Rosenstein BJ, White TB, et al. Guidelines for diagnosis of cystic fibrosis in newborns through older adults: cystic fibrosis foundation consensus report. *J Pediatr* 2008;153(2):S4–14.

Forbes BA, Sahm DF, Weissfeld AS, eds. *Bailey and Scott's diagnostic microbiology*. 12th ed. St. Louis: Mosby Elsevier; 2007.

Hayward CPM, Moffat KA. Laboratory testing for bleeding disorders: strategic uses of high and low-yield tests. *Int J Lab Hematol* 2013;35:322–33.

Jorgensen JH, Pflaller MA, eds. Manual of clinical microbiology. 11th ed. Washington, DC: ASM Press; 2015.

Keohane EM, Smith LJ, Walenga JM, eds. *Rodak's hematology: clinical principles and applications*. 5th ed. St. Louis: Elsevier; 2016.

Kujovich JL. Evaluation of anemia. *Obstet Gynecol Clin North Am* 2016;43:247–64.

Laposata M. *Laboratory medicine: the diagnosis of disease in the clinical laboratory*. New York: McGraw-Hill; 2010.

Mair J. High-sensitivity cardiac troponins in everyday clinical practice. *World J Cardiol* 2014;6(4):175–82.

McKee JR, Wall T, Owensby J. Impact of complete blood count sampling time change on white blood cell and absolute neutrophil count values in clozapine recipients. *Clin Schizophr Relat Psychoses* 2011;5:26–32.

McKenzie SB, Williams JL, eds. *Clinical laboratory hematology*. 3rd ed. Boston: Pearson; 2015.

Miller JM. *A guide to specimen management in clinical microbiology*. 2nd ed. Washington, DC: ASM Press; 1999.

Strasinger SK, Di Lorenzo MS. *Urinalysis and body fluids*. 5th ed. Philadelphia: FA Davis; 2008.

Travis WD. Classification of lung cancer. *Semin Roentgenol* 2011;46:178–86.

# 8

# Interpretation of Blood Gases

*Richard Wettstein and Craig L. Scanlan*

## KEY TERMS

| | | |
|---|---|---|
| acidemia | calibration | hyperventilation |
| alkalemia | dead space ventilation | hypocapnia |
| analytic error | dyshemoglobin | hypoventilation |
| anemia | hypercapnia | hypoxemia |
| anion gap | hyperoxemia | hypoxia |

Care of patients with cardiopulmonary disorders often requires precise knowledge of their oxygenation, ventilation, and acid-base status. This information is obtained by blood gas and oximetry analysis. Respiratory therapists (RTs) must know when and how to obtain these measurements and be able to accurately interpret them.

This chapter focuses on the interpretation of arterial blood gas results. Table 8.1 provides the normal ranges for arterial blood gas measurements.

Peripheral venous blood reflects local metabolism and is of no value in assessing lung function. On the other hand, mixed venous blood samples from the pulmonary artery and more recently central venous catheter blood gases can be used to evaluate overall tissue oxygenation. Use of mixed venous blood and central catheter blood for this purpose is discussed in Chapter 14.

## INDICATIONS FOR BLOOD GAS AND OXIMETRY ANALYSIS

Blood gas analysis is indicated if the patient's symptoms, medical history, physical examination, or laboratory data suggest abnormalities in respiratory or acid-base status. Blood gas analysis also can help evaluate treatment effects and thus be used whenever significant changes occur in therapy that affect oxygenation, ventilation, or acid-base balance.

### TABLE 8.1 Sample Reference Ranges for Arterial Blood Gas Parameters

| Parameter | Symbol | Reference Ranges |
|---|---|---|
| Partial pressure of oxygen | $Pa_{O_2}$ | 80-100 mm Hg (room air) |
| Hemoglobin content | Hb | Males: 14-18 g/dL Females: 12-15 g/dL |
| Hemoglobin saturation | $Sa_{O_2}$ | >95% |
| Carboxyhemoglobin saturation | COHb | <3% (nonsmokers) |
| Methemoglobin saturation | metHb | <1.5% |
| Oxygen content | $Ca_{O_2}$ | 16-20 mL/dL |
| Hydrogen ion concentration (negative log) | pH | 7.35-7.45 |
| Partial pressure of carbon dioxide | $P_{CO_2}$ | 35-45 mm Hg |
| Plasma bicarbonate | $HCO_3^-$ | 22-26 mmol/L |
| Base excess | BE | ±2 mmol /L |

*BE*, Base excess; $HCO_3^-$, plasma bicarbonate concentration; $P_{CO_2}$, partial pressure of carbon dioxide; *pH*, hydrogen ion concentration in blood; $P_{O_2}$, partial pressure of oxygen; $S_{O_2}$ oxyhemoglobin saturation.

Blood oxygenation can be assessed by arterial blood gas (ABG) analysis, hemoximetry, pulse oximetry, and transcutaneous $P_{O_2}$ monitoring (mainly in infants and children). Ventilation can be assessed by ABGs, transcutaneous $P_{CO_2}$ monitoring, or capnography. An ABG is required for accurate assessment of acid-base status. Table 8.2 outlines the key indications for these measurements, as recommended by the American Association for Respiratory Care.

## SAMPLING AND MEASUREMENT

Blood gas sampling and measurement approaches can be broadly classified as being invasive or noninvasive. Invasive approaches require sampling of blood by needle puncture or indwelling catheter. Noninvasive approaches measure blood gas parameters by sensors on the skin or evaluation of exhaled gases.

### Invasive Blood Sampling

If the goal is to accurately evaluate oxygenation, ventilation, and acid-base status, analysis of an arterial blood sample is the gold standard against which other measures are compared. Samples are obtained by percutaneous needle puncture of an artery or from an indwelling arterial catheter. Measurement of arterial pH, $Pa_{CO_2}$, and $Pa_{O_2}$ typically is provided by a blood gas analyzer, which also calculates the $HCO_3^-$ and $Sa_{O_2}$ values. Standard blood gas analyzers do not measure actual $Sa_{O_2}$ or Hb content and cannot detect the presence of abnormal hemoglobins such as carboxyhemoglobin (COHb). Measurement of normal and abnormal hemoglobin (Hb) content and actual saturation usually requires sample analysis by hemoximetry (CO-oximetry).

### Arterial Puncture

An arterial blood sample may be obtained from the radial, brachial, dorsalis pedis, or femoral arteries. The radial artery is preferred because it is readily accessible, easy to stabilize, and seldom results in serious complications due to the collateral circulation provided by the ulnar artery. Box 8.1 outlines the key steps involved in obtaining an arterial blood sample via percutaneous puncture.

Fine points involved in arterial puncture include checking coagulation-related tests, assessing for collateral circulation before and after the procedure, and proper technique to minimize pain and complications.

Coagulation-related laboratory tests should be checked to assess for risk for bleeding. Specifically, low platelet counts or increased bleeding times (high prothrombin time, partial thromboplastin time, or international normalized ratio values) indicate an increased risk of bleeding. This requires the RT to maintain pressure on the puncture site for longer than usual to prevent bleeding. See Chapter 7 for more detail on these tests.

In terms of infection control, standard precautions are a must. Given that blood splashes can occur during arterial puncture, in addition to wearing gloves, clinicians should wear a face shield and consider using a gown to protect the skin and clothing (see Chapter 1). When expelling any air bubbles from the sample, one also must avoid discharge of blood droplets into the environment. This important step is accomplished by either (1) using a filter cap on the syringe or (2) expelling the bubble-containing portion of the sample slowly into sterile gauze pad contained in a sealable plastic bag.

When the radial artery is selected, a modified Allen test must be performed to evaluate the adequacy of collateral circulation to the hand (Fig. 8.1). To perform this test, the patient is instructed to make a tight fist. Then both the radial and ulnar arteries are compressed. Have the patient open and relax the hand, which should reveal a blanched palm and fingers. Next release the pressure on the ulnar artery while

observing the patient's hand for color changes. If collateral flow is adequate, the patient's hand will "pink up" within 5 to 15 seconds—a positive Allen test. A positive result confirms adequate collateral flow and that the radial artery is an acceptable sampling site. If the test is negative (the hand does not pink up rapidly), the radial artery is not an acceptable site for puncture. In such cases the other wrist is evaluated, or another site such as the brachial artery is used.

After the sample is obtained and the puncture site stabilized, the sample is either sent to the laboratory or analyzed at the bedside using a point-of-care analyzer. When using a point-of-care analyzer, the instrument needs to be properly

---

**TABLE 8.2   Indications for Blood Gas and Oximetry Analysis**

| Method | Indications |
| --- | --- |
| Arterial blood gas analysis | Evaluate ventilation ($Pco_2$), acid-base (pH, $Pco_2$, and $HCO_3^-$), and oxygenation ($Po_2$) status |
| | Assess the patient's response to therapy and/or diagnostic tests (e.g., $O_2$ therapy, exercise testing) |
| | Monitor the severity and progression of a disease process |
| Hemoximetry (CO-oximetry) | Determine actual blood $O_2$ saturation (as opposed to that computed with a simple blood gas analyzer) |
| | Measure abnormal hemoglobins levels (e.g., COHb, metHb) |
| Pulse oximetry | Monitor the adequacy of oxyhemoglobin saturation |
| | Quantify the response of oxyhemoglobin saturation to therapeutic intervention or to diagnostic procedure (e.g., bronchoscopy) |
| | Comply with mandated regulations or recommendations by authoritative groups (e.g., anesthesia monitoring) |
| | Screen infants for critical congenital heart diseases |
| Transcutaneous monitoring ($Ptco_2$, $Ptcco_2$) | Continuously monitor the adequacy of arterial oxygenation and/or ventilation |
| | Continuously monitor for excessive arterial oxygenation (hyperoxemia) |
| | Quantify real-time changes in ventilation and oxygenation due to diagnostic or therapeutic interventions |
| | Screen infants for critical congenital heart diseases |

---

**BOX 8.1   Key Steps in Obtaining an Arterial Blood Sample by Needle Puncture**

1. Verify doctor's order.
2. Review chart for diagnosis, anticoagulant therapy, coagulation-related tests, $Fio_2$, and ventilator settings.
3. Gather, assemble, and check required equipment (arterial blood gas kit).
4. Wash hands, and apply standard/transmission-based precautions as appropriate.
5. Identify patient (using two identifiers); introduce self.
6. Explain procedure, and confirm patient understanding.
7. Palpate pulses on both sides to select best site (use nondominant arm if possible).
8. Perform Allen test if radial artery selected (see Fig. 8.1); if negative, repeat on other arm.
9. Prepare the site by rubbing with a 70% isopropyl alcohol solution for at least 30 seconds.
10. Position puncture site by extending wrist 30 degrees over supporting towel.
11. Slowly insert needle bevel up at 45 degrees or less until flash of blood is observed; readjust angle if necessary. If the angle needs to be adjusted pull the needle back until the bevel is visible just under the skin. Change the angle to intersect with the palpated pulse.
12. Obtain sample; remove needle, immediately apply pressure with sterile gauze.
13. Follow sharps procedure to shield needle, e.g., apply automatic capping device.
14. Maintain pressure on site for 3 to 5 minutes; 10 minutes or longer if patient has bleeding disorder or uses anticoagulants.
15. Check puncture site for bleeding, swelling, discoloration, return of proximal and distal pulses.
16. Use gauze pad or venting cap to expel air bubbles from sample (Occupational Safety and Health Administration guidelines).
17. Mix sample with anticoagulant by repeatedly rolling sample between hands and inverting syringe.
18. Label sample with date, time, patient ID, $Fio_2$, ventilator settings; place in sealed container for transport (not required for point-of-care analysis).
19. Dispose of infectious waste; wash hands.
20. Record pertinent data in chart and departmental records.
21. When the results are available notify appropriate personnel, and make any necessary recommendations or modifications to the care plan.
22. Recheck puncture site after 20 minutes if patient is on anticoagulant therapy or has a bleeding disorder.

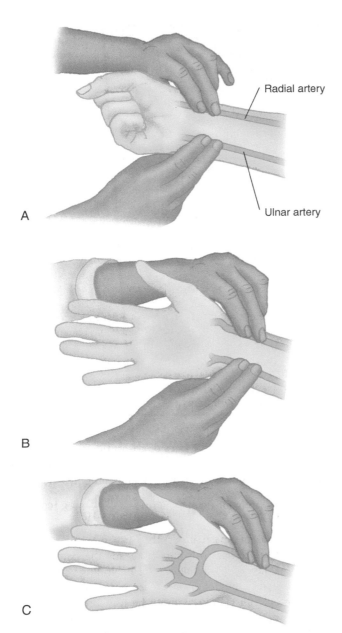

**FIG. 8.1** Assessment of collateral circulation before radial artery sampling. **A,** Patient clenches fist while examiner obstructs radial and ulnar arteries. **B,** Patient gently opens hand while pressure is maintained over both arteries. **C,** Pressure over ulnar artery is released, and changes in color of patient's palm are noted. (From Kacmarek RM, Stoller JK, Heuer, AJ: *Egan's fundamentals of respiratory care,* ed 11, St. Louis, 2017, Mosby-Elsevier.)

prepared before obtaining the blood sample. Normally, this involves verifying its power-up operation, inserting the needed cartridge, and confirming internal calibration. After the sample is obtained and any air bubbles are removed, it should be thoroughly mixed and injected into the cartridge within 2 to 3 minutes, depending on the manufacturer, and the sample should **not** *be placed on ice.* If the analysis results fall outside the analyzer's reportable ranges (results "flagged"), the remaining sample should be sent to the central laboratory for analysis.

Of course, the RT should never wait for the repeat results if the findings indicate a life-threatening problem. For example, if the bedside results indicate oxygen levels below the analyzer's reportable ranges and the patient is cyanotic, the RT should immediately start oxygen administration or raise the $Fio_2$ while awaiting test results from the central laboratory.

### Indwelling Catheter (A-Line)

Arterial puncture causes trauma, so an indwelling arterial catheter, or A-line, should be used when frequent sampling is necessary. As a result of the potential hazards of hemorrhage and bloodstream infection, A-lines require careful management, and their use generally is limited to unstable patients in the intensive care unit.

The A-line catheter is connected to a pressurized heparin infusion set that incorporates a pressure transducer, flush device, and sampling port that is accessed either through a three-way stopcock or a closed reservoir. Fig. 8.2 depicts the design and operation of a typical three-way stopcock sampling port.

The preparatory and follow-up steps for obtaining and processing a blood sample from an A-line are similar to those for radial arterial puncture, though an Allen test is not needed. For patient safety it is important to confirm adequate perfusion distal to the cannulation site. This can be observed by a continuous blood pressure measurement, with a satisfactory arterial waveform (see Chapter 15 for details on assessing arterial pressure waveforms). After gathering the needed equipment, the RT can proceed to obtain the sample using the applicable procedure, as outlined in Table 8.3.

Recently, closed reservoir arterial line blood sampling systems are becoming increasingly popular. In addition to using a standard arterial line sample syringe, these systems employ a special sealed sampling port and incorporate a reservoir syringe to collect and flush back into the patient, essentially all blood withdrawn, except for the actual sample used for analysis. These systems eliminate the need for a waste syringe and wasted blood, thereby conserving the patient's blood. Because of their closed system design, these systems also reduce the potential for line contamination and better protect against exposure to blood-borne pathogens than the stopcock method.

### Noninvasive Measurements

Noninvasive blood gas analysis uses external skin sensors to measure relevant parameters. Pulse oximetry is the most common noninvasive method for ABG-related measurements. An alternative approach, transcutaneous $Po_2/Pco_2$ monitoring, is used primarily for infants and children.

### Pulse Oximetry

Pulse oximetry is a noninvasive technique for measuring oxygen saturation ($Spo_2$) of hemoglobin (Hb) in the blood. When compared with analysis of arterial blood Hb saturation by invasive sampling and CO-oximetry ($Sao_2$) among patients with good perfusion, most pulse oximeters are accurate within 2% with oxygen saturations equal to or greater than 90%. As oxygen saturation falls $Spo_2$ accuracy also

**FIG. 8.2** A three-way stopcock in a vascular line system showing the various positions used. A, Normal operating position with flush solution going to the patient and the sample port closed. B, Position to draw a blood sample from the vascular line (closed to flush solution). C, Position to flush sampling port (closed to patient). In any intermediate position, all ports are closed. (From Kacmarek RM, Stoller JK, Heuer, AJ: *Egan's fundamentals of respiratory care*, ed 11, St. Louis, 2017, Mosby-Elsevier.)

becomes less reliable necessitating the use of CO-oximetry to accurately determine oxygen saturation of hemoglobin.

As the "fifth vital sign," pulse oximetry is commonly used throughout the hospital, outpatient clinics, physician offices, sleep centers, and in the home care setting to titrate oxygen therapy and adjust oxygenation for patients on mechanical ventilation.

Pulse oximeters use the spectrophotometric principle of light absorption. The standard device probe transmits two wavelengths of light—red and infrared—through capillary beds such as the earlobe or digit. A fairly constant level of light is absorbed by the tissues and venous blood. Periodically an increased amount of light is absorbed due to the arterial

| TABLE 8.3   Procedures for Obtaining Blood Samples from an Arterial Line (Adult Patient) | |
|---|---|
| **Three-Way Stopcock Sampling** | **In-line Closed Reservoir Sampling** |
| Swab sample port with alcohol | Slowly draw blood into the reservoir to the needed fill volume |
| Attach waste syringe and turn stopcock off to flush solution/bag | |
| Aspirate 5-6 mL blood (at least 6 times the system "dead" volume) | Close the reservoir shutoff valve |
| | Swab sample port with alcohol |
| Turn stopcock off to port | Attach the blunt/needle-less sampling syringe to the valved sampling port |
| Remove waste syringe, properly discard | |
| Secure heparinized syringe to port, reopen stopcock, collect sample | Aspirate the needed volume of blood |
| | Open the reservoir shutoff valve |
| Turn stopcock off to port, remove syringe | Slowly depress reservoir plunger to reinfuse blood into patient |
| Flush line until clear | |
| Turn stopcock off to patient, briefly flush sampling port, reswab with alcohol | Reswab port and flush line until clear |
| Turn stopcock off to port and confirm restoration of arterial pulse pressure waveform | Confirm restoration of arterial pulse pressure waveform |

pulse. This yields variable rates of absorption for oxygenated Hb ($HbO_2$) and reduced Hb (HHb). The oximeter compares these differences in light absorption and computes the $Spo_2$:

$$\text{Pulse saturation (}Spo_2 \text{ as \%)} = \frac{HbO_2}{HbO_2 + HHb} \times 100$$

Computed in this manner, the $Spo_2$ often is called the *functional saturation*. This simply means the percentage of the normal hemoglobin that is actually binding with oxygen.

Abnormal hemoglobin or dyshemoglobins, such as carboxyhemoglobin (Hbco), cannot be measured by standard pulse oximeters. CO-oximeters and some advanced blood gas analyzers, using at least four wavelengths of light, are able to accurately measure dyshemoglobins. The $Sao_2$ measured by a CO-oximeter is called the *fractional saturation* because it compares the proportion of Hb saturated with oxygen with the total amount of Hb present, including any abnormal hemoglobin:

$$\text{CO-oximeter } Sao_2 = \frac{HbO_2}{HbO_2 + HHb + \text{Dyshemoglobins}} \times 100$$

Because CO-oximeters measure the total complement of Hb and standard pulse oximeters do not, *in the presence of abnormal hemoglobin, pulse oximetry will overestimate the true $Sao_2$.* Other factors that can result in erroneous estimation of $Sao_2$ using pulse oximetry are summarized in Table 8.4. To detect the presence of abnormal hemoglobin (such as in a burn patient suspected of CO poisoning), obtain an arterial blood sample, and analyze it using a

| TABLE 8.4 | **Common Factors Causing Erroneous $SpO_2$ Readings (Compared with CO-Oximetry)** | |
|---|---|
| **Factor** | **Potential Error** |
| Presence of COHb | Falsely high $SpO_2$ |
| Presence of metHb | Falsely low $SpO_2$ if $SaO_2$ > 85%<br>Falsely high $SpO_2$ if $SpO_2$ < 85% |
| Vascular dyes (e.g., methylene blue) | Falsely low $SpO_2$ |
| Dark skin pigmentation | Falsely high $SpO_2$ (3%-5%) |
| Nail polish | Falsely high $SpO_2$ (especially black) |
| Poor local perfusion (vasoconstriction and/or hypothermia) | Possible loss of signal, falsely low $SpO_2$ (may be falsely high in sepsis) |
| Motion artifact | Unpredictable spurious readings or false alarms |
| Ambient light | Varies (e.g., falsely high $SpO_2$ in sunlight); may also cause falsely high pulse reading |

CO-oximeter. New portable multiwavelength pulse oximeters are available that provide relatively accurate noninvasive measurement of common dyshemoglobins at the bedside. Advances in sensor design have decreased the errors associated with motion artifact and ambient light. More problematic are the errors that occur due to poor peripheral perfusion. In these cases, placement of a reflectance (as opposed to an absorption-type) probe on a core body site such as the forehead or chest will provide more accurate estimates of Hb saturation.

When accuracy is essential, with critically ill patients, $SpO_2$ should be compared to simultaneous CO-oximetry analysis. The discrepancy between the $SaO_2$ and $SpO_2$ can then be used to "calibrate" the pulse oximetry reading. For example, if the $SpO_2$ reading is 93% and CO-oximetry analysis reveals a $SaO_2$ of 90%, subtracting 3% from the subsequent $SpO_2$ measurements may provide a better estimate of arterial oxygen saturation.

Pulse oximetry has dramatically reduced the need for arterial blood sampling. However, it should never be substituted for blood sample analysis when the clinical situation demands a complete assessment of oxygenation. In addition, because pulse oximeters only provide oxygenation data, abnormalities in ventilation ($PCO_2$) or acid-base balance ($pH/HCO_3^-$) can go undetected. Standard pulse oximeters do not measure the amount of circulating Hb in the blood, so anemia may be missed if not separately assessed. Finally, as a result of the relationship between Hb saturation and $O_2$ partial pressures, pulse oximetry is of limited utility for detecting abnormally high $PO_2$ values (hyperoxemia). RTs should be extra careful when using pulse oximetry to monitor oxygenation in newborn infants at risk for retinopathy of prematurity (ROP), one cause of which is hyperoxemia. An $SpO_2$ less than 93% to 95% has been shown to reduce the risk of ROP.

## Transcutaneous Analysis

A typical transcutaneous sensor includes an $O_2$ and $CO_2$ electrode and a heating element. The heating element warms the underlying skin to 40°C to 42°C, which increases blood flow and thus "arterializes" the area. Warming also increases skin permeability and enhances diffusion of $O_2$ and $CO_2$ from the capillaries, through the skin, into the electrolyte gel under the sensor. These electrodes measure the gas pressures in the gel using the same electrochemical principles used in blood gas analyzers.

Transcutaneous gas analysis generally has been limited to use with infants and small children in need of continuous monitoring of oxygenation and ventilation (see Chapter 12 for details). However, with the notable exception of monitoring for hyperoxemia, transcutaneous measurement of oxygen ($PtcO_2$) monitoring been replaced by pulse oximetry. This is because the accuracy of $PtcO_2$ is highly dependent on the adequacy of perfusion. Low cardiac output, peripheral vasoconstriction, and dehydration all decrease capillary flow, which lowers $PtcO_2$. And as with $PaO_2$, $PtcO_2$ does not fully reflect total oxygen content of the blood.

On the other hand, the transcutaneous measurement of carbon dioxide ($PtcCO_2$) can be reliably measured in patients in most age groups, making it a good choice for the continuous noninvasive monitoring of ventilation. $PtcCO_2$ monitoring is particularly useful when capnography is unavailable or impractical, such as during noninvasive ventilation. In properly calibrated systems with good sensor placement, $PtcCO_2$ values will fall within 3 to 5 mm Hg of the measured $PaCO_2$.

As a result of the lengthy setup, calibration, and stabilization times needed by transcutaneous monitors, they have no place in assessing patients during emergencies. In these cases, pulse oximetry is the first choice for assessing oxygenation, followed by arterial sampling and point-of-care ABG analysis to obtain a complete picture of oxygenation, ventilation, and acid-base balance.

## Capnography

Capnography involves the measurement of $CO_2$ concentrations or partial pressures in the expired gases and their real-time graphic display during breathing. Measurement is based on $CO_2$ absorption of light in the infrared spectrum in proportion to its concentration. A capnograph employs a light source and photodetector that measures changes in the intensity of infrared light passed through an analysis chamber.

The primary application of capnography is to monitor patients during general anesthesia, mechanical ventilation, or resuscitation. As a noninvasive substitute for $PaCO_2$ to assess ventilation, we generally use the end-tidal partial pressure of $CO_2$ ($PETCO_2$), although %$CO_2$ can also be used. Normally, the $PETCO_2$ is about 2 to 5 mm Hg less than the $PaCO_2$. Ventilation/perfusion (V/Q) imbalances can alter the difference between the $PaCO_2$ and $PETCO_2$, and these imbalances are common in patients with respiratory disorders; therefore we normally focus on trending of the end-tidal $CO_2$ levels when using capnography for continuous monitoring. On the other

**TABLE 8.5   Classification of Hypoxemia**

| Pao$_2$ (mm Hg) | Relative Severity |
|---|---|
| 60-79 | Mild |
| 40-59 | Moderate |
| <40 | Severe |

hand, discrete breath analysis can be used to identify abnormal events such as extubation or rebreathing. Chapter 14 provides more detail on the use of capnography to monitor patients in intensive care.

## ASSESSMENT OF OXYGENATION

A complete assessment of arterial blood gas parameters indicating the state of patient oxygenation includes the arterial partial pressure of oxygen (Pao$_2$), hemoglobin content (Hb) and Hb saturation (Sao$_2$, Spo$_2$), and arterial O$_2$ content (Cao$_2$).

### Partial Pressure of Oxygen (Pao$_2$)

REFERENCE RANGE : 80 to 100 mm Hg breathing room air

The Pao$_2$ is the pressure exerted by dissolved oxygen in the arterial blood. The Pao$_2$ reflects the lung's ability to transfer O$_2$ from the inspired gas into the circulating blood. Thus the Pao$_2$ depends on both environmental factors (O$_2$ concentration and barometric pressure) and lung function. The Pao$_2$ measurement provides clinical significant information as it allows the evaluation of hyperoxia, normoxia, and hypoxemia.

### Hypoxemia: Severity and Causes

Hypoxemia simply means a low oxygen level. It exists when the Pao$_2$ is below 80 mm Hg. The Pao$_2$ level determines whether hypoxemia is classified as mild, moderate, or severe. See Table 8.5.

Causes of hypoxemia include hypoventilation, V/Q mismatch, pulmonary shunting, diffusion defect, and breathing gas with a low partial pressure of oxygen (Pio$_2$). Table 8.6 summarizes these causes, identifies some example conditions, and specifies how to differentiate among them. V/Q mismatch is the most common cause of hypoxemia, whereas pure diffusion defects are rarely seen.

---

**SIMPLY STATED**

Hypoxemia exists when a patient's Pao$_2$ is below 80 mm Hg (the lower boundary of the normal range). It most often results from V/Q mismatching.

---

Hypoxemia is often first suggested by the patient complaining of shortness of breath, especially with exertion. Common clinical manifestations also include tachycardia, tachypnea, hypertension, mental confusion, and cyanosis.

Although universally used as a measure of pulmonary gas exchange, the Pao$_2$ provides only a limited picture of patient oxygenation. Indeed, dissolved oxygen represents only 1% to 2% of the total oxygen normally transported to the tissues. A full picture of patient oxygenation requires assessment of Hb content and saturation, total O$_2$ content, and cardiac output, as these combined determine oxygen delivery to the tissues.

### Alveolar Air Equation

Assuming normal lung function and taking into account the environmental factors, we can compute the partial pressure of oxygen in the alveoli (P$_A$o$_2$) using the alveolar air equation:

$$P_A o_2 = F_{IO_2}(P_B - P_{H_2O}) - (Paco_2 \times 1.25)$$

Where P$_A$o$_2$ = partial pressure of oxygen in the alveoli; Fio$_2$ = fraction of inhaled oxygen; P$_B$ = barometric pressure; P$_{H_2O}$ = water vapor pressure in alveoli, 47 mm Hg at body temperature and pressure, saturated with mater vapor (BTPS); Paco$_2$ = arterial partial pressure of CO$_2$ (assumed to approximate the alveolar Pco$_2$); and 1.25 = factor based on the ratio of CO$_2$ production to O$_2$ consumption (respiratory quotient). For example, the P$_A$o$_2$ of a patient breathing room air (Fio$_2$ = 0.21) at sea level (P$_B$ = 760 mm Hg) with a Paco$_2$ of 40 mm Hg would be computed as follows:

$$P_A O_2 = 0.21(760 \text{ mm Hg} - 47 \text{ mm Hg}) - (40 \times 1.25)$$
$$= (0.21 \times 713 \text{ mm Hg}) - 50 \text{ mm Hg}$$
$$= 149.7 \text{ mm Hg} - 50 \text{ mm Hg}$$
$$= 99.7 \text{ mm Hg} \approx 100 \text{ mm Hg}$$

Even in healthy lungs gas transfer is imperfect, so not all of the O$_2$ in the alveoli diffuses into the pulmonary capillaries. How much O$_2$ diffuses across the alveolar/capillary membrane into the blood depends on both age and the presence of disease. In children and young adults with normal lungs breathing at sea level, there exists on average a 10–mm Hg gradient between the P$_A$o$_2$ and Pao$_2$, yielding a normal Pao$_2$ in the 90– to 100– mm Hg range. This difference—called the alveolar-arterial oxygen tension gradient and abbreviated as P(A-a)o$_2$—increases with age, due to a progressive loss of lung function. For patients breathing room air, this increase in P(A-a)o$_2$ is estimated by multiplying their age by 0.3. For example, we would estimate the P(A-a)o$_2$ of an otherwise healthy 70-year-old patient as being 0.3 × 70, or about 20 mm Hg. This would yield an expected Pao$_2$ for this patient of about 100 − 20 = 80 mm Hg. Recent studies suggest that the age-associated increase in P(A-a)o$_2$ levels off at about 70 years of age, making 80 mm Hg the lower limit of the Pao$_2$ reference range for essentially all age groups breathing air at sea level. For individuals living at high altitude, this lower boundary for Pao$_2$ decreases in direct proportion to the decrease in barometric pressure.

### Hemoglobin (Hb) and Hb Saturation (Sao$_2$, Spo$_2$)

REFERENCE RANGES : Hb males, 14–18 g/dL;
Females, 12–15 g/dL ; Sao$_2$/Spo$_2$ > 95 %

Normally, more than 98% of the O$_2$ in arterial blood is bound to hemoglobin. How much oxygen Hb carries in a given

## TABLE 8.6   Causes of Hypoxemia

| | | | DIFFERENTIAL ASSESSMENT | |
|---|---|---|---|---|
| Type of Hypoxemia | Underlying Cause | Clinical Examples | P(A-a)o$_2$ | Response to O$_2$ therapy |
| Hypoventilation | Rise in P$_A$CO$_2$ reduces P$_A$O$_2$ (alveolar air equation) | Drug overdose<br>Neuromuscular disorders | Normal[a] | Marked |
| V/Q mismatch | Blood flows through underventilated regions of the lung | COPD<br>Asthma | Increased | Marked |
| Pulmonary shunting | Blood flows by alveoli that are not ventilated, does not pick up any oxygen | Atelectasis<br>Pneumonia<br>Pulmonary edema<br>ARDS | Increased | Minimal |
| Diffusion defect | Impaired gas transfer across alveolar-capillary membrane | Interstitial lung diseases (e.g., pulmonary fibrosis, sarcoidosis) | Increased | Marked |
| Low Pio$_2$ | Decreased Pio$_2$ lowers P$_A$O$_2$ | Altitude sickness<br>Equipment failure | Normal | Marked |

*ARDS,* Acute respiratory distress syndrome; *COPD,* chronic obstructive pulmonary disease.
[a]Normal P(A-a)o$_2$ but P$_A$O$_2$ decreased in proportion to rise in P$_A$CO$_2$. Breathing room air, the two gas partial pressures normally sum to about 140 mm Hg. Thus with pure hypoventilation, if the P$_A$CO$_2$ rises from 40 to 70 mm Hg (+30 mm Hg), the P$_A$O$_2$ should fall by a roughly comparable amount, that is, from 100 to 70 mm Hg.

volume of blood depends on (1) the total hemoglobin concentration and (2) what proportion of HB is bound to oxygen (Sao$_2$). The Sao$_2$ in turn depends on the Pao$_2$ and a number of other factors affecting O$_2$ binding with hemoglobin.

It is important to note that the Sao$_2$ reported by standard ABG analysis is a calculated value and that the Spo$_2$ represents only the functional saturation of normal Hb with O$_2$. To obtain true Sao$_2$ values requires the use of a CO-oximeter.

Each gram of normal hemoglobin has the capacity to bind with 1.34 mL O$_2$.[a] With an average Hb content of 15 g/dL, this means that each 100 mL of blood has the potential for carrying about 20 mL O$_2$ (1.34 mL/g × 15 g/dL = 20.1 mL/dL). If the Hb content is lower than normal (as in anemia), the maximal O$_2$ carried is reduced proportionately. For example, if a patient's Hb were to drop by 50% from 15 g/dL to 7.5 g/dL, the O$_2$ carrying capacity of Hb would also be reduced in half, from about 20 mL/dL to about 10 mL/dL. For this reason, a complete assessment of patient oxygenation must include Hb content, as determined by either CO-oximetry or a complete blood cell count (CBC).

Sao$_2$ is a measure of how well Hb molecules are "filled" with O$_2$. The primary factor determining Sao$_2$ is the blood Pao$_2$. The oxyhemoglobin dissociation curve quantifies the relationship between Pao$_2$ and Sao$_2$ (Fig. 8.3). This curve is composed of an upper flat portion and a lower steep portion, with a Pao$_2$ of 60 mm Hg and Sao$_2$ of 90% marking the dividing point between the two. On the flat portion, as the Pao$_2$ drops 40 mm Hg from 100 mm Hg down to 60 mm Hg, the Sao$_2$ decreases very little, by only

about 5% to 7%. On the other hand, when the Pao$_2$ falls below 60 mm Hg onto the steep portion of the curve, the Sao$_2$ decrease is much more precipitous. For example, on this portion of the curve, a decrease in Pao$_2$ of only 20 mm Hg (from 60 to 40 mm Hg) causes a 15% to 20% drop in Sao$_2$.

In patients with normal Hb content, if the Sao$_2$ drops below 80% (equivalent to a Pao$_2$ of about 50 mm Hg), the amount of desaturated Hb in the capillaries is sufficient to cause central cyanosis, the bluish discoloration of the capillary beds observed most easily around the lips and oral mucosa. However, because cyanosis requires an absolute quantity of desaturated Hb (about 5 g/dL HHb), if the total Hb content is low (anemia), this sign may not be apparent, even if the hypoxemia is severe.

### SIMPLY STATED

To relate Pao$_2$ to Sao$_2$, use the "40-50-60/70-80-90" rule: Hb saturations of 70%, 80%, and 90% are associated with Po$_2$ values of 40, 50, and 60 mm Hg, respectively. Hb saturations must always be interpreted with knowledge of Hb content. With normal Hb content, the goal is to keep the Sao$_2$ at or above 90%, which corresponds to a Pao$_2$ of 60 mm Hg or higher.

In addition to Pao$_2$, Sao$_2$ is affected by a number of other factors, the most important of which are body temperature, blood pH, and Paco$_2$ (Box 8.2). Alkalosis, hypocapnia, hypothermia, and the presence of fetal Hb and carboxyhemoglobin shift the oxyhemoglobin dissociation curve to the left, resulting in a higher Sao$_2$ for a given Pao$_2$. Shifts to the

---

[a]Many sources promote 1.39 mL O$_2$/g Hb. Mathematically this is correct, but most respiratory texts use the more conventional 1.34 mL O$_2$/g Hb.

**FIG. 8.3** Oxygen dissociation curve of blood at a pH of 7.40, showing variations at three temperatures. For a given oxygen tension, the lower the blood temperature, the more the hemoglobin holds onto oxygen, maintaining higher saturation. (From Kacmarek RM, Stoller JK, Heuer, AJ: *Egan's fundamentals of respiratory care*, ed 11, St. Louis, 2017, Mosby-Elsevier.)

---

**BOX 8.2 Factors Influencing the Oxyhemoglobin Dissociation Curve**

**Shift to Left (Increase in Hemoglobin-Oxygen Affinity)**
Increased pH
Decreased $CO_2$
Decreased body temperature
Decreased 2,3-diphosphoglycerate (2,3-DPG)[a]
Fetal hemoglobin
Carboxyhemoglobin

**Shift to Right (Decrease in Hemoglobin-Oxygen Affinity)**
Decreased pHs
Increased $CO_2$
Increased body temperature
Increased diphosphoglycerate

[a]2,3-DPG is reduced in stored blood. Patients receiving blood transfusions will be expected to have shift to the left in the oxyhemoglobin dissociation curve.

---

left cause oxygen to bind more tightly to Hb, which facilitates $O_2$ uptake in the lungs but can impair $O_2$ unloading at the tissues. Conversely, acidosis, hypercapnia, and fever shift the curve to the right and result in lower $Sao_2$ values for the same $Pao_2$. Shifts to the right result in decreased oxygen affinity for Hb. Although this facilitates unloading of $O_2$ at the tissues, it can impair uptake in the pulmonary capillaries.

## Dyshemoglobins

REFERENCE RANGE: COHb < 3% (nonsmokers); metHb < 1.5%

Abnormal hemoglobin such as COHb and metHb affect oxygenation in much the same way as anemia. Every gram of Hb chemically bound to a molecule other than $O_2$ is equivalent to an absolute reduction of 1 g/dL of circulating Hb. For example, if a smoke inhalation patient with normal Hb content has a COHb saturation of 40%, it would be as if he had only 9 g/dL circulating Hb, instead of 15 g/dL.

As already noted, the presence of carboxyhemoglobin shifts the oxyhemoglobin dissociation curve to the left, further impairing oxygenation by inhibiting the unloading of oxygen at the tissues. Normal COHb levels for nonsmokers are less than 3% and have a minimal impact on oxygenation. Smokers typically exhibit COHb levels in the 5% to 10% range. Higher levels of COHb occur with inhalation of fire smoke or engine exhaust. In such cases, the $Sao_2$ (which must be measured by CO-oximeter) will be significantly reduced; the conscious patient may complain of headache, dyspnea, and nausea; and signs of hypoxemia such as tachypnea and tachycardia may be present. However, because carboxyhemoglobin is cherry red in color, cyanosis does not occur. At COHb levels above 40%, visual disturbance, myocardial damage, coma, and, eventually, death may occur.

Primary treatment for patients suffering from CO poisoning is high-flow oxygen via nonrebreathing mask.

With severe CO poisoning (COHb > 25%), hyperbaric oxygen is often initiated. This reduces the COHb half-life by a third, while also providing enough oxygen dissolved in the blood (6 mL $O_2$/100 mL of blood) to maintain tissue oxygenation.

Another common dyshemoglobin is methemoglobin (metHb). MetHb is a variant of hemoglobin in which the iron in the heme group has been oxidized from its normal $Fe^{2+}$ (ferrous) state to the $Fe^{3+}$ (ferric) state, which is incapable of binding with $O_2$. Increased levels of metHb (methemoglobinemia) have the same effect as an absolute anemia, causing a reduction in $Cao_2$.

As many as one in five patients evaluated with traditional CO-oximetry exhibits a metHb above the reference range. Methemoglobinemia can be inherited or acquired by exposure to Hb-oxidizing agents. Environmental exposure to nitrates, nitrites, aniline, or benzene can induce methemoglobinemia, as can inhaling fumes containing nitric oxide (NO). Patients treated with inhaled NO are susceptible to acquired methemoglobinemia. More common is methemoglobinemia caused by the administration of cardiac medications (nitroglycerin, nitroprusside), local anesthetic agents (benzocaine, prilocaine, lidocaine), and selected antibiotics (dapsone, sulfonamides).

The $Pao_2$ in patients with methemoglobinemia generally is normal, and standard pulse oximetry cannot measure metHb; therefore detection requires either laboratory CO-oximetry or multiwavelength pulse oximetry. As a result of its dark reddish-brown color, metHb levels as low as 15% can cause cyanosis. The presence of central cyanosis in patients with normal $Pao_2$ strongly suggests methemoglobinemia. Signs and symptoms similar to those due to CO poisoning occur at metHb levels in the 25% to 50% range. With metHb above 50%, patients may develop cardiac arrhythmias, severe central nervous system (CNS) depression, and profound metabolic acidosis leading to death if left untreated. Treatment involves removing the causative factors and administering a reducing agent such as methylene blue. Supplemental $O_2$ therapy is used to maximize the $O_2$ saturation of the remaining normal hemoglobin but is of little value. In severe cases, the use of hyperbaric oxygen has been reported, which provides enough dissolved oxygen to maintain tissue oxygenation.

### SIMPLY STATED

CO poisoning represents double trouble for tissue oxygenation. It reduces the oxygen-carrying capacity of the Hb and inhibits unloading of oxygen at the tissues.

## Arterial $O_2$ Content ($Cao_2$)

REFERENCE RANGE : 16 to 20 mL/dL

$Cao_2$ represents the total oxygen content in the arterial blood, measured in mL/dL. It consists of both physically dissolved $O_2$ and that bound to Hb. The vast majority of $O_2$ carried in the blood is bound to Hb; therefore a normal

$Cao_2$ requires a normal red blood cell count and a normal Hb level.

$Cao_2$ is calculated by adding the mL of dissolved $O_2$ and the mL of $O_2$ bound to Hb. Dissolved $O_2$ is computed by multiplying the solubility coefficient of $O_2$ in plasma at 37°C (0.003 mL/dL/mm Hg) times the $Pao_2$. At a normal $Pao_2$ of 100 mm Hg, the dissolved $O_2$ would therefore be calculated as follows:

$$\text{Dissolved } O_2 = 0.003 \text{ mL/dL/mm Hg} \times 100 \text{ mm Hg} = 0.3 \text{ mL/dL}$$

The volume of $O_2$ bound to Hb is computed by multiplying the Hb content by its oxygen carrying capacity (1.34 mL/g) by the $Sao_2$. If we have 15 g/dL Hb, 97% saturated with oxygen, the amount of $O_2$ carried on Hb would be as follows:

$$\text{Chemically bound } O_2 = 15 \text{ g/dL} \times 1.34 \text{ mL/g} \times 0.97 = 19.5 \text{ mL/dL}$$

By adding the dissolved and bound we determine the $O_2$ content:

$$Cao_2 = 0.3 \text{ mL/dL} + 19.5 \text{ mL/dL} = 19.8 \text{ mL/dL}$$

Knowledge of $Cao_2$ is critical because it is one of two major factors affecting delivery of $O_2$ to the tissues. Thus anything that lowers the $Cao_2$ may decrease the availability of $O_2$ at the tissues. As discussed, a reduction in Hb, either absolute (anemia) or relative (dyshemoglobinemias), is a primary cause of a decrease in $Cao_2$. The other primary cause of a low $Cao_2$ is pulmonary dysfunction resulting in a fall in $Pao_2$ and $Sao_2$.

## $O_2$ Delivery and Hypoxia

In addition to $Cao_2$, $O_2$ delivery to the tissues depends on blood flow or cardiac output (CO). Indeed, we can easily compute $O_2$ delivery to the tissues ($Do_2$) as the product of the two:

$$Do_2 = Cao_2 \times CO$$

With average cardiac output for a normal adult being about 5 L/min, a normal $O_2$ delivery would be computed as follows:

$$Do_2 = 200 \text{ mL/L} \times 5 \text{ L/min} = 1000 \text{ mL/min}$$

Note that the $Cao_2$ is normally 20 mL/dL. Here it is stated in L = 10 dL. 20 × 10 = 200 mL $O_2$/L of blood.

Given a normal resting $O_2$ consumption of about 250 mL/min, the delivery of 1000 mL $O_2$/min provides a reserve sufficient to accommodate differences in metabolism across organ systems and provides some protection against tissue hypoxia.

When the amount of oxygen available to the tissues falls short of metabolic needs, a condition of hypoxia exists. Adequate $O_2$ delivery depends on both adequate $Cao_2$ and cardiac output; therefore a complete assessment of patient oxygenation must take both into account. Clinical signs of an inadequate cardiac output include hypotension, cool extremities, weak or absent peripheral pulses, reduced urine output, and depressed levels of consciousness. More details on the basic assessment of a patient's state of perfusion are provided by physical examination (see Chapter 5) and measurement of blood pressure (see Chapter 4). For critically ill patients, advanced monitoring techniques can provide quantitative assessment of both cardiac output (see Chapter 16) and tissue oxygenation (see Chapter 14).

### SIMPLY STATED

The single most important parameter that reflects the quantity of oxygen carried in the arterial blood is the $Ca_{O_2}$. An adequate Hb concentration must be present for this parameter to be normal.

## ASSESSMENT OF ACID-BASE BALANCE

The average adult produces about 12,000 mmol of acid each day. In combination, the lungs and kidneys ensure proper excretion, maintaining appropriate acid-base balance. The lungs remove the bulk of the acid load through ventilation and $CO_2$ excretion. The kidneys remove a smaller quantity of acid (~1 mm/kg/day) but help restore the buffer capacity of the body fluids by replenishing $HCO_3^-$ levels. Failure of either system can disrupt normal acid-base balance.

Accurate assessment of a patient's acid-base balance is based mainly on interpretation of the arterial pH, partial pressure of carbon dioxide ($Pa_{CO_2}$), bicarbonate concentration ($HCO_3^-$), and base excess (BE).

### pH

REFERENCE RANGE: 7.35 to 7.45

The arterial blood pH is the best indicator of overall acid-base balance. The pH is the negative logarithm of the $H^+$ ion concentration $[H^+]$. The normal $[H^+]$ of arterial blood is 0.00004 mol/L. pH changes this into a more easily remembered number of 7.40. Alterations in pH above or below this normal value can have profound effects on many body systems, especially the CNS.

pH values below 7.35 indicate an abnormally high blood $H^+$ or acidemia. A natural byproduct of metabolism is volatile ($CO_2$) and metabolic acids. Thus the body buffers acids better than bases. However, as acidosis worsens it tends to depress CNS function. For this reason, patients with acidosis may appear lethargic and disoriented. As the acidosis worsens, coma may develop. Significant acidosis may reduce myocardial contractility, cardiac output, and blood flow throughout the body.

pH values above 7.45 indicate an abnormally low blood $H^+$ or alkalemia. The major effect of alkalosis is overexcitability of the CNS and peripheral nerves. This can lead to tetany. Extreme alkalosis also may cause muscular spasms of the extremities, face, and body and cardiac dysrhythmias, and even death.

### Partial Pressure of Carbon Dioxide ($Pa_{CO_2}$)

REFERENCE RANGE: 35 to 45 mm Hg

The $Pa_{CO_2}$ measures the adequacy of ventilation relative to the metabolic production of $CO_2$ by the tissues. The presence of a

$Pa_{CO_2}$ above 45 mm Hg is termed hypercapnia. Hypercapnia occurs when the level of alveolar ventilation is not sufficient to remove $CO_2$ production (hypoventilation). A $Pa_{CO_2}$ below 35 mm Hg is termed hypocapnia. Hypocapnia occurs when alveolar ventilation exceeds $CO_2$ production (hyperventilation).

The $Pa_{CO_2}$ also plays a major role in acid-base balance. $Pa_{CO_2}$ alters $H^+$ and pH according to the following hydration/dissociation equation for carbonic acid ($H_2CO_3$):

$$CO_2 + H_2O \rightleftharpoons H_2CO_3 \rightleftharpoons HCO_3^- + H^+$$

An increase in $Pa_{CO_2}$ (hypercapnia) shifts the equilibrium equation to the right, resulting in an increase in $H^+$ production and a decrease in pH. Acidemia due to an increase in $Pa_{CO_2}$ is called respiratory acidosis or clinically ventilatory failure. A decrease in $Pa_{CO_2}$ (hypocapnia) shifts the equation to the left, lowers $H^+$ production, and causes a rise in pH. Alkalemia due to a decrease in $Pa_{CO_2}$ is called respiratory alkalosis. The kidneys can compensate for respiratory acid-base disorders by adjusting the bicarbonate concentration, as discussed later.

The $Pa_{CO_2}$ is the best measure for evaluating the effectiveness of ventilation and should be interpreted in light of the patient's minute ventilation ($V_E$). A normal $Pa_{CO_2}$ should be accompanied by a normal $V_E$ (5 to 10 L/min in adults). With a normal metabolic rate, an increased $V_E$ normally results in hypocapnia. A normal $Pa_{CO_2}$ in the presence of a higher than normal $V_E$ indicates either an increased metabolic rate (as with exercise) or increased dead space ventilation. Increased dead space ventilation occurs when perfusion to well-ventilated areas of the lungs is reduced, as may occur with a pulmonary embolism. With a normal metabolic rate, any reduction in $V_E$ below normal usually produces hypercapnia. A normal $Pa_{CO_2}$ in the presence of a lower than normal $V_E$ usually indicates a decreased metabolic rate.

### SIMPLY STATED

The best parameter for evaluating the adequacy of ventilation is the $Pa_{CO_2}$. Assessment of $Pa_{CO_2}$ should take into account the patient's minute ventilation ($V_E$).

### Plasma Bicarbonate ($HCO_3^-$)

REFERENCE RANGE: 22 to 26 mmol/L

The plasma $HCO_3^-$ primarily reflects the metabolic component of acid-base balance and is regulated by the renal system. Because $HCO_3^-$ functions chemically as a base, changes in its concentration will cause equivalent directional changes in pH; that is, if the $HCO_3^-$ increases, the pH will rise, and if the $HCO_3^-$ decreases, the pH will fall.

A primary increase in $HCO_3^-$ that causes alkalemia (pH > 7.45) is termed metabolic alkalosis. A primary decrease in $HCO_3^-$ that causes acidemia (pH < 7.35) is termed metabolic acidosis. $HCO_3^-$ levels may also change as a compensatory or secondary response to primary changes in $Pa_{CO_2}$ levels; this usually requires at least 12 to 24 hours to occur, with full compensation taking as long as 3 days or more.

The previously described carbonic acid hydration/dissociation equation indicates that changes in dissolved $CO_2$ levels affect $HCO_3^-$ concentrations. Thus because the $HCO_3^-$ concentration depends in part on $Paco_2$ levels, it is not considered a pure measure of metabolic activity.

## Base Excess

REFERENCE RANGE: ± 2 mmol/L

Base excess (BE) measures changes in total blood buffer base above or below normal. The total quantity of buffer anions in the blood is 45 to 50 mmol/L, or approximately twice that of $HCO_3^-$. Thus $HCO_3^-$ accounts for only about half of the total buffering capacity of the blood. Therefore BE provides a more complete picture of blood buffering. Moreover, unlike $HCO_3^-$, acute changes in $Paco_2$ do not affect BE. For this reason, BE is considered a pure measure of the metabolic component of acid-base balance.

The calculation of BE requires measurements of pH, $Paco_2$, $HCO_3^-$, and hemoglobin content. Hemoglobin is required in the calculation because in its unsaturated form (HHb), it can reversibly bind with $H^+$, thus serving as a blood buffer.

BE is reported as a positive or negative value depending on the direction of buffer base deviation from normal. The larger the BE, the more severe the deviation in the metabolic component. A positive BE indicates either the presence of excess base or excessive loss of acid. A negative BE (sometimes called a *base deficit*) indicates either the presence of excess acid or excessive loss of base.

## Henderson-Hasselbalch Equation

There are two basic types of acid-base disorders: metabolic and respiratory. Metabolic disorders are recognized by abnormalities in plasma $HCO_3^-$, whereas respiratory disorders alter $Paco_2$. The relationship between these two measures and blood pH is defined in the Henderson-Hasselbalch equation:

$$pH = pK + \log_{10}\left(\frac{HCO_3^-\ (renal/metabolic/base)}{Paco_2 \times 0.03\ (lungs/respiratory/acid)}\right)$$

Where pK = 6.1 (an ionization constant) and 0.03 = factor to convert $Paco_2$ to mmol/L (concentration of dissolved $CO_2$).

Assuming a normal $Paco_2$, we compute a normal pH as follows:

$$pH = 6.1 + \log\left(\frac{24}{40 \times 0.03}\right)$$
$$pH = 6.1 + \log\left(\frac{24}{1.2}\right)$$
$$pH = 6.1 + \log(20)$$
$$pH = 6.1 + 1.30$$
$$pH = 7.40$$

Note that for a normal pH, the ratio of $HCO_3^-$ to dissolved $CO_2$ must be 20:1. Any major change in this ratio will result in

an abnormal pH. For example, an increase in $Paco_2$ from 40 to 60 mm Hg increases the concentration of dissolved $CO_2$ to 1.8 mmol/L, which decreases the ratio from 20:1 to approximately 13:1. Based on this decreased ratio of base to acid (due to more acid), we compute a lower pH of 7.23:

$$pH = 6.1 + \log\left(\frac{24}{60 \times 0.03}\right)$$
$$pH = 6.1 + \log\left(\frac{24}{1.8}\right)$$
$$pH = 6.1 + \log(13.33)$$
$$pH = 6.1 + 1.13$$
$$pH = 7.23$$

Clearly, return of the $Paco_2$ to 40 mm Hg (dissolved $CO_2 = 1.2$ mmol/L) would restore the ratio to 20:1 and the pH to 7.4. However, restoration of the pH back to normal could also occur by increasing the $HCO_3^-$ concentration to 36 mmol/L (36:1.8 = 20:1). Thus a pH change due to alteration in one component of acid-base balance can be corrected by a compensatory change in the other component. This example reinforces the concept that pH is not determined by the absolute values of $Paco_2$ and $HCO_3^-$ but by the ratio of the two.

## SIMPLE ACID-BASE IMBALANCES

Most acid-base abnormalities occur as simple disorders. Simple disorders involve a primary abnormality in one component of acid-base balance, either $Paco_2$ or $HCO_3^-$. Simple acid-base disorders also can involve compensatory responses by which the component not primarily affected is altered to restore the pH back toward normal. Thus the presence of a near-normal pH does not rule out the possibility of a primary acid-base disorder but instead may indicate the presence of a compensatory response.

### Respiratory Acidosis

Simple respiratory acidosis is a condition in which there is inadequate ventilation relative to the rate of $CO_2$ production. This results in an elevated $Paco_2$, which causes a fall in pH. In acute respiratory acidosis the $HCO_3^-$ and BE are normal as the kidney's compensatory response (increased $HCO_3^-$) has not occurred. This may be termed *uncompensated respiratory acidosis* or *acute ventilatory failure*.

Respiratory acidosis can occur secondary to a number of respiratory and nonrespiratory abnormalities. Examples include the following:
- Respiratory abnormalities
  - Acute upper airway obstruction
  - Severe diffuse airway obstruction (acute or chronic)
  - Massive pulmonary edema
- Nonrespiratory abnormalities
  - Drug overdose
  - Spinal cord trauma
  - Neuromuscular disease
  - Head trauma
  - Thoracic trauma
  - Gross obesity

Compensation for respiratory acidosis occurs through renal reabsorption of $HCO_3^-$. Partial compensation occurs when the plasma $HCO_3^-$ is above normal, but the pH is still low. If the plasma $HCO_3^-$ is elevated enough to return the pH to its normal range, it is called *fully compensated respiratory acidosis*. Once full compensation occurs, $HCO_3^-$ levels do not rise further, and the pH levels typically remain in the 7.35 to 7.40 range. As a result of the time needed to change $HCO_3^-$ levels, compensated respiratory acidosis also is referred to as *chronic respiratory acidosis* or *chronic ventilatory failure*.

Identifying the expected change in $HCO_3^-$ is useful in determining the degree of compensation. For acute respiratory acidosis, for each 10 mm Hg increase in $Paco_2$, the plasma $HCO_3^-$ increases by 1 mmol/L. Proportionately greater increases in $HCO_3^-$, 5 mmol/L for each 10 mm Hg increase in $Paco_2$, indicate a compensatory response. If the expected compensation is absent, a complicating metabolic disorder may be present.

A quick guide for differentiating between types of ventilatory failure follows these simple steps:
1. If $Paco_2$ is greater than 45 mm Hg and the pH is low, ventilatory failure is present.
2. Determine the type of failure based on $HCO_3^-$ level:
   - If $HCO_3^-$ is less than 30 mmol/L, acute ventilatory failure is present.
   - If $HCO_3^-$ is greater than 30 mmol/L, chronic ventilatory failure is present.
3. If chronic ventilator failure is present and the pH is less than 7.30, acute on chronic ventilatory failure is present. This may occur when patients with moderate to severe chronic pulmonary disease develop an acute pulmonary infection that further compromises their pulmonary function.

Dyspnea is the primary symptom of acute ventilatory failure. Signs include tachypnea, tachycardia, diaphoresis, anxiety, and in severe cases paradoxic abdominal movement. In contrast, with reduced drive to breathe (e.g., narcotic drug overdose), the respiratory rate will be reduced without the sensation of dyspnea.

Acute ventilatory failure also results in a reduction in $Pao_2$, so clinical manifestations of hypoxemia may be present. Patients with severe hypercapnia—$Paco_2$ higher than 70 mm Hg—may become comatose if renal compensation is not present.

High $Paco_2$ levels cause systemic vasodilation. This may cause peripheral vasodilation, an increased cardiac output, leading to warm flushed skin and a bounding pulse. Cerebral vasodilation also occurs, resulting in elevated intracranial pressures, retinal venous distention, papilledema, and headache.

---

**SIMPLY STATED**

Respiratory acidosis is present when the $Paco_2$ exceeds the normal upper limit (45 mm Hg) and causes a low blood pH.

---

## Respiratory Alkalosis

Simple respiratory alkalosis is an abnormal condition in which there is a primary increase in alveolar ventilation relative to the rate of $CO_2$ production (i.e., hyperventilation). The hallmark of acute or uncompensated respiratory alkalosis is a reduction in $Paco_2$ in association with an elevated pH and normal $HCO_3^-$ and BE. Hyperventilation usually is the result of an increased drive to breathe. This occurs with pain, anxiety, and hypoxemia ($Pao_2$ <60 mm Hg) or as a compensatory response to metabolic acidosis. Respiratory alkalosis also may be induced accidentally in patients receiving positive-pressure ventilation. Clinical signs and symptoms associated with acute respiratory alkalosis include tachypnea, dizziness, sweating, tingling in the fingers and toes (paresthesia), and muscle weakness or spasm.

The kidneys compensate for respiratory alkalosis by increasing $HCO_3^-$ excretion. Partial compensation occurs when the plasma $HCO_3^-$ falls below normal, but the pH remains above 7.45. Full compensation occurs when the plasma $HCO_3^-$ decreases enough to return the pH to the high end of the normal range (7.40 to 7.45).

The expected compensatory change in plasma $HCO_3^-$ with respiratory alkalosis depends on the severity and duration of hyperventilation. In acute respiratory alkalosis, for every 5 mm Hg decrease in $Paco_2$, the $HCO_3^-$ decreases by 1 mmol/L. Proportionately greater decreases in $HCO_3^-$ indicate a compensatory response, about 5 mmol/L for each 10 mm Hg decrease in $Paco_2$. If the expected compensation is not present, a complicating metabolic disorder may be present.

## Metabolic Acidosis

Simple metabolic acidosis is an abnormal condition resulting from a net gain in fixed blood acids or reduction in buffer base. The hallmark of metabolic acidosis is a reduced pH associated with a primary decrease in blood buffers, as indicated by a fall in $HCO_3^-$ or BE. Gains in fixed acid load can result from increased metabolic acid production or decreased renal excretion. A reduction in base normally is associated with excessive loss of $HCO_3^-$. Common causes of these two types of metabolic acidosis include the following:

Increase in fixed acids:
- Ketoacidosis (e.g., diabetes/starvation)
- Renal failure (distal tubules/retention of $H^+$)
- Lactic acidosis (shock/anaerobic metabolism)
- Ingestion of acids (e.g., methanol)

Loss of base ($HCO_3^-$):
- Diarrhea
- Pancreatic fistula
- Renal failure (proximal tubules/loss of $HCO_3^-$)
- Hyperalimentation

The anion gap differentiates between metabolic acidosis due to acid gain versus that associated with loss of base. The anion gap is the difference between the concentration of the major serum cations and major anions (the difference being due to unmeasured ions). The most commonly used formula to compute the anion gap is as follows:

$$\text{Anion gap} = [Na^+] - ([Cl^-] + [HCO_3^-])$$

A frequently cited reference range for the anion gap is 8 to 16 mmol/L. It is important to note that the range differs according to whether $K^+$ is included in the formula and the methods used to measure the electrolytes. *For this reason, it is essential that clinicians know the anion gap reference range used in their institution.*

Metabolic acids are buffered by binding with bicarbonate. As metabolic acids increase, the amount of free bicarbonate decreases, resulting in an increased anion gap. On the other hand, when metabolic acidosis is caused by loss of bicarbonate, the anion gap usually remains within the normal range. This is because bicarbonate loss is offset by a gain in chloride. For this reason, metabolic acidosis with a normal anion gap is often termed *hyperchloremic acidosis.*

Acute or uncompensated metabolic acidosis is rarely seen because the compensatory response—a reduction in $Paco_2$ through hyperventilation—tends to occur as the acidosis develops. Indeed, the most common sign of metabolic acidosis is rapid and deep breathing, called *Kussmaul respirations.* The following equation can be used to predict the $Paco_2$ level needed to fully compensate for metabolic acidosis:

$$Paco_2 = [(1.5 \times HCO_3^-) + 8] \pm 2$$

When the $Paco_2$ is higher than predicted, the patient may not have the ability to hyperventilate, which suggests the presence of a primary respiratory abnormality.

As metabolic acidosis worsens, the patient may complain of dyspnea, headache, nausea, and vomiting. Confusion and stupor may follow. Systemic venous constriction may shift blood to the lungs causing pulmonary edema. Dysrhythmias can occur with severe acidosis.

### SIMPLY STATED

Metabolic acidosis puts extra stress on the respiratory system to reduce $Paco_2$ as a compensatory response. This may precipitate respiratory failure in patients with lung disease.

## Metabolic Alkalosis

Simple metabolic alkalosis is an abnormal condition resulting from a net gain in buffer base or loss in fixed acids. The hallmark of metabolic alkalosis is an elevated pH accompanied by an increase in blood buffers, as indicated by a rise in $HCO_3^-$ or BE. Common causes of metabolic alkalosis include the following:

- Hypokalemia or hypochloremia
- Nasogastric suction
- Persistent vomiting
- Diuretic therapy
- Steroid therapy
- Excessive administration of sodium bicarbonate

Certain electrolyte imbalances can lower $H^+$ or increase $HCO_3^-$. Hypokalemia promotes migration of $H^+$ ions into the intracellular fluids in exchange for $K^+$. Hypokalemia increases renal excretion of $H^+$ ions, increasing buffer base. In addition, chloride and bicarbonate ion concentrations tend to be inversely related; thus when hypochloremia is present,

the concentration of $HCO_3^-$ usually rises, causing metabolic alkalosis. Last, gastric suction and vomiting cause loss of stomach acid (HCl) resulting in alkalosis.

Excessive administration of bicarbonate can lead to metabolic alkalosis, which used to be a common occurrence during cardiopulmonary resuscitation. The routine use of sodium bicarbonate no longer is recommended for patients in cardiac arrest, in part because it can produce hypernatremia, elevate $CO_2$ levels, and impair $O_2$ unloading at the tissues.

The expected compensatory response for metabolic alkalosis is an elevation in $Paco_2$, that is, hypoventilation. However, significant hypoventilation tends not to occur in most patients, in part because the hypoxic ventilatory stimulus may supervene.

### SIMPLY STATED

A patient with metabolic alkalosis may tend to hypoventilate, so this acid-base imbalance should be corrected before any attempt to wean from mechanical ventilation is initiated.

Table 8.7 summarizes the anticipated pH, $Paco_2$, and $HCO_3^-$ changes seen in the four simple acid-base imbalances, including the expected compensatory responses.

## COMBINED ACID-BASE DISTURBANCES

Combined acid-base disorders are identified easily because the derangements in $Paco_2$ and $HCO_3^-$ both drive the pH in the same direction—either low (combined respiratory and metabolic acidosis) or high (combined respiratory and metabolic alkalosis).

### Respiratory and Metabolic Acidosis

The hallmark of combined respiratory and metabolic acidosis is the simultaneous presence of an elevated $Paco_2$ and a reduced $HCO_3^-$, which together can dramatically reduce the pH. Even mild hypercapnia ($Paco_2$ = 50 mm Hg) occurring with a moderate reduction in $HCO_3^-$ (15 to 17 mmol/L) results in profound acidosis (pH < 7.15). This combined disorder occurs in a variety of situations, including the following.

#### Cardiac Arrest

During cardiac arrest, both blood flow and ventilation cease, causing tissue hypoxia, lactic acidosis, and $CO_2$ retention.

#### Chronic Obstructive Pulmonary Disease

Patients with moderate to severe chronic obstructive pulmonary disease (COPD) often have chronically elevated $Paco_2$ levels. In these patients, severe electrolyte disturbances, sudden hypotension, renal failure, or anemia can cause a metabolic acidosis to develop "on top" of their chronic respiratory acidosis.

#### Poisoning and Drug Overdose

Some types of poisons and drugs cause respiratory depression even as they are metabolized into strong acids, producing a combined acidosis.

## TABLE 8.7    Summary of Simple Acid-Base Disorders and Expected Compensatory Responses

| Acid-Base Imbalance | pH | $Paco_2$ | $HCO_3^-$ | Expected Compensatory Response |
|---|---|---|---|---|
| **Respiratory Alkalosis** | | | | |
| Uncompensated/acute | ↑ | ↓ | N | For each 10– to 15–mm Hg increase in $Paco_2$, the $HCO_3^-$ increases by about 1 mmol/L |
| Partially compensated | ↑ | ↓ | ↓ | For every 10–mm Hg increase in $Paco_2$, the $HCO_3^-$ increases by |
| Fully compensated/chronic | N | ↓ | ↓ | 5 mmol/L; partial compensation becomes apparent within 12-24 h, with a full response taking up to 72 h or more |
| **Respiratory Acidosis** | | | | |
| Uncompensated/acute | ↓ | ↑ | N | For every 5–mm Hg decrease in $Paco_2$, $HCO_3^-$ decreases 1 mmol/L |
| Partially compensated | ↓ | ↑ | ↑ | $HCO_3^-$ falls 5 mmol/L for every 10 mm Hg fall in $Paco_2$; partial |
| Fully compensated/chronic | N | ↑ | ↑ | compensation becomes apparent within 12-24 h, with a full response taking up to 72 h or more |
| **Metabolic Acidosis** | | | | |
| Uncompensated/acute | ↓ | N | ↓ | Lack of compensation indicates respiratory abnormality |
| Partially compensated | ↓ | ↓ | ↓ | Compensation normally occurs simultaneously with acidosis; |
| Fully compensated/chronic | N | ↓ | ↓ | expected $Paco_2 = [(1.5 \times HCO_3^-) + 8] \pm 2$ |
| **Metabolic Alkalosis** | | | | |
| Uncompensated/acute | ↑ | N | ↑ | Compensation via hypoventilation uncommon; if present $Paco_2$ |
| Partially compensated | ↑ | ↑ | ↑ | usually does not rise above 50-55 mm Hg |
| Fully compensated/chronic | N | ↑ | ↑ | |

$HCO_3^-$, Plasma bicarbonate concentration; *N*, within reference range; *pH*, hydrogen ion concentration in blood; *$Paco_2$*, partial pressure of $CO_2$ in arterial blood; ↑, above reference range; ↓, below reference range.

## Metabolic and Respiratory Alkalosis

The hallmark of combined respiratory and metabolic alkalosis is the simultaneous presence of an elevated $HCO_3^-$ and low $Paco_2$, which together will cause a large rise in pH. The resulting combined alkalosis can be severe and may result in serious complications including life-threatening cardiac arrhythmias. Two clinical situations causing combined respiratory and metabolic alkalosis are noteworthy.

## Critically Ill Patients

Respiratory alkalosis is common among patients undergoing critical care. Causes include anxiety, pain, hypoxemia, hypotension, and neurologic damage. Concurrent metabolic alkalosis may develop as a result of nasogastric suctioning, vomiting, blood transfusions, or antacid therapy.

## Ventilator-Induced Alkalosis

Ventilator-induced alkalosis (also called iatrogenic alkalosis) can occur when patients with compensated respiratory acidosis undergo mechanical ventilation. Typically, these are patients with COPD who have chronically elevated $Paco_2$ levels who develop acute-on-chronic respiratory failure. Their "normal" acid-base state is a compensated respiratory acidosis, and delivery of inappropriately high volumes or rapid respiratory rates may cause a precipitous drop in the $Paco_2$ resulting in respiratory alkalosis. At the same time, the elevated $HCO_3^-$—high due to renal compensation of chronic respiratory acidosis—results in combined alkalosis. This problem can be avoided if initial ventilator

---

### BOX 8.3    Common Causes of Mixed Acid-Base Disorders

- Chronic respiratory acidosis and metabolic alkalosis
  - Ventilatory failure and diuretic therapy
  - COPD patient treated with steroids or ventilation
- Respiratory alkalosis and metabolic acidosis
  - Salicylate intoxication
  - Gram-negative sepsis
  - Severe pulmonary edema

*COPD*, Chronic obstructive pulmonary disease.

---

settings target a $Paco_2$ that is consistent with the patient's elevated "normal" or if the ventilator is adjusted to lower $Paco_2$ slowly.

## MIXED ACID-BASE DISTURBANCES

Mixed acid-base disorders occur when two primary imbalances coexist, with each driving the pH in the opposite direction. These disorders are most common among critically ill patients and generally indicate a poor prognosis. Box 8.3 outlines some of the common causes of mixed acid-base disorders.

### SIMPLY STATED

A normal or near-normal pH in the presence of severe abnormalities in $HCO_3^-$ or $Paco_2$ suggests a mixed acid-base disorder.

Mixed imbalances are difficult to recognize because they can be confused with secondary compensation for a primary disorder. However, in most mixed imbalances, the degree of compensation for what is the presumed primary disorder is greater than the expected response, as previously outlined in Table 8.7. It is important to establish that these are two primary problems, as opposed to a single compensated disorder, to provide appropriate management of both disorders.

## Mixed Metabolic Acidosis and Respiratory Alkalosis

When metabolic acidosis is accompanied by a lower than predicted $PaCO_2$, a concurrent respiratory alkalosis is present (see Table 8.7). In this situation, the pH may be elevated slightly above 7.40 and give the appearance of a compensated respiratory alkalosis. Conversely, this mixed disorder may be diagnosed in a patient with primary respiratory alkalosis when the reduction in plasma $HCO_3^-$ exceeds the predicted amount (see Table 8.7).

## Mixed Metabolic Alkalosis and Respiratory Acidosis

When a patient with respiratory acidosis has a greater than predicted $HCO_3^-$ level (see Table 8.7), a mixed metabolic alkalosis and respiratory acidosis are likely. Conversely, when a patient with a known metabolic alkalosis has $PaCO_2$ above 50 to 55 mm Hg (see Table 8.7), a complicating respiratory acidosis is occurring. A pH of 7.40 occurring simultaneously with significant abnormalities in $PaCO_2$ and $HCO_3^-$ suggests a mixed disorder because normal compensation seldom returns the pH to 7.40.

A typical clinical situation in which mixed metabolic alkalosis and respiratory acidosis may occur is treatment of the patient with COPD who has chronic respiratory acidosis. This type of patient often is treated with diuretics and steroid therapy, which can induce metabolic alkalosis. The complicating metabolic alkalosis may promote further hypoventilation and worsen the clinical picture. Metabolic alkalosis can make weaning patients from mechanical ventilation difficult because it may decrease the patient's ventilatory drive. Recognition and treatment of the metabolic alkalosis are vital to optimizing the patient's respiratory function and may result in a significant reduction in $PaCO_2$.

## ENSURING VALID MEASUREMENT AND USE OF BLOOD GAS DATA

Blood gas results are used to make critical decisions, so measurements must be accurate, their interpretation valid, and their application to patient care correct. Errors in any of these areas can result in poor patient management and unsatisfactory outcomes.

To avoid errors in the measurement and use of blood gas data requires a comprehensive quality assurance program. Such programs are designed to ensure quality in sample acquisition and handling (preanalytic phase: preanalytic errors); calibration, use, and maintenance of the measurement device (analysis phase: analytic errors); and postanalytic reporting (postanalytic errors), interpretation, and use of test results.

### Preanalytic Errors

Blood samples obtained by invasive sampling are analyzed either at the bedside using a point-of-care device or in a central laboratory using a bench-top analyzer. In either case, it is essential that the sample provided for analysis be free of preanalytic errors. Table 8.8 summarizes the common preanalytic errors associated with arterial blood sampling, their effect on measurement, and how to recognize and avoid them.

| TABLE 8.8 | Preanalytic Errors Associated with Arterial Blood Sampling | | |
|---|---|---|---|
| **Error** | **Effect(s)** | **How to Recognize** | **How to Avoid** |
| Air in sample | Lowers $PCO_2$ | Visible bubbles or froth | Discard frothy samples |
| | Raises pH | Low $PCO_2$ inconsistent with patient | Fully expel bubbles |
| | Raises low $PO_2$ | status | Mix only after air expelled |
| | Lowers high $PO_2$ | | Cap syringe quickly |
| Venous blood or venous admixture | Raises $PCO_2$ | Failure of syringe to fill by pulsations | Avoid femoral site |
| | Lowers pH | Patient has no symptoms of hypoxemia | Do not aspirate sample |
| | Can greatly lower $PO_2$ | | Use short-bevel needles |
| | | | Avoid artery "overshoot" |
| | | | Cross-check with $SpO_2$ |
| Excess liquid heparin (dilution)[a] | Lowers $PCO_2$ | Visible liquid heparin remains in syringe | Fill dead space only |
| | Raises pH | before sampling | Collect >2 mL (adults) |
| | Raises low $PO_2$ | | Use dry heparin |
| | Lowers high $PO_2$ | | |
| Metabolic effects | Raises $PCO_2$ | Excessive time lag since sample collection | Analyze within 30 minutes |
| | Lowers pH | | If analysis cannot occur with 30 minutes, place sample in ice slush |
| | Lowers $PO_2$ | Values inconsistent with patient status | |

[a]Rare occurrence, with most arterial blood gas kits now using dry lyophilized heparin.
Modified from Scanlan CL: Analysis and monitoring of gas exchange. In Scanlan CL, Wilkins RL, Stoller JK, editors: *Egan's fundamentals of respiratory care*, ed 7, St. Louis, 1999, Mosby.

## Analytic Errors

Blood gas quality control measures help avoid errors during sample analysis. To minimize analytic errors requires regular calibration of the measurement device. Calibration involves exposing the analyzer to calibration media at two or more known levels of measurement. For example, the calibrating media for a standard blood gas analyzer includes precision mixtures of $O_2$ and $CO_2$ gas (to calibrate the $O_2$ and $CO_2$ electrodes) and buffer solutions with known pH values (to calibrate the pH electrode). During this automated or semi-automated process, the analyzer adjusts its output to correspond exactly to the calibration media's known values.

In addition to automated calibration, analyzers should be subject to regular calibration verification. Calibration verification involves analyzing control media representing at least three levels of the measured parameter. By plotting these data on a chart and using statistical analysis to identify outlier measurements or inappropriate trends, potential malfunctions of the analyzer can be identified and corrected before they affect the accuracy of reported results from patient samples.

An additional component of laboratory quality control is proficiency testing. Proficiency testing involves blind testing of samples distributed by a central site. Once analyzed, results are returned for review and validation. The central site then sends a report back to participating laboratories for inclusion in their quality assurance documentation. Proficiency testing is required to maintain accreditation of laboratories, including blood gas laboratories.

## Postanalytic Errors

In the postanalytic phase, results are provided to the clinician, who interprets them and makes patient management decisions accordingly. Errors in this phase can include incorrect reporting and improper interpretation or use of results. Proper interpretation and use of blood gas results are covered in subsequent sections. However, before results are interpreted and applied to patient management, clinicians should perform both internal and external validity checks on the results reported to them.

### Internal Validity Checks

Application of the Henderson-Hasselbalch equation makes it easy to identify gross errors in blood gas analysis reports. For example, when the pH is greater than 7.45 (alkalemia), either the $CO_2$ must be low or the $HCO_3^-$ high. Likewise, in the presence of elevated $CO_2$ or a decreased $HCO_3^-$, acidemia must be present. If results are not consistent with the relationship established in the Henderson-Hasselbalch equation, they should be deemed inaccurate and not be acted on. Instead, reanalysis should be undertaken.

### External Validity Checks

An important question to ask before making any decisions based on blood gas results is whether the patient's condition is consistent with the results. For example, if a patient presents without cyanosis and is well oriented and in no respiratory distress, a reported $Pao_2$ of less than 50 mm Hg should be suspect (in this case, likely a venous blood sample).

Another validity check is to assess whether the reported $Pao_2$ is attainable on the stated $Fio_2$. If a patient is breathing room air and the sum of the $Pao_2$ and $Paco_2$ exceeds 150 mm Hg, either a measurement or reporting error has occurred. Also, any time the $Pao_2$ is more than 5 times the $O_2$ percentage, the results are suspect (the "rule of 5"). Most likely, the $Fio_2$ is higher than reported, or the $Pao_2$ is inaccurate. For greater accuracy, use the alveolar air equation to determine the $P_{AO_2}$. Any $Pao_2$ that is equal to or greater than the $P_{AO_2}$ is inaccurate.

Discrepancies between measures made by different devices also can occur. For example, a pulse oximeter may indicate a saturation of 85%, but analysis of an arterial sample with a CO-oximeter may indicate an $Sao_2$ of 93%. Such discrepancies are best addressed first by determining which results are most consistent with the patient's condition. If this check fails to resolve the difference, generally one should rely on the most valid analysis results, in this case the CO-oximetry results.

---

### SIMPLY STATED

Rule of 5: if the $Pao_2$ is greater than 5 times the oxygen percentage, the result is suspect.

---

## SYSTEMATIC INTERPRETATION OF BLOOD GASES

To interpret blood gas measurements, oxygenation should be assessed first, followed by a separate evaluation of acid-base balance. This priority is based on the greater sensitivity and more rapid impact that inadequate oxygenation has on organs and tissues than that caused by acid-based imbalances.

### Oxygenation Assessment

#### Step 1

Identify the $Pao_2$, and determine whether it is within an acceptable range. In doing so, be sure to account for the patient's age, $Fio_2$, and barometric pressure. If hypoxemia is present, determine its cause by assessing the $P(A-a)o_2$ or P:F ratio and patient's response to $O_2$ therapy.

#### Step 2

Identify the Hb saturation ($Sao_2$), and determine if it is in an acceptable range. Ideally, this assessment should include the $Sao_2$ obtained by CO-oximetry to determine the impact of abnormal hemoglobin such as COHb and metHb.

#### Step 3

Identify the Hb concentration and $Cao_2$, again ideally through CO-oximetry. Note that $Cao_2$ values reported from laboratories without CO-oximeters are calculated and may not be accurate. As an alternative, use a recent Hb measurement from a CBC report.

#### Step 4

Assess the adequacy of circulation. Remember that oxygen delivery depends on both $Cao_2$ and cardiac output. Basic evaluation of the adequacy of circulation involves assessment of blood pressure and palpation of the extremities for temperature, arterial pulses, and capillary refill (see Chapter 5).

## Acid-Base Assessment

### Step 1

Assess the measured pH. If pH is within its normal range, a normal acid-base status, a completely compensated acid-base disorder, or a mixed acid-base disorder is present. A normal acid-base status is present when the $Paco_2$ and $HCO_3^-$ also fall within their normal ranges. If plasma $HCO_3^-$ and $Paco_2$ are both abnormal with a pH in the normal range, either a fully compensated or mixed acid-base disorder is present.

### Step 2

If the pH is lower than 7.35, the primary imbalance must be an acidosis. Look at $HCO_3^-$ and $Paco_2$ to identify which one is contributing to the acidosis. An elevated $Paco_2$ indicates a primary respiratory acidosis, whereas a decreased $HCO_3^-$ indicates a primary metabolic acidosis.

If pH is greater than 7.45, alkalosis is present. An elevated $HCO_3^-$ level indicates a primary metabolic alkalosis, whereas a decrease in $Paco_2$ below 35 mm Hg indicates a primary respiratory alkalosis.

### Step 3

Once the primary acid-base disorder is identified, assess the degree of compensation (see Table 8.7). An elevation in $HCO_3^-$ compensates for respiratory acidosis, and a decrease in $HCO_3^-$ compensates for respiratory alkalosis. On the other hand, a decrease in $Paco_2$ compensates for metabolic acidosis, and an elevation in $Paco_2$ compensates for metabolic alkalosis.

In general, when the compensatory response is present but incomplete, the pH will remain outside its normal range. This is called *partial compensation*. Full compensation is present when the secondary response restores the pH to normal. When full compensation occurs, the primary abnormality can be identified by determining on which side of the normal mean (7.4) the pH lies. If the pH is on the acid side (7.35 to 7.39), the primary disturbance is likely acidemia. Conversely, if the pH is on the alkaline side (7.41 to 7.45), the primary disturbance is likely alkalemia (see Table 8.7).

Compensation for a primary acid-base disturbance often occurs in a predictable manner. This is particularly true for metabolic acidosis, respiratory alkalosis, and respiratory acidosis. A mixed acid-base problem is likely present when the predicted compensation is not present within the expected time frame.

## KEY POINTS

- Blood gas analysis is indicated if the patient's symptoms, medical history, physical examination, or laboratory data suggest abnormalities in respiratory or acid-base status.
- If the goal is the most accurate evaluation of oxygenation, ventilation, and acid-base status, invasive sampling and analysis of an arterial blood sample are required.
- The radial artery is the preferred puncture site for ABG sampling because it is accessible, is easy to stabilize after puncture, and normally has good collateral circulation.
- Arterial puncture causes trauma, so an indwelling arterial catheter, or A-line, should be used when frequent sampling is necessary.
- Measurement of normal and abnormal Hb content and actual saturation normally requires sample analysis by CO-oximetry.
- Pulse oximeters only provide oxygenation data; abnormalities in ventilation and acid-base balance may go undetected unless measured.
- A measured $Pao_2$ below the predicted range for a patient breathing room air, regardless of the actual $Fio_2$, is called hypoxemia; hypoxia exists when oxygen delivery to the tissues is inadequate to meet their needs.
- Hypoxemia occurs secondary to ventilation/perfusion (V/Q) mismatch, shunt, diffusion defect, hypoventilation, or a reduced partial pressure of oxygen in the inhaled gas ($Pio_2$), with V/Q mismatch being the most common cause.
- Alkalosis, hypocapnia, hypothermia, fetal Hb, and Hbco shift the oxyhemoglobin curve to the left, resulting in higher $Sao_2$ values at the same $Pao_2$ (impaired unloading at the tissues).
- Acidosis, hypercapnia, and fever shift the curve to the right and result in lower $Sao_2$ values for the same $Pao_2$ (improved unloading at the tissues).

- The pH is a reflection of the acid-base status.
- The $Paco_2$ is the best measure for assessing the adequacy of ventilation but should be interpreted in conjunction with knowledge of the patient's minute ventilation.
- The plasma $HCO_3^-$ is primarily a reflection of the metabolic component of acid-base balance and is regulated by the renal system.
- Arterial blood pH is determined by the ratio of $HCO_3^-$ to $Paco_2$, which normally is 20:1.
- Respiratory acidosis is present when the pH indicates acidemia and the $Paco_2$ is higher than normal; respiratory alkalosis is present when the pH indicates alkalemia and the $Paco_2$ is less than normal.
- Metabolic acidosis is present when the pH indicates acidemia and the $HCO_3^-$ or BE is lower than normal; metabolic alkalosis is present when the pH indicates alkalemia and the $HCO_3^-$ or BE is lower than normal.
- When metabolic acidosis is accompanied by a $Paco_2$ that is lower than the predicted level for the degree of acidosis, a respiratory alkalosis is occurring simultaneously. This is known as a *mixed acid-base disorder*.
- Venous admixture, air in the sample, excessive liquid anticoagulant, and ongoing cell metabolism can all lead to preanalytic errors in measurement of blood gas parameters.
- Analytic errors in measurement of blood gas parameters can be minimized by instrument calibration, calibration verification, and ongoing proficiency testing.
- Never act on a blood gas report without first performing internal and external validity checks on the data.

## CASE STUDY

A 52-year-old man is admitted to the hospital after a sudden onset of chest pain and shortness of breath. Thirty minutes after admission to the intensive care unit, the patient suffered cardiac arrest. Cardiopulmonary resuscitation was initiated and was successful after 10 minutes.

Initial examination after resuscitation revealed that the patient was hypotensive with a spontaneous respiratory rate of 40 breaths/min and a heart rate of 120 beats/min. He was comatose, with central cyanosis, cool extremities, coarse inspiratory and expiratory crackles, and weak pulse. The initial blood gas measurements after resuscitation were as follows:

| Parameter | Result |
| --- | --- |
| pH | 7.17 |
| $Paco_2$ | 40 mm Hg |
| $Pao_2$ | 53 mm Hg |
| $Sao_2$ | 85% |
| $Cao_2$ | 11 mL/dL |
| $HCO_3^-$ | 14 mmol/L |
| BE | −14 mmol/L |
| $Fio_2$ | 1.0 |
| P(A-a)$o_2$ | 610 mm Hg |

### Interpretation

The $Pao_2$ of 53 mm Hg is considered moderate hypoxemia; however, considering that the patient is breathing 100%

oxygen, the $Pao_2$ is significantly below the value predicted by the alveolar air equation (>650 mm Hg). The high P(A-a)$O_2$ on 100% $O_2$ indicates that the primary cause of the hypoxemia is shunting. The $Sao_2$ and $Cao_2$ are significantly lower than normal. Because $Cao_2$ is reduced proportionately more than $Sao_2$, the patient must be anemic.

The clinical signs of tissue hypoxia and metabolic acidosis probably are related. The lack of adequate oxygenation and circulation of the arterial blood is resulting in anaerobic metabolism and lactic acidosis. When hypoxemia and the clinical signs of inadequate perfusion occur simultaneously, metabolic acidosis from the production of lactic acid is a possibility.

The pH is well below normal, indicating acidemia. The plasma $HCO_3^-$ is reduced, and the $Paco_2$ is normal, indicating metabolic acidosis as the primary problem. When primary metabolic acidosis is occurring, the expected compensatory change in $Paco_2$ can be calculated by using the following formula:

$$Paco_2 = [(1.5 \times HCO_3^-) + 8] \pm 2$$

$$\text{Expected } Paco_2 = [(1.5 \times 14) + 8] = 29 \pm 2$$

Because the measured $Paco_2$ is higher than this value, a ventilatory disorder is also present. A lack of adequate pulmonary perfusion probably is resulting in an increase in wasted or dead space ventilation.

## CASE STUDY

A 12-year-old boy is brought to the emergency department with chief complaints of shortness of breath and cough. His past medical history was positive for allergies and eczema. His family history includes allergies and asthma. Physical examination revealed the following:

| | |
| --- | --- |
| Pulse | 124 beats/min |
| Respiratory rate | 35 breaths/min |
| Blood pressure | 120/76 mm Hg |
| Temperature | 98.9°F |

The boy is restless and using his accessory muscles to breathe. Bilateral expiratory wheezes are heard on auscultation. His chest appears hyperexpanded. His expiratory phase is prolonged. A complete blood count revealed a slight increase in white blood cells due to eosinophilia. The hemoglobin and hematocrit levels are within normal limits. Arterial blood gas results are as follows:

| Parameter | Result |
| --- | --- |
| pH | 7.49 |
| $Paco_2$ | 30 mm Hg |
| $Pao_2$ | 68 mm Hg |
| $Sao_2$ | 91.5% |
| $Cao_2$ | 16 mL/dL |
| $HCO_3^-$ | 22 mmol/L |
| BE | −1 mmol/L |
| $Fio_2$ | 0.21 |
| P(A-a)$o_2$ | 40 mm Hg |

### Interpretation

The $Pao_2$ and $Sao_2$ are decreased and indicate mild hypoxemia. However, because the $Cao_2$ is within its reference range, anemia must not be present. The slight increase in P(A-a)$o_2$ indicates that the hypoxemia is most likely due to $HCO_3^-$ mismatching. The clinical signs of hypoxemia are evident in the tachycardia and tachypnea. The hypoxemia would be worse if the patient were not hyperventilating.

The pH indicates alkalemia and corresponds to decreased $Paco_2$. The $HCO_3^-$ is normal, so a simple uncompensated respiratory alkalosis is present. The respiratory alkalosis is a result of the tachypnea, which is caused by hypoxemia and anxiety. The patient has an increase in the work of breathing because of diffuse airway obstruction, as evidenced by the expiratory wheezing. It is important to note that, although the arterial blood gas results do not identify any severe abnormalities, the patient's cardiopulmonary system is working hard to maintain these borderline values. The patient's condition could deteriorate rapidly even with appropriate treatment.

## CASE STUDY

A 57-year-old man has a history of chronic cough and sputum production. He was admitted to the hospital for abdominal surgery. On admission, the patient was noted to be using his accessory muscles to breathe, and he appeared mildly short of breath at rest. He had diminished breath sounds bilaterally, increased anteroposterior chest diameter, and increased resonance to percussion. He has an 80 pack-year smoking history. As part of the preoperative evaluation, blood gases were drawn and revealed the following:

| Parameter | Result |
| --- | --- |
| pH | 7.41 |
| $Paco_2$ | 60 mm Hg |
| $Pao_2$ | 66 mm Hg |
| $Sao_2$ | 91.4% |
| $Cao_2$ | 12.2 mL/dL |
| $HCO_3^-$ | 37 mmol/L |
| BE | +11 mmol/L |
| $Fio_2$ | 2 L/min via cannula |

**Interpretation**

Mild hypoxemia is present even though the patient is breathing supplemental oxygen through a nasal cannula. The hypoxemia probably is a result of hypoventilation and V/Q mismatching. With an $Sao_2$ above 90%, the $Cao_2$ should be closer to 20 mL/dL. Because it is lower than normal, anemia is likely.

The pH is within normal range; however, the $Paco_2$ and $HCO_3^-$ are elevated above normal. The initial temptation is to interpret the acid-base status as completely compensated metabolic alkalosis because the pH is on the alkaline side of 7.40. However, in light of the patient's history and physical examination findings, suggestive of COPD, and because patients with normal respiratory systems usually do not hypoventilate significantly to compensate for metabolic alkalosis, the correct interpretation probably is respiratory acidosis and metabolic alkalosis. A mixed acid-base disorder is present. A cause for metabolic alkalosis must be sought to optimize respiratory function before surgery.

## CASE STUDY

A 25-year-old woman has no previous history of cardiopulmonary disease. She was admitted to the hospital complaining of frequent urination, excessive thirst, and nausea for the past 3 days. At the time of admission, she was drowsy but coherent, her skin was warm and dry, and her breathing was extremely deep and rapid. Blood gas and chemistry results were as follows:

| Parameter | Result |
| --- | --- |
| pH | 7.13 |
| $Paco_2$ | 17 mm Hg |
| $Pao_2$ | 110 mm Hg |
| $Sao_2$ | 99% |
| $Cao_2$ | 19 mL/dL |
| $HCO_3^-$ | 5.5 mmol/L |
| BE | −21 mmol/L |
| $Fio_2$ | Room air |
| $Na^+$ | 142 mmol/L |
| $Cl^-$ | 106 mmol/L |

**Interpretation**

The patient's oxygenation status is normal, with the $Pao_2$ over 100 despite being on room air. This is due to the profound hyperventilation (likely Kussmaul respirations), which in reducing the $Paco_2$ has simultaneously elevated the $Pao_2$.

The pH is well below normal (acidemia) and corresponds to the large decrease in $HCO_3^-$ and BE. The $Paco_2$ is significantly reduced, indicating that the respiratory system is attempting to compensate for the severe metabolic acidosis.

The expected compensation for the metabolic acidosis can be calculated as follows:

$$Paco_2 = [(1.5 \times 5.5) + 8] \pm 2$$
$$Paco_2 = [(8.25) + 8] \pm 2$$
$$Paco_2 = 16.25 \pm 2$$

The $Paco_2$ (17 mm Hg) is consistent with the expected compensatory response. However, the metabolic acidosis remains only partially compensated owing its severity and the limited ability of the patient to further increase her ventilation. The anion gap ($Na^+ - [Cl^- + HCO_3^-]$) is 30.5 mmol/L. This result is well above normal (8 to 16 mmol/L) and indicates that the metabolic acidosis is due to acid gain, consistent with a severe diabetic ketoacidosis.

## CASE STUDY

A 38-year-old woman has a positive smoking history but no history of cardiopulmonary disease. She came to the emergency department complaining of right lower quadrant abdominal pain. She is quickly diagnosed with acute appendicitis and taken to the operating room for an emergency appendectomy. The surgery went well. She is brought to the surgical intensive care unit because she is slow waking up from anesthesia. After extubation, she is breathing spontaneously on a 35% air entrainment mask. Her ABG results reveal the following:

| Parameter | Result |
| --- | --- |
| pH | 7.55 |
| $Paco_2$ | 44 mm Hg |
| $Pao_2$ | 210 mm Hg |
| $Sao_2$ | 100% |
| $Cao_2$ | 17.5 mL/dL |
| $HCO_3^-$ | 22 mmol/L |
| BE | −4 mmol/L |
| $Fio_2$ | 0.35 |

## CASE STUDY—cont'd

### Interpretation

Regarding the patient's oxygenation status, her $Pao_2$ is 210 mm Hg and $Sao_2$ is 100%. Although these values look very good, a quick check should be performed before taking action. The rule of 5 should be applied as follows:

$$\% O_2 \times 5 = \text{estimated maximum } Pao_2$$
$$35 \times 5 = 175 \text{ mm Hg}$$

That the patient's $Pao_2$ is higher than the maximum suggests an error. To confirm that this is an error, the $PAo_2$ should be computed:

$$Pao_2 = FiO_2(PB - PH_2O) - (Paco_2 \times 1.25)$$
$$Pao_2 = 0.35(760 - 47) - (44 \times 1.25)$$
$$Pao_2 = 0.35(713) - (55)$$
$$Pao_2 = 250 - 55$$
$$Pao_2 = 195 \text{ mm Hg}$$

Thus the reported $Pao_2$ (210) is greater than the $PAo_2$, which is impossible, so there has to be an error. There are two possible explanations: either the patient was receiving more than 35% $O_2$, or the reported $Pao_2$ is incorrect. If oxygen analysis confirms that the patient is breathing 35%, the laboratory should be called and informed that an error has occurred.

In terms of acid-base balance, the pH is well above the normal range (alkalemia). The $Paco_2$ is at the high end of normal, which will slightly lower the pH. This suggests that alkalosis is not of respiratory origin. The $HCO_3^-$ is on the low end of normal, which will also cause a fall in the pH. Thus considering the combination of slightly elevated $Paco_2$ and a mildly decreased $HCO_3^-$, the pH should be on the acid side of normal. To confirm whether an error has occurred, the $Paco_2$ and $HCO_3^-$ should be entered into the Henderson-Hasselbalch equation:

$$pH = 6.1 + \log [HCO_3^- / Paco_2 \times 0.03]$$
$$pH = 6.1 + \log [22/44 \times 0.03]$$
$$pH = 6.1 + \log 16.67$$
$$pH = 7.32$$

This confirms another potential laboratory error. Based on these validity checks, no patient management decisions should be made on these data until another arterial sample is obtained and sent to the laboratory for retesting.

## ASSESSMENT QUESTIONS

1. What is the common normal range for arterial pH?
   a. 7.25 to 7.35
   b. 7.35 to 7.45
   c. 7.45 to 7.55
   d. 7.55 to 7.65

2. What is the common range for $Pao_2$ breathing air at sea level?
   a. 50 to 60 mm Hg
   b. 60 to 70 mm Hg
   c. 70 to 80 mm Hg
   d. 80 to 100 mm Hg

3. What is the normal range for $Cao_2$?
   a. 16 to 20 mL/dL
   b. 12 to 16 mL/dL
   c. 8 to 12 mL/dL
   d. 4 to 8 mL/dL

4. To evaluate a patient's acid-base status, you would recommend which of the following?
   a. Transcutaneous $Pco_2$
   b. Pulse oximetry
   c. Arterial blood gas
   d. CO-oximetry

5. To measure actual blood $O_2$ saturation, you would recommend:
   a. Transcutaneous $Po_2$
   b. Pulse oximetry
   c. Arterial blood gas
   d. CO-oximetry

6. Which of the following could you use to assess the adequacy of ventilation in an intubated child receiving mechanical ventilation?
   1. Transcutaneous $Pco_2$
   2. Capnography
   3. Pulse oximetry
   4. Arterial blood gas
      a. 1 and 2 only
      b. 1, 2, and 4
      c. 4 only
      d. 1, 2, and 3

7. Continuous noninvasive assessment of patient oxygenation can be provided by which of the following methods?
   1. Transcutaneous $Po_2$
   2. Capnography
   3. Pulse oximetry
   4. Indwelling arterial line
      a. 1 and 3 only
      b. 1 and 2 only
      c. 3 and 4 only
      d. 1, 3, and 4

8. A patient receiving mechanical ventilation requires frequent assessment of oxygenation, ventilation, and acid-base balance. Which of the following would you recommend?
   a. $Ptco_2/Ptcco_2$ monitoring
   b. Continuous pulse oximetry
   c. Continuous capnography
   d. Arterial blood gas sampling through an A-line

9. Before an arterial blood gas sample is obtained, the patient's clotting parameters should be evaluated because:
    a. They may affect the accuracy of the sample $Pao_2$
    b. If reduced, they may hinder filling of the syringe
    c. Bleeding time may be prolonged if they are abnormal
    d. They may affect the accuracy of sample pH

10. Which of the following is the preferred site for arterial puncture?
    a. Radial artery
    b. Femoral artery
    c. Dorsalis pedis
    d. Brachial artery

11. In performing an Allen test on a patient's left wrist before drawing an arterial sample, you note that her hand remains blanched for more than 25 seconds after releasing pressure on the ulnar artery. Which of the following actions would you take at this time?
    a. Insert a catheter into the brachial artery
    b. Repeat the test on the opposite wrist
    c. Report that the sample cannot be obtained
    d. Proceed with sampling through left radial artery

12. Which of the following infection control precautions would you apply when obtaining an arterial blood gas sample?
    a. Standard precautions plus face shield
    b. Contact precautions plus gown
    c. Droplet precautions plus surgical mask
    d. Airborne precautions plus N95 respirator

13. A patient has a measured $Sao_2$ of 82%. What is his approximate $Pao_2$?
    a. 50 mm Hg
    b. 60 mm Hg
    c. 70 mm Hg
    d. 80 mm Hg

14. Which of the following is TRUE regarding standard pulse oximeters?
    a. They measure the fractional saturation of Hb ($O_2$ Hb to total Hb)
    b. In patients with good perfusion, their accuracy is in the 2% to 4% range
    c. Their accuracy increases when the Hb saturation drops below 65% to 70%
    d. In the presence of dyshemoglobins, they tend to underestimate the true $Sao_2$

15. A 5-year-old patient is admitted to the emergency department with suspected smoke inhalation. To assess the oxygenation status, you would recommend:
    a. Standard pulse oximetry
    b. Arterial sample plus arterial blood gas analysis
    c. Transcutaneous $Po_2$
    d. Arterial sample + CO-oximetry

16. Which of the following represents a normal $P(A-a)o_2$ for a 50-year-old woman breathing room air?
    a. 105 mm Hg
    b. 75 mm Hg
    c. 45 mm Hg
    d. 15 mm Hg

17. An 80-year-old patient has a $Pao_2$ of 71 mm Hg. How would you describe this finding?
    a. Normal for his age
    b. Mild hypoxemia
    c. Moderate hypoxemia
    d. Severe hypoxemia

18. A patient breathing 40% $O_2$ has a markedly higher than normal $P(A-a)o_2$, which does not improve when the $O_2$ concentration is increased to 50%. What is the most likely cause of her hypoxemia?
    a. V/Q imbalance
    b. Pulmonary shunting
    c. Hypoventilation
    d. Diffusion defect

19. Which of the following parameters represents the respiratory component of acid-base status?
    a. $Paco_2$
    b. $HCO_3^-$
    c. $Pao_2$
    d. BE

20. Which of the following is the best indicator of metabolic acid-base status?
    a. Plasma $HCO_3^-$
    b. Base excess
    c. Standard $HCO_3^-$
    d. T40 $HCO_3^-$

21. Which of the following ratios of $HCO_3^-/Paco_2$ would result in a pH of 7.40?
    a. 10:40
    b. 25:40
    c. 6:0.82
    d. 15:1

22. Which of the arterial blood gas acid-base reports represents an error?
    a. pH = 7.30, $Paco_2$ = 60 mm Hg, $HCO_3^-$ = 29 mmol/L
    b. pH = 7.40, $Paco_2$ = 25 mm Hg, $HCO_3^-$ = 15 mmol/L
    c. pH = 7.50, $Paco_2$ = 50 mm Hg, $HCO_3^-$ = 20 mmol/L
    d. pH = 7.60, $Paco_2$ = 35 mm Hg, $HCO_3^-$ = 33 mmol/L

23. Which of the following is TRUE regarding respiratory alkalosis?
    a. The $Paco_2$ is less than 35 mm Hg
    b. An increase in $HCO_3^-$ compensates for respiratory alkalosis
    c. It is called completely compensated if the pH is 7.52
    d. It is called partially compensated if the pH is in the normal range

24. A patient has the following arterial blood gas results: pH 7.33, $Paco_2$ 35 mm Hg, 18 mmol/L, BE −7 mmol/L. Based on these findings, the patient has which of the following?
    a. Compensated metabolic acidosis
    b. Uncompensated respiratory acidosis
    c. Uncompensated metabolic acidosis
    d. Compensated respiratory acidosis

25. A 35-year-old, 54-kg woman with congestive heart failure enters the emergency department short of breath. An arterial blood gas sample shows the following results:

pH 7.51, $Paco_2$ 30 mm Hg, $HCO_3^-$ 23 mmol/L, BE +1 mmol/L. These results indicate which of the following?
a. Uncompensated respiratory alkalosis
b. Compensated respiratory acidosis
c. Uncompensated metabolic alkalosis
d. Uncompensated metabolic acidosis

26. Given the following arterial blood gas results, interpret the acid-base status: pH 7.45, $Paco_2$ 25 mm Hg, $HCO_3^-$ 17 mmol/L, BE −6 mmol/L.
a. Compensated metabolic acidosis
b. Uncompensated respiratory alkalosis
c. Uncompensated respiratory acidosis
d. Compensated respiratory alkalosis

27. A 17-year-old man is brought into the emergency department. Vitals are as follows: pulse, 100 beats/min; respiratory rate, 4 breaths/min; and blood pressure, 100/65 mm Hg. The patient was at a party where he was discovered by his friends to be slumped in a chair and unresponsive. Arterial blood gas results are as follows: pH 7.24, $Paco_2$ 68 mm Hg, $HCO_3^-$ 28 mmol/L, BE +1 mmol/L. The patient's acid-base status is classified as which of the following?
a. Uncompensated respiratory acidosis
b. Partially compensated respiratory acidosis
c. Compensated respiratory alkalosis
d. Uncompensated metabolic acidosis

28. An acute increase in $Paco_2$ of 10 to 15 mm Hg causes a corresponding increase in plasma $HCO_3^-$ of how much?
a. 1 mmol/L
b. 2 mmol/L
c. 3 mmol/L
d. 4 mmol/L

29. Which of the following causes metabolic acidosis?
a. Hyperventilation
b. Renal disease
c. Hypokalemia
d. Vomiting

30. Given the following arterial blood gas results, interpret the acid-base status: pH 7.14, $Paco_2$ 55 mm Hg, $HCO_3^-$ 18 mmol/L.
a. Combined respiratory and metabolic acidosis
b. Partially compensated respiratory acidosis
c. Mixed respiratory acidosis and metabolic alkalosis
d. Uncompensated metabolic acidosis

31. Given the following arterial blood gas results, interpret the acid-base status: pH 7.62, $Paco_2$ 30 mm Hg, $HCO_3^-$ 30 mmol/L.
a. Partially compensated metabolic alkalosis
b. Mixed respiratory alkalosis and metabolic acidosis
c. Combined respiratory and metabolic alkalosis
d. Uncompensated metabolic alkalosis

32. A mixed metabolic acidosis and respiratory alkalosis are likely when the pH and $HCO_3^-$ are low and the $Paco_2$ is:
a. Higher than the predicted
b. Within its reference range
c. Lower than the predicted
d. 20 times the concentration

33. Given the following arterial blood gas results, interpret the acid-base status: pH 7.42, $Paco_2$ 56 mm Hg, $HCO_3^-$ 35 mmol/L.
a. Partially compensated metabolic alkalosis
b. Mixed metabolic alkalosis and respiratory acidosis
c. Combined respiratory and metabolic alkalosis
d. Fully compensated respiratory alkalosis

34. The best way to minimize the impact of cell metabolism on analysis of an arterial blood gas sample is to:
a. Use extra heparin in the syringe
b. Analyze the sample within minutes
c. Immediately place the sample on dry ice
d. Fully expel all air bubbles

35. The procedure whereby a blood-measuring instrument is exposed to samples at two or more known levels to ensure accuracy is termed:
a. Proficiency testing
b. Analyzer calibration
c. Preanalytic validation
d. Preventive maintenance

36. The blood gas results from a patient breathing a confirmed $O_2$ concentration of 30% indicate a $Pao_2$ of 250 mm Hg. Based on this datum, it can be concluded that the:
a. Patient has a large pulmonary shunt
b. $Pao_2$ is in the expected range for this $\%O_2$
c. Patient must be at high altitude
d. $Pao_2$ is in error and should be remeasured

*Answer Questions 37 to 40 based on the following blood gas data:*

| | |
|---|---|
| pH | 7.21 |
| $Paco_2$ | 67 mm Hg |
| $HCO_3^-$ | 26 mmol/L |
| BE | +2 mmol/L |
| $Pao_2$ | 53 mm Hg |
| $Sao_2$ | 78% |
| Hb | 10.1 g/dL |
| $Cao_2$ | 10.4 mL/dL |
| Respiratory rate | 25 breaths/min |
| $Fio_2$ | 0.70 |

37. Which of the following is TRUE regarding the patient's $Pao_2$?
a. It is adequate
b. It shows mild hypoxemia
c. It shows moderate hypoxemia
d. It shows severe hypoxemia

38. Which of the following is TRUE regarding the patient's oxygen-carrying capacity?
a. It is normal
b. It is increased
c. It is decreased
d. Unable to determine

39. The acid-base status is classified as:
a. Uncompensated metabolic alkalosis
b. Partially compensated metabolic alkalosis
c. Uncompensated respiratory acidosis
d. Partially compensated respiratory acidosis

40. Which of the following could cause this patient's problem?
    a. Anxiety and fear
    b. Acute airway obstruction
    c. Lactic acid production
    d. Renal failure

## BIBLIOGRAPHY

Adrogue HJ. Mixed acid-base disturbances. *J Nephrol* 2006;**19**(Suppl. 9):S97–103.

Albert TJ, Swenson ER. Circumstances when arterial blood gas analysis can lead us astray. *Respir Care* 2016;**61**(1):119–21. http://dx.doi.org/10.4187/respcare.04556.

American Association for Respiratory Care. Clinical practice guideline. Pulse oximetry. *Respir Care* 1991;**36**(12):1406–9.

American Association for Respiratory Care. Clinical practice guideline. Blood gas analysis and hemoximetry: 2013 revision and update. *Respir Care* 2013. http://dx.doi.org/10.4187/respcare.02786.

American Association for Respiratory Care. Clinical practice guideline. Transcutaneous blood gas monitoring for neonatal and pediatric patients: 2012 revision and update. *Respir Care* 2012;**1149**(9):1955–62.

American Thoracic Society. Patient information series: pulse oximetry. Available at https://www.thoracic.org/patients/patient-resources/resources/pulse-oximetry.pdf.

Andrianopoulos V, Vanfleteren LE, Jarosch I, et al. Transcutaneous carbon-dioxide partial pressure trends during six-minute walk test in patients with very severe COPD. *Respir Physiol Neurobiol* 2016;**233**:52–9. http://dx.doi.org/10.1016/j.resp.2016.08.003.

Barker SJ, Badal JJ. The measurement of dyshemoglobins and total hemoglobin by pulse oximetry. *Curr Opin Anaesthesiol* 2008;**21**(6):805–10.

Brandis K. 2.4 Renal regulation. *acid-base physiology*. Available at http://www.anaesthesiamcq.com/AcidBaseBook/ab2_4.php. (Online Text, Updated April 2016.)

Breen PH. Arterial blood gas and pH analysis: clinical approach and interpretation. *Anesthesiol Clin North Am* 2001;**19**(4):885–906.

Cannesson M, Talke P. Recent advances in pulse oximetry. *F1000 Med Rep* 2009;**1**:66.

Casaletto JJ. Differential diagnosis of metabolic acidosis. *Emerg Med Clin North Am* 2005;**23**(3):771–87: ix.

Comym VC, Macedu YS, Neves EK, et al. Interference of heart and transcutaneous oxygen monitoring in the measurement of bioelectrical impedance analysis in preterm newborns. *J Pediatr (Rio J)* 2016;**92**(5):528–31. http://dx.doi.org/10.1016/j.jped.2016.01.009.

Das J, Aggarwal A, Aggarwal JK. Pulse oximeter accuracy and precision at five different sensor locations in infants and children with cyanotic heart disease. *Indian Ju Anaesth* 2010;**54**(6):531–4.

Fouzas S, Priftis KN, Anthracopoulos MB. Pulse oximetry in pediatric practice. *Pediatrics* 2011;**128**(4):740–52.

Gerdung CA, Adeleye A, Kirk VG. Noninvasive monitoring of CO₂ during polysomnography: a review of the recent literature. *Curr Opin Pulm Med* 2016;**22**(6):527–34.

Gonzalez AL, Waddell LS. Blood gas analyzers. *Top Companion Anim Med* 2016;**31**(1):27–34. http://dx.doi.org/10.1053/j.tcam.2016.05.001.

Goonasekera CD, Goodwin A, Wang Y, et al. Arterial and end-tidal carbon dioxide difference in pediatric intensive care. *Indian J Crit Care Med* 2014;**18**(11):711–5. http://dx.doi.org/10.4103/0972-5229.144011.

Hardie JA, Vollmer WM, Buist AS, et al. Reference values for arterial blood gases in the elderly. *Chest* 2004;**125**(6):2053–60.

Janaillac M, Labarinas S, Pfister RE, et al. Accuracy of transcutaneous carbon dioxide measurement in premature infants. *Crit Care Res Pract* 2016;**8041967**:2016. http://dx.doi.org/10.1155/2016/8041967.

Jing F, Wang J, Li M, et al. The influence of high volume hemofiltration on extra vascular lung water and alveolar-arterial oxygen pressure difference in patients with severe sepsis. *Eur Rev Med Pharmacol Sci* 2015;**19**(20):3792–800.

Jones MB. Basic interpretation of metabolic acidosis. *Crit Care Nurse* 2010;**30**(5):63–9.

Kacmarek R, Stoller JL, Heuer AJ. *Egan's fundamentals of respiratory care*. 11th ed. St. Louis: Mosby-Elsevier; 2017.

Kemper AR, Mahle WT, Martin GR, et al. Strategies for implementing screening for critical congenital heart disease. *Pediatrics* 2011;**128**(5):e1259–67.

Mahle WT, Newburger JW, Matherne GP, et al. Role of pulse oximetry in examining newborns for congenital heart disease: a scientific statement from the American Heart Association and American Academy of Pediatrics. *Circulation* 2009;**120**(5):447–58.

Reddy P, Mooradian AD. Clinical utility of anion gap in deciphering acid-base disorders. *Int J Clin Pract* 2009;**63**(10):1516–25.

Rogers KM, McCutcheon K. Four steps to interpreting arterial blood gases. *J Perioper Pract* 2015;**25**(3):46–52.

Ruckman JS. CO-oximeters. *Biomed Instrum Technol* 2012;**46**(1):61–3.

Sandberg KL, Brynjarsson H, Hjalmarson O. Transcutaneous blood gas monitoring during neonatal intensive care. *Acta Paediatr* 2011;**100**(5):676–9.

Storre JH, Magnet FS, Dreher M, et al. Transcutaneous monitoring as a replacement for arterial Pco₂ monitoring during nocturnal non-invasive ventilation. *Respir Med* 2011;**105**(1):143–50.

Walsh BK, Crotwell DN, Restrepo RD. Capnography/capnometry during mechanical ventilation: 2011 (American Association for Respiratory Care clinical practice guideline). *Respir Care* 2011;**56**(4):503–9.

WHO. *Guidelines on drawing blood: best practices in phlebotomy*. Geneva: World Health Organization; 2010.

Zijlstra WG. Clinical assessment of oxygen transport-related quantities. *Clin Chem* 2005;**51**(2):291–2.

# 9

# Pulmonary Function Testing

*Craig L. Scanlan and Albert J. Heuer*

## LEARNING OBJECTIVES

*After reading this chapter, you will be able to:*

1. Define and cite typical values for and differentiate among the lung volumes and capacities.
2. Compute any lung capacity based on its constituent parts.
3. Specify the indications and contraindications for basic spirometry.
4. Differentiate between the measurement and use of the slow and forced vital capacity.
5. Define the parameters typically derived from a forced vital capacity (FVC) maneuver, plotted as volume versus time.
6. Describe the appropriate use of the peak expiratory flow measure.
7. Define the parameters typically derived from the maximal inspiratory-expiratory flow-volume curves and their use in identifying patterns of ventilatory impairment.
8. Define, describe the utility, and specify how to estimate the maximal voluntary ventilation.
9. Identify the necessary calibration tests and accuracy standards for spirometry equipment.
10. Outline the key procedural elements required to obtain accurate spirometry data.
11. Specify the acceptability and repeatability criteria for FVC measurements.
12. Apply the concept of reference ranges and upper and lower limits of normal to the interpretation of spirometry data.
13. Given a subject's basic spirometry test parameters, classify the results as representing normal function or an obstructive or restrictive ventilatory impairment.
14. Describe how to use basic spirometry to assess for reversibility of an obstructive ventilatory impairment.
15. Specify the indications and contraindications for static lung volume determination.
16. Differentiate among the principles employed, equipment used, and quality assurance standards associated with the three primary methods for measuring functional residual capacity.
17. Compare and contrast the patterns of lung volumes and capacities in normal subjects and those with either an obstructive or restrictive ventilatory impairment.
18. Specify the indications for measuring the diffusing capacity of the lung (DLCO).
19. Identify the equipment needed and test and quality assurance procedures used to measure DLCO.
20. In combination with spirometry and lung volume values, apply DLCO measurements to differentiate among blood/pulmonary vascular disorders and potential causes of restrictive and obstructive ventilatory impairments.
21. Describe three methods used to measure airway resistance and its commonly cited normal reference range.
22. Describe how lung compliance is measured and the commonly cited normal values for lung, thorax/chest wall, and total compliance.
23. Identify the indications for methacholine bronchoprovocation testing, the basic procedure used, and how results are interpreted to classify airway responsiveness.
24. Describe the indications, equipment needed, and quality assurance procedures for measuring expired nitric oxide ($F_ENO$).
25. Apply recommended $F_ENO$ cutoff points to the diagnosis and management of patients with asthma.
26. Outline the basic steps in the 6-Minute Walk Test, specify the cutoff points associated with abnormal functional capacity, and stipulate the percentage change needed to indicate improvement due to medical or surgical interventions.
27. Specify the indications and contraindications for cardiopulmonary exercise testing.
28. Define the measurements made when assessing exercise capacity and their typical values at peak capacity.
29. Apply the results of exercise testing to differentiate among patients with poor conditioning and those with cardiovascular or pulmonary limitations to exercise.
30. Outline the key infection control standards that apply to pulmonary function testing.

## KEY TERMS

6MWD
acceptability
airway hyperresponsiveness (AHR)
airway resistance
anaerobic threshold
back-extrapolated volume
biologic control
breathing reserve
bronchoprovocation testing
calibration
compliance
diffusing capacity
expiratory reserve volume (ERV)
$F_ENO$
flow-volume loop
forced vital capacity (FVC)
forced expiratory flow (FEF)
functional lung volume
functional residual capacity (FRC)

HRmax
inspiratory capacity (IC)
inspiratory reserve volume (IRV)
interstitial lung disease (IDL)
linearity (volume, flow)
lower limit of normal/upper limit of
  normal (LLN/ULN)
maximal expiratory flow-volume
  curve (MEFV)
maximal inspiratory flow-volume
  curve (MIFV)
maximal midexpiratory flow
  ($FEF_{25\%-75\%}$)
maximal voluntary ventilation
  (MVV)
metabolic equivalent of task (MET)
minute volume ($V_E$)
nitrogen washout
$O_2$ pulse

obstructive ventilatory impairment
$PC_{20}$
peak expiratory flow (PEF)
reference range
repeatability
residual volume (RV)
respirometer
restrictive ventilatory impairment
slow vital capacity (SVC)
specific conductance ($G_{aw}$/TGV)
spirogram
switch-in error
thoracic gas volume (TGV)
tidal volume ($V_T$)
total lung capacity (TLC)
vital capacity (VC)
$\dot{V}o_2$max

Pulmonary function testing commonly includes spirometry, static lung volume measurements, and diffusing capacity studies. Pulmonary function testing may also involve measurement of the mechanical properties of the lungs and thorax, such as airway resistance and compliance. Some pulmonary function laboratories also may assess airway hyperresponsiveness using bronchoprovocation testing or exhaled nitric oxide measurements and perform exercise testing.

Because spirometry is commonly performed by respiratory therapists (RTs) at the bedside, this chapter emphasizes the measurement and interpretation of parameters obtained using this assessment method. However, because full comprehension of the role of pulmonary function testing in diagnosis requires some knowledge of the more advanced tests, they will be discussed in brief. Also covered are basic equipment needs, quality assurance procedures, and infection control considerations. This chapter ends with a selection of case studies designed to assist the learner in interpreting pulmonary function data.

## LUNG VOLUMES AND CAPACITIES

Fundamental to understanding pulmonary function testing is knowledge of the lung's volumes and capacities. Fig. 9.1 portrays the four lung volumes and four lung capacities both as a graphic plot of inspired and expired volumes over time (called a spirogram) and as a block diagram. Each measure includes its standard abbreviation, with the spirogram also providing average values for the lung volumes and capacities for a healthy young 70-kg male adult. Reference ranges for these measures vary primarily with the height of the individual but are also affected by gender, age, and race.

As indicated in Fig. 9.1, the four lung volumes (inspiratory reserve volume [IRV], tidal volume [$V_T$], expiratory reserve volume [ERV], and residual volume [RV]) are separate from each other and do not overlap. On the other hand, a lung capacity consists of two or more lung volumes. For example, the total lung capacity (TLC) represents the sum

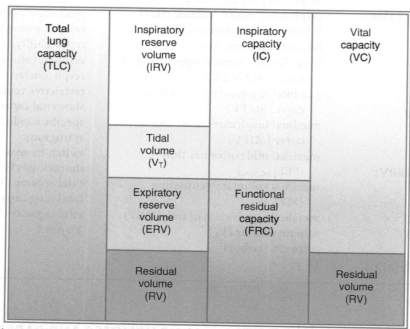

**FIG. 9.1** Lung volumes and capacities. Representation of a simple spirogram and divisions of lung volumes and capacities. (From Kacmarek RM, Stoller JK, Heuer AJ: *Egan's fundamentals of respiratory care*, ed 11, St. Louis, 2017, Mosby.)

of all four lung volumes. As such, lung capacities do over-lap with each other. Note that the residual volume (RV) and the capacities that include it (functional residual capacity and total lung capacity) are not recorded on the spirogram plot in Fig. 9.1. This is because the residual volume remains in the lungs at all times.

Table 9.1 provides functional definitions for each of these volume and capacities.

### SIMPLY STATED

The residual volume and the capacities that include it (FRC and TLC) are not recorded on a simple spirogram because this volume remains in the lungs at all times.

Knowing the tidal volume and rate of breathing (f) allows computation of the volume of gas inhaled or exhaled over 1 minute, called the minute volume or *minute ventilation* and abbreviated as $\dot{V}_E$:

$$\dot{V}_E = f \times V_T$$

Minute volume is commonly measured at the bedside using a simple mechanical or electronic respirometer. For a typical adult breathing at a frequency of 12 breaths per min-ute with an average tidal volume of 500 mL, the minute vol-ume would be computed as follows:

$$\dot{V}_E = 12 \text{ breaths/min} \times 500 \text{ mL/breath}$$
$$= 6000 \text{ mL/min} = 6 \text{ L/min}$$

### TABLE 9.1  Lung Volumes and Capacities

| Measure | Abbreviation | Functional Definition |
|---|---|---|
| **Volumes** | | |
| Tidal volume | $V_T$ | Volume of air inhaled or exhaled during each normal breath |
| Inspiratory reserve volume | IRV | Maximal volume of air that can be inhaled over and above the inspired tidal volume |
| Expiratory reserve volume | ERV | Maximal volume of air that can be exhaled after exhaling a normal tidal breath |
| Residual volume | RV | Volume of air remaining in the lungs after a maximal exhalation |
| **Capacities** | | |
| Total lung capacity | TLC | Maximal volume of air in the lungs at the end of a maximal inhalation (sum of $RV + V_T +$ ERV + RV) |
| Functional residual capacity | FRC | Volume of air present in the lung at end-expiration during tidal breathing (sum of RV + ERV) |
| Inspiratory capacity | IC | Maximal volume of air that can be inhaled from the resting end-expiratory level (sum of $IRV + V_T$) |
| Vital capacity | VC | Maximal volume of air that can be exhaled after a maximal inhalation (sum of $IC + V_T + ERV$) |

Normal minute volumes range between 5 and 10 L/min, depending primarily on the size of the patient. The minute volume increases with fever, pain, hypoxia, acidosis, and increased metabolic rate. It can rise to 60 L/min or more during strenuous exercise.

Also commonly measured at the bedside is the vital capacity. Two different procedures are used, resulting in different measures. If the patient gently but fully exhales from a maximal inspiration, the resulting measure is called a slow vital capacity (SVC). If the patient forcefully empties the lungs from a maximal inspiration, the measure is called the forced vital capacity (FVC).

Typically, the SVC is measured using a respirometer. The SVC measurement can help in assessing perioperative risk because it reflects the patient's ability to take a deep breath, cough, and clear the airways of excess secretions. In general, SVC values lower than 20 mL/kg of predicted body weight indicate an increased risk for postoperative respiratory complications. The SVC also has been used as one of many measures to evaluate a patient's need for mechanical ventilation or readiness to wean. The most commonly cited threshold is 15 mL/kg, with lower values indicating inadequate ventilatory reserve and the need for mechanical ventilatory support.

Measurement of the FVC requires more sophisticated instrumentation capable of nearly instantaneous measurement of airflow. The measurement of FVC and its components is the basis for clinical spirometry.

## SPIROMETRY

Spirometry is the most commonly performed pulmonary function test. Spirometry testing can be conducted in the pulmonary function laboratory, at a patient's bedside, or in an outpatient clinic or doctor's office. Spirometry primarily involves measurement of parameters during patient performance of an FVC maneuver. Spirometry may also include measurement of a patient's maximal voluntary ventilation (MVV).

### Indications and Contraindications

Spirometry is indicated to do the following:
- Detect abnormalities in the lung function suggested by patient history, physical examination, or related diagnostic tests such as chest radiograph.
- Quantify the severity or stage of a known lung disease.
- Follow the course of a patient's disease and response to treatment.
- Assess the risk for perioperative pulmonary complications.
- Evaluate patients for the presence of pulmonary-related disabilities.
- Monitor the effects of exposure to drugs or toxins affecting the lungs.

Relative contraindications for performing spirometry include unstable cardiovascular status, hemoptysis, pneumothorax, and any acute condition that might hinder test performance, such as nausea or vomiting.

### Forced Vital Capacity

The most common spirometry test is the FVC. Table 9.2 summarizes the parameters typically measured and evaluated during this test.

Fig. 9.2 illustrates these parameters on a typical volume-versus-time spirogram. Note that the forced expiratory volume in 1, 3, and 6 seconds ($FEV_1$, $FEV_3$, and $FEV_6$) are all volumes measured at specific times during the forced exhalation. Note also that a normal individual is able to exhale more than 75% of the FVC in 1 second and generally 95% or more in 3 seconds. However, the minimal time needed to ensure a valid FVC measurement is 6 seconds, with some patients requiring more than 10 seconds to fully empty their lungs.

### SIMPLY STATED

A normal individual is able to exhale at least 75% of FVC in 1 second and generally 95% or more in 3 seconds.

Unlike the volume measures, the peak expiratory flow (PEF) and forced expiratory flow ($FEF_{25\%-75\%}$) are represented

| TABLE 9.2 | Parameters Typically Measured during Spirometry | |
|---|---|---|
| Parameter | Abbreviation | Definition |
| Forced vital capacity | FVC | Total volume of air that can be exhaled during a maximal forced expiration effort |
| Forced expiratory volume in 1 second | $FEV_1$ | Volume of air exhaled in the first second after a maximal forced inhalation |
| Ratio of $FEV_1$ to FVC | $FEV_1/FVC$ | Proportion or percentage of the FVC expired during the first second of the maneuver |
| Forced expiratory volume in 3 seconds | $FEV_3$ | Volume of air exhaled in 3 seconds after a forced maximal inhalation |
| Forced expiratory volume in 6 seconds | $FEV_6$ | Volume of air exhaled in 6 seconds after a forced maximal inhalation |
| Peak expiratory flow | PEF | Maximal expiratory flow, typically achieved within 120 ms of the start of the forced exhalation |
| Maximal midexpiratory flow | $FEF_{25\%-75\%}$ | Average flow occurring between 25% and 75% of the FVC |

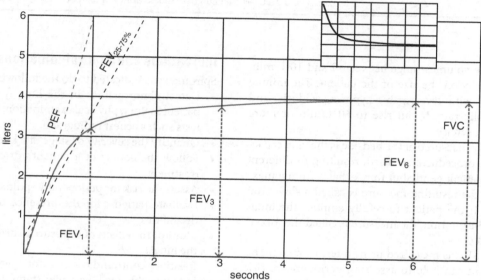

**FIG. 9.2** Parameters measured on a typical volume vs. time spirogram. $FEV_1$, $FEV_3$, and $FEV_6$ are all volumes measured at specific times during the forced exhalation. The PEF and $FEF_{25\%-75\%}$ are flow measures, computed as slopes on the spirogram ($\Delta V/\Delta T$). The *inset* shows an inverted mirror image of the same curve as produced on some spirometers. (Courtesy Strategic Learning Associates, LLC, Little Silver, NJ.)

as sloped lines on the graph. The slope of any line on a graph of volume versus time is flow. The line representing PEF corresponds to the steepest slope of the FVC curve and thus the highest generated flow. The $FEF_{25\%-75\%}$ line is drawn by connecting the two points corresponding to the 25th and 75th percentiles of the FVC. In this example, the FVC is 4 L, so the 25th percentile is reached at 1 L and the 75th percentile occurs at 3 L. Also in this example, as always should be the case, the slope of the $FEF_{25\%-75\%}$ line is less than that plotted for the PEF, signifying what is a progressive decrease in flow throughout the maneuver after the initial PEF blast.

In general, the volume measures obtained by spirometry, including the $FEV_1/FVC$ ratio, are more reproducible than the flow measures. In particular, PEF is very effort dependent. For this reason, it is not given much weight in the overall assessment of pulmonary function.

On the other hand, the PEF is often used by patients with asthma to monitor for evidence of bronchospasm. The test is performed regularly using an inexpensive handheld peak flowmeter. Results are used to help make self-management decisions and incorporated into personal action plans. Typically, these action plans identify 80% to 100% of the patient's personal best peak flow as the green zone, or normal (no special action required); 50% to 80% of the patient's personal best as the yellow zone (requiring self-administration of bronchodilator plus possibly oral steroids); and below 50% of the patient's personal best as the red zone (requiring self-administration of bronchodilator, contacting the doctor, and calling 9-1-1).

**SIMPLY STATED**

PEF is a highly effort-dependent measure and is not particularly useful in diagnosing pulmonary dysfunction. However, it is commonly used by patients with asthma to monitor the severity of bronchospasm and its response to treatment.

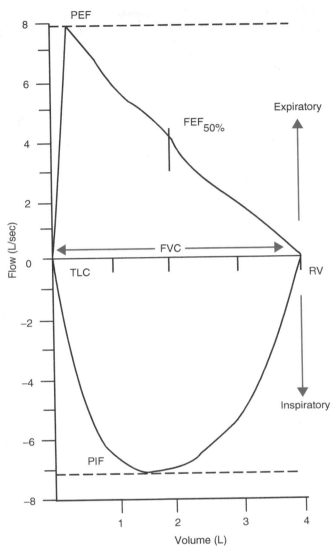

**FIG. 9.3** Example flow-volume loop. Flow in L/s is plotted on the Y-axis and volume in liters on the X-axis. By convention, expiratory flow is plotted upward (positive), and inspiratory flow is plotted downward (negative). (From Mottram C: *Ruppel's manual of pulmonary function testing*, ed 10, St. Louis, 2013, Mosby.)

## Flow-Volume Loops

Most electronic spirometers also can display and record the FVC maneuver as a plot of flow versus volume, typically referred to as a flow-volume loop (Fig. 9.3). To produce a complete flow-volume loop, the patient must be instructed to take a full forced inspiration to TLC before and after the forced exhalation maneuver. The spirometer then records both the inspiratory and expiratory efforts. The expiratory component of the maneuver, called the maximal expiratory flow-volume curve (MEFV), is plotted above the horizontal zero flow line, with the maximal inspiratory flow-volume curve (MIFV) recorded below the zero flow line. The FVC equals the maximal width of the loop along the zero flow line. The PEF equals the maximal positive deflection on the flow axis, with the peak inspiratory flow (PIF) represented as maximal negative deflection on this axis. The FEF at any point in the FVC can also be measured directly. Typically, spirometers record the FEF at

25%, 50%, and 75% of the FVC. For example, the $FEF_{50\%}$ mark on the flow-volume loop in Fig. 9.3 represents the instantaneous forced expiratory flow at 50% of the FVC. Differences in flow between any of these points can also be computed, with the most common being the $FEF_{25\%-75\%}$, which is equivalent to the same measure plotted on a volume-versus-time spirogram.

None of the expiratory measures obtained from a flow-volume loop has proved superior to the $FEV_1$, FVC, $FEV_1/$ FVC, and $FEF_{25\%-75\%}$ obtained by volume-versus-time plots. On the other hand, the shape of the MEFV and MIFV curves can be helpful in detecting certain patterns of disease, as discussed later.

## Maximal Voluntary Ventilation

The MVV is the maximal volume of air a subject can breathe over a specified period of time, usually 12 seconds. The 12-second volume then is multiplied by 5 to extrapolate what could be achieved in 1 minute, with the value expressed in liters per minute. The MVV is affected by the strength of the respiratory muscles, compliance of the lungs and thorax, inspiratory and expiratory airway resistance, and patient motivation and effort. Reference values vary widely, ranging from more than 170 L/min for young adult men to less than 90 L/min for elderly women.

Because one can estimate a patient's MVV by multiplying the measured $FEV_1$ by a factor of 40, this demanding test is no longer included in most standard spirometry protocols. However, the MVV is still used to assess conditions in which ventilatory capacity may be impaired by mechanisms different from those affecting $FEV_1$. For example, some patients with neuromuscular disorders exhibit much larger than expected decreases in their MVV relative to that predicted from their $FEV_1$. The MVV also is used in exercise testing to estimate a subject's breathing reserve (discussed later in this chapter).

### SIMPLY STATED

To estimate a patient's MVV, multiply the measured $FEV_1$ by 40.

## Spirometry Quality Assurance

To obtain valid spirometry data requires accurate instrumentation. However, because FVC maneuvers are technique dependent, obtaining accurate data also depends on the subject being able to perform the maneuvers in an acceptable and reproducible way. Thus there are two major components to spirometry quality assurance: equipment calibration and technique validation.

### Equipment Calibration

The American Thoracic Society (ATS) guidelines specify that spirometers should be capable of measuring volumes of 8 L or more and capturing exhalation maneuvers for at least 15 seconds. Volume accuracy should be at least ±3.5% or ±0.065 L, with the measured flow range between 0 and 14 L per second (−14 to +14 L/s for flow-volume loops). Flow measurements should be accurate within ±5% of the true value over a range

## TABLE 9.3   Calibration Tests for Spirometry Equipment

| Test | Minimum Interval | Action |
| --- | --- | --- |
| Volume | Daily | Calibration check with a calibrated 3-L syringe |
| Volume linearity | Quarterly | 1-L increments with a calibrated syringe over entire volume range |
| Flow linearity | Weekly | Test at least three different flow ranges |
| Software | New versions | Log installation date and perform test using bio-logic controls and known subject |

of $-14$ to $+14$ L per second with a sensitivity (minimal detectable flow) of 0.025 L per second. Spirometers should be able to produce printouts of both volume-time and flow-volume plots.

To ensure spirometry accuracy, regular calibration tests are required. Table 9.3 summarizes these tests as recommended by the ATS and the European Respiratory Society (ERS).

Volume calibration should be performed daily using a calibrated 3-L syringe. The syringe itself must have an accuracy of $\pm 0.5\%$ ($\pm 15$ mL for a 3-L syringe), which is incorporated into the volume accuracy standard ($3.0\% + 0.5\% = 3.5\%$). To assess volume linearity, the syringe should be discharged in three 1-L steps, with each successive volume meeting the 3.5% accuracy standard. To assess flow linearity, the syringe volume should be injected at three different flows, ranging between 0.5 and 12 L per second. With a 3-L syringe, this would equate to injection times between 6 seconds and 0.5 second. The volume at each flow should meet the accuracy standard of $\pm 3.5\%$.

Regular testing using biologic controls also is recommended to assess spirometer performance and accuracy of software computations. A biologic control is a healthy subject for whom quality control data are available. Such data typically include the mean and standard deviation of 8 to 10 reproducible FVC maneuvers measured at different times.

If volume or flow inaccuracy is detected, no tests should be conducted until the cause of the measurement error is corrected. As with any quality assurance program, logs should be maintained to document spirometer calibration, maintenance, and any corrective actions taken.

### Technique Validation

FVC maneuvers are highly technique dependent. For this reason, accurate measurements require proper patient performance of the procedure. Providing clear instructions and eliciting a maximal effort are the keys to ensuring a valid FVC maneuver. In addition, the clinician must be able to recognize and correct any observed errors in technique.

Box 9.1 outlines the key elements in the measurement of FVC using an electronic bedside spirometer. Most elements also pertain to spirometry measurement in the pulmonary function laboratory.

The goal is to obtain at least three acceptable and error-free maneuvers that are repeatable. An acceptable maneuver must

## BOX 9.1   Key Elements in Performance of Forced Vital Capacity Maneuver

- Turn device on, insert mouthpiece/sensor, input sensor data, perform startup test.
- Accurately input all required patient information (height, age, gender, race).
- Have the patient remove candy, gum, and dentures from the mouth.
- Have the patient sit upright or stand with good posture and head slightly elevated (be consistent and record position).
- Demonstrate the procedure using your own mouthpiece/sensor, being sure to show the following:
  - How to hold the sensor steady and avoid jerky motions.
  - How deeply to inhale (completely).
  - How to correctly place the mouthpiece on top of the tongue.
  - How to blast out the breath for as long as possible.
- Use nose clips to prevent patient leaks.
- Have the patient inhale completely and rapidly with a pause of >1 second at TLC.[a]
- Have the patient place mouthpiece/sensor in mouth and obtain tight seal with lips.
- Have the patient perform the FVC maneuver while you observe.
- Have the patient BLAST the breath out, as fast and long as possible.
- Loudly prompt MORE, MORE, MORE, until the subject has exhaled for at least 6 seconds.
- Carefully observe the patient for poor technique and correct as needed.
- Repeat instructions as necessary, coaching vigorously.
- Repeat the procedure until you have three acceptable maneuvers.
- Document the quality of the results, including any validity issues.

[a]To produce a complete flow-volume loop (MEFV + MIFV curves), the patient places the mouthpiece/sensor in mouth before inhalation and must be instructed to take a full forced inspiration to TLC after the forced exhalation maneuver.

be free from artifacts, exhibit a good and forceful start, and achieve complete exhalation. To ensure repeatability, the therapist must confirm that the key volume measures (FVC and $FEV_1$) are free of significant variability. Although many computerized spirometers automatically perform validity checks on each FVC maneuver, the clinician still must manually inspect each plot to confirm that it is acceptable and that the multiple measures are repeatable. A summary of the acceptability and repeatability criteria recommended by the ATS/ERS for FVC maneuvers (plotted as volume vs. time) appears in Box 9.2.

The most common error in obtaining an acceptable FVC is failure to achieve a rapid start to the forced exhalation. This typically is evident when the plotted FVC-versus-time curve is S shaped (like the oxyhemoglobin curve). Alternatively, one can change the spirometer display from volume versus time to flow versus volume and inspect the expiratory curve to determine whether the start of the test was satisfactory. On a flow-volume curve, the PEF should be achieved with a sharp rise and occur close to the point of maximal inflation.

## BOX 9.2  Acceptability and Repeatability Criteria for Forced Vital Capacity Maneuvers

The spirogram is *acceptable* if it meets the following criteria:
- Free from artifacts
  - Coughing/breathing during the maneuver
  - Early termination or cutoff
  - Submaximal effort
- Exhibits a rapid, forceful start
  - Time to peak flow <120 ms
  - Back-extrapolated volume <5% of FVC or 150 mL, whichever is greater
- Achieves complete exhalation
  - Duration of at least 6 s (COPD patients may need >10 s), *or*
  - Attainment of a plateau (<25 mL change in volume for ≥1 s)

Results are *repeatable* if, after three acceptable spirograms have been obtained, the following criteria are met:
- The two largest values of FVC must be within 0.150 L of each other, *and*
- The two largest values of FEV$_1$ must be within 0.150 L of each other

*COPD,* Chronic obstructive pulmonary disease; *FVC,* forced vital capacity; *FEV$_1$,* forced expiratory volume at 1 second.

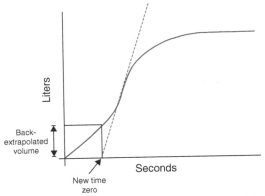

**FIG. 9.4** Calculation of back-extrapolated volume (BEV). Back-extrapolation is used when the spirogram does not exhibit a sharp rise in flow at the beginning of the forced vital capacity (FVC). To compute the BEV, a straight line is drawn through the steepest part of the curve and extended to cross the volume baseline. The point of intersection is the back-extrapolated time zero. The distance from the time zero point to the FVC curve is the BEV. (Courtesy Strategic Learning Associates, LLC, Little Silver, NJ.)

Spirometry software programs typically identify a slow start to forced exhalation by detecting a delay in time to peak flow (>120 ms) or by calculating the back-extrapolated volume. Fig. 9.4 demonstrates how the back-extrapolated volume is calculated, normally by the spirometer's microprocessor. If the back-extrapolated volume is more than 5% of FVC or more than 150 mL, the FVC is unacceptable, and a repeat maneuver is required. On the other hand, if the back-extrapolated volume falls below this quality threshold, the FVC breath still can be used, but with the breath starting point adjusted to the new extrapolated zero time point.

If no acceptable maneuvers can be obtained, results should not be reported; rather, all specific errors encountered should

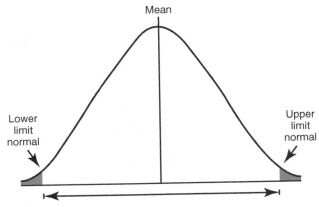

**FIG. 9.5** Determination of upper and lower limits of normal. Ninety-five percent of all values in a normal distribution fall within ±2 standard deviations (SD) of the mean. The boundaries of this range are the lower limit of normal (LLN) and the upper limit of normal (ULN). (Courtesy Strategic Learning Associates, LLC, Little Silver, NJ.)

be documented. Only if three acceptable maneuvers can be obtained, meeting both repeatability criteria, should results be reported. If the initial results are acceptable but are not repeatable, additional testing should be conducted until either the repeatability criteria are met or the patient cannot continue. All reports should contain the therapist's overall assessment of test quality.

### Interpretation of Spirometry Test Results

Interpretation of spirometry test results normally is performed by a trained physician. Assessment involves comparison of the individual patient's data with reference values generated from samples of healthy subjects and review of the applicable plots.

Although other spirometry reference values are available, the preferred prediction equations for subjects 8 to 80 years of age are those established by the National Health and Nutrition Examination Survey (NHANES) III. These equations provide reference ranges for all spirometry parameters based on the subject's height, gender, age, and race.

The pulmonary function community has adopted ±2 standard deviations (SD) from the predicted mean as the normal reference range. With ±2 SD encompassing 95% of the values in a normal distribution (Fig. 9.5), one can define the boundaries of this range as cutoff points, outside of which results are abnormal. These cutoff points are called the lower limit of normal (LLN) and (if applicable) the upper limit of normal (ULN).

For interpretation of tests in which either abnormally low or high values apply, the LLN occurs at the 2.5th percentile and the ULN at the 97.5th percentile. If only abnormally low values are the focus (as with spirometry measures), only the LLN is applicable, which corresponds to values in the distribution below the 5th percentile.

Fig. 9.6 outlines the basic process for interpreting spirometry test results. After ensuring that the test results are valid (three acceptable maneuvers, with two of them being

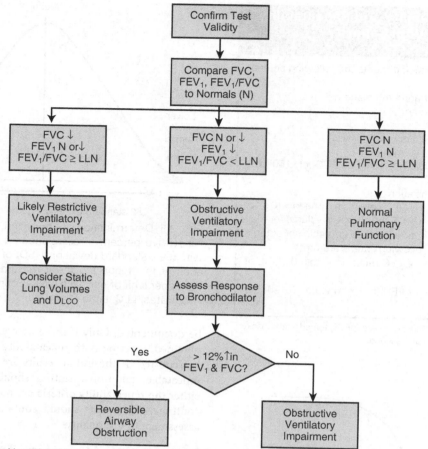

**FIG. 9.6** Algorithm for interpreting spirometry test results. *D*LCO, Diffusing capacity; *FVC*, forced vital capacity; *LLN*, lower limit of normal. (Courtesy Strategic Learning Associates, LLC, Little Silver, NJ.)

repeatable), one compares the patient's FVC, $FEV_1$, and $FEV_1/FVC$ to the predicted reference ranges. If all three values fall within the reference ranges, the results are deemed normal.

If, however, the $FEV_1$ is reduced and the $FEV_1/FVC$ ratio falls below its LLN (below the 5th percentile of predicted), an expiratory flow limitation exists, and the patient is classified as having an obstructive ventilatory impairment. Often, the severity of obstruction is quantified according to magnitude of reduction in $FEV_1/FVC$, as outlined in Table 9.4.

The other major possibility is a reduced FVC, normal or reduced $FEV_1$, and $FEV_1/FVC$ above the LLN (normal or higher than normal). *An $FEV_1/FVC$ above the LLN rules out an obstructive impairment.* However, the presence of a reduced FVC suggests that the patient may have a reduction in lung volume, which would be classified as a restrictive ventilatory impairment.

### SIMPLY STATED

An obstructive ventilatory impairment is characterized by reduced flows, as evident by an $FEV_1/FVC$ ratio lower than the predicted lower limit of normal. A restrictive ventilatory impairment is characterized by decreased lung volumes.

| TABLE 9.4  Severity Classification of Airway Obstruction | |
|---|---|
| **Severity of Obstruction** | **$FEV_1$ (% Predicted)** |
| Mild | 70-74 |
| Moderate | 60-69 |
| Moderately severe | 50-59 |
| Severe | 35-49 |
| Very severe | <35 |

Interpretation is enhanced by review of the graphic plots obtained by spirometry. Fig. 9.7 portrays typical volume-versus-time curves for a normal subject, one with an obstructive impairment and one with a restrictive disorder. Note that the obstructive pattern is characterized by a decrease in the slope of the curve (indicating reduction in expiratory flow) and a longer time to empty the lungs. On the other hand, in the restrictive pattern the lung empties as fast or faster than normal but to a smaller volume.

Inspection of the patient's flow-volume loop can aid in interpretation, especially in identifying the presence and location of large airway obstruction. Fig. 9.8 provides six examples of flow-volume loops representing distinct patterns of abnormal function. Disorders causing generalized expiratory

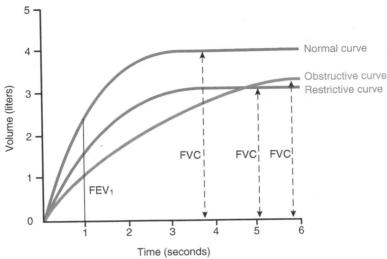

**FIG. 9.7** Forced vital capacity (FVC) curves comparing normal, obstructive, and restrictive disorders. Curves are as they appear on commonly available spirometers with tracings beginning at the bottom left corner. (From Kacmarek RM, Stoller JK, Heuer AJ: *Egan's fundamentals of respiratory care*, ed 11, St. Louis, 2017, Mosby.)

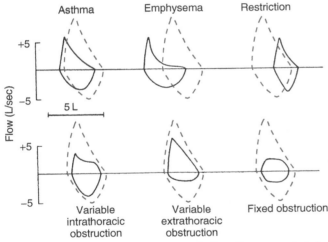

**FIG. 9.8** Patterns of pulmonary dysfunction revealed by flow-volume loops. For comparison, a normal loop is shown with each *(dashed lines)*. See text for details. (From Mottram C: *Ruppel's manual of pulmonary function testing*, ed 10, St. Louis, 2013, Mosby.)

obstruction—such as asthma and emphysema—mainly affect the MEFV curve, with both exhibiting a reduction in peak flow and FEF$_{50\%}$. Note also that the MEFV portion of the loop on the patient with emphysema is markedly concave and positioned left of the normal loop, indicating greater flow obstruction at lower lung volumes, as well as air trapping and hyperinflation. On the other hand, a patient with a restrictive ventilatory impairment typically produces a flow-volume loop with the same shape as normal, but one that is markedly narrower on the volume axis, consistent with the smaller FVC.

The bottom three flow-volume loops in Fig. 9.8 portray different types of *large airway obstructions*. The variable intrathoracic obstruction loop reveals a markedly reduced peak flow on expiration despite near-normal inspiratory flows. This typically is the result of expiratory flow obstruction in the

large airways, as may occur with tracheomalacia or tumors of the trachea or bronchi. The opposite pattern is seen in variable extrathoracic obstruction—that is, reduced inspiratory flow and relatively normal expiratory flow. Vocal cord dysfunction and laryngeal edema are common causes of variable extrathoracic obstruction. An equal reduction in inspiratory and expiratory flows suggests a fixed large airway obstruction. Causes of fixed large airway obstruction include tracheal stenosis, tracheal tumors, and foreign body aspiration.

After the basic pattern is identified, additional testing may be indicated. If the spirometry results indicate that the patient has an expiratory obstructive impairment, the doctor typically will want to determine whether the obstruction is reversible with treatment—that is, if it responds to bronchodilator therapy (see Fig. 9.6). This is accomplished by measuring spirometry values before and after administration of the selected bronchodilator. Normally, the baseline spirometry should be conducted at least 4 hours after any prior use of a short-acting β-agonist (e.g., albuterol) and at least 12 hours after any administration of a long-acting bronchodilator (e.g., salmeterol).

Box 9.3 outlines the key elements in the procedure for assessing reversibility. If, after bronchodilator administration, the FEV$_1$ or FVC increases by more than 12% and at least 200 mL, the obstructive impairment is considered reversible. A lesser response indicates that airflow limitation is not reversible. However, some patients who do not meet the criteria for reversibility may still experience improvement after bronchodilator therapy, such as a decrease in dyspnea. This response likely is due to a decrease in hyperinflation occurring without a significant decrease in airway resistance.

**SIMPLY STATED**

In general, an obstructive ventilatory defect is considered reversible if, after bronchodilator administration, the FEV$_1$ or FVC increases by more than 12% and 200 mL.

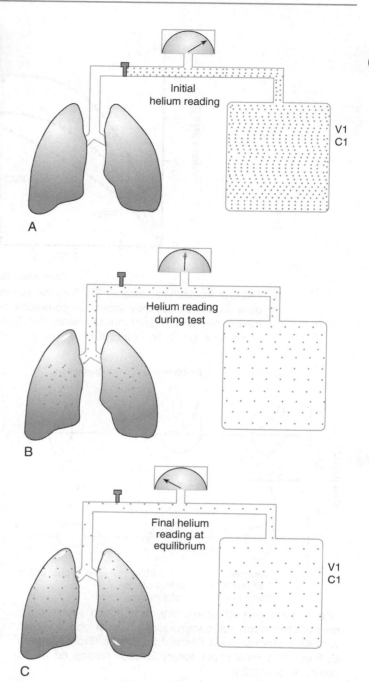

**FIG. 9.9** Closed-circuit helium dilution method for measuring functional residual capacity. Before measurement, enough 100% helium should be added to the system to give a helium reading of about 10%. (From Kacmarek RM, Stoller JK, Heuer AJ: *Egan's fundamentals of respiratory care*, ed 11, St. Louis, 2017, Mosby.)

As indicated in Fig. 9.6, a reduced FVC in the presence of a normal or high FEV$_1$/FVC suggests that the patient may have a reduction in lung volumes. However, this same pattern can occur among patients who fail to completely inhale or exhale during the maneuver. For this reason, confirmation of a reduction in lung volumes and the presence of a restrictive disorder requires measurement of static lung volumes (FRC, RV, TLC). Moreover, if it is suspected that the restrictive condition is due to an interstitial disease processes, most doctors will also request a diffusing capacity study (DLco).

## STATIC LUNG VOLUMES

Static lung volume determination involves measurement of the resting lung volume or FRC. If the FRC is known and the inspiratory capacity (IC) and ERV also are obtained by spirometry, both the RV (FRC − ERV) and the TLC (FRC + IC) can be computed. In general, static lung volume testing is performed in the pulmonary function laboratory.

### Indications and Contraindications

Static lung volume measurements are indicated to do the following:

- Confirm a suspected restrictive disease pattern (low FVC, normal or high FEV$_1$/FVC)
- Assess the impact of or response to medical or surgical interventions such as lung-volume reduction, lobectomy, lung transplantation, and radiation therapy or chemotherapy
- Provide an index of gas trapping (requires comparison of FRC by gas dilution to plethysmographic thoracic gas volume)

Contraindications against performing static lung volume determinations are essentially the same as those previously described for basic spirometry.

### Methods

There are three different methods used to measure FRC: (1) closed-circuit helium dilution, (2) open-circuit nitrogen washout, and (3) body plethysmography. Currently, there is no firm evidence to recommend any one technique over the others. In most cases, the method used will be based on the available equipment and personnel.

### Closed-Circuit Helium Dilution

The closed-circuit helium dilution test is based on the principle that if a known volume and concentration of a gas is added to the patient's respiratory system, it will be diluted in proportion to the lung volume to which it is added (Fig. 9.9). Helium is used because it is an inert gas and is not significantly absorbed

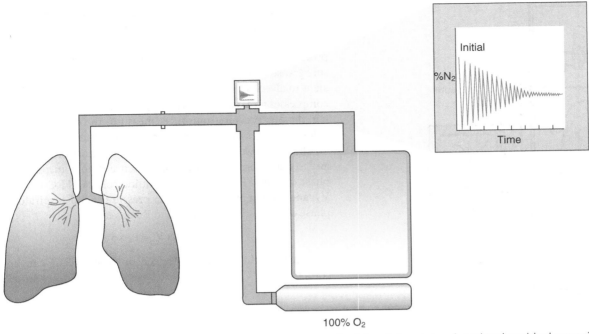

**FIG. 9.10** Open-circuit nitrogen washout method for determining functional residual capacity. (From Kacmarek RM, Stoller JK, Heuer AJ: *Egan's fundamentals of respiratory care*, ed 11, St. Louis, 2017, Mosby.)

from the lungs by the blood. In normal subjects, equilibrium takes about 7 minutes so that oxygen must be added and carbon dioxide ($CO_2$) removed from the system to keep the gas concentrations constant and prevent hypercapnia. After equilibrium is reached, the FRC is calculated as follows:

$$FRC = \frac{(\text{initial He\%} - \text{final He\%}) \times \text{Vapp}}{\text{final He\%}} - V_{Dmech}$$

where Vapp = apparatus volume (volume in the spirometer and connecting tubing) and $V_{Dmech}$ = dead space of the mouthpiece/breathing valve, with the results corrected for BTPS (body temperature and pressure) conditions.

Because helium does not reach areas of the lung distal to any obstruction, the measured FRC reflects only functional lung volume—that is, that in open communication with the airways. The volume of any air trapped in the lungs is not measured.

Measurements normally are made using a volume-displacement (bell or bellows) spirometer. To ensure accuracy, the spirometer capacity should be at least 7 L, and the spirometer should be tested daily for leaks. Ideally, the volume in the empty spirometer and connecting tubing should be ≤4.5 L because the smaller the apparatus volume, the more accurate the measurement. In addition, the breathing valve and mouthpiece should together add less than 100 mL dead space to the system (which is adjusted for in the FRC computation). It is also essential that the test be initiated immediately after the patient normally exhales to FRC. Errors in measurement—called switch-in errors—will occur if the test is initiated at a point either above or below the resting end-expiratory level.

Included with the spirometer should be a helium analyzer with water vapor absorber, a mixing fan, $CO_2$ absorber, and $O_2$ and helium supplies. The helium analyzer should have a range of 0% to 10% with an accuracy of 0.5% of full scale (0.05% for 10% He). Linearity should be checked weekly by two-point calibration with a low gas (room air/0% He) and a known "high" concentration of He (~10%). As with spirometry, regular testing of biologic controls should be part of the quality control program. Biologic control testing has the advantage over standard equipment calibration methods in that it also helps assess the repeatability of the actual procedure used.

### Open-Circuit Nitrogen Washout

Fig. 9.10 depicts the basic principle underlying the nitrogen washout method for measuring FRC. The patient breathes 100% $O_2$, with the expired $N_2$ concentration continuously monitored. The test continues for at least 7 minutes or until all the $N_2$ is washed out of the patient's lungs. Washout is judged complete when the $N_2$ concentration is less than 1.5% for at least three consecutive breaths.

With the total volume and concentration of exhaled $N_2$ known and the knowledge that the air originally in the patient's lungs contained 78% $N_2$, the patient's FRC is computed as follows:

$$FRC = \frac{\text{vol } N_2 \text{ washed out} - \text{vol } N_2 \text{ from tissues}}{\text{starting } N_2\% - \text{ending } N_2\%}$$

The volume of nitrogen washed out during the test is determined either by collecting the entire volume of expired gas and measuring its $N_2\%$ or by computer compilation of

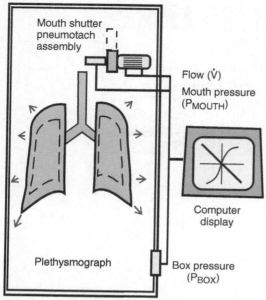

**FIG. 9.11** Body plethysmography method for measuring thoracic gas volume. See text for details. (From Mottram C: *Ruppel's manual of pulmonary function testing*, ed 10, St. Louis, 2013, Mosby.)

the breath-by-breath volume and $N_2\%$. The volume of $N_2$ excreted from the tissues is estimated by equation based on the patient's body surface area.

As with the helium dilution method, accuracy of FRC determination by $N_2$ washout requires an accurate and properly calibrated gas analyzer. The $N_2$ analyzer should have a range of 0% to 100%, with an accuracy of ±0.2% and a rapid response time (<60 ms to a 10% change in $N_2\%$). A two-point calibration should be performed before each patient is tested, with the low gas 100% $O_2$ and the high gas room air (79% $N_2$).

Because a nitrogen washout system simultaneously measures breath-by-breath volumes, the accuracy of volume measurements also must be confirmed daily. Typically, this is done by pumping a calibrated syringe at about the same rates and volumes as expected during patient testing. As with helium dilution, regular (monthly) testing of biologic controls can be used to confirm both equipment function and repeatability of the testing procedure.

Also as with helium dilution, the volume measured by $N_2$ washout is limited to that in open communication with the airways. For this reason, in the presence of significant air trapping, the $N_2$ washout technique will tend to underestimate the actual FRC.

## Body Plethysmography

Fig. 9.11 depicts the concept used to measure lung volumes using a body plethysmograph. The patient sits inside a rigid boxlike enclosure and breathes through a pneumotachometer equipped with a pressure transducer that measures pressure changes at the mouth. The internal box pressure also is measured by a sensitive pressure transducer, calibrated to reflect volume changes inside the enclosure. After the patient completes a normal exhalation, a shutter in the pneumotachometer

closes, occluding the airway. At the same time, the patient gently pants about once per second against the occlusion for 2 to 3 seconds. During the panting maneuver, changes in mouth pressure ($\Delta P$) are recorded by the pneumotachometer's pressure transducer, with the pressure at times of zero flow equivalent to alveolar pressure ($P_{alv}$). Simultaneously, as the patient compresses and decompresses the gas in the lungs while panting, the box pressure transducer measures the corresponding volume changes as the thorax expands and contracts ($\Delta V$).

Thus, we have a starting volume (the unknown FRC = $V_1$) and starting pressure (alveolar pressure before inspiratory phase of pant = $P_1$), as well as an ending volume (FRC + $\Delta V$ = $V_2$) and ending pressure (alveolar pressure at end-inspiratory phase of pant = $P_2$). According to Boyle's law:

$$P_1 \times V_1 = P_2 \times V_2$$

Based on this formula, $V_1$ (the unknown FRC) can be computed as:

$$V_1 = \frac{V_2 \times P_2}{P_1}$$

Expressing pressure and volume as changes from baseline:

$$FRC = \frac{\Delta V}{\Delta P} \times P_2$$

Because the panting creates only small pressure changes around barometric pressure, $P_2$ is assumed to equal $P_B$:

$$FRC = \frac{\Delta V}{\Delta P} \times P_B$$

Thus, the FRC equals the slope of the changes in thoracic volume (measured as changes in box pressure) versus the change in mouth pressure during the panting maneuver, as portrayed on the computer display (see Fig. 9.11).

Unlike the helium dilution and nitrogen washout methods, body plethysmography measures the total compressible gas volume in the thorax, whether or not it is in communication with open airways. When not referenced to any starting point, this volume is called the thoracic gas volume (TGV). When measured from a normal end-inspiratory level, the abbreviation $FRC_{pleth}$ should be used.

In terms of equipment performance, the flow sensor should meet the same accuracy standards as those previously described for spirometers, with the box pressure transducer being accurate to ±0.2 cm $H_2O$ and calibrated daily using volume changes similar in size and frequency to patient panting (usually by a small piston pump delivering 20- to 50-mL stroke volumes). Likewise, the mouth pressure transducer and pneumotachometer should be calibrated daily using both a calibrating manometer (pressure) and syringe (volume).

In regard to procedural quality assurance, sufficient time should be allowed after the patient enters the plethysmograph for the temperature to stabilize. During the panting maneuver, the patient should wear a nose clip (to prevent leaks) and hold the flat of both hands against the cheeks (to prevent error due to oral gas compression and expansion). Typically, the patient is asked to repeat the panting maneuver until at least three

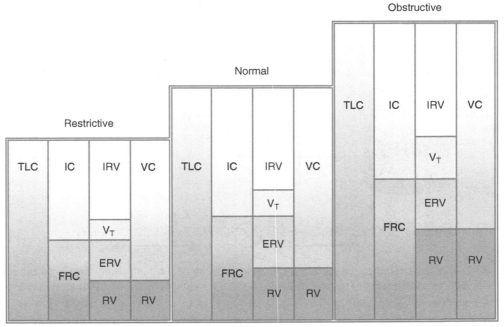

**FIG. 9.12** Changes in lung volumes and capacities characteristic of restrictive and obstructive ventilatory impairments compared with normal. *ERV,* Expiratory reserve volume; *FRC,* functional residual capacity; *IC,* inspiratory capacity; *IRV,* inspiratory reserve volume; *RV,* residual volume; *TLC,* total lung capacity; $V_T$, tidal volume; *VC,* vital capacity. (From Kacmarek RM, Stoller JK, Heuer AJ: *Egan's fundamentals of respiratory care,* ed 11, St. Louis, 2017, Mosby.)

$FRC_{pleth}$ measurements can be obtained that are within ±5% of each other. After the $FRC_{pleth}$ measurements, the shutter is opened, and the patient performs an ERV maneuver, followed by an inspiratory vital capacity (VC) or maximal inhalation from a maximal exhalation.

Overall accuracy (equipment plus procedure) should be assessed at least monthly. One approach is to use a 3- to 4-L glass flask connected both to the pneumotachometer and a large squeeze bulb. Squeezing the bulb simulates the panting maneuver. The average of five such maneuvers should be within ±50 mL or 3% of the known flask volume. Alternatively, two biologic controls should undergo $FRC_{pleth}$ measurement. Values that differ significantly (more than ±10%) from their previously established means indicate either equipment or procedural error.

### Interpretation

Static lung volume measurements are used primarily to confirm the presence of a restrictive ventilatory impairment suggested by spirometry results (low FVC, $FEV_1$/FVC ratio > LLN). As with spirometry, a patient's lung volumes are compared with reference values generated using equations derived from normal subjects, with values outside the 95% prediction interval considered abnormal. Thus an abnormally low FRC, RV, or TLC would be below its LLN, or below the 5th percentile of its predicted value. Based on this interpretation framework, *a patient has a purely restrictive ventilatory impairment if the TLC is lower than its LLN but the $FEV_1$/FVC ratio exceeds its LLN.*

Static lung volumes also have been used to assess for air trapping and hyperinflation in patients with obstructive ventilatory impairments. These abnormalities are associated with an increase in the RV and FRC, with or without an increase in TLC. An increase in the RV occurring with an increase in the TLC (RV/TLC ratio < 35%) is the classic pattern of hyperinflation, sometimes seen in emphysema. An increase in the RV without an increase in the TLC (RV/TLC ratio > 35%) is more consistent with air trapping, as may occur during an exacerbation of asthma. Unfortunately, these patterns often are not so clear-cut, in part because air trapping and hyperinflation are not well-distinguished phenomena. Nonetheless, measurement of the RV in patients with obstructive impairments is potentially useful for monitoring response to therapy (e.g., bronchodilator treatment) and disease progression.

Moreover, knowledge of how lung volumes in restrictive and obstructive disorders differ from normal can be helpful in understanding the nature of these impairments and their differential diagnosis. Fig. 9.12 depicts these patterns compared with normal.

## DIFFUSING CAPACITY OF THE LUNG (D$_{LCO}$)

The diffusing capacity (also called the *transfer factor*) is a measure of the lung's ability to exchange oxygen with the mixed venous blood. Because all methods use low concentrations of carbon monoxide (CO) gas, the abbreviation D$_{LCO}$ is used to refer to this measurement. Several methods can be used to measure CO diffusing capacity. The most commonly used standardized method is the single-breath D$_{LCO}$, or D$_{LCO_{sb}}$.

### Indications

Measurement of D$_{LCO}$ is indicated to do the following:
- Differentiate between interstitial and chest wall/neuromuscular causes of restrictive ventilatory impairments

He/CO analyzers

Spirometer

0.3% CO
10% He
21% $O_2$
Balance $N_2$

End-tidal sampler

Automatic valve

**FIG. 9.13** Apparatus used to measure the diffusing capacity of the lung using the single breath method. See text for details. (From Mottram C: *Ruppel's manual of pulmonary function testing,* ed 10, St. Louis, 2013, Mosby.)

- Evaluate, follow the progress of, and assess the degree of impairment caused by interstitial lung disease (IDL)
- Differentiate between emphysema and other obstructive pulmonary disorders (e.g., chronic bronchitis and asthma)
- Evaluate, follow the progress of, and assess the degree of impairment associated with chronic obstructive pulmonary disorders
- Evaluate pulmonary involvement in systemic diseases (e.g., rheumatoid arthritis, systemic lupus erythematosus)
- Evaluate the effects of chemotherapy, radiation, and selected drugs (e.g., bleomycin, amiodarone) on lung function
- Assess postoperative risk in patients undergoing lung resection or transplantation
- Predict arterial desaturation during exercise in patients with lung disease
- Evaluate the causes of dyspnea in patients with normal spirometry

## Equipment and Quality Assurance

Fig. 9.13 depicts the basic apparatus used to measure $DLCO_{sb}$. The typical test gas contains 0.3% CO mixed with a tracer gas, most commonly helium, with the balance being $O_2$ and $N_2$. The test gas is delivered to the patient through a computer-controlled valve from either a reservoir bag or demand valve. The initial portion of exhaled gas (apparatus and anatomic dead space) is collected by a spirometer, with the remaining end-tidal portion diverted into a sampling system for CO and He measurement.

Volume measurements made by the DLCO apparatus should be accurate within ±3.5% over an 8-L range and checked daily. Both the He and CO analyzers should exhibit linearity, with the maximal error across the range of measurement being no more than ±0.5%. The computer timing mechanism should be accurate to ±1% over 10 seconds. The dead space of the breathing circuit should be less than 350 mL.

Quality assurance testing should be done weekly by performing a DLCO measurement using a 3-L calibrated syringe,

with the resulting DLCO near zero and the measured volume within 3.5% of the syringe volume. This should be supplemented by weekly testing of healthy, nonsmoking biologic controls with known DLCO values.

## Test Procedure and Calculations

Because transfer of CO from the lungs into the blood is affected by existing COHb levels, patients should not smoke on the day of the test. It also is important that there have been no exercise or exertional activities just before the test (which increases blood flow and DLCO). To ensure a resting state, the patient should be seated for at least 5 minutes before the test is conducted, during which time instruction can be provided and the procedure demonstrated.

In the single-breath technique, the patient first fully exhales to RV and then quickly inhales the test gas to TLC (an inspiratory VC). Then the patient performs a relaxed breath-hold with the breathing valve closed. After 10 seconds, the breathing valve opens, allowing the patient to exhale. The initial 0.5 to 0.75 L of the patient's expired gas (dead space) is discarded, with the remainder diverted by the valve to the sampling system for He and CO analysis.

Because at least two acceptable tests are required, a 4- to 5-minute wait between tests is required to wash out any residual CO. Assuming proper equipment function and calibration, a DLCO test is acceptable if the following results are obtained:

- The inspiratory vital capacity exceeds 85% of the patient's largest VC and is inspired in less than 4 seconds
- A stable, relaxed breath-hold is maintained for 10 ± 2 seconds, with no evidence of either active expiratory effort (Valsalva maneuver) or inspiratory effort (Mueller maneuver) against the closed breathing valve
- A smooth, unforced expiration occurs in less than 4 seconds with complete clearance of dead space and proper sampling and analysis of alveolar gas

On completion of an acceptable maneuver, the sample CO concentration ($F_{ACO_T}$) is analyzed, and the "alveolar" CO concentration at the beginning of the breath-hold is computed ($F_ACO_0$). The $D_LCO$ is then calculated as the log ratio of the initial alveolar CO level to that in the end-tidal sample and adjusted for alveolar volume ($V_A$) and breath-hold time (T) using the following equation:

$$D_LCOS_b = \frac{V_A \times 60}{(P_B - 47) \times (T)} \times Ln \frac{F_ACO_0}{F_ACO_T}$$

Computation of both the "alveolar" CO concentration at the beginning of the breath-hold ($F_ACO_0$) and the alveolar volume ($V_A$) is performed using the breath's starting and ending He concentrations (or other tracer gas if used).

Results are reported in milliliters per minute per mm Hg Standard Temperature Pressure Dry (STPD) based on an average of at least two acceptable tests that are repeatable. Tests are repeatable if the results fall within ±3 mL/min/mm Hg of each other or within 10% of the largest observed value. Additional measures in the report typically include the alveolar volume ($V_A$), the ratio of $D_LCO$ to $V_A$, and the average inspiratory vital capacity. In addition, both Hb content and the carboxyhemoglobin levels affect $D_LCO$. The relationship between Hb content and $D_LCO$ is direct; that is, increases in Hb content increase the diffusing capacity. In regard to carboxyhemoglobin, the $D_LCO$ decreases about 1% for each 1% increase in COHb. For these reasons, the $D_LCO$ report should include the Hb-corrected and carboxyhemoglobin-corrected values.

## Interpretation

The most commonly cited normal range for $D_LCO$ is 25 to 30 mL/min/mm Hg. However, as with other pulmonary function tests, interpretation involves comparing the patient's $D_LCO$ measurement with a reference range and its LLN and ULN. Thus an abnormally low $D_LCO$ is one below its LLN, or below the 5th percentile of its predicted value. A reduction in $D_LCO$ below the LLN but above 60% of normal represents a mild impairment. If the patient's $D_LCO$ is less than LLN and between 40% and 60% of predicted, the impairment is considered moderate. A severe impairment exists if the $D_LCO$ is less than LLN and less than 40% of predicted.

Unfortunately, as with lung volume determinations, there are no specific prediction equations for $D_LCO$ that are generally recommended, and variation among different equations is as high as 40%. Moreover, a patient's $D_LCO$ on follow-up may need to fall by 20% to 25% before any clinical impact becomes apparent. Compounding the lack of standard reference values is the fact that $D_LCO$ is affected by so many factors, including the surface area and diffusion characteristics of the alveolar-capillary membrane, blood hemoglobin levels, pulmonary capillary blood flow and volume, and distribution of ventilation and perfusion.

Some clinicians use the $D_LCO/V_A$ ratio to help overcome some of the problems with $D_LCO$ interpretation. However, use of this ratio to support interpretation no longer is recommended. Instead, the $D_LCO$ is interpreted in combination with spirometry and lung volume measures. For example, a low $D_LCO$ in a patient with normal spirometry and lung volumes may indicate anemia, a pulmonary vascular disorder, early ILD,

### TABLE 9.5 Typical $D_LCO$ Results by Disease Category/Disorder

| Disease Category/Disorder | Typical DLCO Findings |
|---|---|
| **Airway Diseases** | |
| Asthma | Normal[a] |
| Chronic bronchitis | Normal |
| Emphysema | Low |
| Bronchiectasis | Low |
| **Interstitial Lung Diseases** | |
| Idiopathic pulmonary fibrosis | Low |
| Collagen vascular diseases | Low |
| Sarcoidosis | Low |
| Drug-induced lung disease | Low |
| **Diseases of Pulmonary Vasculature** | |
| Pulmonary embolic disease | Low |
| Pulmonary hypertension | Low |
| Pulmonary vasculitis | Low |
| Pulmonary hemorrhage | High |
| **Extrapulmonary Diseases** | |
| Respiratory muscle weakness | Low |
| Kyphoscoliosis | Low |
| Obesity | Normal[a] |
| Polycythemia | High |
| Anemia | Low |
| **Other** | |
| Pneumonectomy/lobectomy | Low |
| Congestive heart failure | Low |

[a]High values have also been reported.

or early emphysema. If the $FEV_1/FVC$ ratio exceeds the LLN, but lung volumes are reduced (a restrictive ventilatory impairment), a normal $D_LCO$ suggests a chest wall or neuromuscular disorder, whereas a reduced $D_LCO$ is consistent with an ILD. If spirometry indicates an obstructive airflow impairment that does not respond to bronchodilation, a low $D_LCO$ points to emphysema. Typical $D_LCO$ findings associated with these and other common disorders are summarized in Table 9.5.

### SIMPLY STATED

In patients with restrictive ventilatory impairments, a low $D_LCO$ is consistent with an interstitial lung disease. In patients with obstructive ventilatory impairments, a low $D_LCO$ helps identify emphysema.

## SPECIALIZED TESTS

Specialized assessments conducted in some pulmonary laboratories include measurement of airway resistance and lung compliance, evaluation of airway hyperresponsiveness and inflammation, and selected exercise test protocols. Although normally performed by specially trained personnel, these tests can provide essential information relevant to patient management.

## Airway Resistance

Airway resistance is a measure of the ratio of alveolar pressure ($P_{alv}$) to airflow ($\dot{V}$). There are three methods used to measure airway resistance: plethysmography, the interrupter method, and the forced oscillation technique.

The standard and best validated method for measuring airway resistance is similar to that described for determining TGV by body plethysmograph, with the resulting parameter abbreviated as $R_{aw}$. In this case, the patient first pants with the shutter open as the system plots flow on the Y-axis against box pressure on the X-axis. Then the shutter is closed, and as the patient continues panting, the slope of the box pressure–mouth pressure curve is obtained, as previously described for computing TGV. The ratio of the slopes of the closed-shutter to open-shutter curves is the $R_{aw}$.

The commonly cited reference range for normal $R_{aw}$ in healthy adults is 0.5 to 2.5 cm $H_2O$/L/s. However, $R_{aw}$ varies inversely with lung volume, meaning that as lung volume increases, $R_{aw}$ falls. Unfortunately, this relationship is not linear. However, the reciprocal of $R_{aw}$ is linearly related to lung volume. The reciprocal of $R_{aw}$ is called *conductance* and abbreviated as $G_{aw}$. $G_{aw}$ is computed as follows:

$$G_{aw} = \frac{1}{R_{aw}}$$

$G_{aw}$ normally is adjusted for the volume at which it is measured, which by plethysmography is the TGV. The ratio of $G_{aw}$ to TGV is called specific conductance ($G_{aw}$/TGV), which is useful in measuring the response to interventions affecting airway resistance and lung volumes, such as bronchodilator therapy.

---

**SIMPLY STATED**

Airway resistance ($R_{aw}$) varies inversely with lung volume; as lung volume increases, $R_{aw}$ falls, and as lung volume decreases, $R_{aw}$ rises.

---

Although $R_{aw}$ determined by plethysmography is the gold standard, it requires a cooperative patient able to perform the required maneuvers in a laboratory setting. The interrupted method requires only quiet breathing and can be conducted at the bedside or in the clinic. This method measures tidal airflow and mouth pressure before and after closure of a shutter incorporated into a pneumotachograph. To differentiate it from $R_{aw}$ determined by plethysmography, this measure is called the *interrupter resistance* ($R_{int}$). Reference ranges are available, but current evidence suggests that $R_{int}$ may underestimate $R_{aw}$ as determined by plethysmography, especially if the obstruction is severe.

Like the interrupter method, the forced oscillation technique (FOT) requires only tidal breathing and can be conducted at the bedside or in the clinic. FOT measures resistance by superimposing flow oscillations generated by a loudspeaker on the airways during spontaneous breathing. As the flow changes, so too does the airway pressure. The ratio

of pressure to flow of each of the oscillation frequencies is computed as the respiratory system impedance ($Z_{rs}$). The P/V relationship that occurs in phase with these oscillations is the respiratory system resistance ($R_{rs}$). As with the interrupter technique, reference ranges are available for $R_{rs}$. One major advantage of the FOT method over plethysmography and the interrupted techniques is that it can "partition" a patient's airflow resistance by location. In large airway obstruction, $R_{rs}$ is elevated independent of oscillation frequency. On the other hand, in small airway obstruction, $R_{rs}$ is highest at low frequencies and decreases with increasing frequencies.

## Lung and Chest Wall Compliance

Compliance is defined as the ease of inflation and is measured as volume change per unit pressure change. The total compliance of the respiratory system ($C_{L+T}$) measures the overall distensibility of the lung and thorax together. $C_{L+T}$ can be partitioned into two components: lung compliance ($C_L$) and thorax/chest wall compliance ($C_T$). These two components work in parallel, with the relationship expressed in the following equation:

$$\frac{1}{C_{L+T}} = \frac{1}{C_L} + \frac{1}{C_T}$$

Lung compliance ($C_L$) is measured using a spirometer or other volumetric device to measure volume change and a pressure transducer to measure pressure change. To measure $C_L$, the applicable pressure is the transpulmonary pressure gradient ($P_L$), which equals alveolar pressure ($P_{alv}$) minus the pleural pressure ($P_{pl}$). Pleural pressure is estimated from the pressure within a balloon placed in the esophagus. The subject inhales to TLC and begins a slow exhalation. During exhalation, the volume and pressure are recorded as flow at the airway opening ($P_{ao}$) is interrupted at several descending steps. At times of zero flow, $P_{ao}$ equals $P_{alv}$. Thus, $P_L$ is calculated as $P_{ao} - P_{pl}$. The lung volumes and corresponding transpulmonary pressures are plotted to provide a lung compliance curve. The slope of the curve ($\Delta V/\Delta P$) at any given volume represents the lung compliance, or $C_L$. Typically, the slope between 500 and 1000 mL above the FRC is chosen for the measurement. Because this parameter is based on measurements made at zero flow, it is referred to as the *static* lung compliance. The commonly cited normal static lung compliance for a healthy adult is 0.2 L/cm $H_2O$ or 200 mL/cm $H_2O$.

---

**SIMPLY STATED**

Lung compliance is computed as the lung volume divided by the transpulmonary pressure gradient (alveolar-pleural pressure). Typically, multiple measurements are made and plotted on a curve, with slope of the curve between 500 and 1000 mL above the FRC taken as the patient's measurement.

---

Example lung compliance curves are shown in Fig. 9.14. For reference, the middle curve represents normal static

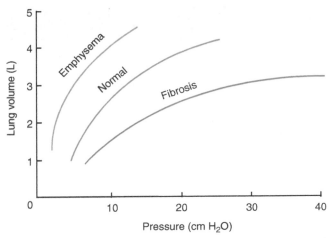

**FIG. 9.14** Example lung compliance curve plotting lung volume vs. transpulmonary pressure. The slope of the curve ($\Delta V/\Delta P$) at any given volume represents the lung compliance, or $C_L$. (Modified from Martin L: *Pulmonary physiology in clinical practice: the essentials for patient care and evaluation*, St. Louis, 1987, Mosby.)

compliance. The lower, flatter curve reflects a stiff lung, as may be observed in pulmonary fibrosis. The upper curve with the greater slope is consistent with greater than normal lung compliance, as can occur in emphysema, owing to loss of elastic recoil.

During the measurement of static lung compliance, the transthoracic pressure gradient ($P_W$) also may be recorded. $P_W$ equals the difference between the alveolar pressure and atmospheric pressure ($P_{alv} - P_B$). Dividing the lung volume by $P_W$ yields the *total compliance* of the respiratory system ($C_{L+T}$). The commonly cited normal total compliance for a healthy adult is 0.1 L/cm $H_2O$ or 100 mL/cm $H_2O$.

Given a patient's lung and total compliance measures, one can then compute thorax/chest wall compliance ($C_T$) using the previously provided compliance equation. The commonly cited normal thorax/chest wall compliance for a healthy adult is 0.2 L/cm $H_2O$ or 200 mL/cm $H_2O$.

## Airway Hyperresponsiveness and Inflammation

Airway hyperresponsiveness (AHR) represents an abnormally exaggerated airway response to a provoking stimulus. The provoking stimulus most often is an inflammatory immune response causing bronchoconstriction, as in asthma.

Two different approaches can be used to assess for AHR. The first is to actually challenge the airways with a provoking agent, a method called bronchoprovocation testing. A newer alternative approach is to assess the actual level of airway inflammation through analysis of an inflammatory marker, exhaled nitric oxide (NO).

## Bronchoprovocation Testing

Bronchoprovocation testing involves exposing a subject to increasing concentrations of a drug agent that can provoke bronchospasm to determine the level at which airway response occurs. The most common drug used is methacholine, a potent cholinergic agent.

Methacholine bronchoprovocation testing is indicated to do the following:

- Rule out a diagnosis of asthma
- Assess the severity of AHR
- Evaluate for occupational asthma
- Assess response to AHR treatment

This test is contraindicated if the patient has severe airflow limitation ($FEV_1$ < 50% predicted or <1.0 L), has had a heart attack or stroke in past 90 days, or has uncontrolled hypertension or a known aortic aneurysm.

Patients scheduled for provocation testing should avoid taking any short-acting inhaled bronchodilator medication for 8 hours before testing, with those receiving long-acting bronchodilators ceasing administration 48 hours in advance.

Two different methods are used for methacholine bronchoprovocation testing: the 2-minute tidal breathing method and the dosimeter method. Laboratories using the tidal breathing method have the patient inhale aerosol from a calibrated jet nebulizer, outputting at a rate of 0.13 mL/min. With the dosimeter method, the device delivers 9 µL of aerosolized solution at the beginning of each of five IC maneuvers that end in a 5-second breath-hold. Regardless of method, a rescue protocol and advanced cardiac life support equipment must be in place to deal with any untoward patient response to the provoking agent.

In both methods, the patient receives an initial normal saline solution (0.9%) aerosol, followed by an $FEV_1$ measurement (the baseline or control). Thereafter, increasing concentrations of methacholine solution are administered every 5 minutes, typically ranging from an initial dose of 0.03 mg/mL up to 16 mg/mL. At each incremental dosage, two repeat $FEV_1$ measurements are made, 30 and 90 seconds after inhalation. At each step, the percentage decrease in $FEV_1$ compared with baseline is computed and plotted on a dose-response curve. The test ends when either the maximal dose of methacholine has been given or the $FEV_1$ has fallen by 20% or more from baseline. In the latter case, the provocative concentration of methacholine resulting in the 20% or greater fall in $FEV_1$ (termed the $PC_{20}$) is computed from the log concentration versus dose-response curve. After the test, the patient normally receives bronchodilator treatment to restore normal airway function, which is confirmed by repeat spirometry.

### SIMPLY STATED

The $PC_{20}$ is the concentration of methacholine that causes a 20% or greater fall in $FEV_1$ during bronchoprovocation testing. Moderate to severe airway hyperresponsiveness is present if the $PC_{20}$ occurs at a methacholine concentration of 1 mg/mL or less.

Regarding the interpretation of PC20, If the $FEV_1$ does not fall by at least 20% with the highest concentration of methacholine, the test is interpreted as negative, and a diagnosis of AHR or asthma can be ruled out. If the $PC_{20}$ occurs at less than 1 mg/mL methacholine concentration, moderate to severe AHR is present, which is consistent with a diagnosis of asthma. $PC_{20}$ values between 1 and 16 mg/mL suggest but do not confirm a diagnosis of asthma.

### Exhaled Nitric Oxide ($F_ENO$) Analysis

NO is a chemical mediator produced by endothelial and epithelial cells, macrophages, and eosinophils. Because it is a gas, NO appears in the exhaled breath, with its concentration increasing in the presence of airway inflammation. For this reason, measurement of the exhaled fraction of NO ($F_ENO$) has been found useful in both diagnosis and management of asthma. Specifically, $F_ENO$ testing is used to do the following:

- Help assess respiratory symptoms (cough, wheeze, dyspnea)
- Help identify the eosinophilic asthma phenotype
- Monitor chronic persistent asthma
- Assess response to and compliance with inhaled steroids
- Guide changes in dosing and discontinuation of inhaled steroids
- Assess whether other factors are contributing to poor asthma control (e.g., sinusitis, anxiety, gastroesophageal reflux disease, continued allergen exposure)

$F_ENO$ typically is measured using chemiluminescence or electrochemical methods. Both provide rapid, real-time sampling during exhalation, with graphic display of $F_ENO$ (similar in concept to capnography). Because NO concentrations are so low, they are measured in parts per billion (ppb). For this reason, NO analyzers used to sample expired gas must have a sensitivity and accuracy of 1 ppb or better and a rapid response time (<500 ms). In addition, NO analyzers should undergo daily two-point calibrations according to the manufacturer's specifications, ideally using a zero-NO gas and one at the high end of the measurement range.

Because many nondisease factors can influence $F_ENO$ levels, it is important to instruct patients before testing to refrain from exercise, alcohol consumption, smoking, and eating for at least 1 hour before testing. In addition, since both steroids and β-agonists alter $F_ENO$ levels, all medications being taken and time of administration should be recorded. Last, because forced expiratory efforts decrease $F_ENO$ levels, NO analysis should be conducted before any spirometry testing.

The basic procedure is simple. The patient inhales NO-free air through the analyzer to TLC and then exhales slowly while the measurement takes place. Key quality considerations in conducting the procedure are outlined in Box 9.4.

---

> **BOX 9.4    Quality Considerations in Measuring Exhaled Nitric Oxide ($F_ENO$)**
>
> - Patient should be seated comfortably in the upright position.
> - Use nose clips only if the patient cannot avoid nasal breathing.
> - Avoid any breath holding preceding the test maneuver.
> - Have the patient do the following:
>   - Exhale normally without the mouthpiece.
>   - Inhale NO-free air through the mouthpiece for 2 to 3 seconds to total lung capacity.
>   - Maintain a steady low expiratory flow for at least 6 seconds (>4 seconds for children).
> - Terminate maneuver once the test is deemed acceptable.
> - Repeat until acceptability and repeatability criteria are met.
> - Allow at least a 30-second interval between maneuvers.

---

$F_ENO$ levels are flow dependent, and measurements must be made at a constant low expiratory flow. The recommended standard flow is 0.05 L per second or 50 mL per second. Typically, this is achieved by having the patient exhale against a fixed resistance, with the monitored flow proportional to the generated back pressure.

Because NO levels in air can be higher than those coming from the lungs, the inhaled gas should contain as little NO as possible. Typically, NO is removed from the inhaled air by exposing it to a filter containing a chemical NO scavenger. NO contamination also can result from gas coming from the nose, which typically has higher NO concentrations than that coming from the lungs. This problem is averted because the back pressure created by the analyzer's expiratory flow resistance closes off the soft palate.

To ensure quality in $F_ENO$ testing, at least three acceptable maneuvers should be obtained. Fig. 9.15 provides an example graphic display of three such maneuvers provided by a rapidly responding $F_ENO$ analyzer on a patient with normal $F_ENO$ levels. Box 9.5 provides the basic acceptability and repeatability criteria for this measurement. The reported $F_ENO$ is the mean value of at least two plateau measurements, the concentrations of which fall within 10% of each other.

The ATS now recommends using cutoff points rather than reference values when interpreting $F_ENO$. This is largely because $F_ENO$ values are not normally distributed in the population, and there is large overlap between mean $F_ENO$ levels in healthy subjects and those diagnosed with asthma. Table 9.6 provides interpretive guidelines based on these recommended cutoff points, which differ for adults and children. Of course, as with all pulmonary function tests, reliance solely on the $F_ENO$ for diagnosis or disease management is inappropriate. $F_ENO$ values should always be interpreted in light of the patient's history, physical

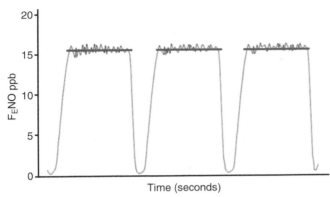

**FIG. 9.15** Graph of exhaled nitric oxide fraction ($F_ENO$) measured over three breaths in a normal subject. Note the consistent plateau levels of about 16 ppb occurring toward the end of each breath, indicating both acceptability and repeatability of the maneuvers. (Courtesy Strategic Learning Associates, LLC, Little Silver, NJ.)

examination, and related diagnostic procedures, including pulmonary function tests.

> ### SIMPLY STATED
>
> An adult patient who reports recurrent episodes of coughing, wheezing, and shortness of breath and who has a measured $F_ENO$ greater than 50 ppb likely has eosinophilic asthma.

## Exercise Tests

Many different protocols involve assessment of a patient's exercise capacity or its effect on body functions. These tests range from simple evaluation of exercise tolerance to complex protocols requiring concurrent assessment of cardiovascular, pulmonary, and metabolism measures. Here, we review the basics involved in the two most common exercise tests, the 6-Minute Walk Test and the treadmill-based cardiopulmonary exercise test.

### 6-Minute Walk Test

The 6-Minute Walk Test measures how far a patient can walk in the specified time, with the resulting distance termed the 6MWD, measured in meters. The test evaluates tolerance for mild exertion and is commonly used to assess a patient's overall functional capacity. Preassessment and postassessment of the 6MWD also can help determine the effect of medical or surgical treatments such as volume reduction surgery or pulmonary rehabilitation. The test is contraindicated in patients with recent myocardial infarction or unstable angina, and caution should be taken with those who are severely hypertensive or have high resting heart rates.

The test should follow the standard protocol published by the ATS. An oxygen source, automated defibrillator, and

> ### BOX 9.5  Acceptability and Repeatability Criteria for $F_ENO$ Maneuvers
>
> - Acceptability criteria for $F_ENO$ maneuvers
>   - Free from any leaks
>   - Exhalation of at least 6 seconds (at least 4 seconds in children <12 years old)
>   - $F_ENO$ plateau at standard flow of 50 mL/s (±10%) held constant for ≥3 s
>   - Variation in $F_ENO$ during the plateau phase is no more than 10%
> - Repeatability
>   - Three maneuvers with $F_ENO$ plateau values within 10% or two maneuvers within 5% of each other

## TABLE 9.6  $F_ENO$ Cutoffs and Related Clinical Considerations for Adults and Children

|  | Low Cutoff | Intermediate Values | High Cutoff |
|---|---|---|---|
| **Adult** | **<25 ppb** | **25-50 ppb** | **>50 ppb** |
| **Child** | **<20 ppb** | **20-35 ppb** | **>35 ppb** |
| Eosinophilic inflammation | Unlikely | Interpret based on clinical context | Likely |
| Response to steroids | Unlikely | Interpret based on clinical context | Likely |
| Diagnostic considerations | Consider other causes of symptoms, e.g., CF, sinusitis, COPD, GERD, anxiety | Be cautious; monitor $F_ENO$ trends | In symptomatic patients (not taking steroids), generally confirms diagnosis of asthma |
| Management considerations for asthmatic patients | • If symptoms persist consider other diagnoses<br>• In asymptomatic patients on inhaled steroids, indicates good compliance with treatment—consider decreasing dose | • In symptomatic patients may indicate persistent allergen exposure, inadequate inhaled steroid dose, poor adherence<br>• In asymptomatic patients indicates adequate inhaled steroid dosing, good adherence | • May indicate poor treatment compliance, poor inhaler technique, inadequate inhaled steroid dose, or steroid resistance<br>• Increased risk for exacerbation; inhaled steroid withdrawal may lead to relapse |

*CF,* Cystic fibrosis; *COPD,* chronic obstructive pulmonary disease; *GERD,* gastroesophageal reflux disease.
Adapted from Dweik RA, Boggs PB, Erzurum SC: An official ATS clinical practice guideline: interpretation of exhaled nitric oxide levels ($F_ENO$) for clinical applications. *Am J Respir Crit Care Med* 184(5):602–615, 2011.

---

**BOX 9.6**   **American Thoracic Society 6-Minute Walk Protocol**

1. Have the patient sit at rest for at least 10 minutes before the test starts.
2. Assemble all equipment—e.g., stopwatch, Borg Scale, recording worksheet.
3. With the patient resting, gather the needed demographic data and record the vital signs.
4. If $SpO_2$ is to be monitored, be sure to record the baseline value.
5. Have the patient stand, and rate his or her baseline dyspnea and exertion levels using the Borg scale.
6. Position the patient at the start line and review the procedure.
7. As soon as the patient starts to walk, begin timing.
8. Remain at the start line while you record completed laps (1 lap = down and back).
9. Each minute, provide encouragement to the patient and specify the time remaining.
10. At exactly 6 minutes, firmly say "Stop!" and place a marker at the stop point.
11. If using a pulse oximeter, record the end-of-walk $SpO_2$ and pulse rate.
12. Have the patient sit in a chair while you repeat the dyspnea and exertion assessment.
13. Record the number of laps and additional distance covered in the final partial lap, if any.
14. Calculate and record the total distance walked, rounding to the nearest meter.

Adapted from American Thoracic Society: ATS statement: guidelines for the six-minute walk test, *Am J Respir Crit Care Med* 166:111–117, 2002.

---

telephone should be available to handle potential emergencies. The walking course should be 30 meters long with a clear start line and turnaround point, marked off every 3 meters. Box 9.6 summarizes the key points in the ATS recommended test protocol.

If the patient complains of chest pain or severe dyspnea, becomes diaphoretic, or develops a pale or ashen appearance, the test should be discontinued, the patient seated and administered $O_2$, and the physician immediately contacted.

Based on existing prediction equations for normal subjects, a 6MWD of less than 350 meters for women or 450 meters for men provides a useful cutoff point for identifying those with abnormal functional capacities. When assessing the effect of a medical or surgical intervention, one should look for at least a 10% to 20% increase in the 6MWD as an indicator of treatment effectiveness.

Although useful as a global assessment of functional capacity, the 6-Minute Walk Test is not diagnostic of any specific condition. It does not measure maximal oxygen uptake or help identify the factors limiting a patient's exercise tolerance. To obtain such information requires a comprehensive cardiopulmonary exercise test.

## Cardiopulmonary Exercise Testing

Cardiopulmonary exercise testing involves analysis of heart and lung function during incremental levels of work, typically performed on a treadmill. The standard workload measure for exercise testing is the metabolic equivalent of task (MET); 1 MET = 3.5 mL $O_2$ consumption per kilogram of body weight, roughly equal to the average resting $O_2$ consumption per minute. Treadmill protocols are designed such that specific speeds and inclinations correspond to specific MET levels. Most exercise protocols increase exercise intensity by 1 to 2 METs at each workload increment.

Exercise testing normally is performed under direct physician supervision in a cardiac, pulmonary, or exercise physiology laboratory. A fully stocked crash cart with defibrillator, oxygen, suction, and airway equipment must be immediately available, with all staff involved in testing proficient in advanced life support.

The classic cardiac electrocardiogram (ECG) stress test measures the patient's 12-lead ECG, heart rate, and blood pressure and is indicated to do the following:

- Diagnose obstructive coronary artery disease (CAD)
- Assess risk and prognosis in patients with a prior history of CAD
- Assess prognosis after myocardial infarction
- Provide the basis for heart patients' activity or rehabilitation prescriptions
- Help evaluate the impact of medical therapies for CAD and congestive heart failure

Measured parameters are carefully monitored at each workload increment, as well as patient symptoms, such as chest pain. ST depression or elevation ($\geq 1$ mm for at least 60 to 80 ms following the QRS) indicates myocardial ischemia and constitutes a positive test result.

When combined with measurement of tidal volume, respiratory rate, $O_2$ consumption, and $CO_2$ production, exercise testing also can be used to do the following:

- Differentiate among factors limiting exercise capacity (cardiac vs. pulmonary)
- Evaluate responses to therapy intended to increased exercise tolerance
- Determine the intensity for exercise training in rehabilitation programs
- Evaluate exercise capacity in heart transplantation candidates
- Assess cardiopulmonary fitness in disability evaluations

The measurements made during exercise capacity testing, their definitions, and their typical values at peak capacity are described in Table 9.7.

The primary criterion for evaluating overall exercise capacity is the $\dot{V}O_2max$. Test results are considered normal if patients can attain their predicted $VO\dot{V}_2max$ and a heart rate at or near their predicted maximum (HRmax) at peak exercise capacity. Normal patients also can readily increase their ventilation in proportion to metabolic demands and maintain normal $SpO_2$ levels during exercise.

---

**SIMPLY STATED**

To estimate the maximal heart rate of a patient at peak exercise capacity, subtract the patient's age from 220.

| TABLE 9.7 | Measurements Made during Testing for Exercise Capacity and Its Limitations | |
|---|---|---|
| Measurement | Definition | Typical Values at Peak Exercise Capacity |
| $\dot{V}O_2$max | Maximal uptake of $O_2$ per minute at peak exercise capacity | Men: 35-90 mL/kg/min<br>Women: 25-75 mL/kg/min |
| Anaerobic threshold | Exercise intensity beyond which progressive increases in blood lactate occur | >40% $\dot{V}O_2$max |
| HRmax | Maximal heart rate at peak exercise capacity | 220 – age |
| Breathing reserve | Proportion of MVV that is unused after reaching maximal minute ventilation at peak exercise | >30% |
| $Spo_2$ | $O_2$ saturation (pulse oximetry) | >88% |
| $O_2$ pulse | Oxygen consumption per heartbeat at peak exercise capacity | Men: >12 mL/beat<br>Women: >8 mL/beat |

*HR*, Heart rate; *MVV*, maximal voluntary ventilation; $\dot{V}O_2$, oxygen consumption.

As a rule of thumb, poor exercise capacity is present if either the $\dot{V}O_2$max is less than 15 mL/kg or the patient cannot achieve a peak exercise level of at least 5 METs. Poor exercise capacity can be due to poor physical conditioning or the presence of a cardiovascular or pulmonary disorder.

Low exercise capacity due to poor conditioning is associated with a low $\dot{V}O_2$max but a normal anaerobic threshold (>40% of the $\dot{V}O_2$max). Poorly conditioned patients also tend to exhibit abnormally high heart rates at peak exercise capacity.

Patients in whom a cardiovascular disorder is the primary factor limiting exercise have a reduced anaerobic threshold, low $O_2$ pulse, and higher than predicted heart rate at peak exercise capacity. The reduced $O_2$ pulse occurs because the diseased heart cannot increase stroke volume sufficiently to meet increased exercise demands.

Patients in whom a pulmonary disorder is the primary factor limiting exercise may have adequate stroke volumes but cannot increase their ventilation sufficiently to meet exercise demands. This limitation is evident as a reduction in breathing reserve. Normal individuals have a breathing reserve of at least 30%, meaning that at peak exercise they are only using about 70% or less of their MVV to meet their metabolic demands. Patients with pulmonary disorders typically exhibit breathing reserves below 30%. In addition, these patients also may exhibit a reduced $Spo_2$ during exercise. This occurs most often in those with advanced COPD and interstitial lung diseases who have marginal arterial oxygen saturation at rest.

Simple exercise testing also may be conducted in the pulmonary function laboratory or outpatient clinic to do the following:
- Assess for exercise-induced bronchospasm and it response to therapy
- Determine whether arterial desaturation occurs with exercise, and titrate needed supplemental $O_2$

The test is used to detect exercise-induced bronchospasm, before and after spirometry is conducted, with a drop of 20% or more in the patient's $FEV_1$ after exercise constituting a positive test.

General contraindications against exercise testing include acute myocardial infarction, uncontrolled heart failure, unstable angina, significant cardiac dysrhythmias, acute pulmonary disorders, and severe hypertension. An exercise test should be terminated if a wide swing in blood pressure occurs, angina or dyspnea becomes severe, a serious dysrhythmia occurs, or the patient becomes dizzy, confused, or cyanotic.

## INFECTION CONTROL

With the increasing use of bacterial filters and disposable breathing circuits and flow sensors, cross-contamination has become less of an issue in pulmonary function testing. Of course, any reusable components such as breathing valves and manifolds should be disinfected or sterilized regularly. The ideal frequency for disinfection or sterilization of reusable components has not been established. However, any reusable components that show visible breath condensation should undergo high-level disinfection or sterilization between patients.

In terms of the methods used to disinfect or sterilize reusable components, it is essential to adhere to the manufacturer's recommendations for processing. This is because some processing methods can cause damage to critical components, such as flow sensors or valve seals. It is important to note that after disassembly, cleaning, and disinfection, nondisposable sensors usually require recalibration before use.

If closed-circuit methods using a volumetric spirometer are employed in testing, the bell or bellows should be flushed with room air at least five times between tests. This is necessary to eliminate the possibility of cross-contamination due to the persistence of droplet nuclei in these systems. In addition, the full breathing circuit, including the mouthpiece, should be decontaminated or changed between patients. When using open-circuit methods in which the patient only exhales into the device, only those elements through which rebreathing occurs need to be decontaminated or changed.

Placement of a disposable bacterial filter between the patient and circuit eliminates the need to regularly decontaminate or change system components. Systems using such filters must still meet the minimal quality assurance standards, as previously discussed. In addition, pulmonary function testing filters must exhibit minimum flow resistance and create little or no back pressure. Specifications proving that their filters have no effect on measurements should be provided by the manufacturer.

To protect oneself from infection, pulmonary function testing should be conducted using standard precautions.

Airborne precautions should be employed when there is potential exposure to infectious agents transmitted by that route, such as tuberculosis. Hands should always be washed between patients and immediately after direct handling of used circuit components, whether reusable or disposable.

## KEY POINTS

- The vital capacity is the maximal volume of air that can be exhaled after a maximal inhalation, typically 4 to 5 L in normal adults and varying primarily with an individual's height.
- Total lung capacity equals the sum of all four lung volumes: $RV + V_T + ERV + IRV$.
- Basic spirometry is indicated primarily to detect abnormal lung function, quantify the severity of disease, and assess a patient's response to treatment.
- Slow vital capacity measured at the bedside using a simple respirometer is used to assess for postoperative risk and need for mechanical ventilation.
- The ratio of $FEV_1$ to FVC ($FEV_1$/FVC) is the proportion of the FVC expired during the first second of the maneuver and is the key spirometry measure used to identify obstructive ventilatory impairments.
- Although effort dependent, the peak expiratory flow (PEF) can be used by patients with asthma to monitor for bronchospasm and help make self-management decisions. Values below 80% of the patient's personal best indicate the need for action.
- The width of a maximal inspiratory-expiratory flow-volume curve is the forced vital capacity or FVC (X-axis); the maximal positive deflection on the flow axis (Y-axis) is the PEF, with the maximal negative deflection on this axis being the peak inspiratory flow (PIF).
- A patient's estimated MVV = measured $FEV_1 \times 40$.
- Spirometer volume measurements should be checked daily and be accurate to ±3.5% of the true value (includes 0.5% syringe inaccuracy); flow measurements should be accurate to ±5% of the true value over a range of −14 to +14 L/s.
- A valid FVC maneuver requires that the subject exhale for at least 6 seconds.
- An acceptable FVC should be free from artifacts; exhibit a rapid, forceful start; and achieve complete exhalation. The results of the test are repeatable if after three acceptable maneuvers the two largest FVC and $FEV_1$ values are within 0.150 L of each other.
- A spirometry value is considered abnormally low if it is below the 5th percentile of the predicted normal, a boundary called the lower limit of normal, or LLN.
- If a patient's FVC, $FEV_1$, and $FEV_1$/FVC all exceed the LLN, results are normal; an obstructive ventilatory impairment exists if the $FEV_1$ is low and the $FEV_1$/FVC ratio is less than the LLN; and the combination of a reduced FVC, normal or reduced $FEV_1$, and $FEV_1$/FVC above the LLN suggests either a restrictive ventilatory impairment or poor effort.
- An obstructive ventilatory defect is considered reversible if, after bronchodilator administration, the $FEV_1$ or FVC increases by more than 12% and 200 mL.
- Static lung volume determinations are used to confirm a restrictive disease pattern, assess the response to medical or surgical interventions, and measure the extent of gas trapping.
- The helium dilution and $N_2$ washout methods for FRC determination only measure lung volume in communication with the airways. The volume of air trapped in the lungs is not measured. Trapped air can only be measured by body plethysmography.
- The classic pattern of a restrictive ventilatory impairment is a reduced TLC due to a reduction in inspiratory capacity and a decrease in FRC or RV, or both.
- The primary indication for measuring DLCO is to help differentiate between interstitial and chest wall or neuromuscular causes of restrictive ventilatory impairments; DLCO measurement also is indicated to evaluate pulmonary involvement in systemic diseases and the effects of chemotherapy, radiation, and selected drugs on lung function.
- A valid single-breath DLCO maneuver requires that the patient inspire quickly to at least 85% of vital capacity, properly hold the breath for at least 10 seconds, and provide a smooth, unforced expiration in less than 4 seconds.
- In patients with restrictive ventilatory impairments, a normal DLCO suggests a chest wall or neuromuscular disorder, whereas a reduced DLCO is consistent with interstitial lung disease.
- The commonly cited reference range for normal airway resistance in healthy adults is 0.5 to 2.5 cm $H_2O$/L per second.
- The slope of the lung volume–versus–transpulmonary pressure curve at any given volume represents the lung compliance.
- The methacholine bronchoprovocation test ends when either the maximal dose of methacholine has been given or the $FEV_1$ has fallen by 20% or more from baseline.
- Moderate to severe airway hyperresponsiveness is indicated when the provocative concentration of methacholine resulting in the 20% or greater fall in $FEV_1$ ($PC_{20}$) is less than 1 mg/mL.
- Measurement of the exhaled fraction of NO is useful in both the diagnosis and management of asthma, including assessing the response to inhaled steroids.
- An $F_ENO$ greater than 50 ppb in symptomatic adults not taking steroids generally confirms the diagnosis of asthma; for patients with asthma, this measure may indicate poor

treatment compliance, poor inhaler technique, or inadequate inhaled steroid dosing.

- When assessing the effect of a medical or surgical intervention, one should look for at least a 10% to 20% increase in the 6MWD as an indicator of treatment effectiveness.
- Cardiopulmonary exercise testing is used to assess coronary artery disease, differentiate between cardiac and pulmonary limitations to exercise, and determine whether arterial desaturation occurs with exercise.
- The primary criterion for evaluating overall exercise capacity is the $Vo_2max$.

- Patients in whom a cardiovascular disorder limits exercise capacity have a reduced anaerobic threshold, low $O_2$ pulse, and higher than predicted heart rate at peak exercise; a reduced breathing reserve is the primary factor limiting exercise in patients with pulmonary disorders.
- Placement of a disposable bacterial filter between the patient and the pulmonary test circuit eliminates the need to regularly decontaminate or change system components.

## CASE STUDY

A 70-year-old man has a chief complaint of severe dyspnea on exertion. The dyspnea has increased gradually over the past several years. He has had severe kyphoscoliosis from his teenage years. He denies a history of cough, sputum production, smoking, working in a polluted environment, or respiratory disease. Physical examination reveals tachypnea, tachycardia, jugular venous distention, ankle edema, and kyphoscoliosis.

### Personal Data
Age: 70 years
Height: 66 inches
Weight: 155 lb
Sex: male

### Spirometry

| Report | Predicted | Observed | Predicted % |
|---|---|---|---|
| FVC (L) | 3.78 | 1.46 | 39 |
| FEV$_1$ (L) | 2.57 | 1.40 | 54 |
| FEV$_1$/FVC | 75% | 96% | — |
| FEF$_{25\%-75\%}$ (L/s) | 2.46 | 2.01 | 82 |

### Lung Volume Studies

| (Body Box) | Predicted | Observed | Predicted % |
|---|---|---|---|
| VC (L) | 3.78 | 1.79 | 47.4 |
| FRC (L) | 2.42 | 2.01 | 83.0 |
| RV (L) | 1.75 | 1.86 | 106 |
| TLC (L) | 5.78 | 3.65 | 63.2 |
| RV/TLC | 30% | 51% | — |

### Interpretation

Spirometry reveals a small FVC and FEV$_1$ with a normal FEV$_1$/FVC ratio and FEF$_{25\%-75\%}$. This suggests that the small FEV$_1$ is caused by restrictive lung disease and small lung volumes rather than by an obstructive impairment with low flows. The lung volume studies demonstrate a small VC and TLC. These findings confirm restrictive lung disease.

The lung function studies are typical for a patient with kyphoscoliosis. Kyphoscoliosis causes a reduction in the size of the thoracic cage and can severely compromise lung expansion and eventually result in pulmonary hypertension (cor pulmonale), which can cause right-sided heart failure, resulting in elevated jugular venous distention and pedal edema.

## CASE STUDY

A 38-year-old man complains of long-standing dyspnea on exertion. His dyspnea has increased over the past year and now occurs with minimal exertion. He denies cough, chest pain, and sputum production. He has a 40 pack-year smoking history. There is no history of exposure to environmental pollutants. Physical examination shows large anteroposterior chest diameter and diminished breath sounds bilaterally.

### Personal Data
Age: 38 years
Height: 76 inches
Weight: 188 lb
Sex: male

| Spirometry Report | Predicted | Observed | Predicted % |
|---|---|---|---|
| FVC (L) | 6.06 | 5.10 | 79 |
| FEV$_1$ (L) | 4.52 | 1.53 | 34 |
| FEV$_1$/FVC | 75% | 28% | — |

### Interpretation
Spirometry reveals a markedly low FEV$_1$ and FEV$_1$/FVC, indicating a severe obstructive ventilatory impairment.

### Discussion
FVC measurement prebronchodilator and postbronchodilator and static lung volume and D$_{LCO}$ measurements would help further evaluate this patient's status. There should be a high index of suspicion for $\alpha_1$-antitrypsin deficiency in this patient given the severity of his lung disease at such a young age.

## CASE STUDY

A 72-year-old woman was admitted to the medical service complaining of weakness and shortness of breath. She recently had been diagnosed with asthma but previously was in good health. Physical examination of the chest revealed markedly diminished breath sounds. There was no wheezing, but crackles were noted at both bases. The admitting chest radiograph revealed the presence of bibasilar atelectasis but was otherwise clear. Her admitting laboratory work was normal. Her blood gas results indicated that her pH was normal, but the $Paco_2$ was 54 mm Hg, with a $Pao_2$ of 58 mm Hg while breathing room air.

After 3 days of standard therapy for asthma that included inhaled bronchodilators and steroids, her respiratory symptoms did not improve. Her $Paco_2$ had increased to 62 mm Hg, and her chest radiograph was unchanged. Her weakness was a little better. Pulmonary consultation was requested.

The consultant requested bedside spirometry. More blood testing was also ordered, including a sedimentation rate and anti–acetylcholine receptor (AChR) antibody.

**Personal Data**
Age: 72 years
Height: 63.5 inches
Weight: 166 lb
Sex: female

| Spirometry Report | Predicted | Observed | Predicted % |
|---|---|---|---|
| FVC (L) | 2.80 | 1.45 | 52 |
| $FEV_1$ (L) | 2.13 | 1.19 | 56 |
| $FEV_1$/FVC | 75% | 82% | — |

**Interpretation**

Results indicate low lung volumes with a normal $FEV_1$/FVC. This indicates restrictive lung disease rather than obstructive lung disease such as asthma.

**Discussion**

Restrictive lung disease may be caused by diseases that decrease lung compliance, such as pulmonary fibrosis; by diseases that "stiffen" the chest wall, such as kyphoscoliosis; by diseases associated with muscle weakness, such as muscular dystrophy; or by neurologic disorders affecting nerve transmission, such as amyotrophic lateral sclerosis or myasthenia gravis. Results in this case confirm a restrictive impairment. Blood testing for antibodies against the neurotransmitter acetylcholine makes the specific diagnosis of myasthenia gravis. As myasthenia gravis worsens, respiratory muscles weaken, and the patient develops hypercapnic respiratory failure ("myasthenia crisis"). This is the reason for the patient's rising $Paco_2$. The patient's chest radiograph findings of small volumes and bibasilar atelectasis are also explained by weakening respiratory muscles, causing an inability to take a deep breath.

## ASSESSMENT QUESTIONS

1. What is the term used to describe the volume of gas that can be exhaled maximally after a full inspiration?
   a. Total lung capacity
   b. Vital capacity
   c. Functional residual capacity
   d. Expiratory reserve volume

2. What volume is obtained by subtracting the VC from the TLC?
   a. Residual volume
   b. Tidal volume
   c. Inspiratory reserve volume
   d. Expiratory reserve volume

3. Which of the following tests would you recommend to quantify the disease severity of a patient diagnosed with asthma?
   a. Basic spirometry
   b. Diffusing capacity
   c. Static lung volumes
   d. Exercise capacity

4. Which of the following slow vital capacity measurements indicates inadequate ventilatory reserve?
   a. 10 mL/kg
   b. 30 mL/kg
   c. 50 mL/kg
   d. 70 mL/kg

5. What percentage of the FVC is normally exhaled in the first second?
   a. 50%
   b. 65%
   c. 75%
   d. 85%

6. What spirometry parameter would you recommend to assist a patient with asthma in monitoring her day-to-day status and need for treatment?
   a. $FEV_1$
   b. PEF
   c. $FEV_3$
   d. FVC

7. Which parameter is represented as the maximal positive deflection on the Y-axis of a standard inspiratory-expiratory flow-volume curve?
   a. PIF
   b. FVC
   c. PEF
   d. $FEV_1$

8. Spirometry results for a patient indicate an FVC of 3.5 L and an $FEV_1$ of 2.5 L. What is this patient's estimated MVV?
   a. 100 L/min
   b. 140 L/min
   c. 80 L/min
   d. 60 L/min

9. In addition to calibration with a 3-L syringe, which of the following methods should be used to validate spirometer performance and accuracy of software computations?
   a. Leak testing of the system
   b. Testing with biologic controls
   c. Random testing of patients
   d. Checking the program code

10. A valid FVC maneuver requires that the subject exhale for at least:
    a. 1 second
    b. 3 seconds
    c. 6 seconds
    d. 10 seconds

11. When performing bedside spirometry, you observe an S-shaped plotted FVC-versus-time curve on the display. Which of the following is the likely problem with this maneuver?
    a. Failure to achieve complete exhalation
    b. Early termination/cutoff of exhalation
    c. Coughing/breathing during the maneuver
    d. Failure to achieve a rapid start to exhalation

12. The upper and lower limits of normal spirometry data are calculated as being how many standard deviations (SD) from the mean?
    a. ±1 SD
    b. ±2 SD
    c. ±3 SD
    d. ±4 SD

13. Bedside spirometry results for a patient indicate an FVC lower than the LLN, with the $FEV_1$ and $FEV_1$/FVC both being higher than the LLN. Which of the following are possible interpretations?
    1. The patient has a restrictive impairment
    2. The results are inconsistent and therefore invalid
    3. The patient is not providing maximal effort
    4. The patient has an obstructive impairment
       a. 1 only
       b. 4 only
       c. 1 and 3
       d. 2 only

14. Which of the following prebronchodilator and postbronchodilator spirometry results is most indicative of a reversible obstructive disorder?
    a. PEF increases 1 L/s
    b. FVC increases 100 mL
    c. $FEV_1$ increases by 15%
    d. FRC increases by 15%

15. Based on their basic spirometry results, which of the following patients would you recommend for static lung volume determination (FRC/TLC measurement)?
    a. Patient A: FVC < LLN, $FEV_1$/FVC > LLN
    b. Patient B: FVC > LLN, $FEV_1$/FVC > LLN
    c. Patient C: FVC < LLN, $FEV_1$/FVC < LLN
    d. Patient D: FVC > LLN, $FEV_1$/FVC < LLN

16. Which of the following tests would you recommend to measure the extent of gas trapping in a patient with emphysema?
    a. Closed-circuit He dilution FRC measurement
    b. Single-breath diffusing capacity of the lung
    c. Open-circuit $N_2$ washout FRC measurement
    d. Body plethysmography measurement of TGV

17. Which of the following are consistent with obstructive lung disease?
    a. Decreased lung volumes and decreased flows
    b. Increased lung volumes and decreased flows
    c. Decreased lung volumes and increased flows
    d. Increased lung volumes and increased flows

18. Which of the following tests would you recommend to help differentiate between interstitial and chest wall/neuromuscular causes of a restrictive ventilatory impairment?
    a. Closed-circuit He dilution FRC measurement
    b. Single-breath diffusing capacity of the lung
    c. Body plethysmography measurement of TGV
    d. Exercise capacity testing with $O_2$ consumption

19. Which of the following would invalidate the results of a single-breath DLCO maneuver?
    a. Patient holding the breath for more than 5 seconds
    b. Patient exhaling smoothly in less than 4 seconds
    c. Patient performing a Valsalva maneuver during breath-hold
    d. Patient inspiring to 90% of best vital capacity

20. After comprehensive pulmonary laboratory assessment, a patient has the following results: FVC < LLN, $FEV_1$/FVC > LLN, TLC < LLN, IC < LLN, DLCO > LLN. Which of the following is the most likely cause?
    a. Pulmonary emphysema
    b. A neuromuscular disorder
    c. An interstitial lung disease
    d. A pulmonary vascular disorder

21. Static lung compliance is computed using which of the following formulas?
    a. Lung volume ÷ transpulmonary pressure gradient
    b. Lung volume ÷ transthoracic pressure gradient
    c. Lung volume ÷ transrespiratory pressure gradient
    d. Transpulmonary pressure gradient ÷ airflow

22. Which of the following patient(s) would you recommend for methacholine bronchoprovocation testing?
    1. A patient who experiences unexplained wheezing at his job site
    2. A patient with a history of nighttime shortness of breath and coughing
    3. A patient with spirometry data indicating severe obstruction ($FEV_1$ < 1 L)
       a. 1 only
       b. 1 and 2
       c. 2 and 3
       d. 1, 2, and 3

23. After progressive step-up to 16 mg/mL methacholine, a patient exhibits a 15% decrease in $FEV_1$ compared with baseline. You would interpret this result as indicating:
    a. Normal airway responsiveness
    b. Borderline hyperresponsiveness
    c. Mild hyperresponsiveness
    d. Severe hyperresponsiveness

24. Which of the following would invalidate the results of an expired nitric oxide ($F_ENO$) maneuver?
    a. Performance after spirometry
    b. Exhalation > 6 s
    c. $F_ENO$ plateau > 3 s
    d. ±5% variation in plateau $F_ENO$

25. An adult patient with recurrent episodes of shortness of breath, wheezing, and coughing has an expired nitric oxide ($F_ENO$) level of 15 ppb. Which of the following diagnosis is *least* likely?
    a. Cystic fibrosis
    b. Eosinophilic asthma
    c. Sinusitis
    d. Gastroesophageal reflux

26. Which of the following patients' 6-Minute Walk Test results indicate an abnormally low functional capacity?
    a. Male patient, 6MWD 500 meters
    b. Female patient, 6MWD 400 meters
    c. Male patient, 6MWD 400 meters
    d. Female patient, 6MWD 500 meters

27. Which of the following are indications for cardiopulmonary exercise testing?
    1. To diagnose obstructive coronary artery disease (CAD)
    2. To differentiate between cardiac and pulmonary limitations to exercise
    3. To determine whether arterial desaturation occurs with exercise
    a. 1 only
    b. 1 and 2
    c. 2 and 3
    d. 1, 2, and 3

28. What would be the estimated maximal heart rate at peak exercise capacity for a 60-year-old man?
    a. 120 beats/min
    b. 140 beats/min
    c. 160 beats/min
    d. 180 beats/min

## BIBLIOGRAPHY

Akker IL, van der Zeijden H, Verheij TJ. Is spirometry essential in diagnosing asthma? Yes. *Br J Gen Pract* 2016;**66**(650):484.

American Thoracic Society. Guidelines for methacholine and exercise challenge testing—1999. *Am J Respir Crit Care Med* 2000;**161**(1):309–29.

American Thoracic Society. ATS statement: guidelines for the six-minute walk test. *Am J Respir Crit Care Med* 2016;**193**:1185.

American Thoracic Society and European Respiratory Society. Standardization of single-breath determination of carbon monoxide uptake in the lung. *Eur Respir J* 2005;**26**:720–35.

American Thoracic Society and European Respiratory Society. General considerations for lung function testing. *Eur Respir J* 2005;**26**:153–61.

American Thoracic Society and European Respiratory Society. Standardization of the measurement of lung volumes. *Eur Respir J* 2005;**26**:511–22.

American Thoracic Society and European Respiratory Society. Standardization of spirometry. *Eur Respir J* 2005;**26**:319–38.

American Thoracic Society and American College of Chest Physicians. ATS/ACCP statement on cardiopulmonary exercise testing. *Am J Respir Crit Care Med* 2003;**167**(2):211–77.

American Thoracic Society and European Respiratory Society. ATS/ERS recommendations for standardized procedures for the online and offline measurement of exhaled lower respiratory nitric oxide and nasal nitric oxide. *Am J Respir Crit Care Med* 2005;**171**(8):912–30.

Brazzale DJ, Upward AL, Pretto JJ. Effects of changing reference values and definition of the normal range on interpretation of spirometry. *Respirology* 2010;**15**(7):1098–103.

Busse WW. What is the best pulmonary diagnostic approach for wheezing patients with normal spirometry? *Respir Care* 2012;**57**(1):39–46.

Chipps BE. Spirometry versus flow volume inspiratory and expiratory loop. *Ann Allergy Asthma Immunol* 2011;**107**(2):183.

Cooper B. Spirometry standards and FEV1/FVC repeatability. *Prim Care Respir J* 2010;**19**(3):292–4.

Cockcroft DW. Airway hyperresponsiveness in asthma: its measurement and clinical significance. *Chest* 2010;**138**(Suppl. 2):18S–24.

D'Urzo AD, Tamari I, Bouchard J, et al. New spirometry interpretation algorithm: Primary Care Respiratory Alliance of Canada approach. *Can Fam Physician* 2011;**57**(10):1148–52.

Dweik RA, Boggs PB, Erzurum SC. An official ATS clinical practice guideline: interpretation of exhaled nitric oxide levels ($F_ENO$) for clinical applications. *Am J Respir Crit Care Med* 2011;**184**(5):602–15.

Enright P. The new all-age spirometry reference equations are the best available for Caucasians, regardless of where they live. *Respirology* 2011;**16**(6):871–2.

Hayes Jr D, Kraman SS. The physiologic basis of spirometry. *Respir Care* 2009;**54**(12):1717–26.

Haynes JM. Comprehensive quality control for pulmonary function testing: it's time to face the music. *Respir Care* 2010;**55**(3):355–7.

Hnatiuk OW. What is the role of PFTs in monitoring adverse effects of surgery, drug treatments, radiation therapy, and during hospitalization? *Respir Care* 2012;**57**(1):75–82.

Kacmarek RM, Stoller JK, Heuer AJ. *Egan's fundamentals of respiratory care.* 11th ed. St Louis: Mosby; 2017.

Kaminsky DA. What does airway resistance tell us about lung function? *Respir Care* 2012;**57**(1):85–96.

Lakshminarasimhachar A, Smetana GW. Preoperative evaluation: estimation of pulmonary risk. *Anesthesiol Clin* 2016;**34**(1):71–88.

Laszlo G. Standardisation of lung function testing: helpful guidance from the ATS/ERS Task Force. *Thorax* 2006;**61**(9):744–6.

Lim KG, Mottram C. The use of fraction of exhaled nitric oxide. *Chest* 2008;**133**(5):1232–42.

Macintyre NR. Spirometry for the diagnosis and management of chronic obstructive pulmonary disease. *Respir Care* 2009;**54**(8):1050–7.

Miller A, Enright PL. PFT interpretive strategies: American Thoracic Society/European Respiratory Society 2005 guideline gaps. *Respir Care* 2012;**57**(1):127–33.

Moore AJ. Spirometer calibration check procedures. *Respir Care* 2007;**52**(3):341–2.

Nickels AS, Lim KG. Evaluation of exhaled nitric oxide's ability to predict methacholine challenge in adults with nonobstructive spirometry. *Ann Allergy Asthma Immunol* 2016;**117**(4):365–369.

Pellegrino R, Viegi G, Brusasco V, et al. Interpretative strategies for lung function tests. *Eur Respir J* 2005;**26**(5):948–68.

Perez-Padilla R, Torre-Bouscoulet L, Vázquez-García JC. Implementing a spirometry program. *Int J Tuberc Lung Dis* 2016;**20**(9):1142.

Petsky HL, Kew KM, Turner C, Chang AB. Exhaled nitric oxide levels to guide treatment for adults with asthma. *Cochrane Database Syst Rev* September 1, 2016;**9**:CD011440.

Pichurko BM. Exercising your patient: which test(s) and when? *Respir Care* 2012;**57**(1):100–10.

Rodriguez-Roisin R, Tetzlaff K, Watz H, et al. Daily home-based spirometry during withdrawal of inhaled corticosteroid in severe to very severe chronic obstructive pulmonary disease. *Int J Chron Obstruct Pulmon Dis* 2016;**22**(11):1973–81.

Quanjer PH, Ruppel GL. Diagnosing COPD: high time for a paradigm shift. *Respir Care* 2011;**56**(11):1861–3.

Ruppel GL. What is the clinical value of lung volumes? *Respir Care* 2012;**57**(1):26–35.

Ruppel GL, Enright PL. Pulmonary function testing. *Respir Care* 2012;**57**(1):165–75.

Stoller JK. Quality control for spirometry in large epidemiologic studies: "breathing quality" into our work. *Respir Care* 2008;**53**(8):1008–9.

Vilozni D, Hakim F, Livnat G, et al. Assessment of airway bronchodilation by spirometry compared to airway obstruction in young children with asthma. *Can Respir J* 2016;**5394876**:2016.

Wang JS. Pulmonary function tests in preoperative pulmonary evaluation. *Respir Med* 2004;**98**(7):598–605.

# Chest Imaging

*Zaza Cohen and Norman McLeod*

## LEARNING OBJECTIVES

*After reading this chapter, you will be able to:*

1. Describe how the chest radiograph is produced.
2. Define the terms *radiolucent* and *radiopaque*.
3. Discuss how the density and thickness of organs and tissues affect their radiographic appearance.
4. Explain how the spatial relationship between the x-ray source, the patient, and the x-ray film affects the magnification of images on the radiograph.
5. Identify the clinical indications for a chest radiograph.
6. Discuss the most common radiographic views used for chest imaging.
7. List the fundamental criteria used in the evaluation of the diagnostic quality of a chest radiograph.
8. Explain the significance of the following special radiographic evaluation signs:
   a. Silhouette sign
   b. Air bronchogram
   c. Deep sulcus sign
   d. Kerley B lines
   e. Coin lesions
9. Discuss the limitations of the standard chest radiographic procedure.
10. Appraise the typical clinical and chest radiographic findings for the following lung disorders:
   a. Atelectasis
   b. Pneumothorax
   c. Hyperinflation
   d. Interstitial lung disease
   e. Congestive heart failure
   f. Pleural effusion
   g. Consolidation
   h. Pneumonia
11. Describe the correct position for endotracheal tube placement as seen on a chest radiograph.
12. Identify the value and limitations of using radiographs to determine the position of tubes and catheters.
13. List the clinical indications for a postprocedure chest radiograph.
14. Explain the technique, indications, and advantages and disadvantages for computed tomography scanning.
15. Discuss the relative uses and indications for magnetic resonance imaging in lung disease.
16. Explain the technique and indications for performing nuclear medicine lung scans.
17. Explain the technique and indications for the use of pulmonary angiography.
18. Discuss the utility of ultrasound, fluoroscopy, and interventional radiology in the diagnosis and treatment of lung diseases.
19. Relate the fundamental principles of radiation safety to the protection of health care workers and patients during radiographic procedures.

## OUTLINE

## KEY TERMS

air bronchogram
anteroposterior (AP) view
apical lordotic view
atelectasis
bronchoscopy
chest radiograph
chest ultrasound
computed tomography (CT)
deep sulcus sign
expiratory view

exudate
fluoroscopy
interventional radiology
Kerley B lines
lateral
lateral decubitus view
magnetic resonance imaging (MRI)
oblique view
pneumothorax
positron emission tomography (PET)

posterior to anterior (posteroanterior [PA]) view
pulmonary angiography
radiolucent
radionuclide lung scanning
radiopaque
silhouette sign
target
thoracentesis
transudate

The discovery of x-rays in 1895 led to significant change in the practice of medicine. For the first time in history, internal anatomic structures could be visualized without the need for surgery or other invasive techniques. The introduction of x-ray technology extended the methods physicians could use to detect disease beyond patient interview and physical examination. The use of radiographic imaging expanded rapidly because the procedures were easy to perform and provided substantial diagnostic information. A few years after the discovery of x-rays, radiology became a hospital-based department and, soon thereafter, a special discipline within the field of medicine.

This chapter begins with a brief description of the physics relevant to the production of radiographs. The use of standard and special views in the assessment of patients with pulmonary disease is presented next. This is followed by a discussion of techniques for interpreting the chest image. The chapter continues with a discussion of some of the more common pathologic abnormalities seen on chest radiographs and their related clinical findings. Additional imaging modalities, such as computed tomography (CT), positron emission tomography (PET) scanning, radionuclide lung scanning, fluoroscopy, chest ultrasound, and magnetic resonance imaging (MRI), as well as the fundamentals of radiation safety, are discussed at the end of the chapter.

## PRODUCTION OF THE RADIOGRAPH

X-rays are high-energy waves that are produced by controlled electrical activity in specially designed vacuum tubes. They make up the high-energy portion of a range of frequencies called the electromagnetic spectrum that includes lower energy waves such as visible light, microwaves, and radio waves. German physicist Wilhelm Roentgen is credited with the discovery of x-rays in 1895. He was studying the effect of passing a high voltage through gases in a glass tube when he observed unexpected activity that he attributed to invisible rays. He called the peculiar radiation he discovered x-rays, "x" for the unknown. Throughout the years, despite extensive scientific investigation of x-rays, the name has not been revised, although in some countries x-rays are referred to as Roentgen radiation.

Medical imaging technology has evolved significantly since x-rays were first used for diagnostic purposes. Today, imaging methods are increasingly computer based and the use of film has declined. The advent of digital image processing revolutionized the way images are acquired, displayed, and stored. In the past, the radiographic image was recorded on a sheet of film that had to be chemically processed (similar to traditional film photography) and then viewed by placing it on a view-box that would provide a background light in a room with subdued lighting. Now, radiographic images are acquired digitally using detectors and can be transferred to a computer database to be viewed electronically or placed in the patient's electronic medical record.

Digital radiography has several advantages over conventional "film" radiography. Once the image is in a digital format it can be enhanced and analyzed in numerous ways. It can also be stored and accessed almost instantaneously via electronic health records (see Chapter 21) and similar secure computer networks. It may be argued that the use of the term *film* is now outdated because the actual film is not used in

**FIG. 10.1** Electric current is generated by the transformer, passes through focusing plates, and arrives at the cathode. Electrons are "boiled off," making a cathode stream. The cathode stream then strikes the anode target and is transformed into x-rays. X-rays leave the sealed vacuum x-ray tube through a window and strike the patient, pass through the patient, and cast a shadow on the image cassette, making an image on the image. (From Scanlan CL, Spearman CB, Sheldon RL: *Egan's fundamentals of respiratory therapy,* ed 5. St. Louis, 1996, Mosby.)

either the production or viewing of the x-ray images. A more generic term that pertains to both analog (film) and digital devices is *image receptor*. Despite this conceptual change, many clinicians continue to use the term *film* when referring to the digital x-ray images. Because of the popularity of this concept, we will continue to refer to x-ray images as the "film" in this chapter.

The production of x-rays requires specialized equipment to ensure consistent high-quality waves, as well as radiation safety (Fig. 10.1). The most important components of the equipment are the vacuum tube where the x-rays originate; the tube housing and beam restricting device that controls the spread of the x-ray beam and projects it in the required direction; the cassette, which captures the image; the transformers that provide the electric power; and the operator's console where the technologist selects the level of penetration of the x-rays, sets the amount of time the patient will be exposed to the beam, and starts the exposure.

The main characteristic of x-rays that is applicable in the field of medicine is the ability to penetrate matter. The amount of penetration depends on the density and thickness of the tissues. Dense substances, such as bone, that significantly absorb x-rays (allow less penetration) are referred to as radiopaque and appear light or white on the x-ray. Conversely, low-density substances such as air-filled lung tissue minimally absorb x-rays and are described as radiolucent, appearing dark or black on the x-ray. Also, the thicker portion of an organ will absorb more x-rays than the thinner portion. Four significant densities recognized on radiographs are those of bone, which is very dense (radiopaque); water, which is less dense; fat, which is mildly radiolucent; and air, which is very radiolucent. Most tissues in the body exhibit x-ray absorption characteristics based on a variation of these four densities.

Some x-rays also *scatter*, or deflect from their original path when they interact with matter. Scattered x-rays mainly occur in the patient's body and are lower in penetrating ability than the primary beam. They increase the radiation exposure of anyone close to the x-ray source during the examination and also reduce the quality of the radiographic image. Methods used to reduce the impact of scattered radiation are discussed at the end of the chapter.

Similar to visible light, x-rays travel in a straight line and diverge or spread out in all directions from the area where they are produced. The fact that the x-ray beam will follow the same path as a corresponding light beam is applied in all modern x-ray equipment. A beam-restricting device using visible light allows the operator to simulate the size and direction of the x-ray beam before the patient is exposed to radiation.

The primary beam exiting the x-ray tube is cone shaped with its apex at the x-ray source. The shape of the beam causes the shadows of the structures it penetrates, such as the heart and great vessels, to appear larger on the image than their actual size. Magnification cannot be totally eliminated, but it is minimized when the object is as close to the image receptor as possible.

One major limitation of all radiographs is that they present a two-dimensional view of a three-dimensional object. Structures on the same horizontal level produce the same shadow on the image whether they are inside or outside of the body. For example, a coin taped to the outside of the patient's chest (either in the front or back) will produce the same shadow as a round lung mass—hence many round-shaped lung masses (or nodules) are called coin lesions. Similarly, nipple shadows often cause concern because they cannot be easily distinguished from lesions originating from lung parenchyma.

X-rays passing through low-density tissue (e.g., lung parenchyma) create a dark area on the image, and dense tissues (e.g., bone) create a white area on the image.

## INDICATIONS FOR THE CHEST RADIOGRAPH EXAMINATION

Various medical imaging techniques are used to show the internal structures of the human body. The chest radiograph is one of the most popular and most useful of these procedures. It provides information that is useful in the following:

- Detecting alterations of the lung caused by pathologic processes
- Determining appropriate therapy
- Evaluating the effectiveness of treatment
- Identifying the position of tubes and catheters
- Observing changes in lung disease
- Assessing the patient after an invasive procedure

The chest radiograph provides important information about the status of the lungs. However, in certain emergency situations treatment should not be delayed while images are produced and interpreted. For example, an undiagnosed pneumothorax may suddenly cause deterioration of a mechanically ventilated patient. If a tension pneumothorax is indicated (discussed in detail later in this chapter), there may not be enough time for an urgent radiograph, and treatment may have to be started solely on clinical grounds. In most instances, a well-trained health care team can coordinate activities to obtain the chest radiograph without delaying assessment and treatment.

Frequently, it is the respiratory therapist (RT) who is at the bedside of the mechanically ventilated patient and is the first person to observe the signs consistent with a pneumothorax or other potentially serious complications. Therefore all RTs must be familiar with the clinical indications for a chest radiograph (Box 10.1). Although RTs cannot order a chest radiograph, they often recommend that one be done to the physician who can then order it, if appropriate.

## RADIOGRAPHIC VIEWS

### Standard and Special Views

The standard examination of the chest consists of two separate radiographic images: one with the x-ray beam projected posterior to anterior (posteroanterior [PA]) and the other with the beam projected from the patient's right side through to the left, with the left side against the image receptor (left lateral). The heart is closer to the film for both PA and left lateral projections, and this minimizes cardiac magnification. The routine PA chest x-ray is done with the patient erect, the patient's anterior chest wall pressed against the cassette, and scapulae (shoulder blades) rotated forward to avoid overlap with lung tissue. For optimal image quality, the distance between the x-ray tube and image receptor is 6 feet (72 inches). This also reduces cardiac magnification and improves image detail. To capture the image,

**BOX 10.1   Clinical Indications for the Chest Radiograph**

**Symptoms**
New or unexplained dyspnea
Cough, sputum, and fever
Chest pain
Hemoptysis

**Medical History**
Recent history of chest trauma
History of aspiration of foreign body
History of tuberculosis
History of chronic obstructive pulmonary disease
Significant smoking history
History of pulmonary fibrosis
Employment history consistent with inhalation of certain dusts

**Physical Examination**
Crackles or wheezes on auscultation
Sudden drop in blood pressure during mechanical ventilation
Unilateral decrease in breath sounds
Extensive use of accessory muscles
Respiratory rate >30 breaths/min at rest
Loud $P_2$ sound
Pedal edema
Cardiac murmurs
Signs of trauma

**Arterial Blood Gas Levels**
Severe hypoxemia
Acute hypercapnia

**Pulmonary Function Tests**
Evidence of air trapping (e.g., increase in residual volume or functional residual capacity)
Reduction in expiratory flows or lung volumes
Reduced diffusing capacity of lung for carbon monoxide

**Postprocedure**
Intubation
Central venous pressure line or pulmonary artery catheter placement
Nasogastric tube placement
Chest tube placement
Thoracentesis
Pericardiocentesis
Bronchoscopy with transbronchial biopsy
Percutaneous needle biopsy of the lung
Abdominal or thoracic surgery

**Other**
Sudden increase in peak airway pressure (with volume-targeted ventilation) during mechanical ventilation
After cardiopulmonary resuscitation
Routinely for mechanically ventilated patients
Routine screening for infectious disease

x-rays are turned on for just milliseconds (1/1000 of a second) to eliminate blur due to the heartbeat. Routine chest images are done on full inspiration; the patient is instructed to "take a deep breath in and hold it" just before the radiograph is taken.

Other views are sometimes required in particular circumstances. Lateral decubitus views are done to see whether pleural fluid is present in the chest. As little as 50 to 100 mL of pleural fluid can be detected with the lateral decubitus view. It is also helpful in the identification of pneumothorax. The lateral decubitus is taken with the x-ray beam directed horizontally and the patient lying on the right or left side. Air tends to rise and water tends to fall; therefore patients with a suspected pneumothorax should be placed on the unaffected side, and patients with suspected pleural fluid should be placed on the side that is affected.

The apical lordotic view is sometimes required for a closer look at the middle lobe or the top (apical region) of the lungs. The x-ray tube is angled upward to project the shadows of the clavicles above the thorax so that they do not overlap the top of the lungs.

Oblique views are done to separate pulmonary or mediastinal lesions from overlapping structures shown in the PA and lateral views (review the limitations of radiographs as two-dimensional views of a three-dimensional object discussed earlier). Oblique views are also done to clarify the location of an abnormality. These views are done with the patient turned 45 degrees to either the right or left, with the anterolateral portion of the chest against the film.

Chest radiographs are usually taken with the patient at full inspiration; however, an expiratory view is helpful in certain situations. For example, a small pneumothorax can be difficult or impossible to detect in a routine inspiratory image. As the patient exhales the lung volume is reduced, but the pleural air volume remains the same. The lung becomes denser, and the pneumothorax occupies a greater percentage of the thoracic volume. These factors result in the pneumothorax being more easily identified.

Recent advances in technology have resulted in CT scans being more readily available. CT provides significantly more information about thoracic structures than routine or special radiographic views. In many instances, these special views have become obsolete and have retained only educational and historical value.

## Portable Chest Image (Anteroposterior View)

Patients in intensive care units are too sick to be transported to the radiology department for the standard radiographic examination. In this situation, chest imaging may be achieved by bringing a mobile radiographic machine to the patient's bedside. The portable radiographs obtained at the bedside have less diagnostic quality in comparison to the standard images done in the radiology department. There is increased cardiac magnification because portable images are done with the cassette placed at the patient's back and the x-ray beam going from front to back producing an anteroposterior (AP) instead of a PA view. Additionally, the distance between the x-ray source and the cassette for bedside examinations is limited to approximately 40 inches instead of 72 inches.

Interpreting the AP chest radiograph is also challenging because often it is not centered, is rotated, is overexposed or underexposed, or is not taken when the patient is in full inspiration. There may be many shadows superimposed on the film caused by bedding, gowns, electrocardiogram (ECG) leads, and tubing. Despite the reduced quality, the clinician may still be able to gather some diagnostic information from the portable images. The AP views are obtained to evaluate lung status, to gain information on how well lines and tubing are positioned, and to see the results of invasive therapeutic maneuvers. Some of the lines and tubes needing evaluation are discussed later under Postprocedural Chest Radiograph Evaluation.

---

### SIMPLY STATED

The standard chest radiograph is taken with the patient's chest pressed against the radiographic cassette. The x-ray passes from back (posterior) to front (anterior), and the resulting chest radiograph is called a PA view. The portable chest radiograph is obtained with the x-ray passing from front (anterior) to back (posterior), producing an AP view.

---

## EVALUATION OF THE CHEST RADIOGRAPH

This section introduces the basic principles of chest radiograph evaluation. Interpreting chest images is a skill obtained only through hours of dedicated practice. The beginner is encouraged to view chest images initially with the help of qualified experts.

Familiarity with the anatomic landmarks seen on normal chest images is extremely helpful in learning to recognize abnormalities. Fig. 10.2 identifies the important landmarks on a normal PA chest radiograph. For additional discussion, see the article by Marano and colleagues.

### Review of Clinical Findings

The clinician will benefit from reviewing the patient's history and physical examination findings before viewing the chest image. This information can provide insight into the abnormalities to be looked for on the chest image.

### Systematic Approach to the Chest Radiograph

The first step in evaluating the chest radiograph is to determine the technical quality of the image. The adequacy of exposure can be judged by looking at the vertebral bodies. The clinician should be able to just about visualize the vertebral bodies through the cardiac shadow. If the vertebral bodies are easily seen, the image is probably overexposed, and the lungs will appear black. Underexposure makes identification of the vertebral bodies more difficult, and the lung fields appear whiter than on a properly exposed image. The pulmonary vascularity and some pulmonary abnormalities may be misinterpreted with overexposure or underexposure.

The chest radiograph should be evaluated to make sure that the patient was not rotated when the chest image was obtained. If the patient is rotated, uniform exposure of both lungs will not be obtained, and one side of the image will be darker than the other. The shadows of the heart and other mediastinal structures may also appear enlarged if the patient is rotated. Patient rotation

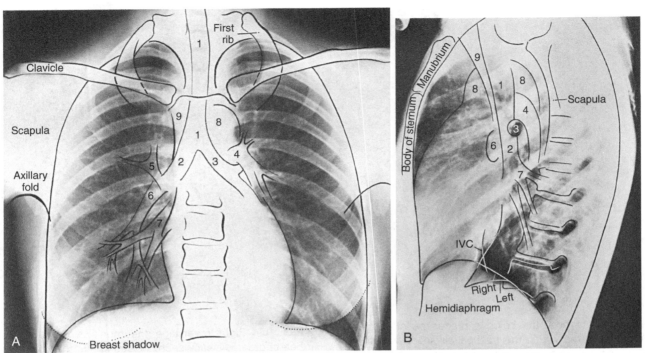

**FIG. 10.2  A,** Posteroanterior projection of normal chest image showing the trachea (1), right main bronchus (2), left main bronchus (3), left pulmonary artery (4), right upper lobe pulmonary artery (5), right interlobar artery (6), right lower and middle lobe vein (7), aortic knob (8), and superior vena cava (9). **B,** Lateral projection of normal chest image showing trachea (1), right main bronchus (2), left main bronchus (3), left interlobar artery (4)—not visible in this view (5), right main pulmonary artery (6), confluence of pulmonary veins (7), aortic arch (8), and brachiocephalic vessels (9). *IVC,* Inferior vena cava. (From Fraser RS, Pare RD: *Diagnosis of diseases of the chest.* Philadelphia, 1970, WB Saunders.)

is assessed by identifying the relationship of the spinous processes of the vertebral column to the medial ends of the clavicles (Fig. 10.3). The spinous processes should be centered between the ends of the clavicles and directly behind the tracheal air shadow. If the medial end of one clavicle appears closer to the spine, the patient probably was rotated.

Finally, the degree of the patient's inspiratory effort is evaluated by counting the posterior ribs visible above the diaphragm. On a PA image, lungs spanning 10 ribs indicate a good inspiratory effort. A poor inspiratory effort may cause the heart to appear abnormally enlarged and increase the density of the lung fields so that they appear too white to allow detection of certain lung abnormalities.

> ### SIMPLY STATED
>
> A good inspiratory effort results in 10 posterior ribs visible above the diaphragm. The depth of the patient's inspiration is assessed to help determine the quality of the chest image.

## Interpretation

Interpretation of the chest image requires a complete understanding of the x-ray principles introduced at the beginning of this chapter. The clinician must remember that x-ray penetration of structures is inversely proportional to the density of the structure, and thus the greater the density, the less the penetration. X-rays that do not penetrate fully are absorbed, resulting in less exposure of the film and the casting of a white shadow on the image.

Normal lung tissue has a low density (air density) so that few x-rays are absorbed, and normal lung fields appear as dark shadows on the chest radiograph. If an area of the lung consolidates (increases in density) because of pneumonia, tumor, or collapse, that area will absorb more x-rays and appear as a white patch on the film. Abnormalities that decrease lung tissue density, such as cavities and blebs, absorb fewer x-rays and result in darker areas on the film.

The heart, diaphragm, and major blood vessels are considered to have the density of water. Water is denser than air, and water densities result in less exposure and therefore whitish-gray shadows on the chest radiograph. The heart, diaphragm, and major blood vessels rarely alter in density but may change in size, shape, and position. Evaluation of the shadows produced on the chest radiograph by these structures allows a clear view of any deviation from normal in position or size.

It is important to note that the lung shadow on a normal chest radiograph is not uniformly black. The pulmonary vessels that are perpendicular to the x-ray plane give round

FIG. 10.3 Note how the spinous processes of the verte-brae are centered within the tracheal air shadow, indicating that the patient was not rotated when the chest image was obtained. Also note the consolidation in the patient's right lung. The infiltrate must be in the right middle lobe because the right heart border is blurred (see description of silhouette sign in text).

FIG. 10.4 Right lower lobe pneumonia. Note how the right heart border is clearly seen, indicating that the infiltrate must be in the lower lobe, which is posterior to the heart. Also note that the right hemidiaphragm is obscured. This provides fur-ther evidence that the consolidation is in the right lower lobe.

shadows, and the vessels that are parallel to the plane give tubular shadows. Therefore the normal lung will appear "pep-pered" with dots and lines that represent pulmonary vas-culature. This appearance is sometimes called *normal lung architecture*. As a result of the absence of the lung vasculature, blebs and the air contained in pneumothorax do not have this particular lung architecture appearance, which makes it eas-ier to distinguish them from the normal lung tissue.

The structures in the chest with the greatest density are the bones, including the ribs, clavicles, scapulae, and vertebrae. They are seen on the radiograph as white shadows. Fractures and changes in position and density of bones may be evalu-ated with a chest radiograph. It should be obtained to evaluate the bony structures of the chest when the patient's history or physical examination suggests chest trauma.

Identification of the abnormalities visible on the chest radiograph requires a systematic review of all the structures shown on it. The sequence in which the structures are evalu-ated is not important as long as all are included. Many experts encourage beginners to develop a habit of evaluating the bony structures and peripheral areas of the radiograph first. This helps prevent overlooking subtle but important abnormali-ties in the less conspicuous areas of the radiograph. Once the peripheral soft tissues and bony structures have been viewed, the lung, mediastinum, heart, and diaphragms are inspected carefully. A system using the alphabet—A to Z—has been rec-ommended to remind the examiner which parts of the chest image to study. This system, starting with A for airway, B for bones, C for cardiac shadow, and so forth, may prove useful

in organizing the approach to reading the chest radiograph. An alternative approach is to follow a comfortable pathway around the chest radiograph. The major goal is to use the same method of complete review in every individual case.

The ability to localize abnormalities within the thorax is aided by special radiographic signs. Two of the most impor-tant radiographic signs are the silhouette sign and the air bronchogram.

### Silhouette Sign

The silhouette sign is useful primarily in determining whether a pulmonary infiltrate is in anatomic contact with another thoracic structure. Normally, the significant differ-ence in density between two adjoining structures will sharply delineate their borders. This allows a person viewing the chest radiograph to see the heart border, the aortic knob, and the diaphragm shadows on the background of radiolucent lung—a natural contrast between the thoracic tissues that makes the chest radiograph a great diagnostic tool. If the lung tissue in contact with heart (or diaphragm) is consolidated, the contrast in densities is lost, and the corresponding heart (or diaphragm) border is blurred (Figs. 10.3 and 10.4). This phenomenon is called the *silhouette sign*.

The heart is located in the anterior thorax, and any infil-trate that obliterates the heart border must also be located in the anterior segments of the lungs (lingula or the right middle lobe). Infiltrates that appear to overlap the heart border on the image but do not affect its sharpness are located in posterior segments and are not in anatomic contact with the heart. An infiltrate in the mid–lung zone on a chest radiograph may be located anteriorly or posteriorly, and the silhouette sign often allows a better localization (a lobe rather than more vague "zone") of the infiltrate. Infiltrates that create a silhouette sign by blurring the diaphragm border are thought to be in the lower lobes.

### Air Bronchogram

The presence of air bronchograms is useful in determining whether an abnormality seen on the radiograph is located within lung tissue. Intrapulmonary bronchi are not normally visible on chest images because they contain air and are surrounded by air-filled alveoli. Bronchi surrounded by consolidated alveoli are visible because the air within their lumina will stand out in contrast to the surrounding consolidation and fluid. In this situation, the bronchi are seen as linear branching air shadows, signifying that the lesion is within lung tissue. Diseases that both consolidate lung tissue and fill the airways will not produce air bronchograms. Therefore the presence of an air bronchogram confirms intrapulmonary disease, whereas the absence of an air bronchogram does not rule it out.

### Limitations

Although the chest radiograph provides important information about the pathologic changes within the thorax, it does have certain limitations. Small lesions and those located in "blind" areas may not be seen. In addition, the chest image is often normal in patients experiencing significant respiratory symptoms. In the setting of asthma with acute bronchospasm, or acute pulmonary embolism (PE), even though the patient may be severely symptomatic, the chest radiograph often appears normal.

## CLINICAL AND RADIOGRAPHIC FINDINGS IN LUNG DISEASES

This section reviews the radiographic findings typical of the more common respiratory disorders. Familiarity with this information is helpful in the interpretation of the chest radiograph. In addition, this section presents the clinical findings typically associated with the different pathologic abnormalities described. In most cases, the most efficient and accurate assessment is achieved when clinical and radiographic findings are used together. The following categories of chest disorders are presented:

- Atelectasis
- Hyperinflation
- Interstitial lung disease
- Congestive heart failure (CHF)
- Pleural effusion
- Consolidation

**FIG. 10.5** This patient's right upper lobe has become consolidated because of a tumor obstructing the right upper lobe bronchus. As a result, pneumonia has developed distal to the obstruction. Note the well-outlined horizontal fissure, slightly rotated up and delineating the inferior boundary of the right upper lobe. The upward displacement of the horizontal fissure suggests atelectasis in the right upper lobe.

### Atelectasis

Loss of air in a portion of lung tissue results in a condition called atelectasis (Fig. 10.5), a word formed from the Greek *ateles* (incomplete) and *ektasis* (extension). Atelectasis may occur as a result of changes in the transpulmonary distending pressure and in such cases is called *compression atelectasis*. It may also be caused by obstruction of one or more airways, which allows distal gas to be absorbed. The latter type of atelectasis may be called *obstructive* or *absorption atelectasis*.

#### Compression Atelectasis

Compression atelectasis is seen in patients with pleural effusion, pneumothorax, hemothorax, and any space-occupying lesion. The degree of pulmonary compromise with compression atelectasis depends on the extent of the problem. Severe atelectasis may shift the mediastinum enough to compromise cardiac output and overall hemodynamic status.

#### Obstructive Atelectasis

Obstructive atelectasis is caused by blockage of an airway so that ventilation of the affected region is absent. Many clinical situations can obstruct an airway, leading to partial or complete lung collapse (atelectasis). Tumor, aspirated foreign body, and mucous plugs are some of the more common causes of obstructive atelectasis.

As long as the airway obstruction remains incomplete, the distal lung will remain inflated. In fact, partial obstruction of a bronchus can lead to hyperinflation of the lung if the obstruction causes a one-way valve effect, allowing air to enter the lung but not escape. Complete obstruction of a larger airway usually leads to atelectasis of the distal lung.

A related form of atelectasis occurs in patients after surgery. It is not uncommon for atelectasis to develop in the postoperative period, especially if the patient has had upper abdominal or thoracic surgery or if the patient is obese or has a history of chronic lung disease. After surgery, lung secretions tend to be retained in the lung because of mucociliary stasis and suppression of coughing and deep breathing. Retained secretions can obstruct multiple small airways, leading to underventilation and microatelectasis in the affected regions.

The physical examination findings of atelectasis vary with the amount of lung involved. With significant loss of lung volume, as occurs with lobar collapse, the findings are striking and usually include the following:

- Rapid shallow breathing
- Decreased to absent breath sounds
- Decreased to absent vocal fremitus
- Decreased resonance to percussion
- Cyanosis
- Shift of the mediastinum toward the affected side

The chest radiograph in most cases demonstrates the loss of lung volume caused by the atelectasis. Collapse of entire segments or lobes produces characteristic densities that show on the chest radiograph. Shift of the trachea, heart, and major thoracic vessels toward the affected side may be seen with lobar atelectasis. The radiographic findings seen with postoperative microatelectasis often are much more subtler or may be absent altogether.

## Pneumothorax

Pneumothorax often causes atelectasis (Fig. 10.6). Pneumothorax is a condition in which air enters the pleural space either externally from a hole in the chest wall or internally from a hole in the lung. This leads to loss of the negative pressure normally found in the pleural space. As a result, the lung's normal elasticity causes it to contract, and the lung collapses.

This is serious enough, but the lung can develop a potentially more serious problem called *tension pneumothorax* (Fig. 10.7). With a tension pneumothorax, the air cannot get out of the pleural space, and pressure builds up. The pressure in the pleural space that's usually negative now becomes positive. This creates ventilatory as well as hemodynamic problems, as the heart cannot properly fill with blood, and cardiac output diminishes. Patients with tension pneumothorax often develop respiratory as well as cardiovascular failure. Not all pneumothoraces develop "tension."

Physical findings with a small pneumothorax may be absent or minimal. With a tension pneumothorax, physical findings are as follows:

- Chest wall: reduction in movement in the chest wall on the side where the pneumothorax has occurred
- Auscultation of the lung: loss of breath sounds or distant breath sounds on the affected side

FIG. 10.6 Good example of pneumothorax involving the right lung. Note the pleural line along the right lateral chest wall where the lung has pulled away from the chest wall as it collapsed toward the hilum.

FIG. 10.7 Portable chest image showing a left-sided tension pneumothorax. Note that the pressure in the left hemithorax has depressed the diaphragm on that side and forced the heart into the right side of the chest. A chest tube must be inserted immediately into the left chest.

- Percussion: increased resonance to percussion on the affected side
- Heart: usually a rapid heart rate (tachycardia) and low blood pressure
- Other: cyanosis, an external wound, or bruising on the affected side
- Absent whispered voice sounds and tactile fremitus

Radiographic changes seen with a tension pneumothorax include shift of the mediastinal structures (the trachea and heart) away from the involved side and deviation of the trachea away from the affected side. Another sign suggestive of pneumothorax is deep sulcus sign as noted in the article by Sabbar and Niles (see Bibliography). A pleural line represents the outer margin of the lung (see Fig. 10.6). It is expected that an experienced clinician (physician, nurse, RT) should be able to diagnose tension pneumothorax on clinical examination and not waste time on obtaining and evaluating radiographs to confirm the diagnosis. The treatment should be started emergently and consists of immediate chest tube placement or needle decompression followed by chest tube placement.

> **SIMPLY STATED**
>
> Tension pneumothorax is a life-threatening condition that is seen on the chest image as extreme hyperlucency on the affected side, with a shift of the mediastinal structures away from the air-filled pleural space.

## Hyperinflation

Lung hyperinflation is seen commonly in patients with emphysema and sometimes in acute asthma. This is seen on chest radiograph as small heart size (Fig. 10.8A), increased AP diameter, a large retrosternal air space (Fig. 10.8B), and flattening of the diaphragm (see Fig. 10.8A and B). The chest radiograph is neither very sensitive nor specific for the diagnosis of chronic obstructive pulmonary disease (COPD) but often provides supporting evidence for the diagnosis. Pulmonary function testing is much more sensitive and specific in the diagnosis of COPD.

The physical examination findings that correlate with the radiographic examination include the following:
- Large barrel chest, with increased AP diameter of the chest wall
- Increased resonance to percussion
- Decreased breath sounds
- Limited motion of low-set diaphragms
- Wheezing (with acute asthma but generally not with emphysema)
- Prolonged expiratory phase
- Rapid respiratory rate
- Use of accessory muscles to breathe

> **SIMPLY STATED**
>
> The severity of the emphysema and pulmonary hyperexpansion in the patient with COPD is often predicted by the size of the retrosternal air space. The larger it is, the more severe the emphysema.

## Interstitial Lung Disease

About 200 different diseases and syndromes can cause interstitial lung disease (Figs. 10.9 to 10.11, Box 10.2). The term *interstitial lung diseases* implies that most of the disease activity is contained within the interstitium (a microscopic anatomic space between the structural elements) of the lung;

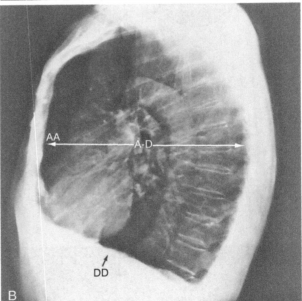

**FIG. 10.8** **A,** Posteroanterior chest image. Note marked hyperinflation with large lung volumes; low-set diaphragm; small, narrow heart; and enlarged intercostal spaces. **B,** Lateral view. Hyperinflation is manifested by increased anterior air space, depressed diaphragm, and increased anteroposterior chest dimensions (barrel chest). *AA,* Anterior air space; *DD,* depressed diaphragm; *A-D,* anteroposterior dimension.

however, this implication is incorrect. Many interstitial lung diseases affect various parts of the lung, including airways, lung parenchyma, the interstitium, and the pleura. A more inclusive name of *diffuse parenchymal lung disease* has been suggested as a replacement for interstitial lung diseases; however, the latter is still commonly used. A simplified classification with a few representative diseases or syndromes causing interstitial lung disease is included to acquaint the reader with the terms (see Box 10.2).

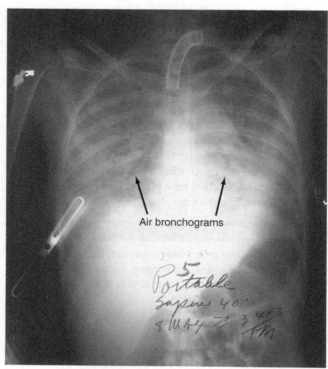

**FIG. 10.11** Typical alveolar filling pattern.

**FIG. 10.9** Theoretical explanation for the development of pulmonary fibrosis. Patients who develop interstitial fibrosis are prone to develop other complications such as pneumothorax, cancer, and pneumonia. (Modified from Simmons DH: *Current pulmonology.* New York, 1981, Elsevier.)

**FIG. 10.10** Severe interstitial fibrosis in the chest. (From Kacmarek RM, Stoller JK, Heuer AJ: *Egan's fundamentals of respiratory care,* ed 11. St. Louis, 2017, Mosby-Elsevier.)

### BOX 10.2   Interstitial Lung Diseases

**Infections**
Influenza
Chickenpox
Pneumocystis

**Exposures**
Asbestosis
Silicosis
Bleomycin
Radiation
Various organic and inorganic dusts

**Neoplastic Causes**
Bronchoalveolar carcinoma
Lymphangitic or hematologic spread of metastases

**Congenital or Familial Causes**
Niemann-Pick disease
Hermansky-Pudlak syndrome

**Systemic Diseases**
Rheumatoid arthritis
Systemic lupus erythematosus

**Idiopathic (Unknown Causes)**
Sarcoidosis
Pulmonary fibrosis

The basic pathologic process associated with pulmonary fibrosis is shown in Fig. 10.9. Some substance (etiologic agent) activates the patient's immune system, and if this process continues the lung begins to scar and become fibrotic. The fibrotic process usually is progressive over a period of months to years. The end result for many of these patients is combined cardiac and respiratory failure.

Initially, the patient with pulmonary fibrosis may notice a dry, nonproductive cough and dyspnea on exertion (DOE). This usually brings the patient in for medical care. The history is probably the most important element in helping to determine what has incited the immune response, causing the lung damage. A history of industrial exposure to silica or asbestos is crucial. A history of systemic symptoms, such as swallowing disorders or joint or muscle pain, may suggest a collagen vascular disease causing the fibrosis.

The pattern seen on the chest radiograph may give a clue to the cause of the abnormality. Examples include large hilar and paratracheal lymph nodes, suggesting sarcoidosis; calcified pleural or diaphragmatic nodules, suggesting asbestosis injury; honeycomb-sized cavities in the lungs, suggesting end-stage pulmonary fibrosis; and large air bronchograms with thick walls, suggesting bronchiectasis.

Physical examination of the patient with interstitial lung disease typically identifies a rapid and shallow breathing pattern. The interstitial fibrosis causes a decrease in lung compliance that results in the patient breathing with a smaller tidal volume ($V_T$). As the $V_T$ decreases, the respiratory rate must increase to maintain adequate ventilation. Auscultation usually identifies fine inspiratory crackles that do not clear with deep breaths or changes in position. The crackles often are more noticeable over the lower lobes. If the interstitial lung disease is severe, hypoxemia and cyanosis may be present.

In the evaluation of a patient with interstitial lung disease, bronchoscopy is commonly done to exclude a few diseases, such as infections, malignancy, and sarcoidosis. In most cases, bronchoscopy does not lead to a final diagnosis, necessitating a surgical lung biopsy.

## Congestive Heart Failure

Early CHF causes the following changes on the chest radiograph (Fig. 10.12):

- Redistribution of pulmonary vasculature with engorgement (cephalization) of the upper lobe vessels. The normal chest image shows the pulmonary blood vessels most prominent in the lower lobes. Left-sided heart failure increases venous pressure, and the increased pressure distends upper lobe vessels that would otherwise carry very little blood.
- Fluid collection in the dependent portions of the lung.
- Increase width of the heart in relation to that of the thorax. Normally, the base of the heart occupies about half of the width of the thorax. In CHF, that ratio increases, and the heart appears larger (see Fig. 10.12). Increase in the width of the shadows of the mediastinal structures is another sign of fluid overload.
- Development of Kerley B lines. These lines, usually seen in the right base, are less than 1 mm thick and approximately 1 to 2 cm in length. They are horizontal and start at the periphery, extending into the lung approximately 1 to 2 cm. They are pleural lymphatic vessels filled with fluid. Kerley B lines are very subtle, often difficult to find

FIG. 10.12 Congestive heart failure with upper lobe redistribution of vasculature markings, especially on the right, increased cardiothoracic ratio, and increased interstitial markings. Cardiac shadow should not be over half of the entire width of the thoracic cage; here it is well over half.

on an actual image, and nearly impossible to reproduce in print. More information on this is available by reviewing the article by Koga and Fujimoto (see Bibliography).

- Miscellaneous signs:
  - Increased interstitial markings caused by fluid collecting around the lymph channels
  - Pleural effusion greater in the right hemithorax than the left hemithorax
  - Enlarged pulmonary artery segments caused by increased pulmonary artery pressure
  - Fluid collection around the vessels causing the margins to appear blurred
  - Increased size of the azygos vein caused by increased venous pressure
  - Fluffy perihilar opacities caused by fluid collection in lung tissue

CHF in patients with severe hyperinflation (especially emphysema) may not result in some of these previously mentioned signs. The development of an enlarged heart may be delayed in patients with emphysema because of the pathologic changes already present in the thoracic cage. With tissue destruction, common in emphysema, redistribution to the upper lobes already may have occurred before CHF develops. Physical examination findings include the following:

- Fine inspiratory crackles
- Rapid heart rate, either regular or irregular in rhythm
- Third heart sound ($S_3$), a consistent finding in CHF
- Jugular venous distention
- Enlarged liver (hepatomegaly)
- Hepatojugular reflex
- Ankle edema (swelling)

## Pleural Effusion

The pleural space usually contains approximately 30 mL of viscous fluid on each side. The major function of this fluid is to lubricate the pleural surfaces and decrease friction between them as the lung moves. Pleural fluid is in constant flux; it is secreted and reabsorbed to maintain its volume and composition. During various pathologic conditions, the amount of fluid in the pleural space may increase, leading to formation of pleural effusion (Figs. 10.13 and 10.14). Usually, 100 mL must be present before the fluid can be seen on the chest radiograph. The fluid can be a clear watery material, caused by the imbalance in hydrostatic pressures (more fluid being secreted under higher pressure or less fluid being reabsorbed under lower pressure). This type of pleural fluid is low in protein content (<3 g/dL) and called a transudate. Alternatively, infection, inflammation, or blockage of the lymphatic flow by tumor can lead to production of fluid with a high protein content (>3 g/dL), called an exudate. Transudates are almost always free flowing, whereas exudates are often loculated, or compartmentalized. Loculated pleural effusions are more difficult to manage because different pockets of fluid do not communicate with each other, making them difficult to drain. Open thoracotomy with decortication (stripping of the pleural surfaces) may be necessary.

The causes of transudative pleural effusion include CHF, hepatic failure, and atelectasis. Each of these causes either low protein in the blood or high pressure within the pleural veins favoring fluid movement into pleural space. The possible causes of exudative pleural effusions are more numerous and include bacterial pneumonia, PE, malignancy, viral disease, tuberculosis, and fungal infections.

Other fluids that collect in the pleural space include blood (hemothorax), a fatty fluid called *chyle* (chylothorax), and pus (empyema or pyothorax). Sometimes there will be a mixture of air, fluid, and blood or pus in the pleural space (hydropneumothorax or pyopneumothorax).

The radiographic findings of pleural effusion depend on the volume of fluid collected in the pleural space. Small volume findings (see Fig. 10.13) are as follows:

- Blunting of the otherwise sharp angle between the chest wall and the point at which the diaphragm touches the chest wall laterally (the costophrenic [CP] angle).
- Small meniscus sign, which is seen when fluid starts to fill the space between the lung and chest wall, forming an opaque white crescent (meniscus) next to the chest wall; partially obscured diaphragm with elevation of the diaphragm from its normal position.

Large (massive) pleural effusion findings (see Fig. 10.14) are as follows:

- Complete or nearly complete whiteout of the involved side
- Complete obscuring of the hemidiaphragm
- Shift of the thoracic organs away from the effusion

FIG. 10.13 A small pleural effusion has developed in the right chest, resulting in a blunted right costophrenic angle and partially obscured right hemidiaphragm.

FIG. 10.14 Large massive pleural effusion involving the left hemithorax. This has caused the x-ray image to appear as a whiteout of the involved side, completely obscuring all structures in the left chest.

It is illustrative to compare the findings of a massive pleural effusion and the mediastinal shift to the contralateral (opposite) side (see Fig. 10.14) to the complete lung collapse and the mediastinal shift to the ipsilateral (same) side (see Fig. 10.17 later in this chapter).

If there is a question as to whether an effusion is present or if the fluid is free to move about, a lateral decubitus image is obtained. This study requires only that the patient lie on

**FIG. 10.15** Patient lying on his side so that pleural effusion fluid has moved to the dependent area of the chest cavity (line indicated by *arrows*). This is called a *lateral decubitus view*. Important information is available from this view: confirmation of the effusion's presence and the fact that the effusion is free and not loculated, or trapped, by adhesions in one area of the chest cavity.

the side suspected of having the pleural effusion while the radiograph is taken. This is called the lateral decubitus view (Fig. 10.15). Free fluid will layer along the new horizontal plane on the lateral decubitus view, and loculated fluid, pneumonia, or tumor will be unchanged from the upright view.

The physical findings with pleural effusion are related to the volume of free fluid in the chest. The patient may complain of pain on inspiration; a dull, heavy feeling in the involved area; coughing; or shortness of breath. Small volumes of fluid are symptom free and undetectable on physical examination. However, when the size of the pleural effusion is significant, the findings may include the following:

- Dullness to percussion in the involved area
- Egophony just above the area of dullness
- Decreased or absent breath sounds on the affected side
- Tachypnea

### Lung Consolidation

Bacterial pneumonia is the most common cause of lung consolidation. The infection causes copious mucous production that fills lung tissue so that it becomes airless but does not collapse. Less common causes of consolidation include obstruction of the airway by aspirated foreign bodies (e.g., peanuts or very small toys) or tumorous growths. Figs. 10.3 and 10.4 show good examples of infiltrates associated with consolidation.

The radiographic signs of consolidation include the following:

- Minimal loss of volume
- Usually lobar or segmental distribution
- Homogeneous density

- Air bronchogram if the airway leading to the consolidated area is open

The physical findings associated with a consolidated lung include the following:

- Reduced resonance to percussion over the involved area
- Bronchophony and bronchial breath sounds
- Fine crackles often heard over the involved area
- Whispered voice sounds increased and egophony present (if airway is patent)
- Tachypnea and fever

## POSTPROCEDURAL CHEST RADIOGRAPH EVALUATION

### Tracheal Intubation

The AP chest image often is used to evaluate the position of the endotracheal (ET) tube to be sure that the inferior tip rests appropriately 3 to 5 cm above the carina after intubation (Fig. 10.16). Although the carina may be difficult to see on some chest images, it is often located at the space between the T4 and T5 vertebrae in many adults. It is also important to note that the position of the ET tube can vary by neck position and can move as much as a total of 4-6 cm as the neck moves from full extension to full flexion. Therefore whenever possible, the chest radiograph should be taken while the patient's neck is in a neutral position.

Accidental placement of the ET tube in the right or left mainstem bronchus or esophagus must be recognized immediately to minimize potential harm to the patient. All manufacturers include a thin radiopaque strip in the wall of the entire length of the ET tube to allow visualization of the

**FIG. 10.16** Pulmonary artery catheter (Swan-Ganz catheter) in its usual position in the right lower lung field. This view does not indicate whether the catheter is anterior or posterior within the chest. The endotracheal tube tip (denoted as "TT") is properly located 3 to 5 cm above the carina. *CT*, Catheter tip; *TT*, tracheal tube.

**FIG. 10.17** Anteroposterior chest image demonstrating placement of the endotracheal tube in the right main stem bronchus *(black arrow)*. The left lung has collapsed because of atelectasis. The central venous pressure line is in good position *(white arrow)*.

tube's precise position in the chest on the radiograph. It must be remembered that the AP chest image helps determine position of the ET tube only on a two-dimensional basis. Therefore an ET tube placed in the esophagus 3 cm above the carina might very well produce a similar (if not the same) shadow on an AP chest image as one placed in the trachea. Therefore it is imperative that other clinical findings, such as capnometry, rise of the chest wall, bilateral breath sounds, absence of gastric sounds, and esophageal detector devices, be used in addition to chest radiographs to ensure proper placement of the ET tube.

Fig. 10.17 shows a common incorrect ET tube placement. Note that the tip of the ET tube has come to rest in the right main stem bronchus, and the mediastinal structures are shifted to the left (ipsilateral or same) side of the lung collapse (see Fig. 10.14 for comparison). Such improper tube placement is more likely due to the right main-stem bronchus being more closely aligned with the trachea and may cause severe hypoxia due to V/Q mismatch (left lung being perfused but not ventilated), overdistention (large tidal volume being delivered to the right lung), or pneumothorax (with additional risk of shock, hypoxia, and even death). After the tube is repositioned, the number of centimeters seen on the tube at the position of the patient's teeth should be noted in the patient record (ventilator-patient flowsheet), the tube carefully secured, and a repeat radiograph obtained for documentation that the tube's malposition has been corrected.

## Central Venous Pressure Line

Evaluation of the CVP line is necessary to be sure that the catheter tip is in the proper position. The catheter is placed into the right or left subclavian or jugular vein and should come to rest just above the juncture of the superior vena cava and the right atrium. During placement of central catheters, it is possible to enter the lung accidentally by passing through the wall of the vein, entering the pleural space, and thus causing the lung to collapse. If fluids are being delivered (e.g., blood replacement or total parenteral nutrition), the fluid will end up in the chest cavity instead of the bloodstream. An AP portable chest image is required immediately after the line is thought to be in position and before fluid is given through the central line.

In Fig. 10.18 the postplacement radiograph shows two CVP lines. Although both appear to be in proper position on the chest radiograph, the catheter "placed" in the right jugular vein missed the vein, entered the pleural space, nicked the lung, and caused a pneumothorax. To make matters worse, fluid delivery was started before the error was

FIG. 10.18 Anteroposterior chest image demonstrating a central venous pressure line in the right jugular vein *(large arrow)*. The line has punctured the vein and entered the right lung. Fluids have been infused into the right pleural space. Note that a left subclavian central venous pressure line is in good position *(small arrow)*.

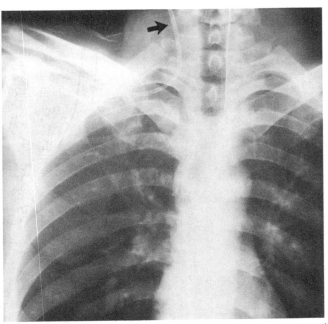

FIG. 10.19 Anteroposterior chest image showing a central venous pressure line in the right subclavian vein. The tip of the line has moved retrograde up the internal jugular vein *(arrow)* and must be repositioned.

discovered. The fluid is seen in the pleural space. A second invasive procedure (chest tube) is now required to relieve the pneumothorax and drain off the fluid. The line placed in the left subclavian vein just above where the superior vena cava and the right atrium join together seems to be in the proper position, but clinical confirmation is necessary before its use.

Radiographs obtained for verification of CVP line placement are at risk for the same limitations as the ones for placement of the ET tube. Therefore it is imperative that physicians, nurses, or other members of the patient care team confirm the intravascular position of the line by aspirating blood from it. Sometimes, when it is unclear whether the line has been placed in the vein or the artery, blood gases are obtained, or pressure tracings are reviewed to ensure proper positioning.

Fig. 10.19 shows another common malpositioning of a subclavian CVP line. It has gone up the neck on the right. Fig. 10.20 shows the venous anatomy in the area of the neck and upper thorax. Every vein shown has the potential to receive a misdirected CVP line.

### Pulmonary Artery Catheter Placement

After the pulmonary artery (Swan-Ganz catheter) is inserted, an AP portable chest radiograph is obtained to identify the position of the catheter tip. This catheter usually stays in the patient for several days, and daily radiographs are used to monitor its position and affect on the pulmonary circulation. Fig. 10.21 shows a pulmonary artery catheter in good position: the right midlung near the hilum.

### Nasogastric Feeding Tubes

The AP chest radiograph is useful to evaluate the position of the nasogastric (NG) feeding tube to ensure that it is located appropriately in the stomach or small bowel. Occasionally, the NG tube can be inserted accidentally into the trachea. In the alert patient, the accidental placement of an NG tube into the trachea causes severe coughing and dyspnea. The patient complains and alerts caregivers to the problem. However, these tubes are often placed in heavily sedated or comatose patients who cannot complain. NG tubes have been placed accidentally into the trachea, down the main stem bronchus, and deep into the lung. This can lead to numerous problems such as pneumonia and pneumothorax.

### Chest Tubes

Chest tubes are large drainage tubes placed into the left or right thorax and attached to a suction device at approximately 20 cm $H_2O$ pressure. The purpose is to drain excess air, blood, pus, or pleural fluid from the pleural cavity.

Placing the chest tube can be very painful for the patient and may require moderate sedation. Pain medication is usually needed as long as the tube remains in the chest. With proper precautions (monitoring the ECG and oxygen saturation [$Spo_2$]), the tube can be placed at the bedside instead of an operating room.

A portable chest radiograph is commonly obtained after the chest tube has been inserted. Fig. 10.22 shows good placement of the tube for the purposes of draining pneumothorax (superior and anterior, as air collects in the gravity nondependent areas). The proper position of the tube is often dependent on the indication for its placement.

**FIG. 10.20** Venous anatomy of the neck. The central venous pressure line is intended to be located in the lower part of the superior vena cava.

**FIG. 10.21** Portable chest image showing good position of the pulmonary artery catheter as it passes through the right side of the heart and into the right pulmonary artery (*long white arrow*). Note the position of the right and left chest tubes (*large black arrows*), endotracheal tube (*black arrow with asterisk*), and nasogastric tube (*small black arrow*). A *short white arrow* points to the left subclavian central venous pressure line in good position.

For example, chest tubes placed for the drainage of pleural fluid would have their tips directed inferiorly and posteriorly (fluid collects in gravity-dependent areas). For loculated fluid collections, the tube may have to be placed by an interventional radiologist (see Interventional Radiology later in this chapter) and properly directed under the ultrasound guidance. Once placed, the tube is sutured in place and heavily bandaged to reduce pain if the patient inadvertently rolls onto the insertion wound. Periodic portable chest radiographs may be needed to ensure that the tube remains in the correct position.

For additional procedures requiring evaluation with an AP portable chest radiograph, see Box 10.3.

### SIMPLY STATED

The chest radiograph is used not only to diagnose lung disease but also to confirm the correct placement of tubes and catheters and the effect of procedures on the lung.

## COMPUTED TOMOGRAPHY

Significant advances in technology have resulted in CT becoming the preferred method for chest imaging in many clinical situations. CT scanning is done by specialized equipment that rotates the x-ray beam in a circular path around the patient. Advanced computers apply complex mathematical techniques to process the CT images from information gathered by detectors during the scan. The images are most frequently displayed as thin transverse sections or slices. High-resolution images showing very fine detail are achieved with slice thicknesses of 1 to 2 mm. Vascular tissue is also enhanced by injecting iodine-based contrast agents intravenously.

**FIG. 10.22** Close-up view of a chest image showing a left chest tube in good position. Note that three distinct lines are seen along the tube. The thicker line in the middle is a radiopaque stripe that allows visualization of the entire length of the tube. The other two lines are the edges of the tube itself; they would not be visible if the tube were accidentally placed in the soft tissues of the chest wall.

Modern equipment uses multiple rows of detectors with the patient table advancing through the x-ray beam during the scan. This method is called spiral or helical CT and captures scan information in a large volume instead of one slice at a time. Anatomy may be viewed from any angle and even shown as three-dimensional structures. The three-dimensional perspective provided by CT is used to guide needle aspirations of tissue masses or catheter placement into body cavities. CT scanning has become indispensable in the medical management of pulmonary disease. However, the major drawback is that it exposes the patient to a significant amount of radiation.

## Lung Tumors

CT scans easily show tissue masses that are hidden by dense tissues on plain radiographs. CT contrast scans help differentiate lymph nodes or tumor masses from blood vessels. High-resolution CT scans can show tissue nodules as small as 2 to 3 mm. CT scans can also provide information regarding the

density of pulmonary nodules. Very dense nodules are likely to contain calcium and are less likely to be cancer.

### Screening for Lung Cancer

Lung cancer remains the second most common type of cancer and the leading cause of cancer death both in the United States and worldwide. Over the past decades, many types of screening modalities have been tried but proven ineffective to reduce the morbidity and mortality associated with lung cancer. A landmark research study known as the National Lung Screening Trial (see Bibliography) showed that screening using low-dose chest CT may increase the survival rate in certain patients at risk for lung cancer. Based on the results of this study, the U.S. Preventive Services Task Force recommends annual screening for lung cancer with low-dose CT in adults ages 55 to 80 years who have a 30 pack-year smoking history and currently smoke or have quit within the past 15 years. Screening should be discontinued once a person has not smoked for 15 years or develops a health problem that substantially limits life expectancy or the ability or willingness to have curative lung surgery.

### Pulmonary Embolism

Currently, CT scanning after administration of intravenous contrast is the test of choice for the diagnosis of suspected PE. A rapid bolus of contrast is typically given, immediately followed by acquisition of CT images. When done properly, this technique leads to near-complete opacification of pulmonary vasculature by the contrast. Many well-done studies allow examination of small segmental and subsegmental branches of the pulmonary artery, so the procedure is often called *CT angiography*. In the presence of a PE, the lumen of the pulmonary vessel with the thrombus will be incompletely opacified, leading to a "filling defect" (Fig. 10.23). In addition to providing vivid images of the pulmonary vasculature, CT scan with contrast also allows examination of the pulmonary

**FIG. 10.23** Computed tomography scan of the chest with intravenous contrast demonstrates multiple filling defects *(arrows)* within pulmonary arteries, indicative of pulmonary embolism. Note that the ascending aorta (AA), descending aorta (DA), and left pulmonary artery (LPA) are all completely opacified with contrast.

parenchyma, leading a physician toward a potential alternative diagnosis, even when there is no evidence of PE. A great deal of emphasis is placed on proper (rapid) administration of the contrast, so many radiology centers will request a dedicated large-bore intravenous line. Patient participation is also important because breath holding during the acquisition of images enhances the overall quality and accuracy of the test. This becomes important in patients with severe dyspnea, who cannot hold their breath even for a few seconds, as well as in patients on mechanical ventilators.

## Chronic Interstitial Lung Disease

High-resolution CT scanning is superior to conventional radiographs in the evaluation of diffuse interstitial lung disease. The CT scan can demonstrate characteristic changes in patients with mild pulmonary fibrosis even when the conventional radiograph appears to be normal. In a few cases, the pattern of abnormality is so specific that a diagnosis can be made without biopsy. However, in most cases, the CT scan shows the nature and extent of the abnormality and suggests the best location for a lung biopsy.

## Acquired Immunodeficiency Syndrome

CT scanning can be useful in the early detection of pneumonias that occur as a result of acquired immunodeficiency syndrome (AIDS). The technique is also useful in detecting abscesses and cavities. The mediastinum also can be evaluated for enlarged lymph nodes caused by infection or the lymphomas seen in AIDS.

## Occupational Lung Disease

The lung diseases resulting from the inhalation of dust, fumes, irritant gases, organisms, and smoke are called pneumoconioses, or extrinsic alveolitis. Inhaling dust and fumes

can cause pulmonary fibrosis. CT scanning is very helpful in identifying the changes seen in the pleura and the lung tissue associated with these occupational lung diseases. They initially cause nodules and subsequently fibrosis, both of which are seen clearly on CT scan. Pleural plaques seen with asbestosis are also readily demonstrated with CT scan.

## Pneumonia

CT scans of the lung are superior to conventional chest radiographs in the visualization of pneumonias and related pathologic changes in the hila and pleura. However, the cost of CT and the risks associated with high radiation exposure have restricted its use in the evaluation of most patients with pneumonia. CT scan is often ordered when radiographic findings do not resolve after clinical improvement, suggesting an alternative etiology (most commonly malignancy). In general, radiographic resolution tends to lag behind clinical resolution by 6 to 8 weeks, so it is advised that a clinician should wait at least 8 weeks until the chest radiograph is repeated or a CT scan is ordered in a clinically stable patient.

## Bronchiectasis

Bronchiectasis is most often caused by repeated infections around the airways. As the infection clears and the concurrent scarring retracts, the airways are pulled widely open. Airways are always adjacent to blood vessels and are usually about the same size as the adjacent blood vessel. Bronchiectasis thus shows up on CT scan as a very characteristic signet-ring pattern with the blood vessel appearing to be a small stone set against the much larger ring of bronchial tissue.

## Chronic Obstructive Pulmonary Disease

CT scans of the emphysematous chest are remarkable in their clarity and detail. The diagnosis of emphysema or COPD using

**FIG. 10.24** Computed tomography slice through the upper lungs in a patient with pulmonary emphysema. Numerous cystic lucencies are present in both lungs. Note the absence of bronchovascular markings within the lucencies. Most of the emphysematous areas are located in a peripheral distribution *(arrows)* along the pleural surface (paraseptal). (From Kacmarek RM, Stoller JK, Heuer AJ: *Egan's fundamentals of respiratory care,* ed 11, St. Louis, 2017, Mosby-Elsevier.)

conventional radiography based on pulmonary hyperexpansion and bullae formation is 65% to 80% accurate. With CT scanning, emphysematous changes, of an even mild to moderate degree, are seen with such ease that diagnosis is made consistently in the high 90% range (Fig. 10.24). It is important to note that the radiographic appearance of COPD often does not correlate with clinical or physiologic measures, such as degree of dyspnea or airflow limitation, on pulmonary function tests.

## MAGNETIC RESONANCE IMAGING

The role of MRI in the diagnosis of lung disease is limited due to the appearance of motion artifacts. Although there may be certain clinical situations in which MRI is superior to CT scan in the diagnosis of lung pathology, such scenarios are rare, especially when CT scans are enhanced with intravenous contrast or with simultaneous CT-PET scanning (see later). Overall, MRIs to demonstrate lung tissue are rarely done. Conversely, cardiac MRI has become a new and exciting method to diagnose heart disease.

Although MRI is not as common as other imaging studies, it is important for the RT to remember that special precautions need to be followed when accompanying a respiratory patient to the MRI unit. Even when the MRI is not fully operational, it emits a powerful magnetic force that can intensely draw to it equipment and devices containing ferrous (iron-containing) metals. In addition, data stored on magnetic strips on computer storage devices and identification cards can be wiped out. Therefore in such settings, special tanks, regulators, ventilators, and other equipment need to be used. Patients should be prescreened for implanted devices, and precautions must be taken to protect data storage devices and identification cards.

**FIG. 10.25** Normal lung perfusion scan. There is no evidence of perfusion defects in the anterior, posterior, oblique, or lateral views of the lungs.

## RADIONUCLIDE LUNG SCANNING

Radionuclide lung scans are obtained by measuring radiation emitted from the chest after radiopharmaceuticals are injected into the bloodstream or inhaled into the lung or both. The two most commonly used lung scans are the V/Q scan and gallium scan. The V/Q scan is useful to study the comparative distribution of ventilation and perfusion and the effects disease may have on these two important functions. The major clinical application of V/Q lung scanning is in the evaluation of patients suspected of having a PE. The concept of the scan relies on the fact that ventilation and perfusion to a given area of the lung should be the same, and therefore the images of ventilation and perfusion scanning should also match (Fig. 10.25). The ventilation scan is compared with the perfusion scan to identify correlation between ventilation and perfusion (Fig. 10.26). When a PE is present, the ventilation scan usually is normal, and the perfusion scan shows a defect in the affected region. In patients with pneumonia, atelectasis, COPD, and many other lung diseases, the relationship between the ventilation and perfusion in a given area is not as straightforward, which leads to V/Q scans that are often difficult to interpret. In comparison, helical CT with intravenous contrast offers superior image quality and additional information for PE diagnosis and has essentially replaced V/Q scanning as the diagnostic test of choice.

**FIG. 10.26** Abnormal ventilation-perfusion scan. The ventilation study **(A)** demonstrates bilateral lung filling without gross defects; however, the perfusion scan **(B)** shows multiple subsegmental perfusion defects of both lungs. These findings are highly suggestive of pulmonary emboli.

Gallium scanning is another radionuclide lung scanning method that is being used less commonly today. The idea of gallium scan is based on the fact that inflamed tissues excessively take up gallium, making certain areas of lung (or the rest of the body) involved in inflammation appear hot. This may be useful in directing the surgeon to the location of the biopsy specimen to be taken in patients with pulmonary fibrosis or other interstitial diseases. Alternatively, gallium uptake in lung hila, mediastinal lymph nodes, and, most important, lacrimal glands could be very helpful in the diagnosis of sarcoidosis.

## POSITRON EMISSION TOMOGRAPHY

PET scanning (Fig. 10.27) uses a glucose analog (fluorine-18-fluorodeoxyglucose) attached to a positron emitter. The patient fasts for several hours, followed by an injection of the radiopharmaceutical labeled "sugar water," and is then asked to remain supine and perfectly quiet for about an hour. Metabolically active tissue will take up the sugar water and thus show hot or black on film. Metabolically inactive tissues will not use much sugar water as fuel and will be cold or clear on film. Tumors and areas of infection increase the local rate of metabolic activity and cause hot spots. This allows the clinician to determine whether a lung mass is metabolically active. Especially helpful are combined CT-PET scans, when both CT and PET images are obtained simultaneously and then superimposed one on another. This allows better correlation between the two imaging studies and determination of whether a lesion seen on CT scan appears malignant or not.

For instance, in the diagnosis of coin lesions of 1 cm or greater, PET scans have shown the ability to readily identify tumors. PET scanning can also demonstrate tumor spread to local and distant tissues, such as lymph nodes in the hilar and mediastinal area, and distant spread to bone and adrenal glands. The brain usually uses glucose exclusively for energy and often appears hot on PET scans. For this reason, PET scanning is not helpful for the diagnosis of brain metastases in most cases.

## PULMONARY ANGIOGRAPHY

Angiography of the pulmonary circulation is rarely used today. In the past, it was generally done only if V/Q lung scanning and CT angiogram were nondiagnostic and the patient was considered to be at risk for PE. Pulmonary angiography is performed by threading an intravascular catheter up a vein to the right side of the heart, past the tricuspid valve and the pulmonary valves, and into the pulmonary artery, and then injecting contrast medium into the pulmonary artery or one of its branches. Angiographic proof of PE is considered to be the identification of one or more filling defects. CT angiography can obtain equal, if not superior, imaging of the pulmonary vasculature. In addition, it does not require placement of a catheter into the pulmonary artery and therefore has essentially replaced pulmonary angiography and V/Q scanning and become the diagnostic test of choice in patients with suspected PE.

### SIMPLY STATED

Widespread availability and the ease of use of helical CT for the diagnosis of suspected PE has essentially made V/Q scanning and pulmonary angiography obsolete.

## CHEST ULTRASOUND

Ultrasound waves are sound waves with frequencies above the upper limit of human hearing. These sound waves are reflected differently by various tissues and structures and give additional methods of imaging the human body. One major difference between ultrasound and electromagnetic waves is that ultrasound is considered harmless to humans, including fetuses, allowing much greater use of ultrasound for pregnant patients. Another feature of the ultrasound is its portability, allowing complete bedside examinations—an important feature for critically ill patients. Portable ultrasound has become nearly as important as the stethoscope in the hands of an experienced emergency department or intensive care unit physician. It allows rapid bedside evaluation of the structure and function of many internal organs. The common chest ultrasound applications in the diagnosis of lung diseases are as follows:

- Visualization of pleural effusion
- Guidance of needle placement during thoracentesis
- Guidance of catheter placement during chest tube insertion
- Guidance of needle placement during central vein line placement

**FIG. 10.27** This series of images shows a coin lesion on routine chest radiograph, a computed tomography (CT) scan of the lesion, and a positron emission tomography (PET) scan. Only the PET scan is able to indicate, with a high sensitivity and specificity, that this lesion is actually cancerous. The routine chest radiograph shows a faint density on the right, behind the right clavicle. The presence of the pacemaker overlying the left chest tends to direct the examiner's eye away from the right upper lobe lesion. The CT scan shows this lesion to be ominous. Is it a cancer or an old scar and thus benign? Two views from the PET scan show this lesion "lights up." It is a cancer.

- Further assessment of a consolidation seen on chest radiograph
- Sniff test for unilateral diaphragm paralysis
- Visualization of pneumothorax
- Visualization of ET tube placement
- Assessment of the heart function (echocardiography)

## FLUOROSCOPY

Fluoroscopy is an imaging technique that projects a continuous x-ray beam through the patient, allowing the visualization of live action much like a radiographic movie. This technique may be used to monitor the progress and location of a needle or a catheter as it is guided into an internal structure to ensure its proper placement. Fluoroscopy is commonly used during cardiac catheterization, bronchoscopy, and many other invasive procedures. During bronchoscopy, it is typically used to establish the position of the bronchoscope or that of the biopsy forceps in relation to the lesion that is not directly seen through the bronchoscope. Although immensely helpful, there are limitations to the use of fluoroscopy. As discussed earlier, x-rays provide two-dimensional images of three-dimensional objects, so a biopsy forceps placed on the outside of the patient's chest, directly above the coin lesion, would appear to be piercing that lesion on fluoroscopy.

One major disadvantage of fluoroscopy is that it emits much greater radiation than is used during conventional radiographs. For this reason, all health care personnel, whether performing, assisting, or observing the fluoroscopic procedure, must wear protective equipment (see Radiation Safety). Similarly, pregnant individuals are instructed to leave the room to avoid exposing the fetus to ionizing radiation.

## INTERVENTIONAL RADIOLOGY

The use of CT, ultrasound, and fluoroscopy allow visualization of, and image-guided access to, nearly every part of the human body. With such precise guidance, needle drainage of a deep tissue abscess is preferred to invasive surgery. This simple concept has led to the development of a whole new subspecialty, called interventional radiology. Today's interventional radiologists offer first-line diagnosis and treatment modalities for a wide variety of diseases. In many instances, interventional radiology procedures have replaced costly and complex surgical interventions with simpler alternatives and provided novel approaches in situations in which no other diagnostic or therapeutic options were available. Commonly performed interventional radiology procedures, as they pertain to lung diseases, are transcutaneous lung biopsy, bronchial artery embolization, ultrasound-guided thoracentesis, and small-bore chest tube placement.

## RADIATION SAFETY

Humans are exposed to radiation from both natural and manmade sources. A routine chest examination (PA and lateral) delivers 0.06 to 0.1 mSv (millisievert) or 6 to 10 mrem (millirem) of radiation. This is equivalent to approximately 2% to 3% of the 3 mSv (300 mrem) of natural background radiation received by an individual who resides in the United States. The amount of radiation increases with more sophisticated studies, such as CT or PET scanning. An annual exposure to more than 100 mSv is considered dangerous to human health. It is therefore extremely important to minimize the level of exposure to ionizing radiation such as x-rays.

Health care workers, including RTs and nurses, are potentially at risk of being exposed to scatter radiation produced during portable procedures performed at the patient's bedside. The exposure can be much greater if one is performing or assisting during fluoroscopy. Typically, the real-time images require more radiation to obtain, and there are often more than 20 images produced during a single procedure such as bronchoscopy.

Occupational exposure to ionizing radiation can be reduced by implementing the three principles of radiation protection—time, distance, and shielding. Whenever possible, limit the amount of time spent in a room where x-rays are being used. Doubling the distance between object and the source reduces the exposure by a factor of ¼ (inverse square law). Finally, during fluoroscopic procedures, use of protective lead aprons to shield the body, neck shields for the thyroid gland, and radiation safety eyeglasses for the lens of the eyes reduces radiation exposure to internal organs.

Health care workers who are frequently exposed to scatter radiation must wear a radiation monitoring device (dosimeter). There are various types of dosimeters, but the most common is the film badge, which is about the size of a modern-day memory card. Individual radiation dose is monitored and a monthly report issued by the radiation safety officer. These reports have to be initialed by the health care worker to verify that they are aware of their radiation dose.

Performance of radiographic procedures on pregnant women requires special consideration. Medical imaging examinations that require the use of ionizing radiation (e.g., x-rays, CT scan, radionuclide scans) are only done during pregnancy if the benefit outweighs the risk. MRI and ultrasound studies do not use ionizing radiation and are generally considered as safe alternatives. During radiographic imaging, even with abdominal shielding, x-rays directed at the thorax will scatter and reach the fetus. The urgency of the test and the information obtained from it often outweigh the health risks of radiation exposure, but each case must be considered by members of the patient care team on an individual basis.

## KEY POINTS

- Dense body tissue (radiopaque) appears white, and air-filled body tissue (radiolucent) appears black on x-rays.
- Image magnification of organs by x-rays is reduced by decreasing the distance between the organ and the film.
- Increasing ventilator pressures may indicate development of a pneumothorax and should prompt an order for a chest radiograph.
- The right main stem bronchus is straighter, wider, and shorter than the left main stem bronchus, making it the usual site for an ET tube placed too deeply, which will usually result in atelectasis of the left lung and overdistention of the right lung.
- CT scans show structural information using x-rays but use digital enhancement to provide much clearer detail and more specific information about density than chest radiographs provide.
- MRI uses a strong magnetic field rather than x-rays to provide images of the body.
- V/Q lung scans are helpful only if they are completely normal or if they are highly suggestive of the presence of pulmonary emboli.
- CT scan of the chest with intravenous contrast has become the diagnostic study of choice in patients suspected for pulmonary embolism.
- PET scan uses a radioactively tagged sugar water injection to demonstrate metabolically active tissue, such as cancer or infection.
- Chest radiograph interpretation requires evaluation of the following:
  - Patient identification
  - Image exposure
  - Patient placement in relation to the film (rotation)
  - Bony structures and other extrapulmonary tissues
  - Trachea and mediastinum
  - Heart and lungs
  - Pulmonary arteries and lung hilum
- The presence of the silhouette sign allows more precise location of the infiltrate.
- Air bronchograms suggest fluid in the lung tissue surrounding patent airways.

## ASSESSMENT QUESTIONS

1. Which of the following tissues is normally the most radiolucent?
   a. Blood
   b. Lungs
   c. Muscle
   d. Fat

2. Which of the following is true regarding the distance between the x-ray source, image, and patient when taking a chest radiograph?
   a. Distance has no effect on the image on the film
   b. As the distance between the source and the patient decreases, magnification increases

c. As distance between the source and patient decreases, the image becomes more sharply focused

d. The distance between the patient and the x-ray machine varies with the size of the patient

3. Which of the following is the standard distance between the x-ray source and the image for a posteroanterior x-ray?
   a. 3 feet
   b. 4 feet
   c. 5 feet
   d. 6 feet

4. A chest radiograph would be most indicated to:
   a. Assess the progression of a patient's pneumonia
   b. Confirm ET tube placement during cardiopulmonary resuscitation
   c. Confirm tension pneumothorax in an unstable patient
   d. Screen for lung cancer in a patient without risk factors for cancer

5. Which of the following is/are true regarding a posteroanterior chest radiograph?
   a. Patient rotation usually is present and makes interpretation difficult
   b. Heart size is subject to less magnification
   c. It is the standard for bedridden hospitalized patients
   d. Lateral image provides little additional information

6. Which of the following views helps to evaluate for the presence of small amounts of free pleural fluid?
   a. Apical lordotic
   b. Expiratory
   c. Anteroposterior
   d. Lateral decubitus

7. Which of the following is a true statement about a portable (anteroposterior) chest radiograph?
   a. Apical areas of the lung are well visualized
   b. It provides the best view for pleural effusion diagnosis
   c. Lateral image is usually obtained in addition
   d. Patient is often not centered on the image

8. Which of the following radiographic findings is associated with a pneumothorax?
   a. Shift of trachea towards the affected side
   b. Increased lung density
   c. Shift of trachea and thoracic structures away from the affected side
   d. Air bronchograms

9. In a properly intubated adult patient, an ET tube tip should be this far from the carina:
   a. 0 to 1 cm
   b. 2 to 3 cm
   c. 3 to 5 cm
   d. 7 to 9 cm

10. After insertion of a CVP line, a chest radiograph is obtained to:
   a. Confirm that the line was placed in the vein, rather than artery
   b. Help with the estimation of central venous pressure
   c. Ensure that the line was not placed in the abdomen

d. Evaluate the position of the line in relation to other thoracic structures

11. In which of the following clinical scenarios is CT scanning most useful?
   a. Interstitial lung disease
   b. Pneumonia
   c. Emphysema
   d. Pulmonary edema

12. An MRI of the chest is most useful for the detection of:
   a. Interstitial lung diseases
   b. Pneumonia
   c. Cardiac diseases
   d. Emphysema

13. In which of the following clinical scenarios is gallium lung most useful?
   a. Lung cancer
   b. Emphysema
   c. Pulmonary embolism
   d. Sarcoidosis

14. Which of the following is the best method to evaluate for the presence of pulmonary embolism?
   a. Lung scan
   b. CT angiography
   c. Standard angiography
   d. MRI

15. The depth of inspiration on an x-ray is considered adequate if the lung shadows span the posterior shadows of this many ribs
   a. 5
   b. 7
   c. 8
   d. 10

16. The significance of the silhouette sign is that:
   a. It allows differentiation between alveolar and interstitial infiltrates
   b. It can aid in detecting pleural effusion
   c. It helps determine the location of a pulmonary opacity
   d. It confirms proper positioning of the ET tube

17. The chest radiograph finding most consistent with tension pneumothorax is:
   a. Increased radiolucency on the affected side
   b. Mediastinal shift toward the affected side
   c. Engorgement of the blood vessels on the affected side
   d. Air bronchograms and silhouette sign of the affected side

18. Which of the following is a radiographic sign of atelectasis?
   a. Enlarged heart
   b. Hilar shift away from atelectasis
   c. Vascular engorgement
   d. Hemidiaphragm elevation

19. The chest radiograph finding most suggestive of heart failure is:
   a. Low and flat diaphragm
   b. Increased cardiothoracic ratio
   c. Tracheal deviation
   d. Increased retrosternal air space on a lateral image

20. The chest radiograph finding most suggestive of pneumonia is:
    a. Silhouette sign
    b. Deep sulcus sign
    c. Coin lesion
    d. Kerley B lines
21. Which of the following chest radiograph findings is consistent with hyperinflation?
    a. Kerley B lines

    b. Enlarged heart
    c. Peripheral pleura line
    d. Large lung volumes
22. Which of the following chest radiograph findings is consistent with a small pleural effusion?
    a. Blunted costophrenic angle
    b. Air bronchograms on the affected side
    c. Peripheral pleural line
    d. Elevated hemidiaphragm

## BIBLIOGRAPHY

Christiani DC. Radiation risk from lung cancer screening: glowing in the dark? *Chest* 2014;**145**:439.

Jarvis C. *Physical examination and health assessment.* 7th ed. St. Louis: Mosby-Elsevier; 2016.

Kacmarek RM, Stoller JK, Heuer AJ. *Egan's fundamentals of respiratory care.* 11th ed. St. Louis: Mosby-Elsevier; 2017.

Koga T, Fujimoto K. Kerley's A, B and C lines. *N Engl J Med* 2009;**360**:1539.

Lichtenstein DA. BLUE-protocol and FALLS-protocol: two applications of lung ultrasound in the critically ill. *Chest* 2015;**147**:1659.

Marano R, Liguori C, Savino G. Cardiac silhouette findings and mediastinal lines and stripes: radiograph and CT scan correlation. *Chest* 2011;**139**:1186.

Mason RL, Broaddus VC, Murray RJ. *Murray and Nadel's textbook of respiratory medicine.* Philadelphia: WB Saunders; 2004.

Moore CL, Copel JA. Point-of-care ultrasonography. *N Engl J Med* 2011;**364**:749.

Moyer VA. Screening for lung cancer: U.S. Preventive Services Task Force recommendation statement. *Ann Intern Med* 2014;**160**:330.

National Lung Screening Trial Research Team. Reduced lung-cancer mortality with low-dose computed tomographic screening. *N Engl J Med* 2011;**365**:395.

Rohner DJ, Bennett S, Samaratunga C. Cumulative total effective whole-body radiation dose in critically ill patients. *Chest* 2013;**144**:1481.

Sabbar S, Nilles EJ. Images in clinical medicine: deep sulcus sign. *N Engl J Med* 2012;**366**:552.

# 11

# Interpretation of Electrocardiogram Tracings

*Albert J. Heuer and Laurel A. Heuer*

## LEARNING OBJECTIVES

*After reading this chapter, you will be able to:*

1. Describe the clinical value of the electrocardiogram (ECG).
2. Describe the clinical findings that indicate the need for an ECG recording.
3. Identify the key components of the electrical conduction system of the heart and the role of each component.
4. Define depolarization and repolarization.
5. Describe the specific electrical activity of the heart associated with each wave and interval of the normal ECG.
6. Identify the normal values for the PR interval and the QRS complex.
7. Identify the ventricular rate and position of the mean QRS vector from an ECG recording.
8. List the steps for ECG interpretation.
9. Describe the ECG criteria for each of the following abnormalities:
   a. Sinus bradycardia
   b. Sinus tachycardia
   c. Sinus dysrhythmia
   d. Premature atrial contraction
   e. Atrial flutter
   f. Atrial fibrillation
   g. Premature ventricular contractions
   h. Ventricular tachycardia
   i. Ventricular fibrillation
   j. Asystole
   k. First-, second-, and third-degree atrioventricular (AV) block
10. Describe the ECG abnormalities associated with chronic lung disease.
11. Identify ischemia, injury, and infarction using the 12-lead ECG tracing.
12. Explain how to assess and help treat patients with chest pain.

## OUTLINE

## KEY TERMS

| | | |
|---|---|---|
| action potential | first-degree AV block | repolarization |
| atrial kick | focus | RR interval |
| automaticity | heart block | ST segment |
| depolarization | hypertrophy | ST-elevation myocardial infarction |
| dysrhythmias | multifocal ectopic impulses | (STEMI) |
| ectopic impulse | QRS complex | |
| escape beat | QT interval | |

Given the hands-on nature of respiratory care, it is important for the respiratory therapist (RT) to have basic knowledge of electrocardiogram (ECG) interpretation. The RT may serve as the first link in the chain of survival for a patient experiencing a cardiac arrest and represent an important part of the medical team providing management of such patients once they are stabilized. Early recognition of a serious cardiac problem may potentially minimize cardiac damage or prevent death. In addition, understanding the significance of the subtle and often progressive aspects of ECG changes enhances the RT's or other clinician's assessment of a patient's cardiopulmonary health and may help optimize interdisciplinary care planning.

This chapter describes the electrophysiology of normal and abnormal ECG tracings. Ultimately, it is intended to explain how to recognize basic and life-threatening ECG patterns that may be observed while performing respiratory care. After a review of cardiac physiology related to the production of electrical activity within the heart, numerous abnormal rhythms (dysrhythmias) are described. Criteria for recognition and possible causes are reviewed for each abnormality presented.

## WHAT IS AN ELECTROCARDIOGRAM?

An ECG (also called an EKG) is an indirect measurement of the electrical activity within the heart. A recording of the electrical currents within the heart is obtained by placing electrodes containing a conductive medium to each extremity and to numerous locations on the chest wall to create a 12-lead ECG. Each specific position of an electrode provides a tracing referred to as a *lead.* The purpose of using 12 leads is to obtain 12 different views of the electrical activity in the heart and therefore a more complete picture.

Current standard of practice in most hospitals calls for patients at risk for cardiac events or dysrhythmias to be initially placed on continuous ECG monitoring using the 3-lead or 5-lead system. These systems use only 3 or 5 leads, placed on the patient's chest, which are less cumbersome and allows for more patient mobility than a 12-lead ECG. Although 3- and 5-lead systems do not provide the level of detail that a 12-lead ECG does, they may help facilitate a rapid assessment of gross abnormalities in the electrical conduction system of the heart. Identification of a rhythm abnormality on a 3-lead or 5-lead tracing often indicates the need to obtain a more detailed 12-lead view of the heart.

## WHAT IS THE VALUE OF AN ELECTROCARDIOGRAM?

The ECG provides valuable information about the cardiac status of a patient presenting with signs and symptoms suggestive of heart disease. For example, if a patient presents with dyspnea and chest discomfort, an ECG can aid in the diagnosis of an ischemic cardiac event. In addition, the ECG may indicate an increased workload on the myocardium as a compensatory response to the chronic dysfunction of another body system such as the respiratory system. Both acute and chronic conditions may have adverse effects on the heart. The severity of such effects (e.g., myocardial infarction, ventricular hypertrophy, or abnormal heart rhythms known as *dysrhythmias*) may be assessed on interpretation of the ECG. The ECG may also be used to monitor the heart's response to treatment or changes in the clinical status of patients with cardiac disease. Therefore several ECGs may be needed over the course of treatment.

It is important to note that the ECG tracing does not measure the pumping ability of the heart. It is not unusual for a patient with a low cardiac output to have a normal ECG tracing. This is because the ECG does not directly depict abnormalities in cardiac structure such as defects in the heart valves or interventricular septum. Another limitation worth noting is that the probability of any patient having an acute problem, such as myocardial infarction, generally cannot be predicted from a resting ECG tracing.

### SIMPLY STATED

The resting ECG does not reflect the pumping ability of the heart or the likelihood that the patient may have a myocardial infarction in the near future.

## WHEN SHOULD AN ELECTROCARDIOGRAM BE OBTAINED?

Because an ECG is noninvasive and does not present a risk to the patient, it is reasonable to obtain an ECG when the patient has signs and symptoms suggestive of an acute or chronic cardiac disorder such as myocardial infarction or congestive heart failure (CHF) (Box 11.1). An ECG is often

## BOX 11.1 Clinical Findings Suggestive of the Need for an ECG

### Medical History

#### Chief Complaints

Chest pain (centrally located and may radiate to the shoulder or back)

Dyspnea on exertion in a patient older than 40 years

Orthopnea

Paroxysmal nocturnal dyspnea

Pedal edema

Fainting spells

Palpitations

Unexplained and persistent nausea and indigestion in a high-risk patient

#### Past Medical History

History of heart disease

History of cardiac surgery

#### Physical Examination

Unexplained tachycardia at rest

Hypotension

Decreased capillary refill

Abnormal heart sounds or murmurs

Pedal edema

Cool, cyanotic extremities

Abnormal heaves or lifts on the precordium

Diaphoresis

Jugular venous distention

Abnormal sensorium

Hepatojugular reflex

Bilateral inspiratory crackles in the dependent lung zones

---

used as an assessment tool to help determine the patient's general health status or as a screening tool before major surgery. An ECG is especially helpful in this situation if the patient is older or has a history of heart disease. If an abnormality is identified early, treatment can be promptly started, thus potentially improving the longer term prognosis. Of course, the process of obtaining the ECG should never delay the initiation of critically needed care such as oxygen therapy, airway placement, or cardiopulmonary resuscitation (CPR).

ECGs can also be useful in alerting the RT of special considerations related to respiratory medications, especially bronchodilators. For example, the RT should consider recommending an anticholinergic bronchodilator such as ipratropium bromide (Atrovent), rather than an adrenergic bronchodilator such as albuterol for patients with certain abnormal heart rhythms (e.g., rapid atrial fibrillation). The rationale for this recommendation is to avoid the effects of increasing the patient's heart rate from $\beta_1$-receptor site stimulation, which may occur to varying degrees with adrenergic bronchodilators. Alternatively, a reduced dose of albuterol (1.25 mg vs. 2.5 mg) may be in order to minimize the side effects of adrenergic bronchodilators on these patients.

## SIMPLY STATED

ECGs can be useful in alerting the RT of special considerations related to respiratory medications. For example, for patients whose ECGs show certain abnormal heart rhythms such as rapid atrial fibrillation, anticholinergic bronchodilators such as ipratropium bromide (Atrovent) should be considered rather than an adrenergic bronchodilator such as albuterol.

It should also be noted that different clinical situations dictate whether a 3-, 5-, or 12-lead ECG is warranted. Suffice to say that 3- or 5-lead ECGs may be adequate for more routine monitoring such as ongoing telemetry or for initial preliminary cardiac screening. However, the most diagnostic value can be gathered from a standard 12-lead ECG. A 12-lead ECG provides a more complete assessment of the electrical activity of the heart by viewing it from 12 different angles. As a result, the focus of this chapter is the 12-lead ECG.

## CARDIAC ANATOMY AND PHYSIOLOGY

Before discussing the interpretation of ECGs, it is important to review the cardiac anatomy and physiology related to electrical activity within the heart. The heart lies inside the thoracic cavity behind the mediastinum and between the lungs. It is made up of four chambers: two upper chambers called *atria* and two lower chambers called *ventricles* (Fig. 11.1). The heart typically is described as having two sides, the right and the left. The right atrium receives deoxygenated blood from large veins, the superior and inferior venae cavae, and directs the blood into the right ventricle via the tricuspid valve. Right ventricular contraction ejects blood through the pulmonic valve into the pulmonary artery, which carries blood to the lungs for oxygenation. The oxygenated blood returns to the left atrium of the heart via the pulmonary veins, where it is directed through the mitral valve into the left ventricle. Left ventricular contraction ejects blood through the aortic valve into the aorta, which branches off into the systemic circulation. Because the left side of the heart pumps blood throughout the entire body, it normally has a significantly larger muscle mass than the right side.

Cardiac muscle is referred to as the *myocardium*. Myocardial contraction occurs as a response to electrical stimulation. For the heart to move blood effectively, stimulation of the myocardium must be coordinated. Initiating and coordinating the electrical stimulation of the myocardium is the responsibility of the electrical conduction system, which is made up of special pacemaker and conducting cells (Table 11.1).

Normally the electrical activity of the heart is initiated in the sinus node, also known as the sinoatrial (SA) node, located in the right atrium (Fig. 11.2). The SA node is a collection of specialized cells capable of spontaneously generating electrical signals. Cells that have the ability to generate electrical activity spontaneously are said to have automaticity. Because the SA node (also known as the sinus node) normally has the greatest degree of automaticity of all the cardiac cells, it usually controls the rate at which the heart beats. In this way, the SA node serves as the primary pacemaker of the heart, discharging at about 60 to 100 beats/min at rest.

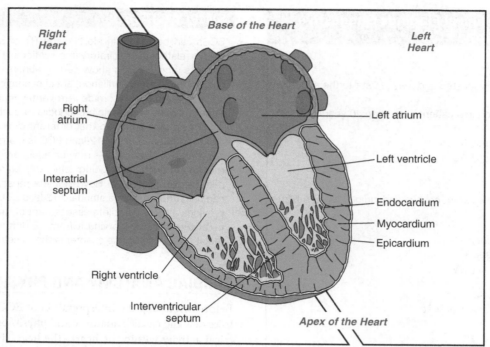

**FIG. 11.1** Anatomy of the heart. (Modified from Wesley K: *Huszar's basic dysrhythmias: interpretation and management*, ed 4, St. Louis, 2011, Mosby.)

| TABLE 11.1 | Types of Heart Cells |
|---|---|
| Pacemaker cells | Specialized cells that have an extensive ability to generate their own electrical activity (automaticity) and provide the electrical power for the heart |
| Conducting cells | Cells that conduct the electrical impulse throughout the heart |
| Myocardial cells | Cells that contract in response to electrical stimuli and pump the blood |

The SA node is strongly influenced by the autonomic nervous system. For this reason, the rate at which the SA node fires can vary significantly. Increased activity of the sympathetic system increases the heart rate. Stimulation of the sympathetic system occurs with stress, anxiety, exercise, hypoxemia, and the administration of certain medications. On the other hand, slowing of the heart rate occurs as a result of vagal stimulation, which is a parasympathetic response.

Once the SA node initiates the electrical signal, the impulse spreads across the atria in a wavelike fashion. The electrical impulse travels through the atria by way of the internodal pathways, also known as *interatrial pathways*, causing depolarization and then contraction. Contraction of the atria just before ventricular contraction (systole) aids in filling the ventricles with blood and accounts for about 10% to 30% of subsequent stroke volume. This atrial contraction is often referred to as the atrial kick.

After the electrical impulse passes through the atria, it reaches the atrioventricular (AV) junction. This junction acts as an electrical bridge between the atria and the ventricles. The

AV junction contains the AV node and the bundle of His (see Fig. 11.2). Once the electrical impulse reaches the AV node, it is delayed for approximately 0.1 second before passing on into the bundle of His. The delay is believed to serve the purpose of allowing more complete filling of the ventricles before ventricular contraction, further adding to the atrial kick. In addition, the AV node can protect the ventricles from excessively rapid atrial rates that the ventricles could not tolerate. Damage to the AV junction, as may occur with a myocardial infarction, usually leads to excessive delays of the electrical impulse passing into the ventricles. This causes a condition known as heart block.

The AV junction normally guides only the electrical impulse from the atria into the ventricles. Under certain circumstances, however, it can also serve as the backup pacemaker. The AV junction has automaticity qualities similar to those of the SA node. If the SA node fails to function properly and does not pace the heart, the AV junction can serve as the pacemaker for the ventricles. When this occurs, the ventricular rate is usually between 40 and 60 beats/min and the ECG reveals a distinct pattern, described later in this chapter (Fig. 11.3).

After the electrical impulse leaves the AV node, it travels rapidly through the bundle of His and then into the left and right bundle branches (see Fig. 11.2). The stimulus travels simultaneously through the bundle branches into the myocardium. At the end of the bundle branches are countless fingerlike projections called *Purkinje fibers*. The Purkinje fibers pass the electrical impulse rapidly throughout the myocardium to create a coordinated contraction of the left and right ventricles.

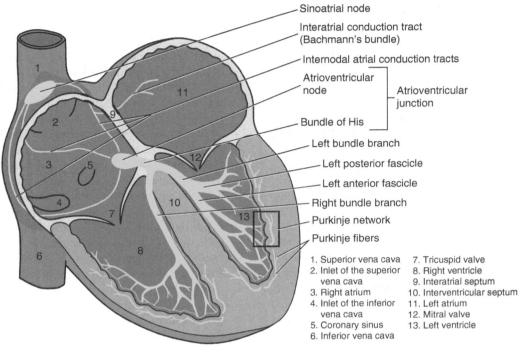

**FIG. 11.2** Electrical conduction system of the heart. (Modified from Wesley K: *Huszar's basic dysrhythmias: interpretation and management,* ed 4, St. Louis, 2011, Mosby.)

Sinoatrial node

Interatrial conduction tract (Bachmann's bundle)

Internodal atrial conduction tracts

Atrioventricular node

Atrioventricular junction

Bundle of His

Left bundle branch

Left posterior fascicle

Left anterior fascicle

Right bundle branch

Purkinje network

Purkinje fibers

1. Superior vena cava
2. Inlet of the superior vena cava
3. Right atrium
4. Inlet of the inferior vena cava
5. Coronary sinus
6. Inferior vena cava
7. Tricuspid valve
8. Right ventricle
9. Interatrial septum
10. Interventricular septum
11. Left atrium
12. Mitral valve
13. Left ventricle

| Pacemaker Site | Rate |
| --- | --- |
| **Dominant Pacemaker** | |
| SA node | 60-100/min |
| **Escape Pacemaker** | |
| AV junction | 40-60/min |
| Bundle branches | 30-40/min |
| Purkinje network | 30-40/min |

AV node
Bundle of His

**FIG. 11.3** Dominant and escape pacemakers. *AV,* Atrioventricular; *SA,* sinoatrial. (Modified from Wesley K: *Huszar's basic dysrhythmias: interpretation and management,* ed 4, St. Louis, 2011, Mosby.)

Because most of the cardiac cells have automaticity characteristics, the heartbeat may be paced by heart tissue other than the SA node. When this occurs, it often indicates that the SA node is not functioning normally or that myocardial tissue is irritated. Any impulse that originates outside the SA node is called an ectopic impulse, and the site from which the ectopic impulse originates is called the focus. Ectopic impulses can originate from foci in either the atria or the ventricles. If the ectopic impulse is generated from different areas of the heart, they will appear different from one another on an ECG and be referred to as multifocal ectopic impulses. When the ectopic impulse results from depression of the normal impulse origin, it is called an escape beat.

The myocardium itself must receive a constant supply of oxygen and nutrients to pump blood effectively. Oxygen and nutrients are supplied to the myocardium via the left and right coronary arteries and their branches. The main coronary arteries arise from the ascending aorta and direct arterial blood into branches that feed various regions of the heart. Blockage of one or more of the coronary vessels leads to regionalized ischemia and tissue death (infarction). The size and location of the region affected by the coronary vessel blockage determine the resulting physiologic and clinical impact. Infarction of a major portion of the left ventricle is likely to cause significant arterial hypotension, abnormal sensorium, and a backup of blood into the pulmonary circulation. Infarction of the tissues associated with pacing the heart (e.g., the SA or AV junction) can lead to significant dysrhythmias and diminished blood flow to all regions of the body.

## CAUSES AND MANIFESTATIONS OF DYSRHYTHMIAS

Disturbances in cardiac conduction are called dysrhythmias. Dysrhythmias can occur even in healthy hearts. Often, minor dysrhythmias produce no symptoms and resolve without any treatment. More serious dysrhythmias indicate significant acute or chronic heart disease. When serious dysrhythmias occur, medication or electrical therapy often is required to increase or decrease the ventricular rate or to suppress an irritable area within the myocardium. Occasionally, surgical intervention or thrombolytic therapy is needed to prevent the progression of injury or infarct, thereby salvaging viable tissue. The application and improved delivery of oxygen often

are key factors in reducing or eliminating cardiac irritability. Causes of dysrhythmias include the following:

- *Hypoxia:* Hypoxia results from inadequate delivery of oxygen to the heart muscle or myocardium and may be caused by hypoxemia or low blood flow known as *ischemia.* Inadequate delivery may be caused by reduced arterial oxygen levels, reduced hemoglobin levels, reduced perfusion (blood flow), or a combination of such factors.
- *Ischemia:* Ischemia results from low blood flow, which can lead to cardiac tissue hypoxia, further resulting in myocardial injury and infarction. Myocardial cells deprived of oxygen neither conduct nor contract well.
- *Sympathetic stimulation:* Physical or emotional stress from fear or anxiety and some medical conditions, such as hyperthyroidism and CHF, can elicit dysrhythmias. Sympathetic stimulation can also result in cardiac ischemia caused by an increased workload on the myocardium without concurrent increase in blood flow such as in the case of diseased coronary arteries.
- *Drugs:* Many prescribed medications taken in nontherapeutic ranges or in the presence of inadequate biotransformation or clearance may produce dysrhythmias. Illegal use of sympathomimetic agents, such as cocaine or methylphenidate (Ritalin), may cause myocardial irritability and even infarction.
- *Electrolyte imbalances:* Electrical activity in the heart results from the exchange of electrolytes within cardiac tissue, known as the action potential. As a result, abnormal serum concentrations of electrolytes, such as potassium, magnesium, and calcium, can cause dysrhythmias.
- *Hypertrophy:* Overdevelopment of the heart muscle (termed hypertrophy) that is due to a genetic disorder or a consequence of increased workload on the myocardium (e.g., pulmonary and/or systemic vasoconstriction, heart valve stenosis) may result in smaller heart chambers and/or abnormal pumping action.
- *Rate:* Rhythms that are too slow or too fast result in inadequate cardiac output. Cardiac output is a product of stroke volume and cardiac rate. Stroke volume is the volume of blood pumped by one ventricle during one beat. Therefore if the heart rate is too slow and the stroke volume is not increased proportionally, the cardiac output will be reduced. On the other hand, if the heart rate is too fast, the ventricles do not have enough time to fill with blood, and stroke volume may be significantly reduced, resulting in poor cardiac output.
- *Stretch:* How much the atrium or ventricle stretches open to accommodate the volume of blood entering and then ejected when the ventricles contract. With all else equal, greater stretch is associated with more stroke volume according to the Frank-Starling law.

## IMPORTANT ABBREVIATIONS AND ACRONYMS

Before coming in contact with a patient, the RT will receive a verbal report from the RT from the preceding shift regarding the patient's clinical status and notable aspects of the patient's medical record (see Chapter 21). It is important to understand the meaning of descriptive terms, abbreviations, and acronyms related to cardiology and ECG interpretation that may be presented while receiving a report or reviewing the medical record. Table 11.2 provides a list of some of the most common cardiology abbreviations and acronyms that may assist in the assessment of the patient's underlying disease process or cardiac conduction abnormalities.

## BASIC ELECTROCARDIOGRAM WAVES

The spread of electrical stimuli throughout the heart by way of the action potential initially causes depolarization of the myocardial cells. Depolarization occurs when a polarized cell is stimulated. Polarized cells carry an electrical charge on their surface; the inside of the cell is more negatively charged than the outside of the cell. The sudden loss of the negative charge within the cell is called depolarization, which is a result of potassium moving out of the cell and sodium moving into the cell. The return of the negative electrical charge is called repolarization (Fig. 11.4) and is a result of potassium moving back into the cell and sodium moving out of the cell. This process of depolarization and repolarization produces waves of electrical activity that travel back and forth across the heart. These waves of electrical activity are represented by waves detected by the ECG electrodes. The magnitude or amplitude of each wave is determined by voltage generated by depolarization of a particular portion of the heart.

Depolarization of the atria corresponds with atrial contraction and creates the initial wave of electrical activity detected on the ECG tracing, known as the *P wave* (Fig. 11.5). Because the atria usually are small, the atria generate less voltage than the ventricles, and the resulting P wave is small. Repolarization of the atria is not seen on the ECG because it usually is obscured by the simultaneous depolarization of the ventricles.

Depolarization of the ventricles corresponds with the ventricular contraction and is represented by the *QRS complex*. Because the ventricular muscle mass is larger than the atria and produces more voltage during depolarization, the QRS complex is normally taller than the P wave in most cases (see Fig. 11.5). Ventricular repolarization corresponds to ventricular relaxation between contractions and is seen as the *T wave*. The T wave is normally upright and rounded.

Just after the T wave but before the next P wave, a small deflection known as the *U wave* is sometimes seen. The U wave is thought to represent the final phase of ventricular repolarization. In most cases the U wave is not seen. The clinical significance of its presence or absence is not fully understood. However, prominent U waves may indicate hypokalemia, sometimes hypercalcemia, thyrotoxicosis, or digitalis toxicity. In addition, when U waves are inverted it may indicate

## TABLE 11.2 Common Cardiology Abbreviations

| | | | |
|---|---|---|---|
| AIJR | Accelerated idiojunctional rhythm | ms | Milliseconds |
| AIVR | Accelerated idioventricular rhythm | mV | Millivolt |
| ARP | Absolute refractory period | NSR | Normal sinus rhythm (see *RSR*) |
| A-tach | Atrial tachycardia | PAC | Premature atrial contraction |
| AV | Atrioventricular | PEA | Pulseless electrical activity |
| BBB | Bundle branch block | PJC | Premature junctional contraction |
| beats/min, bpm | Beats per minute | PJT | Paroxysmal junctional tachycardia |
| BVH | Biventricular hypertrophy | PMI | Point of maximal impulse |
| CABG | Coronary artery bypass graft | PSVT | Paroxysmal supraventricular tachycardia |
| CAD | Coronary artery disease | PTCA | Percutaneous transluminal coronary angioplasty |
| CK-MB | Creatine kinase–myocardial band | | |
| CO | Cardiac output | PVC | Premature ventricular contraction |
| CV | Cardiovascular | PVR | Pulmonary vascular resistance |
| ECG | Electrocardiogram | QTc | QT interval corrected for heart rate |
| EF | Ejection fraction | RAE | Right atrial enlargement |
| EKG | Electrocardiogram (German abbreviation) | RBBB | Right bundle branch block |
| EMD | Electromechanical dissociation (see *PEA*) | RVH | Right ventricular hypertrophy |
| EP | Electrophysiologic | SA | Sinoatrial |
| f wave | Fibrillatory wave | SVR | Systemic vascular resistance |
| F wave | Flutter wave | SVT | Supraventricular tachycardia |
| HR | Heart rate | SSS | Sick sinus syndrome |
| ICD | Implantable cardioverter/defibrillator | TdP | Torsades de pointes |
| IVR | Idioventricular rhythm | VF | Ventricular fibrillation |
| LA | Left atrial | VSD | Ventral septal defect |
| LAE | Left atrial enlargement | VT | Ventricular tachycardia |
| LAP | Left atrial pressure | WAP | Wandering atrial pacemaker (multifocal atrial rhythm) |
| LBBB | Left bundle branch block | | |
| LVH | Left ventricular hypertrophy | WPW | Wolff-Parkinson-White syndrome |
| mA | Milliamperes | 1° AVBL | First-degree AV block |
| MAT | Multifocal (or multiformed) atrial tachycardia | 2° AVBL | Second-degree AV block types I or II |
| MCL | Modified chest lead | 3° AVBL | Third-degree AV block |

ischemia, left anterior descending coronary artery disease, or left ventricular overload.

QRS complexes usually consist of several distinct waves, each of which has a letter assigned to it as a label. This labeling system is needed because the precise configuration of the QRS complex can vary from one lead to the next and from one patient to the next. To establish a standardized labeling system, several guidelines have been developed. If the first deflection of the QRS complex is downward (negative in lead II), it is labeled a *Q wave.* The initial upward (positive) deflection is called an *R wave.* The first negative deflection following an R wave is called an *S wave* (Fig. 11.6). If the QRS complex has a second positive deflection, it is labeled *R′* (R prime), and if a second S wave is also present it is called *S′* (S prime). A negative deflection can be called a Q wave only if it is the first wave of the complex. In clinical practice, each ventricular depolarization complex is called a QRS complex whether it has all three waves or not.

### SIMPLY STATED

The QRS complex is important in evaluating the ECG because it reflects the electrical activity of the ventricles.

### Electrocardiogram Paper and Measurements

The electrical activity of the heart is recorded on paper that has gridlike boxes with light and dark lines running horizontally and vertically and is read from left to right (Fig. 11.7). The light lines circumscribe small boxes (1 × 1 mm), and the dark lines circumscribe larger boxes (5 × 5 mm).

Time is measured on the horizontal axis of the ECG paper. The ECG paper moves through the electrocardiograph at a speed of 25 mm/s. Therefore each small square (1 mm) represents 0.04 second, and each larger square (5 mm) represents 0.2 second. Five large boxes represent 1.0 second; 3- or 5-lead continuous monitoring is usually read in 6-second segments represented by 30 large boxes.

On the vertical axis, voltage, or amplitude, of the ECG waves is measured. The exact voltage of any ECG wave can be measured because the electrocardiograph is standardized so that 1 mV produces a deflection 10 mm in amplitude. Therefore the standard for most ECG recordings is 1 mV = 10 mm. Each small square represents 1 mm.

To measure the amplitude of a specific wave, the isoelectric baseline must be identified. This is the flat line seen just before the P wave or right after the T or U wave (Fig. 11.8). Any movement of the ECG stylus above this line is considered positive; any downward movement is considered negative. To measure the degree of positive or negative amplitude of a specific wave, the isoelectric line is used as a reference point marking zero voltage.

R waves are measured from the isoelectric line to the top of the R wave. Q and S waves are measured from the isoelectric line to the bottom of the wave (see Fig. 11.6). P waves can be either positive or negative and are also measured from the

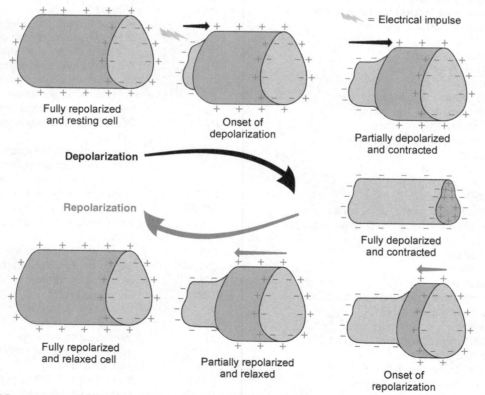

**FIG. 11.4** Depolarization and repolarization of a cardiac cell. (From Wesley K: *Huszar's basic dysrhythmias: interpretation and management,* ed 4, St. Louis, 2011, Mosby.)

isoelectric line to the top (if positive) or bottom (if negative) of the wave.

In addition to the amplitude of any wave, the duration of waves, intervals, and segments can be measured. A *segment* is a straight line between two waves. An *interval* encompasses at least one wave plus the connecting straight line.

The normal P wave is less than 2.5 mm in height and not more than 0.11 second in length. The *PR interval* is an important measurement that provides information regarding conduction time. This interval is measured from the beginning of the P wave, where the P wave lifts off the isoelectric line, to the beginning of the QRS complex (see Fig. 11.5). The PR interval represents the time it takes for the electrical stimulus to spread through the atria and to pass through the AV junction to the ventricles. The normal PR interval is between 0.12 and 0.20 second (3 to 5 small boxes). If conduction of the

impulse through the AV junction is abnormally delayed, the PR interval will exceed 0.2 second. A prolonged PR interval is called **first-degree AV block** and is discussed later in this chapter. An absent P wave may indicate an idioventricular ventricular rhythm and is also described later in this chapter.

The duration of ventricular depolarization is determined by measuring the *QRS interval*. This interval is measured from the first wave of the QRS complex to the end of the last wave of the QRS complex. Normally the QRS interval does not exceed 0.10 second (2½ small boxes). The amplitude of the QRS complex may range from 2 to 15 mm, depending on the lead and the size of the ventricular mass.

A very important segment to evaluate is the ST segment. This segment is the portion of the ECG cycle from the end of the QRS complex (even if no S wave is present) to the beginning of the T wave (see Fig. 11.5). It measures the time from the end of ventricular depolarization to the start of ventricular repolarization. The normal ST segment is isoelectric (no positive or negative voltage) or at least does not move more than

**FIG. 11.5** Normal configuration of electrocardiogram waves, segments, and intervals.

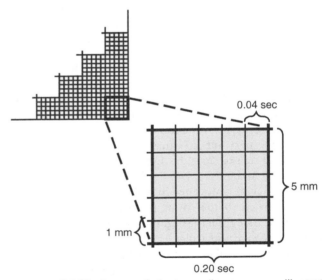

**FIG. 11.7** Gridlike boxes of electrocardiogram paper illustrating the 1-mm and 5-mm boxes.

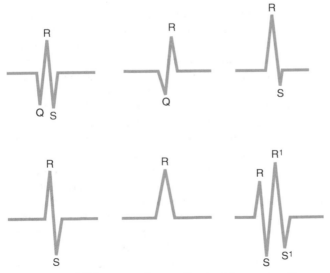

**FIG. 11.6** QRS nomenclature. See text for explanation.

**FIG. 11.8** Isoelectric baseline used for measuring voltage of electrocardiogram waves. (From Goldberger AL: *Clinical electrocardiography: a simplified approach*, ed 8, St. Louis, 2013, Mosby.)

1 mm above or below baseline. Certain pathologic abnormalities, such as myocardial ischemia or injury, cause the ST segment to be elevated or depressed (Fig. 11.9). The duration of the ST segment is not as important as its configuration.

> ### SIMPLY STATED
>
> In patients suspected of having acute myocardial ischemia, the ST segment is important to evaluate. Significant elevation or depression of the ST segment must be recognized and responded to immediately.

The RR interval is useful in identifying the rate and regularity of ventricular contraction. The distance in millimeters is determined from one R wave to the next in successive QRS complexes. This is done for several different RR intervals. ECG calipers can be helpful in making this measurement. The average of the measurements is determined and converted to time. Remember that each large box is equal to 0.2 second, and 5 large boxes equal 1.0 second. If the RR interval is 1.5 seconds, the heart rate is 40 beats/min (60 seconds divided by 1.5 = 40). If the RR interval is 1.0 second, the heart rate is 60 beats/min. If the RR interval is 0.5 second, the heart rate is 120 beats/min. This method for determining the heart rate is easy to apply if the RR interval falls conveniently on one of the numbers just described. Unfortunately, this is not usually the case. Other methods for calculating the heart rate are described later. Marked variation in the RR interval from one interval to the next indicates that the heartbeat is irregular and may be a sign of sinus dysrhythmia, which is described in more detail in the section on dysrhythmia identification.

The QT interval is measured from the beginning of the QRS complex to the end of the T wave (see Fig. 11.5). This interval represents the time from the beginning of ventricular depolarization to the end of ventricular repolarization. The normal values for the QT interval depend on the heart rate. As the heart rate increases, the QT interval normally shortens; as the heart rate decreases, the QT interval increases. As a general rule, the QT interval that exceeds one-half of the RR interval is prolonged if the heart rate is 80 beats/min or less. Common causes of an abnormally prolonged QT interval include hypokalemia

(low potassium), hypocalcemia (low calcium), and the side effects of certain medications such as quinidine.

## Evaluating Heart Rate

If the heart rate is regular, one of the easiest ways of determining the heart rate is to count the number of large (0.2 second) boxes between 2 successive QRS complexes and divide this number into 300. For example, if there is one large box between successive R waves, each R wave is separated by 0.2 second. Over the course of 1.0 second there will be 5 QRS complexes and 300 QRS complexes in 60 seconds. Therefore the heart rate is 300 beats/min. Following this logic:

2 large boxes = rate of 150 beats/min (300/2 = 150)
3 large boxes = rate of 100 beats/min (300/3 = 100)
4 large boxes = rate of 75 beats/min (300/4 = 75)
5 large boxes = rate of 60 beats/min (300/5 = 60)
6 large boxes = rate of 50 beats/min (300/6 = 50)

If the heart rate is irregular, this method will not be accurate because the spacing between QRS complexes will vary from beat to beat. In such cases, the average rate can be determined by counting the number of QRS complexes in a 6-second interval (30 large boxes) and multiplying the number by 10. Because the top of the ECG paper is marked with small vertical dashes every 3 seconds, 6-second intervals are easy to identify.

An increase or decrease in heart rate by more than 20% of the baseline value is generally regarded as a significant change and should be evaluated further. An abnormally slow heart rate may reduce cardiac performance to the point of compromised perfusion. Recall that cardiac output is a product of stroke volume and heart rate. A heart rate below 60 beats/min is referred to as an *absolute bradycardia*. However, bradycardia that may require intervention is relative to the individual patient. For example, a well-conditioned runner may present with a heart rate of 50 beats/min with no signs of inadequate cardiac output. On the other hand, a person with poor myocardial contractility who presents with a heart rate of 50 beats/min is likely to show signs of compromised perfusion or even cardiogenic shock in severe cases. At the other extreme, an adult heart rate greater than 100 beats/min is known as *tachycardia*. An increase in heart rate above 130 to 140 beats/min may compromise cardiac performance. This is because an abnormally rapid heart rate will increase myocardial oxygen demand, possibly to the point of inducing ischemia if the demand exceeds the supply. Additionally, significant tachycardia may further induce ischemia because it shortens the diastolic period, which is the period when most coronary perfusion occurs. In instances of extreme tachycardia where the heart rate exceeds 160 beats/min, the ventricular filling time may be too short to permit adequate refilling, thus reducing cardiac output. In severe tachycardia, the combined effects of increased oxygen demand and decreased cardiac output are potentially dangerous, especially for those patients with preexisting cardiac conditions. Such patients should be monitored carefully and the attending physician notified immediately.

**FIG. 11.9** ST segments. **A,** Normal. **B,** Abnormal elevation. **C,** Abnormal depression.

## ELECTROCARDIOGRAM LEADS

Because the heart is a three-dimensional organ, a more complete picture of the electrical activity in the heart will be obtained if it is viewed from several different angles. The standard ECG uses 12 different leads to provide 12 different views from different angles of the heart. Interpretation of the 12 leads is a little more difficult, but the information obtained is more complete, and abnormalities are not likely to be missed.

The 12 leads can be subdivided into two groups: 6 extremity (limb) leads and 6 chest leads. To obtain the 6 limb leads, 2 electrodes are placed on the patient's wrists and 2 on the patient's ankles. The ECG machine can vary the orientation of these 4 electrodes to one another to create the 6 limb leads. The chest leads are created by attaching 6 electrodes across the patient's chest. The chest leads are discussed after the limb leads are reviewed.

### Limb Leads

The six limb leads are called *leads I, II, III, aV$_R$, aV$_L$, and aV$_F$*. Leads I, II, and III are bipolar. Each lead is created by comparing the difference in electrical voltage between two electrodes. For lead I, the ECG machine temporarily designates the electrode on the left arm as a positive lead and the electrode on the right arm as negative. The measured difference in voltage between these two leads results in lead I. For lead II, the right arm electrode remains negative, and the left leg electrode is positive. Lead III is created by making the left arm negative and the left leg positive.

The other three limb leads (aV$_R$, aV$_L$, and aV$_F$) are called *augmented leads* because the ECG machine must amplify the tracings to get an adequate recording. The augmented leads are created by measuring the electrical voltage at one limb lead, with all other limb leads made negative. For the augmented leads, the ECG machine must augment the recorded voltages by about 50% to get an adequate recording. Lead aV$_R$ is created by making the right arm positive and all the others negative. Lead aV$_L$ calls for the left arm to be positive, and lead aV$_F$ is created by making the left leg positive.

The six limb leads view the heart in a vertical plane called a *frontal plane*. Any electrical activity that is directed up, down, left, or right is recorded by the limb leads (Fig. 11.10). The frontal plane can be envisioned as a giant circle that surrounds the patient and lies in the same plane as the patient. This circle can be marked off in 360 degrees, as shown in Fig. 11.10.

The angle of orientation for each of the bipolar limb leads can be determined by drawing a line from the designated negative lead to the designated positive lead. For lead I, the angle of orientation is 0 degrees; for lead II, +60 degrees; and for lead III, +120 degrees. For the augmented leads, the angle of orientation can be determined by drawing a line from the average of the other three limb leads to the one that is designated as the positive lead. The angle of orientation is −150 degrees for lead aV$_R$, −30 degrees for lead aV$_L$, and 90 degrees for lead aV$_F$.

In review, the limb leads consist of three bipolar leads and three unipolar leads. The three bipolar leads are called leads I, II, and III. The three unipolar leads are called aV$_R$, aV$_L$, and aV$_F$. The abbreviation *a* refers to augmented, *V* to voltage, and *R*, *L*, and *F* to right arm, left arm, and left leg (foot), respectively. The limb leads measure the electrical activity in the heart that occurs in the frontal plane, and each lead has its own specific view or angle of orientation to the heart (Table 11.3).

### Chest Leads

The six chest leads, or precordial leads, are called *leads V$_1$, V$_2$, V$_3$, V$_4$, V$_5$, and V$_6$*. The chest leads are unipolar leads that are placed across the chest in a horizontal plane. Fig. 11.11 shows the correct placement of the six chest leads. The chest leads define a horizontal or transverse plane and view electrical voltages that move anteriorly and posteriorly. Like the limb leads, each chest lead has its own view or angle of orientation. Leads V$_1$ through V$_4$ often are called the *anterior leads* because they view the anterior portion of the heart. Leads V$_5$ and V$_6$ view the left lateral portion of the heart and are therefore called the *left lateral leads* (see Table 11.3). More specifically, leads V$_1$ and V$_2$ are positioned next to the sternum and normally view

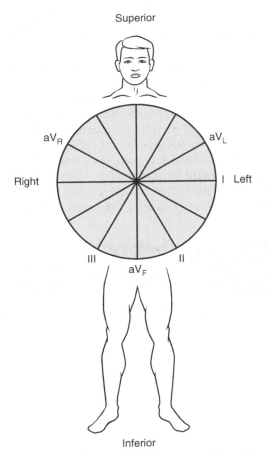

**FIG. 11.10** Frontal plane showing spatial relationships of six extremity leads. (Modified from Goldberger AL: *Clinical electrocardiography: a simplified approach*, ed 8, St. Louis, 2013, Mosby.)

the interventricular septum, leads $V_3$ and $V_4$ are placed on the left anterior chest to view the anterior wall of the left ventricle, and $V_5$ and $V_6$ are positioned on the axillary area of the left chest and therefore view the lateral wall of the left ventricle.

## Evaluating the Mean QRS Axis

The QRS axis represents the general direction of current flow during ventricular depolarization. Although depolarization spreads through the ventricles in different directions, an average or mean direction can be determined. Normally, the mean QRS axis (vector) points leftward (patient's left) and downward, somewhere between 0 and 90 degrees in the frontal plane previously described (Fig. 11.12).

The ECG records a positive (upward) QRS complex when the mean QRS axis is moving toward a positive electrode. When the mean QRS axis is moving toward a negative lead, the QRS complex is negative (downward). Because each of the six limb leads has its own angle of orientation as defined in the hexaxial reference system, a review of the recorded limb leads should identify the mean QRS axis in the frontal plane.

To identify the mean QRS axis, begin by sketching the hexaxial reference system, including labels for the points where the limb leads are located on the circle. Next, identify which limb lead has the QRS complex with the most voltage (positive or negative). This is accomplished by identifying the QRS complex with the largest deflection from baseline. If the largest deflection is positive (R wave), the mean QRS axis points toward the lead with the tallest QRS. If the most voltage is negative (Q or S wave), the mean axis points away from that lead. For example, if the most voltage is found to

be in lead II and it is positive, the mean QRS axis must be about +60 degrees because this is where lead II is located on the hexaxial reference system (see Fig. 11.12). This would be considered a normal axis because it falls between 0 and +90 degrees. If the most voltage is found in lead I and is negative, the QRS axis is approximately 180 degrees because lead I is located at 0 degrees. This would be consistent with right-axis deviation.

In some situations, the most voltage may be equally present in two leads. If two leads exhibit equal positive voltage, the mean axis must fall midway between the two leads. If the most voltage is equally negative in two leads, the mean axis is opposite the midpoint between the two leads.

As mentioned, a normal QRS axis is approximately −35 to +90 degrees. If the axis is found to be between +90 and 180 degrees, right-axis deviation is present. Right-axis deviation is common in patients with cor pulmonale (right ventricular enlargement due to chronic lung disease). In such cases, the QRS complex will be negative in lead I but positive in lead $aV_F$. Leads II and III are both positive in most cases of right-axis deviation; however, lead III will be taller than lead II (Fig. 11.13 and Table 11.4). Right-axis deviation is important to recognize early in the care of the patient because it often indicates significant chronic pulmonary hypertension. This is most often related to chronic hypoxemia from chronic obstructive pulmonary disease (COPD).

Left-axis deviation is present when the mean axis is found to be between −35 and −90 degrees. Left-axis deviation can occur in several different conditions, including left ventricular hypertrophy and blocks of the left bundle branch. In such cases, the QRS complex is positive in lead I and negative in lead $aV_F$. In addition, the QRS complex in lead III will demonstrate negative voltage with left-axis deviation.

| TABLE 11.3 | The 12 Leads of an Electrocardiogram and the Myocardial Wall That Each Set Views |
| --- | --- |
| **Lead** | **View** |
| I, $aV_L$, $V_5$, $V_6$ | Lateral |
| II, III, $aV_F$ | Inferior |
| $V_1$, $V_2$ | Septal |
| $V_3$, $V_4$ | Anterior |
| **Cells and Function** | |
| Pacemaker cells | Specialized cells that have a high degree of automaticity and provide the electrical power for the heart |
| Conducting cells | Cells that conduct the electrical impulse throughout the heart |
| Myocardial cells | Cells that contract in response to electrical stimuli and pump the blood |

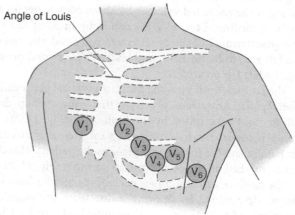

**FIG. 11.11** Position of the six chest leads. $V_1$ is located in the fourth intercostal space right of the sternum. $V_2$ is located in the fourth intercostal space left of the sternum. $V_3$ is placed between $V_2$ and $V_4$. $V_4$ is placed in the fifth intercostal space in the midclavicular line. $V_5$ is placed between $V_4$ and $V_6$. $V_6$ is placed in the fifth intercostal space in the midaxillary line. (Modified from Goldberger AL: *Clinical electrocardiography: a simplified approach*, ed 8, St. Louis, 2013, Mosby.)

If the mean QRS axis is found to be between −90 and −180 degrees, extreme left- or right-axis deviation is present. This condition is not common. When the ECG recording indicates that it may be present, the extremity leads should be checked to make sure they are attached properly.

The same principles of axis evaluation can be applied to the P wave as to the QRS complex. When normal sinus rhythm is present and the atria are normal in size, the P wave is positive in lead II and negative in lead aV$_R$. Therefore the normal P wave is directed toward lead II and away from lead aV$_R$, making the normal mean P wave axis about +60 degrees. In cor pulmonale, right atrial enlargement is common. The ECG will show tall, narrow P waves in leads II, III, and aV$_F$ in such cases.

### SIMPLY STATED

The normal mean axis is somewhere between −35 and +90 degrees. Right-axis deviation indicates that the right ventricle is enlarged; left-axis deviation suggests that the left ventricle is enlarged.

## STEPS OF ELECTROCARDIOGRAM INTERPRETATION

First and most important, the patient's condition must be evaluated. All dysrhythmias should be interpreted and evaluated in accordance with the patient's clinical presentation and medical history. Important signs and symptoms that may be associated with dysrhythmias may include the following:
- Chest pain
- Dyspnea
- Fine, inspiratory crackles in the lower lobes
- Palpitations
- Nausea
- Pale, cool, clammy skin
- Dizziness or syncope
- Sense of impending doom
- Hypotension
- Altered level of consciousness
- Decreased urinary output

Interpretation of dysrhythmias can be accomplished on three levels. The first level is simply identifying ventricular response. The contraction of the ventricles determines the majority of the cardiac output and perfusion of blood to the tissues. The ventricular response is determined by evaluating the QRS complexes and subsequent pulse strength.

Second, dysrhythmias can be placed into categories based on the origin of the impulse formation, which may include the following:
- Atrial
- Junctional
- Ventricular

Third, dysrhythmias can be evaluated based on the electrophysiology (or pathway) of the conduction disturbance. These can be categorized as follows:
- Ectopic beats or rhythms
- Escape beats or rhythms

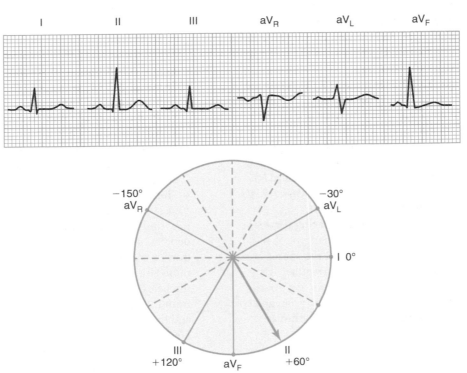

**FIG. 11.12** Normal mean QRS axis of 60 degrees. (Modified from Goldberger AL: *Clinical electrocardiography: a simplified approach*, ed 8, St. Louis, 2013, Mosby.)

**FIG. 11.13** Sample electrocardiogram showing right-axis deviation. Note the positive QRS complex (R wave) in leads II and III and the negative QRS complex (S wave) in lead I. (Modified from Goldberger AL: *Clinical electrocardiography: a simplified approach*, ed 8, St. Louis, 2013, Mosby.)

### TABLE 11.4  Quick Axis Determination

| Lead | Axis |
|---|---|
| I is positive<br>II is positive | Normal |
| I is positive<br>II is negative | Left deviation |
| I is negative<br>II is positive | Right deviation |
| I is negative<br>II is negative | Extreme right deviation |

- AV blocks
- Bundle branch blocks

To make sure that all components of the ECG tracing are reviewed by the RT or other member of the patient care team, a systematic method should be used. It is important to avoid assumptions resulting from quickly glancing at an ECG strip, because they may lead to misinterpretation. Every strip should be read from left to right, and the step-by-step process described here should be followed, generally in the order in which it is listed. The steps are as follows:

1. *Identify the heart rate.* Most modern ECG monitors provide a display of the heart rate. Always take the patient's pulse to verify that the monitor is calculating the heart rate correctly. Note that the monitor may not provide an accurate rate if the rhythm is irregular. If this is the case, a strip should be printed and calculation should be done as mentioned in the section on Evaluating Heart Rate. For adults, rhythms are called *bradycardia* if the rate is below 60 beats/min and *tachycardia* if the heart rate is over 100 beats/min (Table 11.5).

2. *Evaluate the rhythm.* Note whether the spacing between the QRS complexes is equal. Small variations of 0.04 second (40 ms) are considered normal. If the spaces are greater than 0.04 second, the rhythm is irregular. Irregularity may occur randomly or in patterns (e.g., occur every other beat or change with respirations). Irregular rhythms are present with the following dysrhythmias:
   - Ectopic beats
   - Escape beats
   - Second-degree AV blocks
   - Atrial fibrillation
   - Sinus dysrhythmia

3. *Note the presence of P waves.* A normal P wave generally is positive, depending on the lead, and has a rounded shape. Normal P waves are less than 0.11 second (110 ms) wide and less than 2.5 mm (2½ small boxes) tall. Oddly shaped or tall P waves may indicate atrial enlargement or hypokalemia. Normal rhythms will only have one P wave preceding each QRS complex, and each P wave should have the same configuration as the others. If there appears to be more than one P wave preceding a QRS complex, the rhythm may be the following:
   - Atrial flutter
   - Atrial fibrillation (no distinguishable P waves with a chaotic baseline waveform)
   - Second-degree AV block
   - Third-degree AV block

4. *Measure the PR interval.* The normal PR interval is 0.12 to 0.20 second (120 to 200 ms) wide. A PR interval that is wider than 0.20 second indicates a delay in conduction through the AV node, indicating the possibility of a block (see Table 11.5).

5. *Measure the width of the QRS complex.* The normal QRS complex is less than 0.10 second (120 ms) wide. Wide QRS complexes can occur with the following:
   - Bundle branch blocks
   - Ectopic beats originating in the ventricles (premature ventricular contractions)
   - Ventricular dysrhythmias such as ventricular tachycardia, idioventricular rhythm, or premature ventricular complexes
   - Third-degree AV block

6. *Inspect the ST segment in all leads.* ST-segment elevation may indicate myocardial injury whereas ST-segment depression may indicate myocardial ischemia. The portion or wall of the heart that is ischemic can be determined by identifying the leads looking at that portion of the heart (see Table 11.3). The ST segment is measured from the J point: the junction between the QRS complex and the ST segment (see Fig. 11.8).

7. *Identify the mean QRS axis.* Most 12-lead ECG tracings indicate the QRS axis. Normal axis is 0 to +90 degrees. Left-axis deviation is −35 to −90 degrees, and right-axis deviation is +90 to +180 degrees (see Fig. 11.12 and Table 11.4). Box 11.2 lists causes of axis deviation.

**TABLE 11.5 Summary of Normal Values for the Electrocardiogram Interpretation and Common Alterations**

| Variable | Normal Range | Common Alterations |
|---|---|---|
| Rate | 60-100/min | Rates >100 = tachycardia<br>Rates <60 = bradycardia |
| PR interval | 0.12-0.20/s | >0.20 = first-degree AV block |
| QRS interval | <0.10/s | >0.10 = ectopic foci |
| ST segment | Isoelectric | Elevated or depressed = myocardial ischemia |
| T wave | Upright, round, and asymmetric | Inverted with ischemia, tall and peaked with electrolyte imbalances |

8. *Assess the waveform morphology.* Some QRS complexes may have additional deflections. If there is a second deflection, the second portion is called *prime* (see Fig. 11.6). For example, a second R wave would be labeled R′.
9. *Evaluate the Q wave.* A Q wave is considered normal (or physiologic) if it is less than 0.04 second (40 ms) wide and less than one-third the amplitude of the R wave. Q waves that exceed either of these values are considered pathologic and indicate a new or possibly old infarction.
10. *Look for signs of chamber enlargement.* High-voltage R waves in the precordial leads indicate ventricular hypertrophy. Large or abnormally shaped P waves indicate atrial enlargement (see review later in this chapter).

**SIMPLY STATED**

A systematic step-by-step evaluation of the ECG is needed to find all abnormalities.

## NORMAL SINUS RHYTHM

Recognizing abnormal rhythms from an electrocardiographic strip is easier if you have an appreciation for the normal tracing (see Fig. 11.5). The normal sinus rhythm begins with an upright P wave that is identical from one complex to the next. As summarized in Table 11.5, the PR interval is consistent throughout the rhythm strip and is 0.12 to 0.20 second. The QRS complexes are identical and no longer than 0.10 second. The ST segment is flat. The R-R interval is regular and does not vary more than 0.12 second between QRS complexes. The adult heart rate is between 60 and 100 beats/min.

## IDENTIFICATION OF COMMON DYSRHYTHMIAS

This section discusses the characteristics of some of the most commonly seen dysrhythmias. It is always important to treat a symptomatic dysrhythmia, but it is just as important to determine the underlying cause. Some of the most common causes of each dysrhythmia are also discussed.

### Sinus Bradycardia

Sinus bradycardia for adults meets all the criteria for a normal sinus rhythm except for the heart rate, which is less than 60 beats/min. It is important at this point to understand the difference between an absolute bradycardia and a relative bradycardia. Absolute sinus bradycardia is simply a heart rate less than 60 beats/min and may be normal for a particular patient or tolerated well by the patient. For example, a conditioned runner may present with a heart rate of 55 beats/min with no negative cardiopulmonary signs and symptoms. By definition, this is an absolute bradycardia, but it is probably the patient's normal heart rate. On the other hand, a relative sinus bradycardia or a heart rate that is significantly below a patient's baseline is generally not tolerated well because it often compromises cardiac performance. Marked relative sinus bradycardia may result in hypotension, syncope, diminished cardiac output, and shock.

Transient bradycardia may be caused by an increase in vagal tone as a result of direct carotid massage, manipulation of tracheostomy ties or tube, tracheal suctioning, or the Valsalva maneuver. Damage to the SA node, as may occur with a myocardial infarction, can cause a long-term bradycardia. Hypothyroidism, hypothermia, and hyperkalemia, as well as certain drugs, may also result in bradycardia (Fig. 11.14).

### Sinus Tachycardia

Sinus tachycardia is present when the adult heart rate is 100 to 150 beats/min, the SA node is the pacemaker, and all the normal conduction pathways in the heart are followed. Sinus

**BOX 11.2 Causes of Axis Deviation**

**Right Axis**
Left ventricular infarction
Right ventricular hypertrophy
Chronic obstructive lung disease
Acute pulmonary embolism
Infants up to 1 year of age (normal)
Biventricular hypertrophy
Left posterior fascicular

**Left Axis**
Right ventricular infarction
Left ventricular hypertrophy
Abdominal obesity
Ascites or large abdominal tumors
Third-trimester pregnancy
Left anterior fascicular block

**FIG. 11.14** Electrocardiogram tracing of sinus bradycardia.

### Systematic Evaluation

| | |
|---|---|
| Rate | Less than 60 beats/min |
| Rhythm | Regular |
| P waves | Normal configuration; each P wave is followed by a QRS complex |
| PR interval | Less than or equal to 0.2 s in length |
| QRS complex | Less than 0.10 s in width |

**FIG. 11.15** Electrocardiogram tracing of sinus tachycardia.

### Systematic Evaluation

| | |
|---|---|
| Rate | 100 to 150 beats/min |
| Rhythm | Regular |
| P waves | Normal configuration; each P wave is followed by a QRS complex |
| PR interval | Less than or equal to 0.2 s in length |
| QRS complex | Less than 0.10 s in width |

tachycardia may be well tolerated by the patient; however, it increases myocardial oxygen demand and decreases the diastolic period, both of which can lead to myocardial ischemia. Sinus tachycardia results from sympathetic nervous system stimulation and may indicate a significant physiologic problem or be self-limiting and cease once the underlying cause is addressed. Fever, pain, hypoxemia, hypovolemia, hypotension, sepsis, and heart failure are causes of sinus tachycardia. It is especially important for the RT to note that tracheal suctioning, especially if it is performed without adequate oxygenation, can cause sinus tachycardia as a compensatory mechanism to hypoxemia. In addition, many β-agonist bronchodilators and excessive intake of caffeine often increase heart rate (Fig. 11.15).

## Sinus Dysrhythmia

Sinus dysrhythmia is a benign dysrhythmia that meets all the criteria for normal sinus rhythm except that the rhythm is irregular. It usually does not produce symptoms in the patient and requires no treatment. In most cases of sinus dysrhythmia, no abnormality of the heart is present. Often the irregularities are related to the patient's breathing pattern. This suggests that the changes in intrathoracic pressure associated with breathing in and out are causing changes in the tone of the vagus nerve, which may produce mild alterations in regularity of the heart rate.

### Systematic Evaluation

| | |
|---|---|
| Rate | 60 to 100 beats/min, may also present as a bradydysrhythmia (<60 beats/min) |
| Rhythm | Irregular |
| P waves | Normal configuration; each P wave is followed by a QRS complex |
| PR interval | Less than or equal to 0.2 second in length |
| QRS complex | Less than 0.10 second in width |

## Paroxysmal Atrial Tachycardia

Paroxysmal atrial tachycardia (PAT) occurs when an ectopic focus in the atrium overrides the pacemaking function of the SA node and paces the heart, usually at an abnormally rapid rate, generally in the range of 160 to 240 beats/min. It appears on the monitor as a series of normal-looking QRS

**FIG. 11.16** Short run of paroxysmal atrial tachycardia.

## Systematic Evaluation

| | |
|---|---|
| Rate | Generally in the range of 160 to 240 beats/min |
| Rhythm | Regular |
| P waves | Abnormal configuration. May precede the QRS complex or may be hidden within the QRS complex. Usually appear pointed because of combined amplitude with the previous T wave. If observable, each P wave is followed by a QRS complex |
| PR interval | Usually not measurable |
| QRS complex | Less than 0.10 s in width |

complexes, each associated with a P wave. Because of the rapid rate, the P wave may be obscured by the preceding T wave.

Onset of this dysrhythmia is sudden and spontaneous; termination is similarly abrupt. PAT is seen in patients with normal hearts and in those with organic heart disease. The hazard of PAT is that it increases myocardial oxygen demand while decreasing pump effectiveness as a result of the diminished "filling time." PAT may precipitate hypotension or an ischemic episode. PAT is especially dangerous for patients with compromised cardiovascular function, myocardial ischemia, preexisting heart failure, and recent myocardial infarction. Patients with PAT often complain of lightheadedness or palpitation. Occasionally, PAT will cause the patient to faint. Some possible causes of PAT may include emotional stress, mitral valve disease, rheumatic heart disease, digitalis toxicity, or the use of alcohol, caffeine, or nicotine (Fig. 11.16).

### Atrial Flutter

Atrial flutter is a dysrhythmia that produces a very distinctive ECG pattern, usually caused by a rapidly firing ectopic site in the atria that presents as a characteristic sawtooth pattern between normal-appearing QRS complexes. The sawtooth pattern of flutter waves (often referred to as *F waves*) represents the rapid flutter or contraction of the atria on stimulation by a reentry circuit or accelerated automaticity. Atrial flutter results in diminished atrial "filling time," which results in minimal atrial assistance in filling the ventricles. Recall that the term *atrial kick* refers to the contraction of the atria forcing out blood at the latter part of systole and results in about 10% to 30% of cardiac output in a healthy person but is diminished in atrial flutter. A secondary problem with atrial flutter is that the pattern of blood flow in the atria causes areas of diminished blood movement near the atrial walls. This stagnation of blood promotes the formation of thrombi, often referred to as *mural thrombi*, along the wall of the atria. Hence RTs and other members of the patient care team should be mindful that patients with untreated atrial flutter are at higher

risk for pulmonary emboli and stroke caused by the migration of a mural thrombus.

Atrial flutter usually is a short-lived dysrhythmia; it usually deteriorates to atrial fibrillation, or the patient's previous rhythm returns spontaneously. Some possible causes of atrial flutter may include valvular heart disease, myocardial infarction, hypertensive heart disease, cardiomyopathy, myocarditis, and pericarditis (Fig. 11.17).

### Atrial Fibrillation

In atrial fibrillation the electrical activity of the atria is completely chaotic and without coordination because it is arising from multiple ectopic sites within the atria. This results in a quivering of the atrial myocardium and complete loss of atrial pumping ability. Because the atria provide useful assistance in filling the ventricles from the atrial kick, there is a decrease in ventricular filling during atrial fibrillation. In most cases the reduction in cardiac output is not serious enough to produce symptoms, although it reduces cardiac reserve and may limit the normal activities of daily living. Similar to atrial flutter, patients with atrial fibrillation are at greater risk for mural thrombus formation and embolization due to blood stagnation in the atria. As a result, RTs and other clinicians should be on the alert for pulmonary emboli and stroke in such patients. Some possible causes of atrial fibrillation include all of those mentioned under atrial flutter but may also include hyperthyroidism, pulmonary disease, congenital heart or coronary artery disease, or valvular problems.

The ECG tracing shows a chaotic baseline between QRS complexes, with no regular pattern or organization. This irregular baseline is composed of what are called *fibrillatory waves* (f waves) that all have a different configuration because of their origin from different ectopic sites in the atria (Fig. 11.18).

### Premature Ventricular Contractions

Premature ventricular contractions (PVCs) represent ectopic beats originating in one of the ventricles as a result

**FIG. 11.17** Electrocardiogram tracing of atrial flutter.

### Systematic Evaluation

| | |
|---|---|
| Atrial rate | Generally in the range of 180 to 400 beats/min |
| Ventricular rate | Varies but always less than the atrial rate |
| Rhythm | Regular |
| P waves | A uniform sawtooth baseline configuration. The relationship between the flutter waves and the QRS complexes may be regular (e.g., four flutter waves to each QRS complex) or variable |
| PR interval | Not measurable |
| QRS complex | Less than 0.10 s in width |

**FIG. 11.18** Electrocardiogram tracing of atrial fibrillation.

### Systematic Evaluation

| | |
|---|---|
| Atrial rate | Difficult to determine |
| Ventricular rate | Varies but always less than the atrial rate |
| Rhythm | Irregularly irregular |
| P waves | All f waves have a different configuration. The relationship between the f waves and the QRS complexes is irregular |
| PR interval | Not measurable |
| QRS complex | Less than 0.10 s in width |

of irritable foci. QRS intervals of PVCs are generally wider than normal (>0.10 second). PVCs occur in both the normal and the diseased heart. PVCs commonly occur with anxiety or excessive use of caffeine, alcohol, or tobacco. Certain medications, such as epinephrine and theophylline, may also provoke PVCs in patients with normal hearts. Myocardial ischemia is a common cause of PVCs in patients with heart disease. Other causes may include acidosis, electrolyte imbalance, CHF, myocardial infarction, and hypoxia.

A single PVC poses no threat to the patient (Fig. 11.19), but certain configurations of PVCs may signal a serious cardiac problem that may need immediate treatment. Although the idea that PVCs are "warning" dysrhythmias has not been proved by clinical research, the following conditions warrant further investigation and indicate the need for close monitoring of the patient:

- *Increased frequency:* Multiple PVCs occur in 1 minute (Fig. 11.20).

- *Multifocal PVCs:* The QRS complexes of the PVCs have more than one configuration (Fig. 11.21); this indicates that more than one area of the ventricles is irritated.
- *Couplets:* Two PVCs occur in a row.
- *Salvos:* Three or more PVCs occur in a row (sometimes called a *short run of ventricular tachycardia*).
- *R-on-T phenomenon:* The PVC occurs during the downslope of the T wave of the preceding beat; this poses a real danger because it can precipitate ventricular tachycardia (Fig. 11.22).
- Most PVCs occurring in the presence of an acute myocardial infarction.

## Ventricular Tachycardia

Ventricular tachycardia appears on the monitor as a series of broad QRS complexes, occurring at a rapid rate, each without an identifiable P wave. This condition originates from an ectopic focus in the ventricles that may also be associated with enhanced automaticity or reentry. By definition, ventricular tachycardia is

FIG. 11.19 Electrocardiogram tracing of a single premature ventricular contraction.

### Systematic Evaluation

| | |
|---|---|
| Rate | That of the underlying rhythm |
| Rhythm | Underlying rhythm is usually regular but irregular with a PVC |
| P waves | None associated with the PVC |
| PR interval | Not measurable |
| QRS complex | Generally more than 0.10 s in width, abnormal configuration, and premature. T wave after the PVC is deflected in a direction opposite to that of the QRS complex. There is a full compensatory pause after the PVC confirmed by measuring the interval between the normal QRS complex immediately before the PVC and the normal QRS complex immediately after the PVC; it will be double the normal RR interval for that patient |

FIG. 11.20 Electrocardiogram tracing of frequent premature ventricular contractions.

FIG. 11.21 Electrocardiogram tracing of multifocal premature ventricular contractions.

FIG. 11.22 Electrocardiogram tracing of R-on-T phenomenon.

a run of three or more consecutive PVCs. It may be classified as *sustained ventricular tachycardia,* which lasts more than 30 seconds and requires immediate medical attention, or *nonsustained ventricular tachycardia,* which terminates spontaneously after a short burst. The rhythm is regular, and the rate is usually in the range of 100 to 250 beats/min. The majority of patients

deteriorate rapidly with this dysrhythmia; therefore it must be treated as an emergency. Without appropriate treatment, sustained ventricular tachycardia may lead to ventricular fibrillation (described later). When ventricular tachycardia occurs, the patient may become hypotensive and be slow to respond. If cardiac output deteriorates significantly, the patient usually

**FIG. 11.23** Electrocardiogram tracing of ventricular tachycardia.

### Systematic Evaluation

| | |
|---|---|
| Rate | Generally in the range of 100 to 250 beats/min |
| Rhythm | Regular |
| P waves | None associated with the QRS complex. They may occasionally occur because the sinoatrial node is still functioning |
| PR interval | Not measurable |
| QRS complex | Abnormal and greater than 0.10 s in width |

**FIG. 11.24** Electrocardiogram tracing of ventricular fibrillation.

### Systematic Evaluation

| | |
|---|---|
| Rate | None |
| Rhythm | Irregular, chaotic waves |
| P waves | None |
| PR interval | None |
| QRS complex | No waves appear with any regularity on the tracing. There may be occasional low-amplitude waves that appear somewhat like ventricular-origin complexes, but they are sporadic in occurrence and totally irregular |

becomes unresponsive. In addition, such patients in ventricular tachycardia may not have a detectable carotid pulse, in which case the American Heart Association (AHA) Basic Life Support (BLS) and Advanced Cardiac Life Support (ACLS) rescue protocols should be immediately initiated. Ventricular tachycardia is often caused by problems similar to those that cause PVCs. When the heart is hypoxic, as occurs with severe myocardial ischemia, ventricular tachycardia is common and is a sign that the patient needs immediate care (Fig. 11.23).

### Ventricular Fibrillation

Ventricular fibrillation is the presence of chaotic, completely unorganized electrical activity in the ventricular myocardial fibers. It produces a characteristic wavy, irregular pattern on the ECG monitor. Depending on the amplitude of the electrical impulses, it can be mistaken for asystole or ventricular tachycardia. Because the heart cannot pump blood when fibrillation is occurring, the cardiac output drops to zero and the patient becomes unconscious immediately. This dysrhythmia is life threatening and must be treated immediately in accordance with the BLS and ACLS resuscitation protocols,

including chest compressions between each defibrillation attempt. Ventricular fibrillation often is caused by the same factors that precipitate ventricular tachycardia (Fig. 11.24).

### Asystole

Asystole is cardiac standstill and is invariably fatal unless an acceptable rhythm is rapidly restored. In fact, asystole is one of the criteria used for the determination of clinical death. Asystole is recognized on the ECG monitor as a straight or almost straight line. In accordance with AHA resuscitation protocols, the RT or other clinician should quickly assess for a pulse and patient responsiveness early in any rescue effort because what may initially appear to be asystole on an ECG monitor may simply be a disconnection of the ECG leads, which can resemble asystole. In addition, the AHA guidelines call for the confirmation of asystole in more than one lead during resuscitation efforts to ensure that it is not fine ventricular fibrillation. Clinically, asystole is characterized by immediate pulselessness and loss of consciousness. The ECG tracing shows a line that is flat or almost flat, without discernible electrical activity (Fig. 11.25).

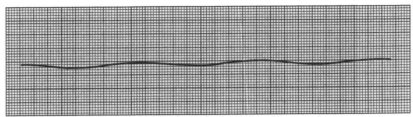

**FIG. 11.25** Electrocardiogram tracing of asystole.

**FIG. 11.26** First-degree atrioventricular block with a PR interval of 0.30.

### Systematic Evaluation

| | |
|---|---|
| Rate | Underlying rhythm rate |
| Rhythm | Regular |
| P waves | Normal sinus configuration, each preceding a QRS complex |
| PR interval | Greater than 0.20 s in length and constant |
| QRS complex | Less than 0.10 s in width |

### SIMPLY STATED

In an apparent case of asystole, the patient's pulse and responsiveness should be quickly checked to confirm whether the patient is indeed pulseless or whether a lead has become disconnected or the equipment has otherwise malfunctioned. Also, asystole should be confirmed in more than one lead during resuscitation efforts to ensure that it is not fine ventricular fibrillation.

## Pulseless Electrical Activity

Pulseless electrical activity (PEA) is not a discrete dysrhythmia but rather an electromechanical condition that can be diagnosed clinically. As the name implies, there is a dissociation of the electrical and the mechanical activity of the heart. In other words, the pattern that appears on the ECG monitor does not generate a pulse. Fortunately, PEA is rare and does not occur without a precipitating event. Tension pneumothorax, cardiac trauma, hypothermia, and severe electrolyte or acid-base disturbances are among the most common causes of PEA. PEA sometimes is seen as a terminal event in an unsuccessful cardiac resuscitation effort.

There is no relationship between the electrical pattern appearing on the ECG monitor or tracing and the mechanical activity of the heart. PEA therefore is any rhythm that does not produce a pulse, with the exception of ventricular tachycardia, ventricular fibrillation, and asystole.

## Atrioventricular Heart Block

*AV heart block* is a general term that refers to a disturbance in the conduction of impulses from the atria to the ventricles

through the AV node. However, the block may be at the level of the AV node or the bundle of His or in the bundle branches. Classification of the AV blocks is based on the site of the block and the severity of the conduction disturbance.

Disturbances in AV conduction can occur as an adverse effect of medications, such as digitalis, or when damage to the conduction system occurs with myocardial infarction. In some cases of complete heart block, the patient may develop symptoms associated with hypotension (fainting and weakness) if the ventricles are beating too slowly. In milder forms of heart block, the patient often is asymptomatic.

### First-Degree AV Block

The mildest form of heart block is first-degree block, which is present when the PR interval is prolonged more than 0.20 second. In first-degree block, all the atrial impulses pass through to the ventricles but are delayed at the AV node. First-degree AV block may or may not compromise cardiac output. It is important to assess the patient as discussed earlier in the section on steps of ECG interpretation. Some potential causes of first-degree AV block include adverse effects of medications such as digitalis, β-blockers, and amiodarone; increased vagal tone; hyperkalemia; myocarditis; and degenerative disease (Fig. 11.26).

### Second-Degree AV Block Type I (Mobitz I)

Second-degree AV block type I, also known as *Wenckebach,* is an intermediate form of heart block that presents with a PR interval that becomes progressively longer (changes in length) until the stimulus from the atria is blocked completely for a single cycle (dropped QRS complex). After the blocked beat, relative recovery of the AV junction occurs, and the

**FIG. 11.27** A, Second-degree atrioventricular block type I.

### Systematic Evaluation

| | |
|---|---|
| Rate | Varies, but ventricular rate is always less than the atrial rate |
| Rhythm | Regular |
| Ventricular rhythm | Irregular |
| P waves | Normal sinus configuration, not always followed by QRS complex |
| PR interval | Varies, lengthens, and then drops a QRS complex |
| QRS complex | Less than 0.10 s in width |

**FIG. 11.27** B, Second-degree atrioventricular block type II.

### Systematic Evaluation

| | |
|---|---|
| Rate | Varies, but ventricular rate is always less than the atrial rate |
| Atrial rhythm | Regular |
| Ventricular rhythm | May be regular if there is a constant conduction ratio or irregular if conduction is not constant |
| P waves | Normal sinus configuration, not always followed by QRS complex |
| PR interval | Normal or prolonged but always constant |
| QRS complex | Less than 0.10 s in width |

progressive increasing of the PR interval starts all over again. The ventricular rhythm is almost always irregular. As with first-degree AV block, second-degree AV block type I may or may not compromise cardiac output; thus it is important to assess the patient in conjunction with rhythm interpretation. Causes of second-degree AV block type I are similar to those of first-degree AV block (Fig. 11.27A).

### Second-Degree AV Block Type II (Mobitz II)

Second-degree AV block type II is a rarer but more serious form of second-degree AV block and is characterized by a series of nonconducted P waves followed by a P wave that is conducted to the ventricles. It is important to note that each time the P wave is followed by a QRS complex, the PR interval is always fixed (not changing in length). This will help differentiate between the two types of second-degree AV block. Sometimes the ratio of nonconducted to conducted P waves is fixed (at 3:1 or 4:1, for example). This block should be considered serious and treated promptly. Common causes of second-degree AV block type II include extensive damage to the bundle branches after an acute anteroseptal myocardial infarction or degenerative disease (Fig. 11.27B).

### Third-Degree AV Block

The most extreme form of heart block is third-degree AV block, which is caused by conduction disturbances below the AV node in the bundle of His (producing a narrow QRS complex) or bundle branches (producing a wide QRS complex). This block does not allow any conduction of stimuli from the atrium to the ventricles. In this situation, the ventricles and atria beat independently of one another. Thus there is no distinguishable pattern between the atria and ventricles. Third-degree AV block may be transient or permanent but is always considered serious and should prompt immediate intervention. Possible causes of transient third-degree AV block may include inferior myocardial infarction, increased vagal tone, myocarditis, and digitalis toxicity. Permanent causes may include hyperkalemia, degenerative disease, endocarditis, or acute anteroseptal myocardial infarction (Fig. 11.28).

### Idioventricular Rhythm

Idioventricular rhythm occurs when the normal pacemaker does not set the pace for the ventricles. In this case, an ectopic focus in one of the ventricles becomes the pacemaker for the ventricles. The intrinsic rate of the ventricular tissue is usually less than 40 beats/min, so the ventricular rate is very

**FIG. 11.28** Third-degree heart block characterized by independent atrial (P wave) and ventricular activity. The atrial rate is always faster than the ventricular rate.

### Systematic Evaluation

| | |
|---|---|
| Rate | Usually less than 60 beats/min but may vary; ventricular rate is always less than the atrial rate |
| Rhythm | Both atrial and ventricular rates are regular |
| P waves | Normal sinus configuration, not always followed by QRS complex |
| PR interval | Varies, no relationship |
| QRS complex | Usually greater than 0.10 s but may also be less than 0.10 s in width |

**FIG. 11.29** Electrocardiogram tracing of idioventricular rhythm.

### Systematic Evaluation

| | |
|---|---|
| Rate | 30 to 40 beats/min or slower, unless accelerated, then it may be between 40 and 100 beats/min |
| Rhythm | Regular |
| P waves | Absent |
| PR interval | None |
| QRS complex | Greater than 0.10 s |

slow (Fig. 11.29). In idioventricular rhythm, the ECG pattern appears as a slow series of wide and bizarre QRS complexes. The slower ventricular rate and the loss of assistance in ventricular filling provided by the atria decrease cardiac output significantly and can lead rapidly to heart failure and more severe dysrhythmias.

There is a variation of idioventricular rhythm called *accelerated idioventricular rhythm*. In accelerated idioventricular rhythm, the rate is in the normal range (40 to 100 beats/min).

### Junctional Rhythm

In a junctional rhythm, an area in the AV junction assumes the pacemaking role and sends impulses down the normal conduction pathways in the ventricles. Because the normal conduction pathways in the ventricles are being used, the QRS complexes appear normal. The P wave may be present or absent. If present, it may appear immediately after the QRS, plainly demonstrating retrograde conduction. In this case the P wave is typically inverted, indicating that depolarization of the atria followed a retrograde path. The P wave may appear before the QRS, but when it does the PR interval is less than normal duration (0.10 second). This indicates that there was not sufficient time for the P wave

to be responsible for initiating the associated QRS complex. Some potential causes of a junctional rhythm may include AV node damage, electrolyte disturbances, digitalis toxicity, heart failure, valvular disease, rheumatic fever, and myocarditis (Fig. 11.30).

## EVIDENCE OF CARDIAC ISCHEMIA, INJURY, OR INFARCTION

Normally, the ST segment is isoelectric, which means that it is in the same horizontal position as the baseline, or isoelectric line. Significant deviations (1 mm) of the ST segment from baseline, either up or down, suggest an abnormality in myocardial perfusion and oxygenation.

Cardiac ischemia is often seen on the ECG as depression of the ST segment (Fig. 11.31) or inversion of the T waves. At this point, there is no permanent damage to the heart, and proper therapy usually reverses any ECG abnormalities. In many cases of myocardial infarction, however, this pattern of ischemia may not be seen because the event has already progressed to the injury phase.

When ischemia persists, the heart muscle can become permanently injured due to inadequate oxygen delivery for a sustained time period. This is known as ST-elevation

FIG. 11.30 Electrocardiogram tracing showing junctional tachycardia.

### Systematic Evaluation

| | |
|---|---|
| Rate | Normal intrinsic junctional rate, 40 to 60 beats/min Accelerated junctional rate, 60 to 100 beats/min Junctional tachycardia, >100 beats/min |
| Rhythm | Regular |
| P waves | Absent or inverted |
| PR interval | Short if present |
| QRS complex | Less than 0.10 s |

FIG. 11.31 Electrocardiogram tracing showing ST-segment depression.

myocardial infarction (STEMI). In cases involving STEMI, the typical manifestation on an ECG tracing is an ST elevation in the leads monitoring the electrical activity of the corresponding injured heart tissue (Fig. 11.32). For example, an acute myocardial injury to the anteroseptal part of the heart will cause ST-segment elevation in the leads that examine the anteroseptal portion of the heart (Fig. 11.33; see Table 11.3). In general, the degree of damage to the heart caused by the ischemia correlates with the degree of ST-segment elevation. In addition, other symptoms including chest pain, often radiating to the neck and jaw, will accompany STEMI.

It can be helpful to identify ST-segment abnormalities by drawing a straight line over the imaginary isoelectric line. This will reveal whether ST-segment elevation or depression is present and to what degree. If the deviation from the isoelectric line is greater than 1 mm, significant changes have occurred and further investigation is appropriate. The patient should be monitored closely when this abnormality is identified.

It should be noted that rapid identification and treatment of STEMI is critical in achieving favorable clinical outcomes. As a result, the AHA has issued specific guidelines for identifying patients with suspected STEMI. In addition to ECG changes, these include chest discomfort, shortness of breath, weakness, diaphoresis, nausea, and lightheadedness, particularly in the presence of a prior cardiac history or other risk factors such as smoking and obesity.

In patients with STEMI, the ST-segment abnormality often resolves when perfusion is restored. However, it should be noted that at some point after myocardial infarction, significant Q waves (0.04 second in length) will be seen on the ECG in the corresponding leads. Q waves may develop within hours of an infarction but may not evolve for several days in some patients. They persist for the remainder of the patient's life.

### SIMPLY STATED

T-wave inversion and ST-segment depression indicate myocardial ischemia. ST-segment elevation indicates that an acute myocardial injury has occurred and indicates the presence of an ST-elevation myocardial infarction, or STEMI.

### ASSESSING CHEST PAIN

The significance of pain as a general clinical finding is discussed in Chapter 3. Pain and distress are subjective to the patient's perception of his or her condition and may be difficult to assess. However, it is essential that signs and symptoms associated with cardiac events be accurately reported both verbally and on the patient's chart. The following sequence will provide you with a reference for assessing these signs and symptoms. Ask the patient the following:

**O** When and how abrupt was the onset of the symptoms?

**P** What provoked the symptoms? (e.g., exercise, sleep, emotional upset)

**Q** How would you describe the quality of the pain? (e.g., sharp, dull)

**FIG. 11.32** Electrocardiogram tracing showing ST-segment elevation with a PVC.

**FIG. 11.33** Twelve-lead ECG tracing showing ST-segment elevation in leads $V_1$, $V_2$, $V_3$, and $V_4$. This pattern is indicative of acute anteroseptal myocardial injury.

**R** Does the pain *radiate* anywhere?
Does anything provide *relief* from the pain?
In what *region* is the pain located?
Does the pain change with deep *respiration*?
**S** Placing severity on a *scale* of 0 to 10, how would you rate your pain?
**T** What is the *time* frame of your symptoms? Is this chronic or acute?
**U** What do *you* think is wrong? Is this different from any previous episodes?

The AHA recommends that for chest pain or associated symptoms not relieved by nitroglycerin, a myocardial infarction should be suspected until proven otherwise. Remember that "time is muscle," and treatment interventions, such as thrombolytic therapy or surgical intervention, should be implemented quickly to minimize damage to the myocardium.

The role of an RT in such cardiac events is to notify the patient's physician, evaluate and optimize oxygen delivery, obtain a 12-lead ECG, and stand by to participate as a member of the cardiac arrest team if needed.

### SIMPLY STATED

For a patient with severe cardiac symptoms, the role of the RT is to quickly notify the physician, optimize oxygen delivery, obtain an ECG, and assist in resuscitation if the patient worsens.

## ELECTROCARDIOGRAM PATTERNS WITH CHRONIC LUNG DISEASE

The majority of patients with COPD have ECG abnormalities. Hyperinflation of the lungs and flattening of the diaphragm are associated with a more vertical position of the heart. This causes a clockwise rotation and contributes to the right-axis deviation associated with COPD. (For quick axis determination, see Table 11.4.) Additionally, chronic pulmonary hypertension is common in patients with COPD and causes an enlargement of the right side of the heart. Enlargement of the right atrium causes the following:

- Rightward deviation of the P-wave axis
- Enlarged positive P waves greater than 2.5 mm in leads II, III, and $aV_F$
- A prominent and negative P wave in lead I
- This syndrome is called *cor pulmonale*. Right ventricular enlargement may be associated with this syndrome and is recognized certain characteristics, including the following:
- Right-axis deviation of the QRS complex
- Increased R-wave voltage in leads $V_1$, $V_2$, and $V_3$

Reduced voltage in the limb leads (I, II, and III) is seen when severe pulmonary hyperinflation (emphysema) is present. This is seen as QRS complexes that are less than 5 mm tall in leads I, II, and III. Reduced voltage in precordial leads $V_5$ and $V_6$ may also be present. The reduced measured voltage appears to be caused by the following two factors:

- Reduced transmission of electrical activity through hyper-inflated lungs
- A mean QRS axis directed posteriorly and perpendicular to the frontal plane of the limb leads, causing decreased voltage on the ECG

Dysrhythmias often are seen in patients with COPD and acute lung disease. Tachycardia, multifocal atrial tachycardia, and ventricular ectopic beats are some of the more common ECG abnormalities seen in COPD. Such dysrhythmias occur as the result of hypoxemia from lung disease and from adverse effects of medications (e.g., bronchodilators) used to treat the obstructed airways. Hypoxemia often worsens during sleep in patients with COPD and increases the prevalence of night-time dysrhythmias.

## SIMPLY STATED

Patients with chronic hypoxemic lung disease often have evidence of right-axis deviation on the ECG. This is seen as a negative QRS in lead I.

## KEY POINTS

- An ECG is an indirect measurement of the electrical activity of the heart.
- The normal electrical conducting pathway of the heart starts with the SA node and then travels through the AV junction, bundle of His, bundle branches, and Purkinje fibers, and finally through the heart muscle known as the *myocardium.*
- The RT should recommend that an ECG be obtained whenever the patient has signs and symptoms (e.g., chest pain) of an acute cardiac disorder such as a myocardial infarction.
- Disturbances in the cardiac conduction system are called *dysrhythmias,* which can be detected with an ECG.
- The RT should remember that dysrhythmias can occur for many reasons, including hypoxemia, myocardial ischemia, sympathetic nerve stimulation, and certain drugs.
- For patients whose ECGs show certain abnormal heart rhythms such as atrial fibrillation, the RT should consider recommending anticholinergic bronchodilators such as ipratropium bromide (Atrovent), rather than an adrenergic bronchodilator such as albuterol.
- On an ECG, the initial wave of electrical activity or P wave signals atrial depolarization, the QRS complex represents ventricular depolarization, and the T wave occurs with ventricular repolarization.
- On ECG paper, time is measured on the horizontal axis, and voltage or amplitude is measured on the vertical axis.
- On ECG paper, each small square represents 0.04 second, and each large square is 0.2 second. Therefore if the interval between R waves (RR interval) is 5 large boxes (1 second) and the rhythm is regular, the rate is 60 beats/min.
- An ECG involves the placement of six leads on the extremities and another six chest leads across the chest to measure cardiac electrical activity from several different angles.
- There are several steps involved in ECG interpretation, including identifying the heart rate, evaluating the rhythm and presence of P waves, and measuring both the PR interval and the QRS complex.
- Sinus tachycardia in an adult is a common dysrhythmia characterized by a heart rate of 100 to 150 beats/min, a regular rhythm, and normal P waves, PR interval, and QRS complex. It may be caused by hypoxemia and selected respiratory medications such as certain β-agonist bronchodilators.
- Sinus bradycardia in an adult is characterized by a regular rhythm and heart rate less than 60 beats/min, as well as normal P waves, PR interval, and QRS complex. This dysrhythmia can be caused by vagal stimulation associated with suctioning or tracheostomy tube manipulation.
- PVCs can occur in a normal heart as a result of causes such as hypoxemia, or they can signal a diseased heart. PVCs can occur several times per minute, two or more in a row, as different shapes tend to be considered more serious.
- Dysrhythmias, such as ventricular fibrillation characterized by chaotic electrical activity or asystole (cardiac standstill), should be considered by the RT as medical emergencies that require immediate and aggressive intervention according to resuscitation protocols.
- In an apparent case of asystole, the RT should quickly assess for a pulse and patient responsiveness early in any rescue effort because what may initially appear to be asystole on an ECG monitor may simply be a disconnection of the ECG leads.
- The AHA guidelines indicate that during resuscitation efforts, asystole should be confirmed in more than one ECG lead to rule out fine ventricular fibrillation.
- Rapid identification and treatment of ST-elevation myocardial infarction (STEMI) is critical in achieving favorable clinical outcomes. As a result, the AHA has issued specific guidelines for identifying patients with suspected STEMI. In addition to ECG changes, these include chest discomfort, shortness of breath, weakness, diaphoresis, nausea, and lightheadedness.
- The role of the RT for a patient experiencing severe chest pain is to notify the physician, evaluate and optimize oxygen delivery, help ensure that a 12-lead ECG is quickly obtained, and be ready to participate as part of the cardiac resuscitation team.

## ASSESSMENT QUESTIONS

1. ECGs are useful to evaluate all of the following *except:*
   a. Impact of lung disease on the heart
   b. Pumping ability of the heart
   c. Severity of the myocardial infarction
   d. Heart rhythm
2. What clinical findings are most suggestive of the need for an ECG?
   a. Headache and flulike symptoms
   b. Orthopnea and chest pain
   c. Fever and cough
   d. Joint pain and swelling
3. For an adult, what is the normal intrinsic rate of the heart's primary pacemaker?
   a. 90 to 110 beats/min
   b. 60 to 100 beats/min
   c. 40 to 80 beats/min
   d. 40 to 60 beats/min
4. What is the normal intrinsic rate of the heart's secondary pacemaker?
   a. 80 to 100 beats/min
   b. 60 to 100 beats/min
   c. 40 to 60 beats/min
   d. 30 to 40 beats/min
5. What does the P wave on the ECG recording represent?
   a. Atrial depolarization
   b. Atrial repolarization
   c. Ventricular depolarization
   d. Ventricular repolarization
6. What does the QRS wave on the ECG recording represent?
   a. Atrial depolarization
   b. Atrial repolarization
   c. Ventricular depolarization
   d. Ventricular repolarization
7. What does the T wave on the ECG recording represent?
   a. Atrial depolarization
   b. Atrial repolarization
   c. Ventricular depolarization
   d. Ventricular repolarization
8. Which of the following is within the normal range for a PR interval?
   a. 0.10 second
   b. 0.20 second
   c. 0.30 second
   d. 0.40 second
9. What is the upper limit of a normal QRS complex?
   a. <0.04 second
   b. <0.08 second
   c. <0.10 second
   d. <0.16 second

10. The QRS complexes are equally spaced with three large boxes between each complex. What is the heart rate?
    a. 150 beats/min
    b. 100 beats/min
    c. 75 beats/min
    d. 60 beats/min
11. A prolonged PR interval is indicative of which of the following?
    a. Sinus dysrhythmia
    b. Sinus bradycardia
    c. Sinus block
    d. AV block
12. An early, widened QRS complex with an inverted T wave and no associated P wave is consistent with which of the following?
    a. PVC
    b. Ventricular tachycardia
    c. Ventricular fibrillation
    d. Ventricular asystole
13. What ECG finding is suggestive of an acute myocardial infarction?
    a. Prolonged PR intervals
    b. Elevated ST segments
    c. Tall, peaked T waves
    d. Narrow QRS complexes
14. What ECG finding is suggestive of cor pulmonale?
    a. Inverted T waves
    b. Elevated ST segments
    c. Right-axis deviation
    d. Small QRS complexes
15. Which of the following statements is true regarding sinus tachycardia?
    a. It is caused by parasympathetic stimulation
    b. It may be caused by a vasovagal response
    c. It is a meaningless clinical finding
    d. It may be caused by fever, fear, or pain
16. For a patient experiencing severe chest pain and other acute cardiac symptoms, the immediate role of the RT is to do which of the following?
    a. Call the respiratory care supervisor
    b. Help ensure that a stat ECG is quickly obtained
    c. Administer a bronchodilator
    d. Notify the nurse and doctor, and be ready to assist the cardiac arrest team

   *For Questions 17 through 26, please list the Rate, Rhythm, P Wave, PR Interval, QRS, and Interpretation for the following tracings.*

**17.**

Rate: _____
Rhythm: _____
P wave: _____
PR interval: _____
QRS: _____
Interpretation: _____

**18.**

Rate: _____
Rhythm: _____
P wave: _____
PR interval: _____
QRS: _____
Interpretation: _____

**19.**

Rate: _____
Rhythm: _____
P wave: _____
PR interval: _____
QRS: _____
Interpretation: _____

**20.**

Rate: _____
Rhythm: _____
P wave: _____
PR interval: _____
QRS: _____
Interpretation: _____

**21.**

Rate: _____
Rhythm: _____
P wave: _____
PR interval: _____
QRS: _____
Interpretation: _____

**22.**

Rate: _____
Rhythm: _____
P wave: _____
PR interval: _____
QRS: _____
Interpretation: _____

**23.**

Rate: _____
Rhythm: _____
P wave: _____
PR interval: _____
QRS: _____
Interpretation: _____

**24.**

Rate: _____
Rhythm: _____
P wave: _____
PR interval: _____
QRS: _____
Interpretation: _____

**25.**

Rate: _____
Rhythm: _____
P wave: _____
PR interval: _____
QRS: _____
Interpretation: _____

**26.**

Rate: _____
Rhythm: _____
P wave: _____
PR interval: _____
QRS: _____
Interpretation: _____

## BIBLIOGRAPHY

Aehlert B. *ECGs made easy*. 5th ed. St. Louis: Elsevier Health Services; 2013.

American Heart Association. *Handbook of emergency cardiovascular care for healthcare providers*. Dallas: American Heart Association; 2015.

Goldberger AL. *Clinical electrocardiography: a simplified approach*. 8th ed. St. Louis: Mosby-Elsevier; 2013.

Huff J. *ECG workout: exercises in arrhythmia interpretation*. 6th ed. Philadelphia: Lippincott Williams & Wilkins; 2011.

Jayasingle R. *ECG workbook*. 1st ed. Philadelphia: WB Saunders; 2012.

Nayeem U Hassan, Dar AM, Wani ML, Rather HA, Ganie FA. A comparative study on the effect of amiodarone and metaprolol for prevention of arrhythmias after open heart surgery. *Int Cardiovasc Res J*. 2013 Mar;7(1):1-4.

Phalen T, Aehert B. *The 12-lead ECG in acute coronary syndromes*. 4th ed. St. Louis: Mosby-Elsevier; 2011.

Tanel RE. ECGs in the ED. *Pediatric Emerg Care*. 2016;32:496.

Thaler MS. *The only EKG book you'll ever need*. 8th ed. Philadelphia: Wolters Kluwer; 2015.

Wesley K. *Huszar's ECG and 12-lead interpretation—Elsevier ebook on Intel education study*. 5th ed. St. Louis: Mosby-Elsevier; 2016.

# 12

# Neonatal and Pediatric Assessment

*Narciso E. Rodriguez*

## LEARNING OBJECTIVES

*After reading this chapter, you will be able to:*

1. Describe the type of information found in the pregnancy, labor, and delivery history and the clinical significance of common perinatal findings.
2. Explain the value of the Apgar scoring system and its interpretation.
3. Identify normal values for the vital signs in newborns and older children and the clinical implications of abnormalities.
4. Describe the clinical implications of retractions, nasal flaring, and grunting in neonates and infants.
5. Summarize the proper technique for auscultation of the neonate and infant.
6. Describe the clinical implications of abnormal breath sounds in infants and children.
7. List potential causes of cardiac murmurs heard during auscultation of the infant precordium.
8. Identify the presence of a pneumothorax using transillumination.
9. Identify normal values for the white and red blood cell counts and partial differential for the infant at birth, 7 days of age, and 14 days of age.
10. List the possible causes of abnormalities in the white and red blood cell counts in the infant.
11. Describe the clinical implications of abnormalities in blood glucose, total protein and albumin, serum enzymes, and electrolytes.
12. Identify normal and abnormal values for arterial pH, $Pao_2$, $Paco_2$, $HCO_3^-$, and base excess at birth, 24 hours after birth, 2 days to 1 month after birth, and 1 month to 2 years after birth.
13. Identify differences in blood gas parameters for capillary blood and arterial blood.
14. Describe the factors that can lead to misleading results from a transcutaneous oxygen monitor.
15. Describe the role of pulse oximetry assessment in the newborn for the detection of critical congenital heart diseases.
16. Describe the lung volumes and lung mechanics that can be measured in newborns, infants, and children and the clinical value of such measurements.
17. Describe the clinical findings that suggest the need for a chest radiograph in infants and children.
18. Identify signs and symptoms of a compromised airway in infants and children with a tracheostomy.
19. List the indications and advantages of flexible bronchoscopy in infants and children.

## OUTLINE

## KEY TERMS

abortion
acrocyanosis
anasarca
anterior fontanel
Apgar score
apnea
ascites
asthma
bradycardia
bradypnea
bronchopulmonary dysplasia (BPD)
bruit
coarctation of the aorta (COA)
cholestasis
cranial sutures
critical congenital heart disease (CCHD)
croup
crying vital capacity (CVC)
epiglottitis
estimated date of confinement (EDC)
extremely low birth weight (ELBW)
fetal hemoglobin (HbF)
gestational age

gravida
grunting
hepatomegaly
hyperbilirubinemia
hyperdynamic precordium
hyperglycemia
hyperthermia
hypoglycemia
hypothermia
hypotonia
impulse oscillometry (IOS)
interrupted aortic arch syndrome
intraventricular hemorrhage (IVH)
intrauterine growth retardation (IGR)
leukocytosis
leukopenia
low birth weight (LBW)
meconium
meconium aspiration syndrome (MAS)
nasal flaring
neonatal abstinence syndrome (NAS)
neutral thermal environment (NTE)

neutropenia
osteopenia of the premature
para
patent ductus arteriosus (PDA)
periodic breathing
pneumoperitoneum
polycythemia
postterm infants
preterm infants
pulmonary interstitial emphysema (PIE)
respiratory distress syndrome (RDS)
retractions
sinus bradycardia
splenomegaly
sudden infant death syndrome (SIDS)
tachycardia
tachypnea
term infants
thrombocytopenia
thrombocytosis
transient tachypnea of the newborn (TTN)
very low birth weight (VLBW)

The fundamentals for assessing the newborn and pediatric patient are a good history, thorough physical examination, and careful attention to selected laboratory and diagnostic information. Although most of the basic principles that apply to adults also apply to newborn and pediatric patients, certain characteristics make their assessment unique for the respiratory therapist (RT). These characteristics include lack of verbal communication skills, tendency to be afraid of strangers (particularly people in white coats), and inability or reluctance to follow directions, to mention just a few. This chapter reviews the respiratory assessment of the newborn and pediatric patient with respiratory disease.

For the purposes of this chapter, a neonate is a full-term newborn up to 28 days old, an infant is less than 1 year old, and a child is between 12 months of age and adolescence. The gestational age of a newborn is usually assigned based on the history and physical examination. Term infants are born between 37 and 42 weeks of gestational age, preterm infants (premature or "preemies") are born at fewer than 37 weeks of gestational age, and postterm infants are born at 42 or more weeks of gestational age. Fetal viability is considered to be between weeks 23 and 24 of pregnancy when the lungs are mature enough to support gas exchange because of the presence of surfactant.

## ASSESSMENT OF THE NEWBORN

### History

A good prenatal history is essential to anticipate the mother's and newborn's immediate needs and make appropriate preparations for resuscitation and initial nursery care of the baby.

The prenatal history is obtained from several sources and covers more than just the medical history of the newborn. Sources include the parents, the mother's labor and delivery (L&D) chart, and the infant's own chart. When the prenatal history is absent or prenatal care was not done the team should prepare for a high-risk delivery.

### Maternal History

The newborn's history begins with the mother's history obtained during her prenatal care. If no prenatal care is noted, the RT should be on the alert for the potential of a high-risk delivery and possible postnatal complications.

The mother's previous pregnancy history can give the RT valuable information. Obstetricians note this information in the mother's medical record using the terms *gravida*, *para*, and *abortion* (G, P, Ab). Gravida stands for the number of pregnancies, para indicates live births, and abortion shows the number of dead infants or embryos. For example, *G2, P1, Ab0* means that this woman is in her second pregnancy, has delivered a living infant, and has not had any abortions. Abortions can be further subdivided into therapeutic (*TAb*) and spontaneous (*SAb*) abortions.

Other maternal factors that may indicate a high-risk pregnancy are listed in Table 12.1. Of special interest is the use of drugs (especially opium-based substances) during pregnancy leading to neonatal abstinence syndrome (NAS). Neonates are being exposed to substances including illicit drugs, prescription drugs, and other legal substances that should not be used during pregnancy because of their potential effects as possible teratogens or their potential to create dependence and thus withdrawal in the neonate. It has been reported that one infant is born every 25 minutes with NAS in the United States.

## Family History

It is important to inquire about family history, as well as maternal history, especially a history of spontaneous abortions during pregnancy and multiple early neonatal deaths. Spontaneous abortions and early neonatal deaths may be clues for genetic diseases or the presence of other risks factors such as alcohol or drug abuse. Prematurity and history of other infants with respiratory problems are important because the

severity of diseases, such as respiratory distress syndrome (RDS), are similar among siblings. RDS is discussed later in the chapter.

## Pregnancy History

In evaluating the infant with respiratory disease, valuable information can be found in the pregnancy, labor, and delivery histories. In the pregnancy history, the interviewer records information about the mother and the fetus. Table 12.2 lists the most common situations during pregnancy that may affect the fetus or the neonate after birth. Any of these conditions may cause significant respiratory distress in the newborn.

The incidence of respiratory disease varies with different gestational ages, and determining when the infant was actually due is important. The interviewer should attempt to identify the date of the mother's last menstrual period (LMP), her estimated date of delivery (this appears as the estimated date of confinement [EDC] on the mother's chart), her obstetric record of uterine growth, and any reports from ultrasound examinations that she may have had.

Infants born prematurely are more susceptible to develop RDS, pulmonary interstitial emphysema (PIE), intraventricular hemorrhage (IVH), and bronchopulmonary dysplasia (BPD). Postterm infants are more susceptible to severe perinatal asphyxia, meconium aspiration syndrome (MAS; discussed later in this chapter), and the development of persistent pulmonary hypertension of the newborn (PPHN).

### Labor and Delivery History

The labor and delivery (L&D) history is obtained to evaluate the well-being of the newborn during the transition from intrauterine to extrauterine life. The newborn must successfully deal with cyclic decreases in uterine blood flow caused by contraction and possible umbilical cord compression, as well as compression of his or her body. The RT should consider fetal heart rate tracings, fetal activity, biophysical profile, and fetal ultrasound, as well as neonatal age, to anticipate possible complications.

### TABLE 12.1   Common Maternal High-Risk Factors

| Classification | Factors |
| --- | --- |
| Medical history | History of hypertension and preeclampsia |
| | Pulmonary disease |
| | Cardiovascular disorders |
| | Seizure disorder |
| | Pregestational diabetes |
| | Smoking and drug use |
| | Infectious and venereal diseases |
| Obstetric history | Cervical insufficiency |
| | Absence of prenatal care |
| | Maternal anemia |
| | History of ectopic pregnancy |
| | Previous cesarean delivery |
| | History of miscarriage or ectopic pregnancy |
| Others | Low socioeconomic status |
| | Minority |
| | Malnutrition |
| | Maternal age <18 years |

### TABLE 12.2   Common Pregnancy Conditions That May Affect the Fetus or Neonate after Birth

| Condition | Consequences |
| --- | --- |
| Gestational diseases (bacterial and viral) | Maternal bacterial and viral infections may affect the infant at birth and for life. |
| | Common viruses linked to congenital infections include cytomegalovirus, herpes, rubella (German measles), parvovirus, varicella (chickenpox), and enteroviruses. |
| | Group B streptococcus (*Streptococcus agalactiae*) is the most common cause of life-threatening bacterial infection in newborns. |
| Vaginal bleeding | The infant must be evaluated at birth for hypovolemia or low hematocrit. |
| Amniotic fluid infection or urinary tract infection | Increased risk for respiratory difficulty and other complications. |
| Maternal traumatic injury | It may compromise the uteroplacental interface and decrease transfer of oxygen and other nutrients to the baby. |
| | It can lead to hemorrhage and low hemoglobin and hematocrit in the newborn infant. |
| Intrauterine growth retardation (IGR) | It may lead to pulmonary hypoplasia, severe malformations, or congenital infection. |

## BOX 12.1   Clinical Findings That Suggest Perinatal Asphyxia during Pregnancy and Labor

- Variable or late heart rate decelerations
- Low biophysical profile score
- Decrease in fetal movement
- Presence of meconium (first feces of an infant) in the amniotic fluid
- Long labor
- Abnormal vaginal bleeding

## TABLE 12.3   Preductal Spo₂ Targets after Delivery

| Time after Delivery | Spo$_2$ Target Range |
|---|---|
| 1 min | 60%-65% |
| 2 min | 65%-70% |
| 3 min | 70%-75% |
| 4 min | 75%-80% |
| 5 min | 80%-85% |
| 10 min | 85%-95% |

## BOX 12.2   Manifestations Indicating Abnormal Transition to Extrauterine Life

- Persistent tachypnea (early symptom), nasal flaring, and grunting
- Fixed bradycardia
- Marked retractions
- Diffuse and persistent fine crackles on auscultation
- Persistent cyanosis (Spo$_2$ <90%) in room air and prolonged requirements for supplemental oxygen (after 2 to 3 hours of age)
- Episodes of prolonged apnea (>20 s) and bradycardia (<80 beats/min)
- Marked pallor or ruddiness (may indicate systemic hypotension)
- Persistent temperature instability after 2 to 3 hours of age
- Poor capillary refill (>3 s) and blood pressure instability
- Unusual neurologic behavior (lethargy, hypotonia, jitteriness)
- Excessive oral secretions, drooling, and choking or coughing spells accompanied by cyanosis
- Hypoglycemia

Modified from Gardner SL, Carter B, Enzman-Hine M, et al: *Merenstein and Gardner's handbook of neonatal intensive care*, ed 8, St. Louis, 2015, Mosby-Elsevier, pp 565-643.

## TABLE 12.4   Apgar Scores

| Sign | Score 0 | Score 1 | Score 2 |
|---|---|---|---|
| Heart rate | Absent | <100 beats/min | >100 beats/min |
| Respiratory effort | Absent | Gasping, irregular | Good |
| Muscle tone | Limp | Some flexion | Active motion |
| Reflex irritability | No response | Grimace | Cry |
| Color[a] | Body pale or blue, extremities blue | Body pink, extremities blue | Completely pink |

[a]Skin pigmentation and race may affect this evaluation. In this case, assess oral mucosa and nail beds for a more accurate assessment. Beware of acrocyanosis in hands and feet, as explained later in this section.

Box 12.1 lists clinical findings that suggest perinatal asphyxia during pregnancy and labor. The RT should also look for information that might suggest an infection in the infant or the mother. This information might include maternal fever, high maternal white blood cell (WBC) count, tender uterus, rupture of the amniotic membranes for more than 24 hours, foul-smelling or colored amniotic fluid, and fetal tachycardia.

A healthy fetus is capable of withstanding the challenges of labor. However, when the fetus is compromised or the labor is dysfunctional, the fetus can be taxed beyond capacity. This stress can place the fetus at risk for further compromise, including but not limited to asphyxia, intrauterine growth retardation (IGR), and intrauterine death (stillborn). Box 12.2 lists some of the more significant clinical manifestations signaling abnormal transition to extrauterine life.

The delivery history should include the method of delivery for the infant: vaginal or cesarean section; spontaneous, forceps, or vacuum extraction; or low, middle, or high forceps. Neonates who have trouble during labor and delivery are more likely to be delivered by vacuum extraction, middle or high forceps, or cesarean section. Some cesarean deliveries are performed because the infant is positioned in such a manner that vaginal delivery would be high risk, not because the infant is in trouble. Infants born by cesarean section are at greater risk for respiratory diseases, such as transient tachypnea of the newborn (TTN), caused by a failure to reabsorb fetal lung fluid after birth. It is also helpful to know what type of anesthetic the mother had for delivery (e.g., narcotics, local, epidural, spinal, or general). Narcotics and general anesthetics may enter the fetus's bloodstream and produce respiratory depression in the newborn. Spinal anesthetics may lower the mother's blood pressure, thus compromising the oxygen supply to the fetus.

The failure of the neonate to achieve target preductal saturations after delivery should also be considered as an abnormal sign indicating the presence of fetal asphyxia or the presence of a critical congenital heart disease (CCHD). Preductal target saturations by pulse oximetry are listed in Table 12.3.

The most standard objective measurement of the newborn's well-being during the perinatal period is the Apgar score. The Apgar score is a simple, quick, and reliable means to assess and document the newborn's status immediately after birth. It assigns the infant points for the presence of five specific physical criteria (Table 12.4). Most infants are evaluated and assigned Apgar scores at 1 and 5 minutes. However, if the infant is having difficulty during the transition to extra-uterine life, Apgar scores can be assigned more often and over a longer time span. For example, a sick infant may have 1-, 2-, 5-, 10-, 15-, and 20-minute Apgar scores. The process of assigning an Apgar score must not delay the initiation of resuscitative measures.

The Apgar score is useful in identifying neonates who may need further resuscitation and assistance. Those who are adjusting well to extrauterine life usually have 1-minute scores of 7 to 10 but may still show acrocyanosis (bluish coloration of hands and feet due to immature peripheral circulation), irregular respirations, or hypotonia (decreased muscle tone). Such neonates usually require only routine newborn care such as drying, temperature maintenance, and clearing of the airway. These neonates may occasionally require supplemental oxygen or positive pressure ventilation (PPV) via bag-mask ventilation (BVM) for a brief period. Moderately depressed infants with 1-minute scores of 4 to 6 may need more than routine care and often require an increased fraction of inspired oxygen (Fio$_2$) with BVM ventilation. Most infants respond well to this therapy and improve in a few minutes. Infants who have 1-minute scores of 0 to 3 are severely depressed and need extensive medical resuscitation that may include intubation and mechanical ventilation.

Although the 1-minute Apgar score is a useful tool in screening infants who might require resuscitation, the 5-minute Apgar score is a better predictor of the infant's neurologic outcome. For preterm and term infants, neonatal survival increases with increasing Apgar scores; low 5-minute scores (e.g., 0 to 3) are associated with the highest risk for neonatal morbidity and mortality.

### SIMPLY STATED

Newborns are evaluated at 1- and 5-minute intervals after birth with the Apgar score. This score calls for evaluation of the infant's color, heart rate, respiratory rate, muscle tone, and reflex irritability (normal score is 7 to 10, moderate depression is 4 to 6, and severe depression is 0 to 3).

### Postnatal History

After the delivery, the clinician should document the magnitude of the infant's resuscitation, presence of disease, treatment of disease, length of the hospital stay, condition at discharge, and problems that have developed since the infant was last seen. For most infants, all of this information is normal, and the postnatal history is brief.

All newborns require some form of resuscitation. The simplest resuscitation required is clearing the airway (mouth first!) and drying the skin. It is important to document whether the infant required only this simple intervention; a more significant intervention with blow-by oxygen, manual ventilation with bag and mask, or intubation; or chemical resuscitation with the administration of drugs to support cardiac output. How did the infant respond to resuscitation? Was the response immediate or slow?

**FIG. 12.1** Events leading to neonatal death. (Courtesy Narciso Rodriguez.)

If the infant is still hospitalized, the only further information needed for an adequate assessment is what diseases the infant has, what treatment has been initiated, and what the response to treatment has been. If the infant has been discharged and is now being readmitted, seen again in a practice office, or seen at home, the clinician must inquire about the infant's condition since discharge. Was the infant still sick at the time of discharge? Did the infant require continuing treatment at home? How is the infant doing with the current treatment? What kind of problem does the infant have now?

### Fetal Assessment

Useful information about the future well-being of the infant can be determined from the prenatal assessment of the fetus. This information could include but is not limited to the following:

- Fetal movement monitoring
- Genetic karyotyping during amniocentesis and biophysical profile to assess fetal growth and development
- Lecithin-to-sphingomyelin (L/S) ratio
- Presence of phosphatidylinositol (PI) and phosphatidylglycerol (PG) to assess lung maturity
- Fetal monitoring tracings and nonstress tests (NSTs) to assess for proper neurologic development

Fetal movement monitoring is easily accomplished using three widely available tools: maternal observation, fetal ultrasound, and fetal Doppler ultrasound. The simplest of these tools is having the mother keep a log of the timing, strength, and duration of the fetal movements for a period of time. Fetal ultrasound and Doppler ultrasound provide more quantifiable data but for shorter periods. Having a history of decreased fetal movement should alert the clinician to the possibility of the fetus being in trouble. This could indicate prenatal asphyxia and impending death or the possibility of severe neuromuscular disease, in which the newborn will be unable to support spontaneous independent respiration after birth. See Fig. 12.1 for a representation of the events leading to neonatal death.

The biophysical profile is an ultrasound evaluation of fetal breathing, body movement, tone, reactive heart rate, and

## TABLE 12.5   Biophysical Profile

| Biophysical Variable | Normal (Score 2) | Abnormal (Score 0) |
|---|---|---|
| Breathing | At least 30 s of sustained FBMs observed over a 30-min period | Fewer than 30 s of sustained FBMs observed over a 30-min period |
| Movements | At least three discrete body/limb movements in a 30-min period | Absent or less than three movements in a 30-min period |
| Tone | At least one movement of a limb from a position of flexion to one of extension, with a rapid return to flexion | Fetal limb in extension with no return to flexion with movement |
| FHR | Two or more episodes of acceleration of ≥15 beats/min and of >15 beats/min associated with fetal movement within 20 min | One or more episodes of acceleration of fetal heart rate or acceleration of <15 beats/min within 20 min |
| AFV | At least a single amniotic fluid pocket measuring 2 × 2 cm in two perpendicular planes | No amniotic fluid pocket that measures at least 2 × 2 cm in two perpendicular planes |

*AFV,* Amniotic fluid volume; *FBMs,* fetal breathing movements; *FHR,* fetal heart rate.
Adapted from Oyelese Y, Vintzileos AM: Uses and limitations of the fetal biophysical profile, *Clin Perinatol* 38(1):47-64, 2011.

amniotic fluid volume that predicts the presence or absence of fetal asphyxia and, ultimately, the risk for fetal death. Like the Apgar score, each of these parameters has a maximum score of 2 and a minimum score of 0. The score for a normal fetus is 8 to 10. With lower biophysical profile scores, the chance of significant fetal and newborn problems increases (Table 12.5). These potential problems include IGR, significant fetal acidosis, stillbirth, and neonatal death (see Fig. 12.1).

Amniocentesis also allows for the evaluation of the L/S ratio to assess pulmonary lung maturity. The L/S ratio is the ratio of two surfactant phospholipids: lecithin and sphingomyelin. Increasing levels of lecithin indicate improving maturation of the lung's surfactant system. Like lecithin, the presence of Phosphatidylinositol (PI) and Phosphatidylglycerol (PG) is usually indicative of advancing lung maturation. In general, L/S ratios of less than 2:1 and the absence of PG are associated with high risks for RDS.

Fetal monitoring is a continuous graphic method of recording the fetal heart rate and uterine contractions. Various patterns (fetal tachycardia, variable decelerations, and late decelerations) are signs that a fetus may be in trouble in the uterine environment. Knowing that a fetus has any of these heart rate patterns should alert the health care team that this infant may need a more extensive resuscitation and more careful evaluation after birth.

The fetal NST is a method of evaluating the stability of the fetus's physiology within the uterine environment. The NST monitors the acceleration of the fetal heart rate in response to fetal movement. A healthy fetus has a minimum of an increase in heart rate of at least 15 beats/min in response to fetal movement. To be considered reactive, the fetus needs to have a minimum of two accelerations exceeding 15 beats/min in 20 minutes for term pregnancies. A fetus is considered nonreactive when it fails to have heart rate response in two consecutive 20-minute periods. Nonreactivity may be associated with prolonged fetal sleep states, immaturity, maternal ingestion of narcotics and sedatives, and fetal cardiac or neurologic anomalies. A fetus that is nonreactive is at greater risk for serious complications and fetal death. This will prompt the obstetrician to consider the possibility of an accelerated or operative delivery

(cesarean). Knowing that a fetus has a nonreactive NST should alert the health care team that this infant may need a more extensive resuscitation and more careful evaluation after birth.

## Physical Examination of the Newborn and Infant

Unlike the adult patient, the nonverbal neonate communicates primarily by behavior. Through objective physical observations and evaluations, the clinician can interpret this behavior into information about the individual neonate's condition during the postnatal period.

Examination of a newborn is based on three of the four classic principles of physical examination as described in Chapter 5: inspection, palpation, and auscultation. To accomplish this, the newborn should be initially placed in a prone position. Percussion is rarely used in examining newborns because of their small cavity and organ sizes and the possibility of injury. Therefore percussion is not described in this chapter. Careful inspection reveals clues about the type and severity of respiratory disease. It is important to inspect the overall appearance of the infant carefully because respiratory pathology in the newborn is often manifested by extrapulmonary signs. Palpation is useful in assessing growth and gestational age and in determining the cause of respiratory distress and the severity of side effects from the lung disease and its treatment. As in the adult, auscultation is used to define characteristics of the disease process occurring in the lung. However, statements about the internal location of the pathologic process must be made with greater caution in newborns because localization by auscultation is difficult in the small chest cavity.

### Growth and Gestational Age Assessment

Preterm infants are also classified based on their birth weight, as follows:

- **Low birth weight (LBW):** less than 2500 g
- **Very low birth weight (VLBW):** less than 1500 g
- **Extremely low birth weight (ELBW):** less than 1000 g

Newborn classification based on birth weight and gestational age is a valuable tool in predicting possible

**NEWBORN MATURITY RATING & CLASSIFICATION**

ESTIMATION OF GESTATIONAL AGE BY MATURITY RATING

Symbols: X - 1st Exam  O - 2nd Exam

Gestation by Dates _____ wks

Birth Date _____ Hour _____ am / pm

APGAR _____ 1 min _____ 5 min

## NEUROMUSCULAR MATURITY

| | -1 | 0 | 1 | 2 | 3 | 4 | 5 |
|---|---|---|---|---|---|---|---|
| Posture | | | | | | | |
| Square Window (wrist) | >90° | 90° | 60° | 45° | 30° | 0° | |
| Arm Recoil | | 180° | 140°-180° | 110°-140° | 90°-110° | <90° | |
| Popliteal Angle | 180° | 160° | 140° | 120° | 100° | 90° | <90° |
| Scarf Sign | | | | | | | |
| Heel To Ear | | | | | | | |

### MATURITY RATING

| score | weeks |
|---|---|
| -10 | 20 |
| -5 | 22 |
| 0 | 24 |
| 5 | 26 |
| 10 | 28 |
| 15 | 30 |
| 20 | 32 |
| 25 | 34 |
| 30 | 36 |
| 35 | 38 |
| 40 | 40 |
| 45 | 42 |
| 50 | 44 |

## PHYSICAL MATURITY

| | -1 | 0 | 1 | 2 | 3 | 4 | 5 |
|---|---|---|---|---|---|---|---|
| Skin | sticky; friable; transparent | gelatinous; red; translucent | smooth; pink; visible veins | superficial peeling &/or rash; few veins | cracking; pale areas; rare veins | parchment; deep cracking; no vessels | leathery; cracked; wrinkled |
| Lanugo | none | sparse | abundant | thinning | bald areas | mostly bald | |
| Plantar surface | heel-toe 40-50 mm: -1 <40 mm: -2 | >50 mm; no crease | faint red marks | anterior transverse crease only | creases ant. 2/3 | creases over entire sole | |
| Breast | imperceptible | barely perceptible | flat areola; no bud | stippled areola; 1-2 mm bud | rasised areola; 3-4 mm bud | full areola; 5-10 mm bud | |
| Eye/Ear | lids fused loosely: -1 tightly: -2 | lids open; pinna flat; stays folded | sl. curved pinna; soft; slow recoil | well-curved pinna; soft but ready recoil | formed & firm; instant recoil | thick cartilage; ear stiff | |
| Genitals male | scrotum flat; smooth | scrotum empty; faint rugae | testes in upper canal; rare rugae | testes descending; few rugae | testes down; good rugae | testes pendulous; deep rugae | |
| Genitals female | clitoris prominent; labia flat | prominent clitoris; small labia minora | prominent clitoris; enlarging minora | majora & minora equally prominent | majora large; minora small | majora cover clitoris & minora | |

Scoring system: Ballard JL, Khoury JC, Wedig K, Wang L, Eilers-Walsman BL, Lipp R. New Ballard Score, expanded to include extremely premature infants. *J Pediatr* 1991;119:417-423.

### SCORING SECTION

| | 1st Exam=X | 2nd Exam=O |
|---|---|---|
| Estimating Gest Age by Maturity Rating | _____ weeks | _____ weeks |
| Time of Exam | Date _____ Hour _____ am/pm | Date _____ Hour _____ am/pm |
| Age of Exam | _____ Hours | _____ Hours |
| Signature of Examiner | _____ M.D./R.N. | _____ M.D./R.N. |

**FIG. 12.2** Ballard gestational age scoring system. (From Ballard JL, Khoury JC, Wedig K, et al: New Ballard Score, expanded to include extremely premature infants, *J Pediatr* 119: 417-423, 1991.)

complications in the postnatal period and neonatal diseases. In any gestation, the poorest outcome is seen in infants born with marked IGR.

Based on their weight and gestational age, newborn infants are further classified as follows:

- Appropriate for gestational age (AGA): weight is appropriate for the gestational age.
- Small for gestational age (SGA): smaller than expected, the weight falls below the 10th percentile for the gestational age.
- Large for gestational age (LGA): heavier than expected, the birth weight is above the 90th percentile for the gestational age.

Gestational age is assigned by the maternal dates, fetal ultrasound, and gestational assessment examination. Assessment of gestational age should be done to assign a newborn classification, determine neonatal mortality risk, assess for possible morbidities, and quickly initiate the proper interventions to address the identified risk factors.

Most women know approximately when they conceive. This is frequently confirmed by an early fetal ultrasound examination. Sometimes the mother does not know the date of conception, or there is significant disagreement between the maternal dates and the fetal ultrasound. In those situations, the gestational age assessment can be performed with a gestational assessment tool.

The original assessment tools were developed by Dubowitz and Dubowitz. These tools have been modified and validated over many years. Most nurseries currently use a Ballard examination (Fig. 12.2), which is a modification of the Dubowitz

| TABLE 12.6 | Ratio of Surface Area to Body Mass | | |
| --- | --- | --- | --- |
| | Surface Area (m²) | Mass (kg) | Area/Mass (m²/kg) |
| Adult male | 1.7 | 80 | 0.02 |
| Term infant | 0.25 | 3.5 | 0.07 |
| 28-week-old infant | 0.15 | 1.0 | 0.15 |

examination. Gestational age assessment should be performed for all newborns.

The Ballard examination is divided into two sections: neuromuscular maturity and physical maturity. The infant's neuromuscular and physical characteristics are scored by matching the infant's characteristics to the table's descriptions and then marking the table. Each column of the table has a numeric value ranging from −1 to +5. The numeric values for all of the marked cells are added together. It is important that a cell is marked in each row. The sum is then compared with the maturity scale, and a gestational age is assigned. The Ballard examination is accurate to within 2 weeks of the gestational age.

### Vital Sign Assessment

*Body Temperature.* The range of normal body temperature in the newborn does not differ from that in the adult. Humans maintain body temperature by balancing heat production with heat loss. The newborn loses much more heat to the environment than the older child or adult, largely because heat loss is determined by the ratio of the surface area of the body to the total body mass (Table 12.6). The neonatal surface area–to–mass ratio is more than 3 times the surface area–to–mass ratio of an adult male. For premature neonates, the problem becomes even more significant owing to the lack of brown fat tissue and a very low surface area–to–mass ratio. Brown fat tissue, which is present in a full-term neonate, is a major source of heat production for the newborn and helps to maintain internal body temperature. A 28-week gestational age neonate has a body surface area of approximately 0.15 m² and a body mass of 1 kg. This results in a surface area–to–mass ratio of 0.15 m²/kg, which is more than 6 times greater than that of an adult male. Therefore newborn term and preterm infants lose heat easily and are extremely dependent on the environment to help them maintain a neutral thermal environment (NTE). An NTE is the environmental temperature at which the infant's metabolic demands and therefore oxygen consumption are the least (Fig. 12.3).

Neonates, like all physical objects, lose heat to the environment by one of four mechanisms: conduction (touching a cold or wet object), convection (gas blowing over the skin surface), evaporation (liquid evaporating from the skin surface), and radiation (attempting to warm a cold surface not in contact with the skin). All these mechanisms must be considered when helping newborns deal with their environment.

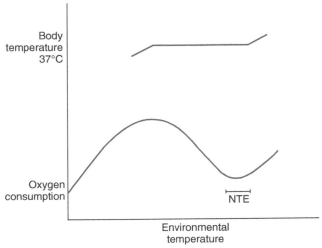

FIG. 12.3 Effect of environmental temperature on oxygen consumption and body temperature. *NTE,* Neutral thermal environment.

### SIMPLY STATED

Newborns are very prone to heat loss because of their high ratio of surface area to body mass. Maintaining an NTE is essential to avoid stressing the infant and causing "cold stress."

Hyperthermia is a core body temperature of more than 37.5°C, or 99.5°F. Hyperthermia in the newborn usually is caused by environmental factors. The infant may be wrapped in too many clothes, placed too close to a heater, or placed in an isolette or radiant warmer that is too warm. It is uncommon, although not rare, for an infant with hyperthermia to have an infection.

Hypothermia is a core body temperature of less than 36.5°C, or 97.7°F. Hypothermia is a more common and significantly more serious sign of infection in the newborn than in the older child or adult. Hypothermia probably occurs because the newborn is unable to maintain normal heat production or there is an increase in heat loss caused by environmental factors around the neonate. The newborn, in contrast to the adult, does not shiver when hypothermic.

**Assessment of Body Temperature.** The most common methods to measure temperature are axillary and rectal temperatures. In addition to noting body temperature, the clinician should also note the temperature of the infant's environment. Most sick infants are placed in an NTE (see Fig. 12.3). If the environmental temperature leaves the neutral thermal range, the infant usually can maintain a stable body temperature but at the cost of a significant increase in oxygen consumption. NTEs are defined for an infant based on weight and gestational and chronologic age.

*Heart Rate.* The normal heart rate for newborns is between 100 and 160 beats/min. Their heart rate is age and size dependent and is usually a function of the developmental age of the neonate. The normal resting heart rate is higher in premature infants than in a full-term newborn. The resting

**FIG. 12.4** Position of brachial and femoral pulses in the newborn.

heart rate also decreases with increasing chronologic age. Newborns and infants cannot significantly change their cardiac output by increasing stroke volume (volume of blood ejected from the heart with ventricular contraction) because their stroke volume at rest is normally more than 90% of maximal stroke volume. Neonates and infants increase their cardiac output by increasing their heart rate. However, too high a rate (>180 beats/min) may impede ventricular refill and lead to cardiovascular collapse and shock in the small infant or child.

Tachycardia in the newborn is a heart rate greater than 160 beats/min, and bradycardia is a heart rate of less than 100 beats/min. Tachycardia in the newborn can be caused by crying, pain, decrease in the circulating blood volume, drugs, hyperthermia, and heart disease. Bradycardia can be caused by hypoxia, Valsalva maneuver (often occurs during crying), heart disease, hypothermia, vagal stimulation (e.g., passing a nasogastric tube), **CCHD**, and certain drugs. In addition, there are a few infants with sinus bradycardia (a normal variant) and resting heart rates between 70 and 100 beats/min.

**Assessment of Heart Rate.** The pulse usually is evaluated at the brachial or femoral artery because of the small size of the radial arteries. To evaluate the brachial pulse, the clinician places his or her index finger pad over the brachial artery just above the elbow, with the baby in a supine position. The femoral artery pulse can be assessed at the groin, about halfway across the thigh (Fig. 12.4). On a newborn, the pulse can also be felt at the base of the umbilical cord. This is the preferred site in the L&D room during assessment and during resuscitation of the neonate.

*Respiratory Rate.* The normal respiratory rate for neonates and infants is between 30 and 60 breaths/min and is a function of the developmental age of the infant. The normal respiratory rate decreases as gestational age increases. Infants' respiratory rates are higher than those of older children and adults because of mechanical properties of their chest walls and airways. Infants' chest walls are more compliant, leaving them more prone to excessive inward movement of the chest (*retractions*, discussed later in this chapter) on inhalation. As a result, infants normally breathe rapidly and shallowly to help avoid retractions and chest wall collapse.

Tachypnea is a respiratory rate greater than 60 breaths/min, and bradypnea is a respiratory rate of less than 30 breaths/min in an infant (<40 breaths/min in a newborn). In newborns and infants, tachypnea can be caused by hypoxemia, metabolic and respiratory acidosis, CCHD, anxiety, pain, hyperthermia, and crying. Bradypnea is not a normal physiologic response in newborns. Bradypnea can be caused by certain medications (e.g., narcotics), hypothermia, and central nervous system diseases, and it may be an important clinical sign of the imminent respiratory decompensation from fatigue of the newborn with significant lung disease. Nonintubated infants with lung disease usually are tachypneic. As the disease progresses and the infant or child tires from the increasing work of breathing, bradypnea occurs just before ventilator respiratory failure.

All newborns display an irregular breathing pattern. Respiratory rates that exceed 60 breaths/min but normalize over the next several hours may indicate TTN.

Another common respiratory pattern of infants is apnea, or the cessation of respiratory effort. Apnea is a pathologic condition in which breathing ceases for longer than 15 to 20 seconds. Apnea may be accompanied by cyanosis, bradycardia, pallor, and hypotonia. More than six events of apnea accompanied by bradycardia in an hour (A&Bs) should be further investigated and their cause properly treated or addressed. A phenomenon known as periodic breathing also exists in newborns. During periodic breathing, the infant has multiple episodes of respiratory pauses or short apnea interspersed with normal-appearing ventilation. This pattern of breathing may continue for several minutes to several hours. All episodes of apnea must be investigated to establish the cause.

**Assessment of Respiratory Rate.** The respiratory rate can be obtained by visually observing chest motion or counting respirations while listening with a stethoscope. Visual observation provides a respiratory rate closer to the infant's resting rate. However, because the normal infant breathes rapidly with a small tidal volume, visualization of all of the true breaths may be difficult. If the RT or other member of the patient care team thinks this is a possibility, the respiratory rate should be assessed by listening with a stethoscope. The infant is likely to respond

| TABLE 12.7 Normal Newborn Blood Pressures in the First Hours of Life | | |
|---|---|---|
| Birth Weight (g) | Systolic (mm Hg) | Diastolic (mm Hg) |
| 501-750 | 50-62 | 26-36 |
| 751-1000 | 48-59 | 23-36 |
| 1001-1250 | 49-61 | 26-35 |
| 1251-1500 | 46-56 | 23-33 |
| 1501-1750 | 46-58 | 23-33 |
| 1751-2000 | 48-61 | 24-35 |
| 2001-3000 | 59 | 35 |
| >3000 | 66 | 41 |

Adapted from Hegyi T, Carbone MT, Anwar M, et al: Blood pressure changes in premature infants. I. The first hours of life, *J Pediatr* 124:627-633, 1994.

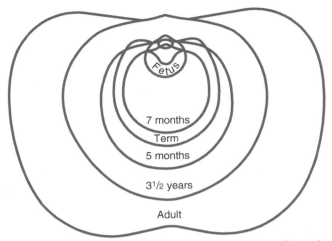

**FIG. 12.5** Changes in anteroposterior chest configuration with age.

to the touch of the stethoscope with a temporary increase in respiratory rate. The chest piece of the stethoscope must be warmed before placing it on the baby's chest.

The infant's respirations are assessed for rate, regularity, and depth. Many premature infants have normal rates but very irregular breathing patterns, which may include brief periods of apnea as described before. In addition, infants with significant lung disease may have normal respiratory rates but tidal volumes so small that they have minimal effective ventilation. Gasping respiratory efforts are never to be considered normal respiratory patterns in newborns.

*Blood Pressure.* The normal values for blood pressure depend on the size of the infant or neonate, with pressures decreasing with lower weights (Table 12.7). Usually, a term neonate's systolic blood pressure should be no higher than 70 mm Hg, with diastolic pressure no higher than 50 mm Hg. Normal pulse pressure (the difference between systolic and diastolic blood pressure) in a term infant is between 15 and 25 mm Hg.

**Assessment of Blood Pressure.** There are two common methods of determining blood pressure in newborns: use of a blood pressure cuff (sphygmomanometer) and direct arterial pressure monitoring. The more common method is to use a blood pressure cuff. The other common method for obtaining blood pressure in newborns is the direct measurement of pressure through an arterial cannula, also known as an arterial pressure catheter usually inserted through the umbilical artery (see Chapter 15). In the newborn, it is important to measure the blood pressure in all four extremities after birth. A difference in blood pressure between upper and lower extremities can be an indication of a CCHD such as coarctation of the aorta (a narrowing of the ascending or descending aorta in a newborn).

### Morphometric Measurements

In newborns there are three important measurements, two of which are not usually thought of in the physical examination of adults: weight, length, and head circumference. There are standard tables of normal growth for all gestational and developmental ages for these measurements. These measurements provide important clues to assessing the infant's past nutritional environment and current state and predicting the

infant's long-term growth. They are also essential to determine whether IGR has occurred during fetal development.

### Lung Topography

The infant's lungs are situated in the chest much as in the adult, but the infant's chest has a greater anteroposterior (AP) diameter than the adult's chest. The AP diameter of the infant's chest decreases proportionally and becomes more like the adult configuration with growth (Fig. 12.5). The imaginary lines and thoracic cage landmarks are the same in infants as in adults (see Chapter 5).

### Techniques of Examination
#### Inspection

Inspection is probably the most important and often the most neglected portion of the physical examination of a newborn. The infant should be unclothed and in a supine position initially in a quiet environment. The clinician should look first at the infant's overall appearance to identify level of illness, presence of malformations, and whether the infant's body position is appropriate for the gestational age (Fig. 12.6). The full-term neonate at rest flexes the arms and legs into a fetal position. Premature infants at earlier gestational ages have less muscle tone, and their extremities are less flexed at rest.

The RT should also look at the infant's skin to see whether the infant is cyanotic. Some caution must be used in interpreting these findings. Infants with hypothermia or infants with polycythemia (hematocrit level >65%) may have bluish extremities, yet they are not really hypoxemic. The mucosal color of infants who are preterm and immature with thin skin can look quite pink when they are really hypoxemic. The color of the mucous membranes in the mouth and tongue and the nail beds in the extremities give a more reliable indication of the infant's true level of oxygenation. Acrocyanosis, which is peripheral cyanosis of the hands and feet during the first 24 to 72 hours of life, is normal and is due to immature development of peripheral capillary beds.

The effort involved in breathing and the breathing pattern should be noted, especially the regularity of respirations.

**FIG. 12.6** Progression in body position with gestational age. **A**, A 26-week infant. **B**, A 28-week infant. **C**, A 32-week infant. **D**, A 36-week infant. **E**, A 40-week term infant.

An infant with respiratory distress characteristically exhibits tachypnea (discussed earlier), retractions, nasal flaring, and sometimes grunting.

*Retractions.* Sinking inward of the skin around the chest wall during inspiration (termed retractions) occurs when the lung's compliance is less than the compliance of the chest wall or when there is a significant airway obstruction. Thus retractions are a sign of an increase in the work of breathing. The diaphragm contracts during inspiration, lowering the negative pressure in the intrapleural space. In the normal respiratory system, the lung is the most compliant structure and will inflate to relieve this negative pressure. Furthermore, in a healthy infant the chest wall is as compliant as the lungs. Any lung disease that causes a decrease in compliance can cause the lung to become less compliant than the chest wall. The chest wall then represents the most compliant structure in the respiratory system and collapses inward in response to the increasing negative intrathoracic pressure generated by diaphragmatic contraction.

Retractions tend to be in different locations, depending on the cause of the respiratory distress. Three common points of collapse are the intercostal area (between the ribs), the subcostal area (below the lower rib margin), and the substernal area (below the bottom of the sternum). A fourth point of collapse is the supraclavicular area (above the clavicles) (Fig. 12.7).

Infants with lung disease tend to have retractions toward the center of the body (substernal and subcostal). Infants with heart disease tend to have intercostal retractions on the sides of their bodies because their large hearts prevent backward motion of the sternum. Finally, infants with obstructed airways tend to have large suprasternal retractions due to the pronounced use of accessory respiratory muscles.

**FIG. 12.7** Retractions commonly occur in these areas: intercostal (A), subcostal (B), substernal (C), and supraclavicular (D).

be achieved through their nose. Nasal flaring is an attempt by the infant to achieve airway dilation to decrease airway resistance, increase gas flow, and achieve a larger tidal volume. It is generally an attempt to compensate for increased work of breathing.

> ### SIMPLY STATED
>
> Nasal flaring is a cardinal sign of respiratory distress and increased work of breathing in the infant.

> ### SIMPLY STATED
>
> Retractions in the infant generally indicate a decrease in lung compliance, and a serious increase in the work of breathing or airway resistance, or both. Further assessment and monitoring of the infant are necessary.

*Nasal Flaring.* The dilation of the alae nasi during inspiration is called nasal flaring. Infants are obligatory nose breathers, and the minute ventilation they require must

*Grunting.* Grunting is a sound heard at the end of expiration just before rapid inspiration. Grunting is caused by closure of the glottis during expiration in an attempt to provide increased positive end-expiratory pressure and to maintain lung volume and functional residual capacity (FRC). The infant accomplishes this by occluding the airway with glottic closure and actively exhaling against the closed glottis after the end of inspiration. The grunting sound is

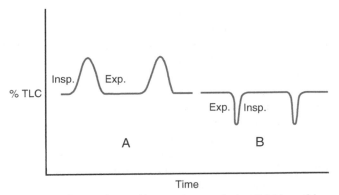

**FIG. 12.8** Comparison of lung volumes during tidal breathing: A, Adult. B, Grunting infant. *exp.,* Expiratory; *insp.,* inspiratory; *TLC,* total lung capacity.

produced when the infant suddenly opens the glottis and quickly exhales, inhales, and again closes the glottis (Fig. 12.8). Grunting is typically heard in infants with diseases that decrease lung volume (e.g., RDS).

*Precordium.* While observing the respiratory pattern and effort, the clinician should look at the precordium (area over the heart) for any increase in motion. Increased motion is present if the chest wall is visibly lifting or moving as the heart contracts. This increase in motion, or hyperdynamic precordium, is an indication of increased volume load on the heart, usually secondary to a left-to-right shunt of blood through the ductus arteriosus or any other shunt. If a preterm newborn has a patent ductus arteriosus (PDA), the anatomic connection between the aorta and pulmonary artery remains open and blood from the aorta flows into the pulmonary artery, which can cause congestive heart failure and pulmonary edema. The presence of a hyperdynamic precordium is a clue that the infant's respiratory distress may not be completely of pulmonary origin and requires further evaluation.

### Palpation

In infants, palpation is an important tool for physical assessment. However, the use of palpation in the physical examination of infants is directed less at the lungs than at other organ systems that may influence pulmonary function.

The easiest organ to palpate is the skin. Palpation of the skin can give the clinician valuable information about the infant's cardiac output and fluid volume status, both of which are clinically important in the evaluation of the infant's pulmonary status.

The three aspects of the skin that are useful in evaluating cardiac output are the skin perfusion, skin temperature, and peripheral pulses. To check the skin perfusion, or capillary refill, the clinician should gently blanch the infant's skin at the palm of the hands and feet and note how long it takes for the blanched area to recover its color. Capillary refill is checked on the trunk and extremities. Capillary refill should be less than 3 seconds and will be greater than 3 seconds if the infant has a low cardiac output or decreased peripheral perfusion.

The clinician should keep in mind that other pathologic states, such as acidosis, hypoxemia, hypoglycemia (low blood glucose), and hypothermia, can decrease blood flow to the skin and prolong capillary refill.

An approximation of the infant's skin temperature can be determined by feeling the skin. The dorsum, or back side, of the examiner's hand and fingers is more sensitive to temperature than the front side or palmar surface. Infants with hypothermia, low cardiac output, shock, or any abnormality that decreases skin blood flow have skin that feels cool.

Comparing the central and peripheral arterial pulses gives the clinician valuable clues about the infant's cardiac output. A careful clinician should be able to palpate the pulses of the radial, brachial, posterior tibial, and dorsalis pedis arteries. The infant should be examined closely for a decrease in cardiac output if these pulses are not easily palpable or if there is a large discrepancy between them and the central arterial pulses of the femoral or axillary arteries. The clinician should also look for any discrepancies between the intensity of the pulses in the upper and lower extremities. As previously mentioned, if pulses in the lower extremities are weaker than those in the upper extremities, the infant may have an aortic obstruction such as coarctation of the aorta or interrupted aortic arch syndrome.

### SIMPLY STATED

Palpation of the infant for skin temperature, capillary refill, and quality of peripheral pulses is helpful in determining the general quality of cardiac output and perfusion.

Finally, the clinician can achieve a rough idea about the fluid volume of the infant by feeling the turgor or fullness of the infant's skin. Infants with low fluid volume have a loss of skin turgor. This is manifested by "tenting," or gathering of the skin when it is lightly pinched together.

Palpation of the abdomen may be helpful in assessing an infant's pulmonary status. An infant's abdomen and abdominal organs move significantly with respiration because the diaphragm is the major source of power for respiration and an infant's abdominal wall musculature is relatively weak. Anything that impedes the motion of the abdomen or its organs hinders the infant's respiration. Liver or spleen enlargement (hepatomegaly or splenomegaly, respectively); enlargement of other organs, such as kidneys, bladder, or bowel; or intraabdominal tumors can impede abdominal motion and affect respiration. Distention of the abdomen by fluid (ascites), air (gaseous bowel distention), or pneumoperitoneum (free air in the abdomen) also impedes abdominal motion. Some of these conditions above are found in Necrotizing enterocolitis (NEC) discussed later on the chapter.

Gentleness is important when palpating an infant's abdomen. The liver should be soft and mobile and palpable on the right side of the abdomen parallel to and 1 to 2 cm below the costal margin. The spleen may be palpable as a soft tip below the left costal margin at the anterior axillary line. The kidney can be palpated in the immediate newborn period by compressing it between one hand placed under the posterior flank and the other hand firmly pressing in from the anterior abdominal wall. In infants with significant chronic cholestasis (internal obstruction to bile flow), the liver and spleen may be so large that their lower edge may be close to the pelvis and would be missed if the clinician started palpation in the midabdomen.

Major central nervous system diseases, such as Intracraneal Ventricular Hemorrhage (IVH) and hydrocephalus, are causes of respiratory problems in preterm infants. The clinician should evaluate the tension of the anterior fontanel (the soft spot on top of the infant's head). Infants who have had a major IVH or hydrocephalus may have a full, tense fontanel. In addition, the cranial sutures (junctions between two skull bones) may be widely separated in these conditions. The anterior fontanel would be depressed in a newborn with mild to severe hypovolemia.

## Auscultation

The last of the classic techniques routinely used in newborn examination is auscultation. Auscultation is the least definitive of the three examination techniques discussed, but this does not mean it is unimportant. Auscultation yields the best information if the infant is quiet; therefore auscultation is the first examination performed after inspection. Auscultation should be performed with a warm chest piece that has a small (1.0- to 1.5-cm diameter) diaphragm and bell. This allows for maximal localization of the findings. For auscultatory examination of the lungs, the infant is ideally in the prone position. However, because most neonates are in a supine position or on one side, the RT should try to complete most of the examination before moving the infant. If the infant's position does not allow an adequate examination, the clinician should gently move the infant to a more desirable position. Normal infant breath sounds are bronchovesicular in character and harsher than in the adult. The techniques for use of the stethoscope and the types of adventitious lung sounds heard are the same as in the adult (see Chapter 5).

The clinical significance of breath sounds in the infant and small child is similar to that in the adult. The mechanisms and significance of breath sounds are explained in detail in Chapter 5. The infant's thoracic cage is small, and sound is transmitted easily; therefore breath sounds usually are not entirely absent. A decrease in breath sounds implies a decrease in gas flow through the airways, as it may occur in RDS, atelectasis, pneumothorax, or in a pleural effusion. Wheezing implies gas flow through constricted airways; infants with BPD may have wheezing. Crackles usually imply excess fluid or secretions in the lung (pulmonary edema) or the presence of pneumonia. Crackles may also be heard in neonates with RDS. A loud ripping sound like the separation of Velcro often is associated with the presence of pulmonary interstitial emphysema.

In addition to listening for the breath sounds, the clinician should listen for the presence of cardiac murmurs. The presence of a murmur does not mean that the infant has heart disease, but it may mean that the infant requires further diagnostic evaluation. Almost all infants have physiologic murmurs such as physiologic pulmonary stenosis or a venous hum. The pathologic murmurs that are characteristic of the newborn period are often caused by a PDA, ventricular septal defect, tricuspid insufficiency, or a major CCHD.

The abdomen is another area of the body where auscultation may help in pulmonary assessment. The abdomen should be auscultated when there is a question about whether an infant is properly intubated. Loud sounds of air movement are heard over the stomach during inspiration if the endotracheal tube is in the esophagus. The presence of a bruit (a murmur-like sound) in the liver or neck should raise the question of whether the infant has an arteriovenous malformation in the liver or in the head. This type of malformation can cause respiratory distress because of high-output heart failure.

### Transillumination

Transillumination is a technique often used in examining the chest of neonates and small infants but not an older child or adult. It can be used in small infants because their chest wall is thin enough to shine a light through. The source is usually a bright fiberoptic light, which is placed against the chest wall in a dark room. Normally, this produces a lighted halo around the point of contact with the skin. In the presence of a pneumothorax or pneumomediastinum, the entire hemithorax lights up, dispersing the light in an irregular shape (Fig. 12.9). This technique is quick and allows rapid treatment of a serious condition. The procedure should be performed by a clinician who is familiar with the technique because some fiberoptic lights can cause cutaneous burns, and it is possible to be misled by the area of transilluminance.

## Clinical Laboratory Data

Two crucial issues face anyone who wants to use the clinical laboratory in pulmonary assessment of newborns. The first and most obvious issue is that the normal values for clinical laboratory tests may be different between newborns and adults. The magnitude of these differences depends on the laboratory test in question. However, to complicate this issue further, the normal values may depend on the gestational or chronologic age of the newborn or infant. The second, less obvious issue is the relationship between the test sample volume and the neonate's or infant's blood volume.

An infant's blood volume is approximately 80 to 110 mL/kg of body weight, with premature infants tending to have higher volume per weight. Depending on the severity of the illness or condition, most infants can tolerate an acute blood loss of no more than 10% of their blood volume at any given time. This means that for a 0.5-kg infant, all of the laboratory tests should require no more than 5.5 mL of blood. The infant will need replacement volume if the laboratory tests require more than this amount. A corollary of this issue is that even if the infant can tolerate the volume loss, it may not be practical or technically feasible to withdraw the sample volume. Infants have small vessels that tend to be fragile, and often it is not possible to draw large volumes by venipuncture or arterial puncture.

**FIG. 12.9** Transillumination of a pneumothorax.

| High-intensity flexible light source | | | | | |
| Reflected light "glowing" on surface of thorax | | | | | |
| Abnormal finger of reflected light indicating a pneumothorax | | | | | |

**TABLE 12.8    White Blood Cell, Neutrophil, and Platelet Counts of Very Low-Birth-Weight Infants during the First 6 Weeks of Life**

| Day of Life | n | PERCENTILES | | | | |
|---|---|---|---|---|---|---|
| | | 10 | 25 | 50 | 75 | 90 |
| **WBCs (10⁹/L)** | | | | | | |
| 3 | 376 | 4.8 | 7.1 | 9.5 | 14.4 | 24.5 |
| 12-14 | 180 | 8.1 | 9.7 | 12.3 | 15.2 | 19.8 |
| 24-26 | 233 | 7.2 | 8.5 | 10.4 | 12.4 | 14.6 |
| 40-42 | 212 | 6.8 | 7.7 | 9.1 | 11.0 | 13.0 |
| | | | | | | |
| **Neutrophils (10⁹/L)** | | | | | | |
| 3 | 334 | 1.5 | 2.7 | 4.7 | 8.2 | 14.8 |
| 12-14 | 161 | 2.2 | 3.1 | 4.6 | 6.8 | 10.6 |
| 24-26 | 205 | 1.3 | 1.9 | 2.9 | 4.0 | 5.3 |
| 40-42 | 175 | 1.0 | 1.4 | 2.2 | 3.1 | 4.6 |
| | | | | | | |
| **Platelets (10⁹/L)** | | | | | | |
| 3 | 558 | 95 | 140 | 204 | 285 | 355 |
| 12-14 | 372 | 142 | 216 | 318 | 414 | 499 |
| 24-26 | 394 | 171 | 242 | 338 | 443 | 555 |
| 40-42 | 370 | 189 | 275 | 357 | 456 | 550 |

n, Number of infants involved in calculating values; WBCs, white blood cells.
From Martin RJ, Fanaroff AA, Walsh MC, editors: *Behrman's neonatal-perinatal medicine: diseases of the fetus and infant*, ed 10, St. Louis, 2015, Mosby-Elsevier.

## Hematology

The WBC count in infants tends to be higher than in an older child or adult. Normal values vary with the chronologic age of the infant. Table 12.8 indicates typical values for WBCs, neutrophils, and platelets for VLBW infants at selected intervals during the first 6 weeks of life. In general, infants closer to delivery have higher WBC counts. Over the first week of life, total WBCs tend to fall to a plateau that is just slightly higher than the normal values for adults.

Leukocytosis, or a WBC count greater than 15,000/mm³, usually is a reflection of the infant's environment rather than of infection, as in the older child or adult. When evaluating an infant with a high WBC count, the clinician should consider infection as well as crying, hyperthermia from excess wrapping or high environmental temperature, and other environmental stresses. Leukopenia, particularly neutropenia (absolute neutrophil count <2000/mm³), is a more ominous sign. Usually, neutropenia indicates an infection and implies that the infant may be developing an overwhelming infection. The neutropenia from infection can be caused by one of two mechanisms: peripheral consumption of neutrophils or failure to produce and release neutrophils from the bone marrow.

There is still a great deal of debate about whether the newborn's leukocytes function as well as those of an older person.

**TABLE 12.9    Red Blood Cell Parameters of Very Low-Birth-Weight Infants during the First 6 Weeks of Life**

| Day of Life | *n* | PERCENTILES | | | | |
|---|---|---|---|---|---|---|
| | | 10 | 25 | 50 | 75 | 90 |
| **Hemoglobin (g/dL)** | | | | | | |
| 3 | 559 | 12.5 | 14.0 | 15.6 | 17.1 | 18.5 |
| 12-14 | 203 | 11.1 | 12.5 | 14.4 | 15.7 | 17.4 |
| 24-26 | 192 | 9.7 | 10.9 | 12.4 | 14.2 | 15.6 |
| 40-42 | 150 | 8.4 | 9.3 | 10.6 | 12.4 | 13.8 |
| **Hematocrit (%)** | | | | | | |
| 3 | 561 | 39 | 43 | 47 | 52 | 56 |
| 12-14 | 205 | 34 | 39 | 44 | 48 | 53 |
| 24-26 | 196 | 29 | 32 | 39 | 44 | 48 |
| 40-42 | 152 | 26 | 28 | 33 | 38 | 44 |
| **Corrected Reticulocytes (%)** | | | | | | |
| 3 | 283 | 1.9 | 4.2 | 7.1 | 12.0 | 20 |
| 12-14 | 139 | 0.5 | 0.8 | 1.7 | 2.7 | 5.7 |
| 24-26 | 140 | 0.5 | 0.8 | 1.5 | 2.6 | 4.7 |
| 40-42 | 114 | 0.6 | 1.0 | 1.8 | 3.4 | 5.6 |

*n*, Number of infants involved in calculating values.
From Martin RJ, Fanaroff AA, Walsh MC, editors: *Behrman's neonatal-perinatal medicine: diseases of the fetus and infant*, ed 10, St. Louis, 2015, Mosby-Elsevier.

It is fair to say that even a term newborn's response to infection is not optimum, but why this is and what cellular or immunologic function is involved are still being investigated.

### SIMPLY STATED

In the infant, significant leukocytosis (WBC >15,000/mm³) is more often the result of environmental stress (e.g., hyperthermia) than infection, as it is in the older child or adult. Neutropenia (absolute neutrophil count <2000 neutrophils/mm³) is a serious condition and needs to be evaluated immediately.

The normal values for the red blood cell (RBC) count, hematocrit, and hemoglobin depend on chronologic age. In utero, the fetus is stimulated to produce a large number of RBCs by the low partial pressure of arterial oxygen ($Pao_2$). This stimulus is withdrawn at the time of birth. The normal newborn severely limits or ceases the production of RBCs until a new stimulus is received. Anemia is the normal physiologic stimulus for this. In healthy term infants, this "physiologic" anemia occurs between 6 and 8 weeks of age. In healthy preterm infants, the lowest decrease in hemoglobin occurs between 8 and 12 weeks. Infants who have received transfusions have a 4- to 6-week delay in onset of RBC production. After an infant begins RBC production, hematocrit and hemoglobin levels rise slightly above the level of an adult and remain there throughout childhood. Table 12.9 indicates typical values for hemoglobin, hematocrit, and corrected reticulocytes (%) for VLBW infants at selected intervals during the first 6 weeks of life.

Platelet counts often are obtained in newborns and infants when they are being evaluated for thrombocytopenia, disseminated intravascular coagulation (DIC), or other bleeding disorders. Normal values are between 100,000 and 350,000/mm³; however, most clinicians will not transfuse infants with platelets unless the count is less than 25,000/mm³ and the infant is bleeding. Thrombocytopenia (platelet count <100,000/mm³) may be a sign of DIC from severe infection or one of many other causes. Thrombocytosis (platelet count >350,000/mm³) usually is not a clinical problem in the newborn. Thrombocytosis can be seen in infants with iron deficiency anemia or hemolytic anemia, during recovery from thrombocytopenia, and in infants whose mothers have inflammatory collagen vascular disease. Thrombocytosis can also be seen in infants after cardiac transplantation. A high-normal value in infants is not well established, but clinical symptoms are not usually seen until the platelet count exceeds 1 million.

The normal values for coagulation tests, such as partial thromboplastin time (PTT), prothrombin time (PT), and fibrinogen, are listed in Table 12.10. Values for mean corpuscular volume, mean corpuscular hemoglobin, mean corpuscular hemoglobin concentration, and reticulocyte count (see Table 12.9) in infants are close to the normal values for adults. Mean corpuscular volume and reticulocyte counts are higher in the immediate newborn period but decrease over the first few months of life to normal adult levels.

### Blood Chemistry

Blood glucose probably is the most frequent blood chemistry determination made in newborns. This simple test is of tremendous importance because hypoglycemia is as detrimental to the developing newborn's brain as hypoxia. The exact levels and length of time necessary to cause damage to the central nervous system have not been determined, so most physicians treat an infant with a glucose level of less than 40 mg/dL (<20 mg/dL in preterm infants). There are easy methods for approximating serum glucose at the bedside by point-of-care testing. These methods are used as screening tests, and any abnormalities found are confirmed with serum glucose levels obtained in the clinical laboratory.

Hypoglycemia can be caused by a variety of metabolic disturbances, including infection, hyperinsulinemia secondary to maternal diabetes mellitus, and inadequate glycogen stores secondary to SGA. Although only symptomatic treatment is usually needed, an extensive evaluation of the infant's glucose control mechanisms is often necessary. Hyperglycemia, or blood glucose greater than 125 mg/dL in a term infant (>150 mg/dL in a preterm infant), is most often iatrogenic. However, hyperglycemia is also one of the early signs of septicemia in infants. The problems with hyperglycemia from diabetes mellitus are rare in this age group.

Total protein and albumin are useful tools in evaluating the nutritional status of the ill newborn. They may also give helpful clues for evaluating the cause of pulmonary edema (Table 12.11). Colloid osmotic pressure usually is not measured in infants because the sample volume required is large.

### TABLE 12.10   Normal Coagulation Test Values

| Category | Partial Thromboplastin Time (s) | Prothrombin Time (s) |
|---|---|---|
| Preterm infant (1500-2500 g) | 21.7-51.2 | 10.0-16.2 |
| Term infant, 1 day | 37.1-48.7 | 11.6-14.4 |
| Term infant, 5 days | 34-51.2 | 10.9-15.3 |

From Martin RJ, Fanaroff AA, Walsh MC, editors: *Behrman's neonatal-perinatal medicine: diseases of the fetus and infant*, ed 8, St. Louis, 2006, Mosby.

### TABLE 12.11   Normal Values for Blood Chemistries

| Determination | Value |
|---|---|
| Sodium (mmol/L) | 133-149 |
| Potassium (mmol/L) | 5.3-6.4 |
| Chloride (mmol/L) | 87-114 |
| Total carbon dioxide (mmol/L) | 19-22 |
| Total protein (g/dL) | 4.8-8.5 |
| Albumin (g/dL) | 2.9-5.5 |
| **Bilirubin (mg/dL)** | |
| 24 hours | 1.0-6.0 |
| 48 hours | 6.0-8.0 |
| 3-5 days | 4.0-15.0 |

From Martin RJ, Fanaroff AA, Walsh MC, editors: *Behrman's neonatal-perinatal medicine: diseases of the fetus and infant*, ed 10, St. Louis, 2015, Mosby-Elsevier; and Meites S, editor: *Pediatric clinical chemistry: a survey of normals and instrumentation, with commentary*, Washington, DC, 1992, American Association for Clinical Chemistry.

The serum enzymes that are so useful in adults are much less useful in newborns and the pediatric age group. For many of the enzymes, normal values have not yet been established, and the clinical significance of abnormal values often is unknown. Lactate dehydrogenase (LDH), aspartate transaminase (AST), and alanine transaminase (ALT) are used when evaluating liver function. Creatine phosphokinase (CPK), also known as creatine kinase (CK), and its isoenzymes are useful in determining myocardial injury. Alkaline phosphatase is useful in evaluating bone growth and the adequacy of an infant's nutrition.

Serum drug level determinations are becoming increasingly useful during the newborn period. As a result of their small size, there is a narrow difference between therapeutic and toxic doses of most medications for infants. The need to obtain drug levels has always been present, but it has been practical only as improving technology has permitted smaller sample volumes. Drug levels for antibiotics (vancomycin, gentamicin, and other aminoglycosides), anticonvulsants (phenobarbital and phenytoin), antiarrhythmics, caffeine, and theophylline are often used. Digitalis and cyclosporine levels are used less often.

Serum bilirubin determination is often used in evaluating newborns. Probably more than 70% of infants have a bilirubin determination during the first week of life. There are many causes for hyperbilirubinemia during the newborn period. Some abnormalities in bilirubin metabolism are likely to affect pulmonary function. First is hyperbilirubinemia from any cause that requires treatment by phototherapy. Second is hyperbilirubinemia caused by hemolytic disease that requires an exchange transfusion. An exchange transfusion is a procedure in which the infant's blood is replaced with donor blood by cyclically withdrawing the infant's blood and gradually transfusing donor blood. Finally, the most severe and most rare is hyperbilirubinemia associated with severe hemolytic disease and hydrops fetalis (abnormal accumulation of fluid in 2 or more fetal compartments). In this disorder, the hyperbilirubinemia is not the fundamental problem. The infant has anasarca (massive total body edema) with pleural effusions and abdominal ascites that may cause profound respiratory failure.

Electrolytes, blood urea nitrogen (BUN), and serum creatinine determinations are all useful laboratory tests for newborns. The normal values depend on the infant's chronologic age, nutritional status, and fluid status. They are generally similar to adult values, with serum potassium being slightly higher and BUN and creatinine levels lower. These values are useful in a variety of clinical situations, from assessing the infant's fluid status to evaluating renal function (see Table 12.10).

Calcium and phosphorus levels are indirectly important in the evaluation of a newborn with chronic lung disease. Infants with BPD or other chronic lung diseases have increased work of breathing and increased metabolic and nutritional needs. The metabolism of calcium and phosphorus is a valuable clue to the nutritional status of the chronically ill infant. A chronically ill infant with poor nutrition has low levels of calcium and phosphorus and an increased risk for developing rickets. Osteopenia of the premature (a rickets-like disease caused by chronically low phosphorus intake) may worsen the infant's pulmonary status by increasing the chest wall compliance secondary to a decrease in the mineralization of the ribs and decreasing the infant's depth of respiration secondary to pain from rib fractures.

## Microbiology

The sputum analysis that is useful in adults is not possible in newborns. Until a child is about 6 years old, sputum is swallowed and not expectorated. However, if the infant is intubated, samples can be obtained with sterile suction catheters through the endotracheal tube. In an older infant or young child, samples may be obtained from the stomach through nasogastric tubes. Samples obtained from the stomach should be interpreted with caution. Even samples obtained through the endotracheal tube may reflect bacterial colonization rather than infection. In addition to the Gram stain, culture, and sensitivity, a polymorphonuclear neutrophil (PMN) count is useful. High PMN counts in tracheal or stomach samples are strongly suggestive of infection rather than colonization.

## Newborn Blood Gases

Monitoring the blood gas status of newborns is performed either by analysis of the gas in a blood sample or by transcutaneous monitoring ($P_{TC}$). Analysis of blood samples is performed on blood obtained from arterial, capillary, or venous sources. The clinician must consider the limitations of the different techniques and sources of the blood when drawing clinical conclusions from blood gas results on neonates, infants, and children alike.

## Fetal Hemoglobin

The newborn's oxygen-carrying mechanism is significantly different from that of the older infant, child, or adult. The presence of **fetal hemoglobin (HbF)** has significant effects on the transport of oxygen. HbF meets the needs of the fetus in the oxygen-poor environment of intrauterine life. The fetal hemoglobin curve is shifted to the left of the adult hemoglobin (HbA) curve (Fig. 12.10). Thus HbF has a higher affinity

for oxygen than HbA. This means that HbF absorbs oxygen more readily but also releases it more slowly. The half-life for RBCs with HbF is about 45 days. Thus a newborn infant will typically have a significant portion of the RBC population with HbF until about 60 to 90 days of life.

## Arterial Blood Gases

Arterial blood samples are the most reliable source for blood gas analysis in newborns. Normal values in newborns depend on the age of the infant when the blood is drawn (Table 12.12). Once infants are beyond the transitional period after delivery (usually 4 to 12 hours), their arterial oxygen ($Pa_{O_2}$), carbon dioxide ($Pa_{CO_2}$), and pH values should be similar to those of the older child or adult. During the transitional period, $Pa_{O_2}$ is lower, $Pa_{CO_2}$ is higher, and pH is lower compared with later in the newborn's development. Sick infants who require supplemental oxygenation or mechanical ventilation often have values for $Pa_{O_2}$, $Pa_{CO_2}$, and pH that are not quite normal for this age but are accepted because of the complications that result from oxygen therapy and mechanical ventilation.

The fact that an arterial blood sample provides the most reliable source for blood gas analysis in newborns must be weighed against the problems associated with arterial puncture in newborns and young infants. Arterial puncture is technically possible, but it requires good technique and often extra assistance. Newborns and young infants have small arteries and are notoriously uncooperative, moving their extremities and making the arterial puncture difficult. This also increases the risk for arterial damage. In addition, arterial blood does not always reflect the resting state for the newborn or young infant because the discomfort associated with the puncture usually causes the baby to cry. Infants who are crying change their ventilation in one of two patterns: they either hyperventilate or hold their breath and stop ventilating. Either of these changes in ventilation rapidly alters the values for oxygen, carbon dioxide, and pH in the blood.

In the newborn, the placement of an umbilical arterial catheter (UAC) allows the clinician to obtain arterial blood samples without altering the infant's physiology in the immediate newborn period. This is useful in evaluating sick infants without causing them the pain and discomfort of percutaneous arterial puncture. UACs are widely used in neonatal intensive care units. The use of these catheters presents some significant risks such as embolization, thrombosis, vasospasm, and infection. Their use by experienced personnel minimizes these risks.

## Capillary Blood Gases

Many nurseries and pediatric units obtain blood gas samples by capillary puncture because of the risk and the technical expertise involved in obtaining arterial blood gas (ABG) samples. Although the results require special consideration, less technical expertise and fewer people are required to do a capillary blood gas (CBG) than an arterial puncture. In general, capillary samples are obtained by puncturing the skin of the

**FIG. 12.10** Oxygen hemoglobin dissociation curves for fetal and adult hemoglobins. Fetal hemoglobin $P_{50}$ is approximately 18.6. Adult hemoglobin $P_{50}$ is approximately 27.

## TABLE 12.12   Normal Values for Arterial Blood Gases in Infants at Room Air

| Age | pH | Pao$_2$ (mm Hg) | Paco$_2$ (mm Hg) | HCO$_3^-$ (mmol/L) | Base Excess |
|---|---|---|---|---|---|
| Newborn | 7.25-7.35 | 50-70 | 26-40 | 17-23 | -10 to -2 |
| 24 hours | 7.30-7.40 | 60-80 | 26-40 | 18-25 | -4 to +2 |
| 2 days to 1 month | 7.32-7.43 | 85-95 | 30-40 | 16-25 | -6 to +1 |
| 1 month to 2 years | 7.34-7.46 | 85-105 | 30-45 | 20-28 | -4 to +2 |

Unpublished data from author's laboratory and data from Meites S, editor: *Pediatric clinical chemistry: a survey of normals and instrumentation, with commentary*, Washington, DC, 1992, American Association for Clinical Chemistry.

infant's warmed heel. Fingers and earlobes can also be used for obtaining capillary samples.

When the values of capillary carbon dioxide tension (Pcco$_2$) and pH are compared with those obtained by arterial sample, Pcco$_2$ is 2 to 5 mm Hg higher and pH is 0.01 to 0.03 units lower. These small differences are inconsequential in most clinical situations. However, when the values of the capillary oxygen tension (Pco$_2$) are compared with those obtained by arterial samples, the differences are not so slight. Unfortunately, there is no fixed ratio for Pao$_2$/Pco$_2$. An infant with a Pco$_2$ of 50 mm Hg may have a Pao$_2$ of 50 to 90 mm Hg or higher. The only statement that can be made about Pao$_2$ by knowing only Pco$_2$ is that Pao$_2$ is probably higher than Pco$_2$. Pulse oximetry or transcutaneous oxygen monitoring should be used to monitor the oxygenation status if needed.

When capillary blood gas sampling is appropriate, the person drawing the sample and the person evaluating the results need to remember the underlying problems that must be overcome in obtaining the sample. A capillary sample that closely reflects arterial blood must be obtained from a warmed extremity (skin temperature should be approximately 39°C, or 102°F). Caution must be used in warming the extremity so that the infant is not burned and the warming device does not cool and secondarily cool the extremity if left in place for too long. All the values will be unreliable if the extremity is edematous, acrocyanotic, or not warmed or if the infant has poor peripheral circulation. In addition, because this procedure, like arterial puncture, is painful, it reflects the infant's condition during crying, which may be vastly different from rest. Finally, if there is difficulty obtaining the sample, the results may reflect air or tissue contamination rather than the infant's true status.

### SIMPLY STATED

Capillary blood samples from the infant usually reflect Pco$_2$ and pH values reasonably close to those of arterial blood; however, the Po$_2$ of capillary blood is often significantly below that of arterial blood and should not be used for clinical decision making. To assess Po$_2$ accurately an ABG should be drawn.

### Venous Blood Gases

Venous blood samples can also be obtained for gas analysis. These are useful in computing the oxygen extraction or carbon dioxide production of tissues (see Chapter 14). Great care should be exercised if using venous blood samples for routine

gas analysis. The values obtained by this method may be very misleading.

### Noninvasive Monitors

One of the most significant advances in monitoring sick newborns has been the development of transcutaneous oxygen and carbon dioxide monitors. These monitors give caregivers up-to-date information that would otherwise be unavailable. In newborn intensive care units, these devices can be used around the clock to monitor sick infants and for trending.

*Transcutaneous Oxygen Monitors.* Transcutaneous oxygen pressure (tcPo$_2$) monitors measure electrical current that is directly proportional to the number of oxygen molecules present in the electrode (e.g., the Clark electrode). The tcPo$_2$ electrode measures oxygen present in the underlying capillaries and tissue of the skin and not Pao$_2$ directly, but tcPo$_2$ usually approximates Pao$_2$, with tcPo$_2$ slightly lower than Pao$_2$. Any condition that decreases blood flow under the electrode, such as acidosis, shock, hypovolemia, or hypoglycemia, can cause tcPo$_2$ to be falsely lower than Pao$_2$.

The tcPo$_2$ monitor is a good method of evaluating the physiologic changes that occur with blood gas sampling. The pain of blood gas sampling can cause changes in the infant's resting condition. The infant can produce an increase in Paco$_2$ and a decrease in Pao$_2$ by becoming apneic. If the infant cries and hyperventilates, the Paco$_2$ might decrease and the Pao$_2$ might increase. The person obtaining the sample should note the tcPo$_2$ value three times: before disturbing the infant, at the beginning of blood flow, and 40 to 60 seconds after completion of sampling. These three values can then be used to assess the infant's resting condition, the physiologic changes the procedure caused, and the correlation between Pao$_2$ and tcPo$_2$.

In a neonate with a CCHD or heart condition, the position of the Ptco$_2$ electrode will also allow for the comparison of preductal and postductal Po$_2$ values. The right upper chest just below the right clavicle is the recommended site for the preductal electrode position. Any other position in the body is considered postductal except the right arm.

*Transcutaneous Carbon Dioxide Monitors.* Transcutaneous carbon dioxide pressure (tcPco$_2$) electrodes are used clinically. Similar to the tcPo$_2$ electrodes, they measure the gas present in the underlying skin and not gas present in the blood. The tcPco$_2$ electrode has merit as a trend monitor for carbon dioxide.

There are still problems with both tcPo$_2$ and tcPco$_2$. Both techniques use heated electrodes, which must be repositioned every 2 to 4 hours. The heater element in the electrode can cause burns. The tape used to secure the electrode may tear the fragile skin of a preterm infant during repositioning. The monitors have slow response times and are subject to multiple skin perfusion artifacts. Other than difficulty validating the $tcPO_2$ and $tcPCO_2$ against the patient's arterial values, the most common problem with transcutaneous monitoring is air leaks around the adhesive ring. Air leaks always cause a dramatic fall in $tcPCO_2$. If the leak is large, the $tcPO_2$ and $tcPCO_2$ values will mimic those in room air ($PO_2 \sim 150$ mm Hg; $PCO_2 \sim 0$ mm Hg). In these cases, you should reapply the sensor using a new adhesive ring.

New available technologies in blood gas monitoring have improved some of these drawbacks and have made transcutaneous gas monitoring a more reliable source for clinical information and decision making in the neonatal intensive care unit.

*Pulse Oximeters.* Pulse oximetry has become a useful monitoring tool and a standard of care in neonatal and pediatric medicine. Pulse oximeters measure the changing transmission of red and infrared light through a pulsating capillary bed to identify the saturation of the hemoglobin. They overcome many of the problems of the transcutaneous monitors. The oximeter is not heated; therefore it does not require repositioning and does not cause burns. It has a much faster response time, and it does not require tight taping to the skin. (See Chapter 14 for a further discussion of pulse oximeters.)

Pulse oximetry screening for CCHD is recommended for all newborns. Pulse oximetry screening during the first 48 hours of life can identify some infants with a CCHD before they show any signs.

A finding of oxygen saturation of less than 95% in both extremities warrants a repeat screen (after 1 hour) to reduce false-positive results. A second finding of less than 95% warrants a third screen. A positive pulse oximetry screen is defined as a greater than 3% absolute difference in oxygen saturation between the right hand and foot on three measures, each separated by 1 hour. A negative screen was defined as a finding 95% or higher in either extremity with 3% or less absolute difference in oxygen saturation between the upper and lower extremities. Once identified, babies with a CCHD can receive specialized care and treatment that could prevent death or disability early in life.

### SIMPLY STATED

Pulse oximetry screening is a low-cost and safe procedure that when performed both preductally and postductally can detect 100% of infants with pulmonary duct-dependent circulation (e.g., PDA). When combined with routine clinical examination during the first 24 hours of life before hospital discharge, it may also detect infants with CCHD and has a higher detection rate than physical examination alone.

## Pulmonary Function Testing
### Volumes

Pulmonary function can be tested in newborns and small infants. In the past few years, standard computerized equipment for infant pulmonary function testing has become available. This has taken pulmonary function testing in this age group out of the realm of the research laboratory and made it available to the clinician. Although nurseries that measure pulmonary function usually are still found in major teaching and research institutions, now small institutions without major research support can be involved in pulmonary function testing. A variety of technologies that compute pulmonary functions exist. These devices are capable of traditional lung mechanics, active and passive exhalation mechanics, and FRC measurements using either helium dilution or nitrogen washout techniques. New techniques are being developed to measure FRC that use ultrasonic washout methods.

The fundamental difference between newborn and adult pulmonary function testing is the patient's ability to cooperate. The ability of adults and children to perform standard pulmonary function tests depends on the patient's ability to follow simple commands, which typically occurs at age 5 or 6 years old. The tests performed on infants must be reproducible without patient cooperation.

Three volumes can be measured easily in newborns independent of their cooperation: FRC, thoracic gas volume (TGV), and crying vital capacity (CVC). However, a certain degree of caution must be exercised when interpreting the results of these tests. The range of normal values is great, and all three tests are subject to error. To compare the results of these tests for two babies or even for the same baby at different times, the results must be described against a standard unit. Usually, this is done with the body weight in kilograms (e.g., milliliters of gas per kilogram), body length in centimeters (e.g., milliliters of gas per centimeter), or body surface area (e.g., milliliters of gas per square meter).

FRC is measured by two methods: closed-system helium dilution and open-system nitrogen washout. Both methods are available with the computerized pulmonary function machines. TGV requires the use of a plethysmograph and measures all of the gas in the thoracic cavity whether it is communicating with the airway or not. By comparing the TGV with the FRC, the clinician can determine the presence of trapped gas in the thorax. The use of plethysmography in infants and children is very difficult and is not typically available in most centers.

CVC is the measurement of tidal volume while the infant is crying. It is useful in following infants who have lung diseases that cause changes in FRC (e.g., RDS) in whom it is difficult to measure FRC. CVC does require that the infant be able to cry vigorously, which may be difficult for sick infants.

A method of measuring distribution of ventilation is available using a nitrogen washout curve. The lung clearance index (LCI) obtained from a multiple breath tracer gas washing or washout curve is the most frequently reported measure of ventilation inhomogeneity in infants because it is clearly defined and easy to comprehend from expired nitrogen concentrations obtained during a nitrogen washout test. The LCI can be used to evaluate what percentage of the lung is ventilating effectively. This measurement does not require active cooperation and can be performed in ventilated and sedated infants.

The most important clinical lung volume measurement is the FRC. The lung mechanics are affected if the FRC is either too high or too low, so it is imperative that clinicians be able to regulate FRC. In either situation (high or low FRC), the compliance decreases, the resistance increases, and $PaCO_2$ is significant elevated. Low FRC can also cause the $PaO_2$ to drop significantly.

RDS causes the FRC to be decreased. Meconium aspiration syndrome (MAS) and PIE are diseases in which FRC is increased. Diseases such as pneumonia and BPD may have either decreased or increased FRCs, depending on the current stage of the disease and the respiratory support being used.

## Mechanics

*Compliance.* Compliance is a measure of the distensibility of the lung. It is calculated by dividing change in volume by change in pressure and requires measurement of tidal volume and transpulmonary pressure. Tidal volume can be measured in newborns by either pneumotachography or plethysmography. Plethysmographs are tricky to use with infants because making an airtight seal around the face is difficult. In addition, plethysmographs for infants are all custom made. Therefore most nurseries measure tidal volume by pneumotachography.

Transpulmonary pressure is the difference between alveolar pressure and pleural pressure. It is approximated by measuring airway and esophageal pressure in intubated infants and esophageal pressure in nonintubated infants. Either an air-filled balloon or saline-filled catheter in midesophagus can be used. Tidal volume is integrated from the pneumotachometer signal, a pressure-volume loop is constructed, and the compliance of the lung is calculated. The compliance of the chest wall can also be measured by changing the two pressure sources from airway minus esophageal to esophageal minus atmospheric pressure.

Compliance is significantly lower in infants with RDS. Compliance begins to improve dramatically with the return of surfactant function in the lung. Compliance is also lower in infants with BPD, PIE, and pneumonia.

*Resistance.* Resistance is a measure of the inhibition of gas flow through airways. It is calculated by dividing change in transpulmonary pressure by change in flow. These measurements are obtained with the same equipment used for compliance.

Resistance is elevated in infants with MAS and BPD. The airway resistance in infants with MAS remains elevated for several weeks until the chemical inflammatory phase of the disease is resolved. Infants with BPD will probably have increased airway resistance all of their lives.

*Work of Breathing.* The work of breathing (WOB) is the cumulative product of the pressure generated and the volume at each instant of the respiratory cycle. It is usually calculated by calculating the area between the pressure-volume curve and the volume axis or by electrically integrating the pressure and volume signals using an esophageal catheter.

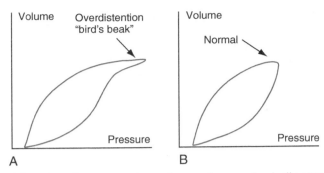

**FIG. 12.11** Pressure-volume loops of a mechanically ventilated infant showing overdistention (A) and normal inflation pressures (B).

**FIG. 12.12** Volume-time curves of a mechanically ventilated infant show air leak around the endotracheal (ET) tube (A) and no air leak (B).

Airway resistance is the major contributor to the area of a pressure-volume loop, and work of breathing is increased in the diseases that have major resistive components: MAS and BPD.

*Lung Mechanics with Mechanical Ventilators.* The newer, more sophisticated infant ventilators can measure the mechanical properties of the respiratory system in the newborn during mechanical ventilation. These new ventilators allow the clinician to match the settings of the ventilator with the individual needs of the infant. It is possible to diagnose overdistention (Fig. 12.11), air leak (Fig. 12.12), short inspiratory time (Fig. 12.13), and other dysfunctional ventilator-patient interactions. These ventilators are capable of synchronizing the mechanical cycle with the infant's spontaneous breaths.

Newer modes of ventilation, such as airway pressure release ventilation-assist (APRV), neurally adjusted ventilatory assist (NAVA), and closed-loop ventilation, among others, will respond to the patient's chest and lung mechanics, as well as to physiology parameters as determined by the mode and the clinician. These newer modes provide lung-protective strategies, improve patient-ventilator synchrony, and optimize gas exchange and lung volumes in neonates and infants. They also provide a plethora of clinical data regarding the infant's lung and the patient-ventilator interface, helping to fine-tune the ventilatory management of neonates and children.

## Chemoreceptor Response

Sudden infant death syndrome (SIDS) has stimulated a tremendous amount of research into the way infants

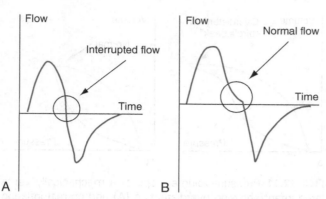

**FIG. 12.13** Flow-time curves of a mechanically ventilated infant show interrupted inspiratory flow secondary to inadequate inspiratory time (A) and normal inspiratory flow with adequate inspiratory time (B).

control respiration. Some investigators have shown that newborns have a blunted response to hypercapnia and a severely diminished or paradoxic response to hypoxia. Many nurseries have the ability to look at carbon dioxide and oxygen responses. These studies are usually performed by measuring tidal volume, minute ventilation, end-tidal oxygen and carbon dioxide, and transcutaneous oxygen levels. The infant's minute ventilation is then plotted against $Paco_2$ or $Fio_2$ to assess the infant's ventilatory response to increased $Paco_2$.

## Radiographs

Chest radiography is discussed in detail in Chapter 10. However, radiographic views and the methods for obtaining radiographs are significantly different between infants and older children. In the older pediatric patient, the preferred position for taking x-ray films is upright. Infants cannot be placed upright easily, and they dislike being forced to lie on their stomachs; thus most chest x-ray films are taken with the infant in the supine position, lying on the x-ray film. The x-ray beam passes from the front to the back of the infant (AP view). Most adult radiographs are taken in the posteroanterior (PA) view, which minimizes distortion and enhances the quality of the film.

The typical views used to evaluate an infant's lung are AP and lateral chest films. As in the older patient, these two views allow the clinician to see all areas of the lung in a standard presentation. It is important that the viewer approach the reading of these films systematically. The viewer should evaluate the airways, including the larynx, trachea, and major bronchi, for deviation from external masses or pressure, for filling defects from internal masses or hypoplasia, and for normal location in the chest.

Occasionally, decubitus films of the chest and abdomen are helpful in evaluating the status of the newborn. They can be useful in detecting the presence of fluid or air in the pleural space. Inspiratory and expiratory chest films are also useful in evaluating the presence of a foreign body. Most aspirated foreign bodies are radiolucent and will not show in a chest radiograph. However, in an expiratory film, the lung area below the

mechanical obstruction will remain hyperinflated when compared with an inspiratory film on the same patient, letting the clinician know the probable position of the foreign body.

Chest radiographs should be done in infants who have unexplained tachypnea, cyanosis, abnormal breath sounds, malformations of the chest or airway, or an overall generalized sick appearance. In addition, any infant who has a significant worsening of clinical status should have a chest radiograph. This might include infants who suddenly have an increase in respiratory rate, the appearance or worsening of retractions, or a sudden increase in $Paco_2$. Less obvious, but equally important, is the need to obtain a chest radiograph in mechanically ventilated infants who suddenly improve clinically. This is especially true for infants who are being mechanically ventilated with high-frequency ventilators, which can make physical assessment much more difficult (e.g., breath sounds cannot be evaluated).

The two classic newborn lung diseases are RDS and MAS. RDS is a disease of inadequate surfactant production. The immature alveoli have increased surface tension and collapse. The chest radiograph of these infants is fairly typical. It includes a diffuse, hazy ground-glass appearance; air bronchograms extending out to the periphery of the lungs; and low lung volumes (Fig. 12.14). MAS is primarily an airway disease. The stressed mature fetus passes meconium into the amniotic fluid and then with gasping respirations inhales the meconium-laden amniotic fluid into its lungs. The disease has two phases: an early mechanical phase and a late chemical phase. The chest radiograph shows a typical pattern of mixed atelectasis and local emphysema (Fig. 12.15).

TTN is another disease that has diagnostic radiographs. In TTN, the amniotic fluid in the lung is incompletely resorbed at the time of delivery. The characteristic chest radiograph shortly after birth shows diffuse streakiness and fluid in the major and minor fissures. This is impossible to distinguish from the chest radiograph of pneumonia. The characteristic of TTN is the rapid resolution of the disease. By 24 hours of age, the newborn's chest radiograph is typically normal (Fig. 12.16). A description of radiologic findings for additional neonatal and pediatric pathologies can be found in Table 12.13.

Other imaging techniques available for the assessment of the fetus and neonate are high-resolution ultrasound, rapid-sequencing magnetic resonance imaging (MRI), and even three-dimensional computed tomography (CT). These techniques provide exquisite detail regarding the fetus and the intrauterine environment.

**FIG. 12.14** Anteroposterior (A) and lateral (B) chest radiographs of a preterm infant with respiratory distress syndrome. Both views show diffuse, hazy ground glass appearance, air bronchograms, and low lung volumes.

**FIG. 12.15** Anteroposterior chest radiograph of a term infant with meconium aspiration syndrome (MAS). This view shows the typical pattern of mixed atelectasis and local emphysema. An endotracheal tube is seen in good position.

Imaging advances in fluoroscopy, ultrasound, MRI, and CT continue to provide improved care of the neonate. Fluoroscopy can quickly identify life-threatening abnormalities of the gastrointestinal tract such as meconium ileus and esophageal atresia. Ultrasound remains essential in neonatal imaging of the brain, chest, and abdomen because of the lack of radiation, the portability, and the lack of sedation requirements. MRI-compatible incubators have improved the safety of performing the examination on unstable infants. Multidetector CT with multiplanar reconstruction and three-dimensional volume rendering are infrequently used in neonates because of the high radiation exposure; however, they can quickly provide critical information in the unstable infant with pulmonary or vascular abnormalities.

**FIG. 12.16** Two anteroposterior chest radiographs of an infant with transient tachypnea of the newborn (TTN). **A,** First day of life. **B,** Second day of life.

**TABLE 12.13    Most Common Radiologic Findings in the Neonatal and Pediatric Population**

| Disease | Pathology | Description |
|---|---|---|
| BPD | This is a complication from a combination of respiratory distress, mechanical ventilation, and high concentration of oxygen over a prolonged period of time (>28 days). | X-ray findings of stage four BPD may show multiple pneumothoraces, in a sponge-like "honeycomb pattern" with flattened diaphragm. |
| PIE | Occurs when air is present outside the normal airways within the interstitium of the lung; it may develop into a pneumothorax or pneumomediastinum. | CXR findings show air trapping with barrel chest or increased AP diameter and irregular "bubbles" in the hilar area radiating outward. |
| Pneumonia | Commonly caused by lower respiratory tract infections. Viruses are the most common cause in children. | CXR may resemble RDS/BPD and have bilateral infiltrates and diffused lung markings. Consolidation of a lobe or segment is very rare in neonates. |
| Tetralogy of Fallot | CCHD consisting of four specific malformations: VSD, malpositioned aorta, pulmonary stenosis, and right ventricular hypertrophy | Echocardiogram and CXR show a "boot-shaped heart." Pulmonary congestion may appear with patchy infiltrates and increased vascular markings. |
| Transposition of the great vessels | Reversal of the origin of the aorta and the pulmonary artery, so the right ventricle leads to the aorta and the left to the pulmonary artery. | Echocardiogram and CXR show an "egg-shaped heart," as well as the transposed vessels. |
| Congenital diaphragmatic hernia | Results from the absence or incomplete development of one of the hemidiaphragms, allowing the abdominal organs to enter the thorax. | CXR shows abdominal organs in the thoracic area and atelectasis; 90% of hernias occur on the left. |

*AP,* Anteroposterior; *BPD,* bronchopulmonary dysplasia; *CCHD,* critical congenital heart disease; *CXR,* chest x-ray; *PIE,* pulmonary interstitial emphysema; *RDS,* respiratory distress syndrome; *VSD,* ventricular septal defect.

## Apnea Monitoring

Apnea monitoring is designed to warn of life-threatening respiratory and cardiac events, most often in neonates. Apnea monitors use two electrodes placed on the chest wall to detect respiratory movements through changes in electrical impedance, with most units also able to detect heart rate through the electrocardiogram signal.

Apnea monitoring is indicated in neonates at risk for recurrent apnea, bradycardia, and hypoxemia. This procedure may also be considered for infants

- Receiving drug therapy (e.g., caffeine) for a history of apnea and bradycardia
- With bronchopulmonary dysplasia, especially those requiring supplemental oxygen

- With symptomatic gastroesophageal reflux
- Born to a substance-abusing mother if clinically symptomatic
- With a tracheostomy or an airway abnormality that increases the risk for obstruction
- With neurologic or metabolic disorders affecting respiratory control

Apnea monitoring is often done within a hospital or clinic but continues to be performed from the home once the patient is discharged. In the case of home monitoring (see Chapter 20), it is essential that the parents and all other caregivers receive proper training on the apnea monitoring equipment and on responding to actual episodes of apnea and bradycardia, before the patient is discharged.

# ASSESSMENT OF CRITICALLY ILL INFANTS

## Airway

Evaluation of airway patency in newborns is not as easy as it is in adults and older children. Infants with obstructed airways still have chest wall motion, and with chest auscultation they may even make noises that could be misinterpreted as breath sounds. The clinician needs a thorough knowledge of normal newborn breath sounds and chest wall motion to be able to evaluate airway patency in infants.

Even experienced clinicians can be deceived about the adequacy of the airway in intubated infants because the signs usually used in the older patient may not be reliable in the newborn. For example, an infant whose right main stem bronchus is intubated may still have breath sounds in the left hemithorax, as well as left chest wall motion. This can occur because of the short tracheal lengths (<10 cm) and the increased compliance of the chest wall. The clinician must be careful to compare all of the lung fields when auscultating. A misplaced endotracheal tube creates a subtle difference in breath sounds, particularly in the apices, which can be picked up by the careful clinician.

The synchrony of spontaneous ventilation rate compared with mechanical ventilation rate is more important than its frequency in the newborn. An infant who exhales during the inspiratory phase of the ventilator can generate tremendous intrathoracic pressures, potentially damaging the lung. Asynchronous breathing between the infant and the ventilator usually is seen during the hours and days immediately after intubation and the start of mechanical ventilation. The clinician must watch the infant's chest wall motion while listening to the ventilator cycle to document this asynchronous breathing. An inward motion of the chest or absence of an outward motion of the chest wall during mechanical inspiration may indicate that the infant is breathing asynchronously with the ventilator.

One major cause of neonate/infant ventilator asynchrony is the trigger setting in the ventilator, also called ventilator sensitivity. Mechanical ventilators use a variety of triggers for the infant to control the initiation of the breath. These triggers are volume (through either pneumotachography or hot-wire anemometry), abdominal wall motion, thoracic impedance, and flow triggering. The important characteristics that must be present for any of the systems to be useful are sensitivity to small changes and rapid response time.

The airway pressures monitored in infants are the peak inspiratory pressure (PIP), mean airway pressure (MAP), positive end-expiratory pressure (PEEP), and, occasionally, esophageal pressure. These pressures are interpreted like their counterparts in the adult intensive care unit (see Chapter 14).

Static airway pressure, intrapleural pressure, lung volume, and expired gas analysis generally are not used in the clinical management of newborns. Airway resistance and lung compliance are being used clinically more often with the advent of reproducible, easy-to-use neonatal pulmonary function equipment.

## Tracheostomy

Special assessment consideration should be given to the infant or older child who has undergone a tracheotomy procedure. Congenital defects, acquired airway lesions, tracheal malacia, neuromuscular disorders, and ventilator dependency are the most common indications for this procedure in the infant population. Emphasis should be put on assessment of airway patency and signs of distress to prevent short- and long-term complications. Caregiver education and monitoring of the child play an important role in preventing complications.

Factors to consider when assessing risk for complications in a child with a tracheostomy include age, size of the tracheostomy, degree of airway obstruction, behavior of the child, underlying airway pathology, presence of other medical conditions, and social environment. Common signs and symptoms that may indicate airway patency compromise include rattling or "noisy" secretions, thick and inspissated secretions, inability to cough and clear secretions, silent cough, absent or diminished breath sounds, lack of air movement felt around the tracheostomy or mouth, increased work of breathing, and pallor or cyanosis. For some high-risk tracheostomy patients who have a history of airway instability, 24-hour home nursing monitoring may be necessary.

## Hemodynamic Assessments

Hemodynamic monitoring in the critically ill infant is in some ways easier and in other ways more difficult than in the adult. The presence of patent umbilical vessels makes cannulation of the aorta and inferior vena cava simple. However, cannulation of the pulmonary artery is difficult and usually must be performed in a cardiac catheterization laboratory in specialized centers. In addition, the newborn may have varying degrees of right-to-left shunt, depending on the pulmonary vascular resistance, with the presence of a PDA and a patent foramen ovale. This makes calculation of cardiac output difficult if not impossible.

Cannulation of the umbilical artery and vein is a routine practice in most nurseries. The technique for such a cannulation is easy, and although there are risks to indwelling central catheters, they can be minimized by using a good technique and appropriate indications. In addition, many nurseries are now using percutaneous cannulation of radial arteries and subclavian veins in neonates. The indications for umbilical artery catheterization include a source for frequent ABG sampling, continuous blood pressure monitoring, and large-scale blood replacement (e.g., exchange transfusion). The indications for umbilical venous catheterization include central venous pressure monitoring and large-scale blood replacement. The course of the umbilical artery and vein is shown in Fig. 12.17.

These two methods of hemodynamic monitoring are susceptible to many of the same problems that exist in adults and older children. Signal damping is a major concern for several reasons: the small internal lumina of the catheters involved, softer materials used in catheter production, and development of fibrin sleeves. Infections, thrombus formation, embolization, and arteriospasm are also major concerns when

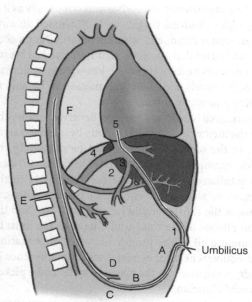

FIG. 12.17 Lateral radiograph and diagram of the course of umbilical venous and arterial catheters. Umbilical venous catheter enters through umbilicus, passes through 1, umbilical vein; 2, portal vein; 3, ductus venosus; and 4, inferior vena cava and stops in 5, right atrium. Umbilical arterial catheter enters through umbilicus, passes through A, umbilical artery; B, hypogastric artery; C, internal iliac artery; D, common iliac artery; and E, abdominal aorta and stops in F, thoracic aorta.

using these monitoring methods. Newer and safer methods of monitoring hemodynamic parameters noninvasively (see Chapter 14) have been developed for adults but have not crossed over yet to the neonatal and infant population.

## ASSESSMENT OF THE OLDER INFANT AND CHILD

### History

The history of the older infant and the child combines that of the newborn and the adult. The parents remain the major source of information about the infant or child until adolescence. Until age 2 years, it is important to include the birth history as part of the evaluation of these patients. The clinician assessing the patient must begin to include a review of systems in the historical assessment at 3 months of age. The review of systems may not be of great benefit before this.

It is important to differentiate acute from chronic problems. When did the symptoms begin? How rapidly have the symptoms progressed? Is the child truly sick or just not feeling well?

The clinician inquiring about the pulmonary symptoms in an older infant or child is limited to signs that are visible or audible to the parent. Historical information about coughing, wheezing, cyanosis, purulent nasal discharge, frequent colds or infections, and change in behavior is easy to obtain. Dyspnea, chest pain, night sweats, and other symptoms that are not observable by the parent may be impossible

to document. It should be remembered that hemoptysis and sputum expectoration do not occur in children. Most children swallow any mucus, blood, or purulent material that might be generated by the upper or lower airway.

In addition to experiencing the usual respiratory symptoms, the older infant and child often have extrapulmonary symptoms caused by pulmonary disease. The careful clinician queries parents about these symptoms. The most obvious of these signs is general activity. Infants and children who are sick act differently from well babies and children. The parents or guardians are the best judges of an infant's or a child's normal behavior. The clinician must be alert to a parent's statement that the child is acting differently, particularly not eating or not playing. The interviewer should inquire about the infant's feeding habits if the parents do not bring this up.

Gastrointestinal upset is a common complaint in infants and children and can lead to dehydration and hypovolemia. Vomiting and diarrhea are major causes for hospitalization in this age group. Many people who take care of infants and children forget that vomiting and diarrhea may be manifestations of pneumonia or other pulmonary diseases. In addition, diseases such as cystic fibrosis and gastroesophageal reflux may have gastrointestinal and pulmonary symptoms.

Finally, an infant or child who does not maintain growth appropriate for developmental age (failure to thrive) should be investigated for an underlying chronic pulmonary disease. In this age group, such diseases include asthma, cystic fibrosis, gastroesophageal reflux, foreign body aspiration, chronic infection (e.g., sinusitis, cytomegalovirus, tuberculosis, sarcoidosis, histoplasmosis, coccidioidomycosis, bronchiectasis, lung abscess, and empyema), nonasthmatic allergic pulmonary diseases, neuromuscular disease affecting the chest wall, and immotile cilia syndrome.

## Physical Examination

The components of the physical examination discussed in Chapter 5 are the basis for the physical examination of an older infant or child. Observation, palpation, percussion, and auscultation should be used to localize the disease process within the patient's body. The uniqueness of the physical examination in the older infant or child is in the order in which the examination progresses. It is most important to gain the infant's or child's trust and cooperation. The clinician should first examine the parts that upset or frighten the infant or child the least, saving for last the parts of the examination that are upsetting or frightening. If possible, the clinician should make a game out of the examination.

Asthma is especially common in children and adolescents. Various age-specific questionnaires and other similar diagnostic tools can be helpful to RTs and other clinicians in assessing the presence of this disease and the extent to which it is, or is not, well controlled. These tools generally rely on a combination of information from the patient's history as well as findings from direct patient assessment.

If these criteria are not met, the child's asthma would be classified as *not well controlled*. In these situations the treatment regimen should be intensified or "stepped up," and the patient should be reassessed in 2 to 6 weeks.

---

**SIMPLY STATED**

If asthmatic children display daytime symptoms one or more times per week or nighttime symptoms more than one to two times per month, they are using their short-acting bronchodilator more than once per week, or their activities are limited as a result of their condition, their asthma should be classified as *not well controlled*. As a result, the RT should recommend that their treatment plan be modified and that they be reassessed within 2 to 6 weeks.

---

Asthma is an increasingly prevalent disease in children of all ages beyond infancy. Asthma is a chronic airway disease that is caused by airway inflammation and hyperresponsiveness to irritants. The typical symptoms include intermittent dry cough and expiratory wheezing. Young children may report nonfocal chest pain. Older children may report shortness of breath and chest tightness. Severe exacerbations may include airflow obstruction that can be life threatening. In 2007 the National Institutes of Health (NIH) issued its third Expert Panel Report detailing the guidelines for the diagnosis and management of asthma. According to these guidelines, the functions of assessment and monitoring for asthma are closely linked to the concepts of severity, control, and responsiveness to treatment. Both severity and control include the domains of current impairment and future risk of the asthmatic patient. The ultimate goal of treatment is to enable a patient to live symptom free, and an initial assessment of the severity of the disease allows an estimate of the type and intensity of treatment needed to achieve this goal.

The following are some criteria used to assess and classify asthma patients as being well controlled (or not):

- Daytime symptoms ≤ days per week, *and*
- Awakenings at night from asthma ≤1/month if <12 years old, or ≤2/month if ≥12 years old, *and*
- No limitation to exercise, *and*
- Use of short-acting β-adrenergic bronchodilators ≤2 days/week, *and*
- Less than or equal to 1 course of oral corticosteroids per year, *and*
- Forced expiratory volume in 1 second ($FEV_1$) ≥80% predicted, *and*
- $FEV_1/FVC$ ≥85% (for patients up to 19 years old).

Two other major respiratory diseases in the young child are croup and epiglottitis. Croup is usually a viral disease affecting the trachea and small airways in children. Croup tends to appear in children between 3 months and 5 years old, but it can happen at any age. Some children are prone to croup and may get it several times. The child may have cold symptoms, such as a stuffy or runny nose, for a few days and may also have a fever. These symptoms progress to a loud, seal-like barking cough; rapid or difficult respiration; and grunting or wheezing while breathing. In severe cases, the child may develop stridor (high-pitched squeaking noise during inspiration) or cyanosis. An AP neck radiograph usually shows a narrowed subglottic airway (termed the *steeple sign*). The symptoms of croup often worsen when the infant is upset or crying and at night. Scoring systems have been developed to help quantify the degree of illness with croup. These scoring systems often can be used with minimal disturbance of the sick and often anxious child. A scoring system developed by Leipzig and colleagues has been widely used for children with croup (Table 12.14). It has been independently validated and has been shown to be a reliable score. A score greater than 5 is an indication of impending airway obstruction.

Epiglottitis is usually a bacterial disease that causes significant edema and inflammation of the epiglottis. Epiglottitis is now very uncommon because the *Haemophilus influenzae* type B (Hib) vaccine is a routine childhood immunization. The disease was once most often seen in children ages 2 to 6 years. Rarely, epiglottitis can occur in adults. The child with epiglottitis presents with drooling, dysphasia, and respiratory distress. All these symptoms come from the swelling and inflammation of the epiglottis. These children are usually febrile and appear sick and anxious. They often have stridor. They usually do not cough. Epiglottitis can be a life-threatening disease that should be treated as an emergency. The child with epiglottitis should not be disturbed until the airway is secured. However, if a lateral film is done, it will show a swollen epiglottis blocking the upper airway (usually called the *thumb sign*).

**TABLE 12.14** Croup Assessment Scoring System

| | CROUP SCORE | | | |
|---|---|---|---|---|
| | 0 | 1 | 2 | 3 |
| Stridor | None | Faintly audible | Easily audible | — |
| Sternal retraction | None | Minimal | Obvious | — |
| **Respiratory rate (breaths/min)** | | | | |
| 0-5 kg | <35 | 36-40 | 41-45 | >45 |
| 5.1-10 kg | <30 | 21-24 | 25-30 | >30 |
| >10 kg | <20 | 21-24 | 25-30 | >30 |
| **Pulse rate (beats/min)** | | | | |
| <3 months | <150 | 151-165 | 166-190 | >90 |
| 3-6 months | <130 | 131-145 | 146-170 | >170 |
| 7-12 months | <120 | 120-135 | 136-150 | >150 |
| 1-3 years | <110 | 111-125 | 126-140 | >140 |
| 3-5 years | <90 | 91-100 | 101-120 | >120 |

The respiratory rate is adjusted for body weight and the pulse rate for age.
From Jacobs S, Shortland G, Warner J, et al: Validation of a croup score and its use in triaging children with croup, *Anaesthesia* 49(10):903-906, 1994.

## Clinical Laboratory Data

Older infants, children, and adolescents tend to have a narrower range of normal values on both clinical laboratory and blood gas laboratory tests. Their normal values tend to reflect the normal values seen in adults. Although some laboratory tests show a wide divergence from adult values (e.g., growth hormone and others), in most clinical situations the normal values for adults can also be used for children.

Other special tests are occasionally used in this age group for the diagnosis of diseases that have a major pulmonary component. Sweat chloride is the most prominent of these. This test is used to diagnose cystic fibrosis. It is simple to perform, but laboratories often obtain erroneous results because of poor methods or techniques. Sweat chloride levels higher than 60 mmol/L are considered indicative of cystic fibrosis. However, levels as low as 39 mmol/L have also been recommended as a threshold for cystic fibrosis diagnosis.

## Blood Gases

The older infant and child present a unique problem in obtaining and interpreting blood gases. Their arteries are still small, and arterial puncture is not easy. Most of these patients vigorously object to having an arterial puncture performed even if they are sick. Therefore more than one person is usually required to obtain the sample. As in the newborn, the older infant and child can quickly change ABG values by crying and hyperventilating. The clinician interpreting the ABG sample should be aware of the patient's disease, as well as what conditions existed when the sample was obtained.

Pulse oximetry is more reliable in this age group than is transcutaneous monitoring. There is a greater difference between arterial and transcutaneous gas values because of the increased thickness of the skin and subcutaneous tissue. However, transcutaneous monitoring is still useful as a trending device to identify changes in the patient's status. It is also useful in estimating the true arterial gas value because the value may have changed during the sampling process.

## Pulmonary Function Testing

Beyond the newborn and young infant stage, standard pulmonary function testing is not possible until the child is 5 years of age. There are two important points to remember when doing pulmonary function tests on a child. First, the validity of the results is directly related to the child's cooperation. Children in the 5- to 8-year age range can have remarkably short attention spans and be frustratingly uncooperative. Second, the lungs of the child are still growing, and the results of pulmonary function tests must be adjusted to body size.

Pulmonary function testing is particularly useful in children with asthma. Machines are now available for clinical use in the outpatient setting. These allow rapid diagnosis of expiratory collapse. Most of these systems use a forced exhalation, measuring peak expiratory flow. With increasing bronchospasm, the child has progressively lower peak flows and a scooped rather than linear expiratory flow pattern (Fig. 12.18).

Impulse oscillometry (IOS) is a fairly new technique being used for the diagnosis and management of respiratory and allergic diseases in children. IOS measures respiratory function during normal breathing by transmitting mixed-frequency rectangular pressure impulses down the airways and measuring the resultant pressure and flow relationships, which describe the mechanical parameters of the lungs. This technique requires little patient cooperation because only tidal volume breaths are required, and children as young as 2 years old can be readily examined. Thus measurement of pulmonary resistance in preschool-age children can be used to diagnose and manage respiratory diseases. Currently, this innovative technique has produced excellent results for pediatric pulmonary function assessment.

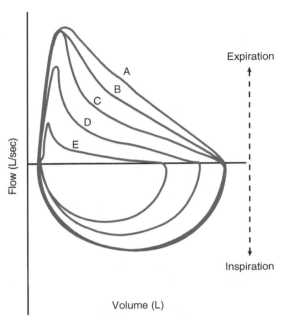

**FIG. 12.18** Forced expiratory flow-volume loops in asthmatic children showing **(A)** normal flow and **(B to E)** progressive worsening of flow with airway constriction.

## Pediatric Bronchoscopy

Traditionally, rigid bronchoscopy (see Chapter 17) has been the bronchoscopic technique of choice to use in infants and children throughout the years. However, the development of smaller, more flexible bronchoscopes has led to the widespread use of this procedure in the pediatric population. Pediatric flexible bronchoscopy is now performed by many medical specialists in a variety of settings and is becoming a major tool for the evaluation of several respiratory disorders. Some of the indications of flexible bronchoscopy in children include stridor, wheeze, cough, radiographic abnormalities, foreign body aspiration, hemoptysis, and inhalation injury.

## Radiographs

As the infant becomes older and progresses through childhood, radiographs become easier to obtain and interpret. After the child can sit erectly, it becomes possible to take a PA chest radiograph. Chapter 10 covers most of the chest radiograph techniques and interpretation that can also be applied to the older child.

A lateral view of the neck can help distinguish between croup and epiglottitis. Subglottic narrowing is present in laryngotracheobronchitis, and supraglottic narrowing with a large thumb-shaped epiglottis is present with epiglottitis, as mentioned in the previous section (Fig. 12.19).

**FIG. 12.19** Lateral neck radiograph demonstrating an enlarged epiglottis *(arrow)*. (Courtesy Lionel Young, MD, Loma Linda University Children's Hospital, Loma Linda, California; from Wilkins RL, Dexter JR: *Respiratory disease: principles of patient care*, Philadelphia, 1993, FA Davis.)

## KEY POINTS

- The newborn's history is obtained from several sources and covers more than just the medical history of the infant. Sources include the parents, the mother's labor and delivery chart, and the infant's chart.
- Obstetricians note the mother's previous pregnancy history in the mother's medical record using the terms *gravida, para,* and *abortion.* Gravida is a pregnant woman, para is a woman who delivers a live infant, and abortion is the delivery of a dead infant.
- In evaluating the infant with respiratory disease, valuable information can be found in the pregnancy, labor, and delivery histories. An infant delivered in the presence of infection has an increased risk for respiratory difficulty.
- The biophysical profile is an ultrasound evaluation of fetal breathing, body movement, tone, reactive heart rate, and amniotic fluid volume. Like the Apgar score, each of these parameters has a maximum score of 2 and a minimum score of 0. The score for a normal fetus is 8 to 10.
- The labor history is obtained to evaluate the well-being of the infant during the transition from intrauterine to extrauterine life.
- The delivery history should include the method of delivery for the infant: vaginal or cesarean section; spontaneous, forceps, or vacuum extraction; or low, middle, or high forceps. Infants with uncomplicated deliveries are usually born by spontaneous or low forceps vaginal deliveries.
- The most standard objective measurement of the newborn's well-being is the Apgar score. This is a simple, quick, and reliable means of assessment. It assigns the infant points for the presence of five specific physical criteria: color, reflex irritability, muscle tone, respiratory effort, and heart rate.
- The Apgar score is useful in identifying infants who need resuscitation. Infants who are adjusting well to extrauterine life usually have 1-minute scores of 7 to 10. Infants who have 1-minute scores of 0 to 3 are severely depressed and need extensive medical care such as intubation and mechanical ventilation.
- The range of normal body temperature in the newborn does not differ from that in the adult.
- Newborn term and preterm infants lose heat easily and are extremely dependent on the environment to help them maintain body temperature.
- Hypothermia is a core body temperature of less than 36.5°C, or 97.7°F. Hypothermia is a more common and significantly more serious sign of infection in the newborn than in the older child or adult.
- Most sick infants are placed in an NTE, which is the environmental temperature at which the infant's metabolic demand and therefore oxygen consumption are the least.
- The normal pulse rate for infants is age and size dependent, is usually between 100 and 160 beats/min, and is a function of the developmental age of the infant.
- Tachycardia in the newborn can be caused by crying, pain, decrease in the circulating blood volume, drugs, hyperthermia, and heart disease.

- The normal respiratory rate for infants is between 30 and 60 breaths/min and is a function of the developmental age of the infant.
- In newborns, tachypnea can be caused by hypoxemia, metabolic and respiratory acidosis, CCHD, anxiety, pain, hyperthermia, and crying.
- The normal values for blood pressure depend on the size of the infant, with pressures decreasing with lower weights. Usually, a term infant's systolic blood pressure should be no higher than 70 mm Hg, with diastolic pressure no higher than 50 mm Hg.
- Inspection is probably the most important and often the most neglected portion of the physical examination of a newborn.
- Retractions (sinking inward of the skin around the chest wall during inspiration) occur when the lung's compliance is less than the compliance of the chest wall or when there is a significant airway obstruction.
- Nasal flaring is the dilation of the alae nasi during inspiration. Nasal flaring is an attempt by the infant to achieve airway dilation to decrease airway resistance, increase gas flow, and achieve a larger tidal volume.
- Grunting is a sound heard at the end of expiration just before rapid inspiration. Grunting is the infant's attempt to increase gas volume in the lung by holding back pressure in the airway.
- Capillary refill is checked on the trunk and extremities. Capillary refill should be less than 3 seconds and will be greater than 3 seconds if the infant has a low cardiac output.
- A decrease in breath sounds implies a decrease in gas flow through the airways, as in RDS, atelectasis, pneumothorax, or pleural effusion.
- Wheezing implies gas flow through constricted airways; infants with BPD may have wheezing.
- Crackles usually imply excess fluid or secretions in the lung (pulmonary edema) or the presence of pneumonia. A loud ripping sound like the separation of Velcro often is associated with the presence of pulmonary interstitial emphysema and atelectasis.
- Leukocytosis, or a WBC count greater than 15,000/mm³, usually is a reflection of the infant's environment rather than of infection, as in the older patient.
- Leukopenia, particularly neutropenia (an absolute neutrophil count of <2000/mm³), is a more ominous sign. Usually, neutropenia indicates an infection and implies that the infant is being overwhelmed.
- The normal values for the RBC count, hematocrit, and hemoglobin depend on the chronologic age of the infant. Blood glucose probably is the most frequent blood chemistry determination made in newborns. This simple test is of tremendous importance because hypoglycemia, or low serum glucose, is as detrimental to the developing newborn's brain as hypoxia.
- Monitoring the blood gas status of newborns is done by analysis of the gas in a blood sample, by transcutaneous monitoring, or by pulse oximetry.

- Normal ABG values in newborns depend on the age of the infant when the blood is drawn.
- Once infants are beyond the transitional period after delivery (usually 4 to 12 hours), their arterial oxygen ($Pao_2$), carbon dioxide ($Paco_2$), and pH values should be similar to those of the older child or adult.
- The $tcPo_2$ electrode measures oxygen present in the capillaries and tissue of the skin and not $Pao_2$, but $tcPo_2$ usually approximates $Pao_2$, with $tcPo_2$ slightly lower than $Pao_2$. Any condition that decreases blood flow under the electrode, such as acidosis, shock, hypovolemia, or hypoglycemia, can cause $tcPo_2$ to be falsely lower than $Pao_2$.
- The fundamental difference between newborn and adult pulmonary function testing is the patient's ability to cooperate.
- Crying vital capacity is the measurement of tidal volume while the infant is crying. It is useful in following infants who have lung diseases that cause changes in FRC (e.g., RDS), in whom it is difficult to measure FRC.
- The most important clinical lung volume measurement in the infant is the FRC. The lung mechanics are affected if the FRC is either too high or too low, so it is imperative that clinicians be able to regulate FRC.
- Compliance is significantly lower in infants with RDS. This begins to improve dramatically with the return of surfactant function in the lung. Compliance is also lower in infants with BPD and pneumonia.
- Chest radiographs should be done in infants who have unexplained tachypnea, cyanosis, abnormal breath sounds, malformations of the chest or airway, or a sick appearance. In addition, any infant who has a significant worsening of clinical status should have a chest radiograph.
- The chest radiograph of infants with RDS shows a diffuse, hazy ground-glass appearance; air bronchograms extending out to the periphery of the lungs; and low lung volumes.
- Impulse oscillometry (IOS) is a PFT technique that can measure oscillatory resistance in the airways and can be helpful in diagnosing allergic respiratory dysfunction in infants and children unable to fully cooperate during PFT.
- Asthmatic children with daytime symptoms one or more times per week or nighttime symptoms more than one to two times per month, who are using their short-acting bronchodilator more than once per week, or whose activities are limited as a result of their condition, have asthma that is *not well controlled*, and their treatment plan should be modified.
- In a child with croup, an AP neck radiograph will show a narrowed subglottic airway, usually called the steeple sign.
- If a lateral film is done in a child with epiglottis, it will show a swollen epiglottis blocking the upper airway, usually called the thumb sign.

## ASSESSMENT QUESTIONS

1. What range of gestational weeks is considered term?
   a. 32 to 36
   b. 34 to 40
   c. 37 to 42
   d. 38 to 44
2. You are looking at the chart of your patient, and in the maternal history you see the following: G3, P2, Ab0. The correct interpretation of the abbreviation is that:
   a. The mother is in her third pregnancy
   b. The mother is in her second pregnancy
   c. The mother has delivered three healthy children
   d. The mother has had one abortion
3. Which of the following conditions is commonly associated with an infant born early in gestation?
   a. Meconium aspiration
   b. RDS
   c. Transient tachypnea of the newborn
   d. Perinatal asphyxia
4. All of the following are part of the biophysical evaluation of the fetus using ultrasound *except*:
   a. Reactive heart rate
   b. Body tone
   c. Amniotic fluid volume
   d. Body temperature
5. What Apgar parameter usually deteriorates first in the hypoxic infant?
   a. Respiratory effort
   b. Heart rate
   c. Muscle tone
   d. Skin color
6. Infants needing extensive medical resuscitation at birth will have Apgar scores in the range of which of the following?
   a. 11 to 13
   b. 7 to 10
   c. 4 to 6
   d. 0 to 3
7. Which of the following is a common cause of hypothermia in the infant?
   a. Infection
   b. Heart failure
   c. Atelectasis
   d. Liver disease
8. What is the upper limit of normal range for heart rate in the newborn?
   a. 120 beats/min
   b. 140 beats/min
   c. 160 beats/min
   d. 180 beats/min
9. All of the following are a typical cause of tachypnea in the newborn *except*:
   a. Hypothermia
   b. Hypoxemia
   c. Respiratory acidosis
   d. Pain

10. In what position should a newborn infant be placed to perform a physical examination?
    a. Prone
    b. Supine
    c. Fowler
    d. Trendelenburg

11. All of the following can account for the presence of chest retractions in a newborn *except:*
    a. Airway obstruction
    b. Decreased lung compliance
    c. Increased work of breathing
    d. Hyperthermia

12. What is indicated by a capillary refill time longer than 3 seconds in an infant?
    a. Normal cardiopulmonary function
    b. Respiratory failure
    c. Decreased cardiac output
    d. Renal failure

13. What effect does abdominal distention have on respiration?
    a. Impedes diaphragm movement
    b. Decreases airway resistance
    c. Decreases work of breathing
    d. Produces periodic apnea

14. Transillumination of an infant's chest may be helpful in diagnosing which of the following conditions?
    a. Pneumothorax
    b. Pneumonia
    c. Meconium aspiration syndrome
    d. Transient tachypnea of the newborn

15. Leukopenia in the infant indicates what type of infection?
    a. Overwhelming infection
    b. Chronic infection
    c. Acute infection
    d. Local infection

16. What clinical problem is associated with low serum levels of calcium and phosphorus?
    a. Acute hypoxia
    b. Liver failure
    c. Poor nutrition
    d. Renal failure

17. What is the normal range for $Pao_2$ at birth?
    a. 40 to 60 mm Hg
    b. 50 to 70 mm Hg
    c. 60 to 80 mm Hg
    d. 70 to 90 mm Hg

18. Which parameter demonstrates the largest difference when comparing capillary blood with arterial blood?
    a. $Po_2$
    b. $Pco_2$
    c. pH
    d. $HCO_3^-$

19. Which of the following conditions is least likely to cause a falsely low $ptco_2$ reading?
    a. Acidosis
    b. Shock
    c. Hypovolemia
    d. Hyperthermia

20. All of the lung volumes are easily measured in the newborn *except:*
    a. Thoracic gas volume
    b. Residual volume
    c. FRC
    d. CVC

21. Which of the following findings is not an indication for a chest radiograph in an infant?
    a. Cyanosis
    b. Unexplained tachypnea
    c. Abnormal breath sounds
    d. Periodic apnea

22. What lung disease of newborns is caused by inadequate surfactant production and leads to a decrease in compliance, as well as a diffuse, ground-glass appearance on the chest radiograph?
    a. RDS
    b. MAS
    c. Infant asthma
    d. TTN

23. All of the following are indications for umbilical artery catheterization in infants *except:*
    a. A source for frequent arterial blood gas samples
    b. Continuous blood pressure monitoring
    c. Accurate cardiac output monitoring
    d. Large-scale blood replacement

24. For older infants and children, all of the following are chronic pulmonary diseases that can cause developmental delays *except:*
    a. Cystic fibrosis
    b. MAS
    c. Bronchopulmonary dysplasia
    d. Bronchiectasis

25. Which of the following is not a recommended method for gaining the trust of young children about to have a physical examination?
    a. Make a game out of the examination
    b. Ensure they are sedated
    c. Start by examining parts that are least likely to upset them
    d. Distract them by letting them play with the stethoscope

26. An acute viral disease affecting the trachea and small airways of young children, causing fever, barking cough, grunting, and wheezing, is known as:
    a. Epiglottitis
    b. Croup
    c. RDS
    d. Asthma

27. An acute bacterial infection causing significant edema and inflammation to the tissue around a child's glottis, often leading to dysphasia and severe respiratory distress, is known as which of the following?
    a. Croup
    b. RDS
    c. Epiglottitis
    d. Asthma

28. Which of the following is a chronic disease caused by airway inflammation and resulting in intermittent wheezing

and dry cough, as well as the possible complaint of chest pain or shortness of breath by an affected child?

a. Asthma

b. Cystic fibrosis

c. Croup

d. Bronchiectasis

29. At about what age does standard pulmonary function testing become possible in children?

a. 2 to 3 years old

b. 3 to 4 years old

c. 5 to 6 years old

d. 8 to 9 years old

30. All of the following factors are considered signs of airway compromise in an infant with a tracheostomy airway *except:*

a. Absence of airflow

b. Silent cough

c. Capillary refill time of <3 seconds

d. Copious, inspissated secretions

## BIBLIOGRAPHY

Dalili H, Sheikh M, Hardani AK, et al. Comparison of the combined versus conventional Apgar scores in predicting adverse neonatal outcomes. *PLOS One.* February 12, 2016;11(2):e0149464.

Fanaroff AA, Martin RJ, Walsh MC, eds. *Behrman's neonatal-perinatal medicine: diseases of the fetus and infant.* 10th ed. St. Louis: Mosby-Elsevier; 2015.

Garbutt JM, Conlon B, Sterkel R, et al. The comparative effectiveness of prednisolone and dexamethasone for children with croup: a community-based randomized trial. *Clin Pediatr.* 2013;52(11):1014–1021.

Gardner SL, Carter B, Enzman-Hine M, Hernandez JA. *Merenstein and Gardner's handbook of neonatal intensive care.* 8th ed. St. Louis: Mosby-Elsevier; 2015.

Hess DR. Respiratory mechanics in mechanically ventilated patients. *Respir Care.* 2014;59(11):1773–1794.

Kattwinkel J, Bloom RJ, eds. *American Academy of Pediatrics and American Heart Association textbook of neonatal resuscitation.* 7th ed. Elk Grove Village, IL: American Academy of Pediatrics; 2016.

Kliegman RM, Marcdante KJ. *Nelson essentials of pediatrics.* 7th ed. Philadelphia: Elsevier-Saunders; 2015.

Mahle WT, Newburger JW, Matherne GP, et al. Role of pulse oximetry in examining newborns for congenital heart disease: a scientific statement from the American Heart Association and American Academy of Pediatrics. *Circulation.* 2009;120:447.

Michl RK, Tabori H, Hentschel J, et al. Clinical approach to the diagnosis and treatment of cystic fibrosis and CFTR-related disorders. *Expert Rev Respir Med.* 2016 Oct 12:1–10.

Narayanan S, Funkhouser E. Inpatient hospitalizations for croup. *Hosp Pediatr Mar.* 2014;4(2):88–92.

Patrick SW, Davis MM, Lehmann CU, et al. Increasing incidence and geographic distribution of neonatal abstinence syndrome: United States 2009 to 2012. *J Perinatol.* 2015;35(8):650–655.

Perretta J. *Neonatal and pediatric respiratory care: a patient case method.* 1st ed. Philadelphia, PA: FA Davis; 2014.

Raouf S, Sheikhan F, Hassanpour S, et al. Diagnostic value of non stress test in latent phase of labor and maternal and fetal outcomes. *Glob J Health Sci.* 2014;7(2):177–182.

Sasidharan K, Dutta S, Narang A. Validity of New Ballard Score until 7th day of postnatal life in moderately preterm neonates. *Arch Dis Child Fetal Neonatal Ed.* 2009;94:F39.

Scanlan C, Heuer AJ. *Comprehensive respiratory therapy exam preparation guide.* 2nd ed. Burlington, MA: Jones & Bartlett Learning; 2015.

Schmalisch G, Wilitzki S, Bührer C, et al. The lung clearance index in young infants: impact of tidal volume and dead space. *Physiological Measurement.* 2015;36(7):1601.

Tennant C, Friedman AM, Pare E, et al. Performance of lecithin-sphingomyelin ratio as a reflex test for documenting fetal lung maturity in late preterm and term fetuses. *J Matern Fetal Neonatal Med.* 2012;25:1460–1462.

Walsh BK. *Perinatal and pediatric respiratory care.* 4th ed. St. Louis: Mosby-Elsevier; 2015.

Wanger J. *Pulmonary function testing: a practical approach.* 3rd ed. Burlington, MA: Jones & Bartlett Learning; 2012.

Whitaker K, Eberle P, Trujillo L. *Comprehensive perinatal and pediatric respiratory care.* 4th ed. Stamford, CT: Cengage Learning; 2015.

Wilkins RL, Hodgkin JE, Lopez B. *Fundamentals of lung and heart sounds.* 3rd ed. St. Louis: Mosby-Elsevier; 2011.

Wiberg N, Källén K, Herbst A, et al. Relation between umbilical cord blood pH, base deficit, lactate, 5-minute Apgar score and development of hypoxic ischemic encephalopathy. *Acta Obstet Gynecol Scand.* 2010;89:1263.

# 13

# Older Patient Assessment

*Tracy Davis and Albert J. Heuer*

## LEARNING OBJECTIVES

*After reading this chapter, you will be able to:*

1. Describe several techniques for reducing communication barriers with older adult patients.
2. Describe how patient loss of vision and hearing affect geriatric assessment efforts.
3. Identify techniques health care providers can use to compensate for hearing or vision loss in patients.
4. Identify age-related structural and physiologic changes in the cardiovascular and pulmonary systems.
5. Describe why older adults have a depressed immune system.
6. Describe pulmonary and cardiac assessment techniques.
7. List specific diagnostic tests that have altered age-related normal values.
8. Describe how functional ability relates to level of health, both actual and perceived.

## OUTLINE

## KEY TERMS

ageism
congestive heart failure (CHF)
crepitus
fremitus

immunosenescence
isolated systolic hypertension (ISH)
ototoxicity
presbycusis

presbyopia
pseudohypertension
tinnitus

The purpose of this chapter is to introduce the respiratory therapist (RT) to many age-related changes in older adult patients. Many health care professionals are focused on the treatment of acute illnesses and conditions. Clinicians need to use a different perspective when assessing and managing elderly patients and the chronic conditions associated with old age.

Communicating with older adults in the health care environment can be challenging owing to hearing loss, vision loss, gradual declines in language production, and dementia.

However, effective communication is a necessary component of patient care. Chapters 1 and 2 of this text describe various strategies that can be used to help optimize communication and overall outcomes with all patient populations, including older adults. When possible, older patients should be encouraged to share in medical decision making. Including patients in the decision-making process can increase trust, enhance patient and provider satisfaction, and increase patient adherence to medical recommendations.

**SIMPLY STATED**

It is important for RTs and other clinicians to understand the major age-specific physiologic changes that can occur with the aging process, including but not limited to a decline in pulmonary function.

It is also important for the RTs and other members of the patient care team to understand age-specific physiologic and structural changes in organ systems that pertain to older adults. Such changes may be apparent in general appearance, vital signs, and diagnostic tests, including pulmonary function test results (see Chapter 9). In addition, realizing that older adults have depressed immune systems and may present with unusual signs and symptoms is especially important to their disease management.

The "graying of America" will increase the number of older adults seeking medical attention. Over the next 30 years, the population of older adults will dramatically increase. Currently, it is estimated that approximately 44.7 million people living in the United States are age 65 or older. It is projected that by 2050, the number of people over age 65 will reach 83.7 million—double that of the current population of those over 65. Additionally, the older adult population is becoming more and more diverse. For example, in 2014 there were approximately 4 million non-Hispanic African American older adults; however, that number is expected to increase to 10 million by 2050. In 2014 older adults spent 13.4% of their total expenditures on health, more than all other consumers. Additionally, the rate of visits to emergency departments by senior citizens in the United States is growing faster than in any other age group. This translates to an increase in the need for clinicians, including RTs, who are knowledgeable about aging and the diverse aging population.

**SIMPLY STATED**

More than 50% of patients requiring the services of cardio-pulmonary professionals are age 65 years and older.

## PATIENT-CLINICIAN INTERACTION

The importance of patient-clinician interaction cannot be overstated. Chapter 1 discusses the stages of patient-clinician interaction. The same general techniques for establishing rapport with patients hold true for older adults, but one important difference that must not be overlooked with older patients is time. Gathering data from older patients takes more time. Wise and efficient use of time can make a difference between just recording vital signs and really assessing the patient. Having a plan before making contact with the patient allows the clinician to gather a better history and physical data, in the most efficient manner. Keep in mind that older adults who are institutionalized may be weakened by chronic or acute conditions. Asking an older patient to do unnecessary repeated maneuvers, performing unnecessary manipulations, and exposing his or her skin for long periods of time may exacerbate these conditions. Performing a structured assessment in a calm, unhurried, and respectful manner is fundamental to good geriatric patient assessment.

**SIMPLY STATED**

To maximize efficiency and conserve energy of older patients and those who are especially ill, it is important to use an organized approach to clinical assessment.

## Principles of Communication

Many young clinicians in their daily lives seldom interact with older adults. There may be a tendency to associate aging with illness and death. The connection of aging with chronic illness and death may lead to ageism, or discrimination against older adults. Ageism in the health care setting can lead RTs and other members of the patient care team to listen to older patients less carefully, spend less time addressing their concerns, and treat them mechanically, without compassion. If clinicians approach their patients with an ageist attitude, communication is hindered.

### Reducing Communication Barriers

Communication implies two things: the message has been delivered, and the message has been understood. When older patients know what clinicians are asking and why, they are usually more compliant.

There are many potential barriers that hinder patient-provider communication. Sensory deficits, such as hearing or visual impairment, are obvious barriers. Physical barriers related to poorly fitted dentures, nonfunctional hearing aids, or surgical removal of vocal cords may make it impossible for patients to talk. Aphasia, related to stroke, head trauma, or dementia (e.g., Alzheimer's disease), might affect both speech and processing of language, as can the adverse effects of many medications. Emotional barriers often manifested as depression can block communication efforts. Other emotional events, such as the loss of a loved one, the death of a spouse, or even being relocated to a health care institution against the patient's wishes, may be obstacles to effective communication.

Although determining the exact cause of the communication barrier is beyond the scope of therapists, there are a few interventions that may help bridge the gap. It is always important to approach older adults in a caring manner. A smile, a pat on the hand, and a kind word while making eye contact are usually successful forms of nonverbal communication. When addressing the patient, use his or her last name preceded by the appropriate title (e.g., Ms., Mr., Dr.). Using the patient's last name shows respect and promotes an atmosphere of equality. Call the patient by his or her first name only if you are given permission. Calling patients "sweetie" or "dear" is too familiar, and may be interpreted as condescending, and should be avoided.

Be aware of the environment. If the room is too hot, too cold, or too dark or if sunlight from a window is blinding your patient, his or her discomfort may affect your assessment. Introduce yourself clearly, both by name and by department. Give the patient your full attention. Let him or her know that you are performing an important job. Tell the patient you look forward to working with him or her, and encourage the patient to ask questions as they arise. If the patient seems confused, a gentle reminder of your role and goal may reassure him or her; repeat questions or information as needed. Eliminate or reduce background noise and interruptions when possible. Taking a few seconds to do this up front will save time later.

Approach the patient, and position yourself at eye level (Fig. 13.1). Maintain an unhurried pace, but keep the assessment structured in a logical manner so that all subjective and objective data can be recorded. An unorganized, unstructured, and hurried approach to assessment can be counterproductive. When asking your patient a question, wait for his or her answer—it may take the older patient a little longer to process what you've said. Try not to put words in the patient's mouth. Older adults function better when they do not feel rushed.

## Communicating with Older Adults with Dementia

In the early stages of some forms of dementia, changes in communication may not be noticeable, or the person might repeat stories or have difficulty finding certain words. As the disease progresses, the affected person may begin to use familiar words repeatedly, invent new words to describe familiar objects, easily lose his or her train of thought, revert back to a native language, have difficulty organizing words logically, and/or speak less. To help the person with dementia communicate, be patient and supportive (i.e., let the person know that you are listening and trying to understand); offer comfort and reassurance (e.g., encourage the person to continue to explain his or her thoughts); avoid criticizing, correcting, and arguing; offer a guess (i.e., if the person uses the wrong word or cannot find a word, try guessing the right one); encourage unspoken communication (i.e., ask the person to point or gesture); and limit distractions.

**FIG. 13.1** Patient-clinician interaction: elderly people may need very little, but they need that little so much. (From Sorrentino SA: *Mosby's textbook for long-term care nursing assistants*, ed 6, St. Louis, 2010, Mosby-Elsevier.)

# AGE-RELATED SENSORY DEFICIT

Although research confirms the presence of age-related decremental changes in vision and hearing, it is important to remember that not all older adults are hard of hearing or visually impaired.

## Hearing Impairment

Mild hearing impairment begins in the 40s and slowly worsens as we get older. Hearing impairment affects approximately 16.1 million people or almost two-thirds of those over 70 years of age in the United States. It is estimated that by 2030, 35 to 40 million older adults will have significant hearing loss.

Presbycusis, an age-related, progressive, bilateral hearing loss, is the most common cause of auditory impairment in the United States. The hearing loss associated with presbycusis is usually greater for high-pitched sounds; however, as the loss progresses it can become more difficult to hear low-pitched sounds. There are many causes of presbycusis; most commonly it occurs from changes in the inner ear of a person as he or she ages, but it can result from changes in the middle ear or from complex changes along the nerve pathways to the brain. It is estimated that presbycusis affects 40% of those 75 and older. The burden of hearing loss is significant and is associated with poorer hearing-related quality of life, depression, cognitive decline, impaired activities of daily living, increased falls, and increased hospitalization.

Tinnitus is the perception of sounds in one or both ears without an auditory stimulus. Millions of Americans experience tinnitus, often to a debilitating degree, making it one of the most common health conditions in the country. The Centers for Disease Control and Prevention (CDC) estimates that 15% of the general public and 30% of seniors experience some form of tinnitus. Tinnitus may be described as ringing, buzzing, roaring, or chirping in the ears. Depending on the severity of symptoms, tinnitus can result in mental status changes ranging from mild irritation to depression and suicidal thoughts. Tinnitus can be a result of ototoxicity; therefore drug-induced hearing impairment should always be considered in older adults. Ototoxicity is defined as a damaging effect on the eighth cranial nerve or in the organs of hearing or balance. The diminished hearing capacity that clinicians observe in institutionalized patients may be inflated by ototoxicity. Many prescription and over-the-counter medications can cause ototoxicity, including medications used to treat serious infections, cancer, and heart disease.

## Assessing for Hearing Impairment

Simple and accurate methods assess the presence or absence of hearing loss. Some that are commonly used are the whispered voice, a tuning fork, finger rub, a portable audioscope, and the Hearing Handicapped Inventory for the Elderly–Screening (HHIE-S) Questionnaire. If the RT suspects that a patient may have significant hearing loss, he or she should inform the nurse and other appropriate members of the patient care team to collectively determine whether further action is appropriate.

## Compensating for Hearing Impairment

If a hearing loss is suspected, ask clearly, "Can you hear me?" while facing the patient. If no documented hearing loss exists on the chart, discuss with the nurse the possibility of accumulated earwax or ototoxicity. If the patient has a hearing aid, make sure that it works and that it is in place. If there is no hearing aid, consider using an amplification device, if available. Face the patient and speak slowly and clearly, keeping the entire mouth visible—unless an isolation mask is required. Lower the pitch of your voice and do not shout—shouting makes the voice pitch even higher and is embarrassing to the patient.

## Vision Impairment

Visual impairment is one of the most significant changes associated with aging. Vision is an important part of performing activities of daily living (ADLs) and interaction with society. The patient care team must consider the effect visual impairment has on the geriatric population, including ability to drive a car, read newspapers and books, and identify common objects or people. Given the importance of vision and the impact of vision loss on the patient's well-being, it is important for the clinician to understand the most common causes of vision impairment.

Presbyopia, a normal age-related change in the lens of the eye, usually results in correctable farsightedness. Although presbyopia can occur in adults as early as age 40, it is much more common in older adults. More serious disorders of the eye that frequently affect older patients and are often the cause of blindness include cataracts, glaucoma, diabetic retinopathy, and age-related macular degeneration. A cataract is a cloudy or opaque lens that limits visions by interfering with light passing through the lens. Glaucoma is particularly dangerous because it progresses slowly with no symptoms. Glaucoma occurs when there is an increase in intraocular pressure, as a result of improper drainage of intraocular fluid. Diabetic retinopathy is a visual problem associated with diabetes. Chronically high blood sugar from diabetes is associated with damage to the tiny blood vessels in the retina, leading to diabetic retinopathy. Diabetic retinopathy can cause blood vessels in the retina to leak fluid or bleed, which distorts vision. Age-related macular degeneration (AMD) is a disease that blurs the sharp, central vision needed for "straight-ahead" activities such as reading and driving. AMD affects the macula, the part of the eye that allows you to see fine detail.

Visual impairments can have significant functional implications for older adults. Thus RTs need to be aware of assessment techniques and compensatory strategies when caring for patients with visual impairments.

### Assessing for Vision Impairment

To determine the level of vision loss in older adults, evaluation by an optometrist or ophthalmologist who specializes in low vision is necessary. An evaluation of visual acuity, however, is probably not necessary for providing many forms of respiratory care. Vision impairment generally places the patient at higher risk for falling. As a result, once a clinician suspects that a patient may have a vision problem, especially one that has not previously been detected, appropriate members of the patient care team should be informed, and additional interventions should be considered.

### Compensating for Vision Loss or Impairment

Consistency and safety are of primary importance for hospitalized patients with low vision. Waste baskets, chairs, and bedside tables that are moved around the room for the convenience of the caregivers may pose a hazard for those with visual impairments. Knowing which side of the bed that this patient is used to getting out on will help in properly organizing the hospital room. Paper handkerchiefs, a hairbrush, or a telephone moved from where the patient has placed them will be missed. If the patient wears eyeglasses, make sure they are clean and properly positioned. Older adults with low vision may be able to read words that are enlarged and in bold print. Medicine bottle lids can be marked with a single large letter indicating the name of the medication for when the patient is discharged from the hospital. Words written with puff paint can help patients distinguish between different metered-dose inhalers (MDIs). Older patients with low vision will require increased illumination. Halogen lighting, if available, provides more illumination than incandescent bulbs. Enhancing contrast also enables older adults with low vision to locate and identify objects.

When patients are blind, verbal communication is extremely important. Speak clearly, and thoroughly explain the procedures you are going to perform until comprehension is evident. If it becomes necessary to move a patient with vision loss, tell him or her what you are going to do, offer an arm as a support and guide, and let the patient initiate the movement.

> **SIMPLY STATED**
>
> Communication barriers that result from sensory deficit may hinder geriatric assessment and compromise patient safety.

## AGING OF THE ORGAN SYSTEMS

The effect of aging on specific organ systems varies widely from one person to another. We spend about one-fourth of our lives growing up and another three-fourths growing old. Simple observation will attest to the fact that we do not all age at the same rate. Organ systems also age independent of one another. Lifestyle choices and environmental factors influence organ system functioning. The combination of these external factors, along with aging and disease processes, alters the body's organ systems in both structure and function.

### Age-Related Changes

A brief review of age-related changes in the cardiovascular and pulmonary systems may be helpful before the assessment of an older adult patient. Keep in mind that the following information reflects average changes with age. In older adults, deviation from average is more common than not. Aging and disease processes also tend to overlap in producing similar signs and symptoms. When evaluating older patients, it is important to understand and recognize the differences.

## Cardiovascular System

Diseases of the heart and blood vessels are common in elderly patients. The widespread prevalence of coronary artery disease has presented a challenge for researchers engaged in studying the effect of normal aging on the heart. Evidence regarding aging and human cardiovascular function is generally limited by the need to measure serial cardiac anatomy and physiology noninvasively. Cardiovascular changes have been studied in aging animals; however, translation of animal data to humans cannot be presumed. Many older adults do have some measure of cardiac hypertrophy, but it is generally accepted that in the absence of disease, there is minimal alteration in the size of the heart. As a result of decreased contractile properties in the heart and blood vessels, there is an age-related increase in systolic blood pressure and an elevated left ventricular afterload, which results in left ventricular wall thickening. Arterial walls stiffen with age. Blood vessels lose elastin and smooth muscle fibers and gain collagen and calcium deposits. Left ventricular systolic function remains relatively stable with no significant changes in resting left ventricular ejection fraction, cardiac output, or stroke volume. Left ventricular diastolic function, however, is reduced; this is most likely a result of structural changes in the left ventricular myocardium. The early left ventricular diastolic filling rate progressively slows after age 20 years. With age, the ratio of early left ventricular diastolic filling rate to the atrial filling component declines.

There is an age-related increase in elastic and collagen tissue in the cardiac conducting system, heart, and arteries, causing the vessels to become more rigid and thick. Researchers have noted a pronounced reduction in the number of pacemaker cells in the sinoatrial (SA) node, estimated by one author to be as high as a 90% decline in SA node cell numbers. Research indicates pronounced decline in the number of pacemaker cells after age 60; furthermore, less than 10% of the number seen in young adults remains.

The consequence of these age-related losses is an increase in cardiac arrhythmias. Atrial fibrillation (AF) is the most common cardiac arrhythmia; approximately 2.7 million people are living with AF. Pressure receptor sensitivity declines with age. As a result, older adults have a blunted compensatory response to both hypertensive and hypotensive stimuli.

Calcification of heart valves (i.e., aortic stenosis) is more prevalent in elderly people. In elderly patients, the predominant causes of valvular heart disease are degenerative calcification, myxomatous degeneration, papillary muscle dysfunction, and infective endocarditis. Age-related aortic stenosis usually begins after age 60; however, symptoms often do not show up until age 70 or 80.

Congestive heart failure (CHF) results from when valvular disease, systemic hypertension, cardiomyopathy, or ischemic heart disease cause left ventricular function to decline. When untreated, this can further result in blood backing up into the pulmonary vessels, increased pulmonary vascular pressures and leaking of fluid (transudate) across the alveolar-capillary membrane and into the alveoli. The incidence of CHF doubles for each decade of life between 45 and 75 years, usually develops gradually and progresses over time. Left ventricular failure or CHF can ultimately result in right ventricular failure or biventricular failure. Left- and right-sided failures will both result in reduced cardiac output and an increased heart rate. Some other symptoms left or right heart failure are summarized in Box 13.1. Other clinical manifestations of both left and right heart failure are discussed more in Chapter 16.

---

**SIMPLY STATED**

In persons older than 65 years of age, CHF is the most common medical diagnosis.

---

## Pulmonary System

There are a number of age-related physiologic changes in the pulmonary system. Structurally, the trachea and bronchi become more rigid with age. Smooth muscle fibers in the lungs are progressively replaced with fibrous connective tissue. Alveolar septa gradually deteriorate. Although the number of alveoli does not change, loss of alveolar walls increases the size of the alveoli and reduces surface area for gas exchange. The alveolar-capillary membrane thickens, causing a reduction in diffusion of pulmonary gases. Aging lungs have less elastic recoil. The chest wall becomes stiffer, probably as a result of ossification of the cartilage-rib juncture and progressive dorsal kyphosis. Although loss of elasticity of lung tissue actually increases lung compliance, the rigidity of the thoracic cage reduces compliance enough to result in an overall decrease in lung compliance. The stiffer chest wall and reduction in elastic recoil are factors in an age-related

---

**BOX 13.1    Symptoms of Left-Sided versus Right-Sided Congestive Heart Failure**

**Left-Sided Failure**
- Exertional dyspnea, orthopnea
- Possible nocturnal dyspnea
- Cheyne-Stokes breathing
- Pale, cool skin
- Arrhythmias
- Fatigue
- Restlessness, irritability
- Shortened attention span

**Right-Sided Failure**
- Edema
- Distended neck veins
- Cyanosis
- Dyspnea
- Arrhythmias
- Hepatomegaly
- Occasional ascites

increase in functional residual capacity (FRC) and residual volume (RV).

Physiologically, aging alters both ventilation and gas exchange. Changes in ventilation and gas distribution are primarily related to the altered lung and chest wall compliance. The balance of inward forces (elastic recoil) and outward forces (chest wall and muscles of ventilation) determines lung volumes at rest. At about 55 years of age, respiratory muscle strength begins to weaken. The strength of the diaphragm for a 55-year-old is only about 75% of that for a healthy young adult. The important functional changes that take place with aging of the pulmonary system are reductions in elastic recoil and ventilatory muscle strength. The central control of these activities also changes with increasing years. Cardiac and pulmonary responses to decreased oxygen and elevated carbon dioxide levels diminish with age. Thus the changes in ventilation and respiration with aging emerge as a complex picture. In the absence of disease, age-related changes in the lungs are inconsequential. However, the combination of age-related and disease-related pulmonary changes puts the patient at risk for increased morbidity and mortality.

## Pulmonary Defense Mechanisms

Aging not only alters physiologic functioning of the lung (ventilation and respiration) but also affects the protective function of the lungs. With increasing age, the epithelial cells of the mucous membranes that line the tracheobronchial tree show degenerative changes. The number of cilia is reduced, and ciliary activity slows down. There is a decrease in the phagocytic activity of the macrophages in the mucous membrane. Combined, these changes lead to a reduction in mucociliary clearance. In addition, the loss of an effective cough reflex contributes to the increased susceptibility of older patients to lung infections.

Institutionalized older adults are subject to some conditions that may result in a reduced level of consciousness. Neurologic disorders and pharmacologic agents, such as narcotics or sedatives, can effectively blunt the cough reflex. Aspiration is always a concern. Patients with dysphasia, impaired esophageal motility, or reflux disease are at added risk when the cough mechanism is not working properly.

## Immunity

Humoral immunity, which takes place in bodily fluids, is associated with antibody production and B lymphocytes. T cells are primarily related to cell-mediated immunity and constitute about 70% of the lymphoid pool in the blood. Cell-mediated immunity involves a variety of activities designed to restrain or destroy cells that the body recognizes as harmful. With age comes a decrease in cell-mediated immunity. This age-related decline in cellular immunity correlates with an increased frequency of secondary (reactivation) tuberculosis in elderly patients. The acute antibody response to extrinsic antigens, such as pneumococcal and influenza vaccines, is also reduced in old age. Immunizations, although not as effective in older adults, are still strongly recommended.

Research regarding the clinical implications of immunosenescence, which is aging of the immune system, is confounded by a number of factors. Within subpopulations of older adults, there is considerable heterogeneity of the immune response. Genetic factors may play a role, as may environmental pollutants, socioeconomic status, and nutrition. Even efforts to increase immune function (nutritional supplements or booster vaccines) may not be equally effective in older adults. Although increased rates of infection and malignancy are associated with the dysregulated immune response common in older adults, these changes have not been causally related to the increased incidence of disease. What does seem reasonable to presume, however, is that the age-related changes in the immune system may impair the older patient's ability to effectively repel bacterial infections and may make them more susceptible to increased morbidity and mortality from pneumonia, sepsis, or other bacterial growths. Furthermore, changes in the cardiac system may result in the blunting of the tachycardiac response to hypoxia or sepsis. Some aging organ systems lose the ability to compensate for injury to other organ systems.

## Unusual Presentations of Illness

What you see in a 40-year-old patient presenting with an acute condition or exacerbation of a chronic disease may differ from the presenting symptoms of an 80-year-old patient with the same disease. The variations in signs and symptoms can make it difficult to diagnose such common occurrences as pneumonia or a heart attack. Furthermore, some older adults will misinterpret their symptoms, assuming the aches and pains are simply due to old age.

Inflammation is one of the body's first responses to infection or injury. It was once believed that in older adults the diminished febrile response, mild leukocytosis, and weakened local inflammatory response were related to the aging process. New evidence has shown that the same lack of immune response occurs in younger adults with multiple illnesses.

### Pneumonia

In a patient with pneumonia, typical presentations are cough, fever, and purulent sputum production. These signs can be deceptively subtle in older adults, particularly a lack of an elevated temperature. With a lower base temperature and a reduced ability to mount a febrile response, older adults with pneumonia may be quite ill before the cause is detected. Some older patients with an infection may simply complain of a poor appetite, fatigue, lack of ability to perform daily activities, a generalized weakness, altered mental status, and lethargy. Extrapulmonary symptoms, such as nausea, vomiting, diarrhea, myalgia, and arthralgia, are common. The most sensitive sign of pneumonia in an elderly adult is an increased respiratory rate (>28 breaths/min).

Chest radiographs may be helpful in diagnosing pneumonia, but this is not the case if the patient is dehydrated. The pneumonic infiltrate may be obscured by pulmonary edema or may not be detectable on the chest film until 24 to 48 hours after the patient has been rehydrated.

Sputum specimens collected for culture and sensitivity are recommended to avoid empiric therapy with a broad-spectrum antibiotic. Unfortunately, obtaining a good sputum specimen from an older debilitated patient can be challenging. For patients who do not respond to therapy or who relapse after an initial response to therapy, collecting sputum by transtracheal aspiration or a bronchoscopy may be considered. Depending on the pathogenic organism, blood cultures have a diagnostic yield of only about 10% to 20%.

## Myocardial Infarction

Although the incidence of death from myocardial infarction (MI) or heart attack has been reduced over the past 30 years, MI remains an important cause of morbidity in the older population. About 66% of cardiovascular disease deaths occur in people age 75 and older. Unfortunately, the clinical presentation of heart attack may be altered by advanced age. The most common symptom in younger adults is chest pain, but this symptom decreases with age or may not be present at all. Complaints of shoulder, throat, and abdominal pain are common. Other atypical symptoms that can accompany a heart attack include acute confusion, weakness, fatigue, and dizziness. If a patient complains of dizziness the health care professional should suspect heart problems as a result of the degeneration of the cardiac conduction fibers. Because of the potential of an atypical presentation and silent MI (i.e., MI with few symptoms), thorough evaluation is essential. For example, in patients with certain types of neuropathies such as those associated with diabetes, chest pain may not be a symptom of an MI. In these cases, clinical findings such as fatigue, diaphoresis, and electrocardiogram changes must be relied on to make the diagnosis.

## Asthma

It is estimated that approximately 6.9% of adults older than 65 years of age have asthma. However, in 2013 the asthma death rate was highest among people 65 or older. Asthma, unfortunately, is often misdiagnosed or underdiagnosed in the older patient population. Underdiagnosis of asthma may be related to the underuse of objective measurement instruments such as spirometers and peak flowmeters. Also, asthma is often considered a disease of young adults and perhaps is often overlooked. Other potential confounding factors may be associated with normal age-related pulmonary changes and a blunted perception of symptoms. It is possible that when asthma and chronic obstructive pulmonary disease (COPD) occur simultaneously, only the COPD is diagnosed. Common symptoms of asthma include coughing, shortness of breath, wheezing, and chest tightness. Elderly asthmatic patients are less likely to have a history of allergic disease, less likely to have nocturnal or early morning symptoms, more likely to have a poor immediate response to bronchodilator therapy, and more likely to have a later onset of symptoms. Wheezing, however, remains common. A diagnosis of asthma should be considered in elderly patients with wheezing or dyspnea.

### SIMPLY STATED

The diagnosis of asthma should be considered in older adults who are wheezing.

## Chronic Obstructive Pulmonary Disease

COPD is a progressive disease that makes it hard to breathe. There are two forms of COPD. One is emphysema, which is characterized by the loss of lung elastic recoil, which further results in air trapping. Emphysema is also associated with damage to the alveolar capillary membrane, resulting in moderate to mild hypoxemia and the retention of $CO_2$ in the arterial blood, known as hypercapnia (see Chapter 8). The other form of COPD is chronic bronchitis, which results in excessive mucus from inflamed and hyperactive mucosa and cells within it. Cigarette smoking is the leading cause of COPD. Most people who have COPD smoke or used to smoke. Long-term exposure to other lung irritants—such as air pollution, chemical fumes, or dust—also may contribute to COPD.

Early on, the signs and symptoms of COPD may not be apparent. However, as the disease progresses, most COPD patients will demonstrate shortness of breath, coughing that produces large amounts of mucus, wheezing, chest tightness, and other symptoms. Other clinical findings may include arterial blood gases that indicate chronically high arterial $CO_2$ or hypercapnia and mild to moderate hypoxemia (see Chapter 8) and chest x-rays that indicate signs of hyperinflation (see Chapter 10).

## HIV/AIDS and Associated Complications

The number of older adults living with and newly diagnosed with human immunodeficiency virus (HIV) is increasing substantially. According to the CDC, people over age 55 accounted for a quarter of the 1.2 million people living with HIV in 2012. Furthermore, in 2013 people over 50 accounted for 37% of the deaths related to acquired immunodeficiency syndrome (AIDS). Older adults have the same risk factors for HIV (e.g., unprotected sex and/or sharing needles), and many older adults remain sexually active and some use intravenous drugs. Older adults are more likely than younger people to be diagnosed with HIV infection late in the course of the disease process. Delayed diagnosis means a late start to treatment, the potential for substantial damage to the immune system, and shorter survival after diagnosis. HIV affects many systems of the body, including the immune, respiratory, and cardiovascular systems. As HIV disease progresses, immune system symptoms can include cough, fever, swollen lymph nodes, fatigue, shortness of breath, and weight loss. HIV increases the risk of colds, influenza, and pneumonias and can lead to opportunistic lung diseases. As the disease progresses people with HIV are susceptible to tuberculosis and a disease called *Pneumocystis jiroveci* (formerly *carinii*) pneumonia (PCP or PJP). PJP causes trouble breathing, cough, and fever. Additionally, HIV raises the risk of pulmonary arterial hypertension, which places a strain on the heart.

All health care providers should be aware of the possibility of having undiagnosed HIV or AIDS and should recommend HIV screening as a part of routine health care or when presenting with symptoms associated with the disease.

> **SIMPLY STATED**
>
> Older adults are susceptible to HIV/AIDS, and thorough health care should include prompt HIV screening when a patient presents with symptoms associated with the disease.

## PATIENT ASSESSMENT

Patient assessment is the foundation of good patient care. Patient assessment represents a skill that is crucial to caring for elderly people. Vital signs, such as temperature, pulse, blood pressure, and respiratory rate, as well as lung sounds and breathing patterns, are noninvasive windows to the health status of the patient. Given today's climate of managed care, protocols, and clinical practice guidelines, strong assessment skills are vital to good patient care and cost-effective disease management.

One component of assessment that is occasionally overlooked is taking a patient's complete medical history. In the case of acute-onset dyspnea, a good history and physical examination can establish the diagnosis most of the time. Another means of facilitating physical assessment is to conceptualize the anatomy. Having a basic knowledge of anatomy and understanding how disease alters both anatomy and physiology are key to accurate assessment.

### Vital Signs

Chapter 4 describes techniques involved in obtaining and interpreting vital signs. However, it is important for the RT and other members of the patient care team to keep in mind that age-specific considerations apply when assessing vital signs in elderly patients. The means by which certain vital signs are obtained, normal ranges, and their clinical significance for older adults are often different from other patient populations.

### Temperature

As a result of decreased metabolism, the loss of muscle mass, and a reduction in vasoconstriction, older adults have an altered ability to regulate body heat. Older adults usually have lower body temperatures. In patients older than 90, body temperatures of 96°F and 97°F are not uncommon. Simply taking temperatures in older adults may be a challenge. Oral thermometers are not useful if the elderly patient cannot easily keep his or her mouth closed for 2 or 3 minutes.

The axillary method may not be accurate, particularly in a thin older adult with a loss of underarm body tissue. Rectal temperatures are accurate but necessitate turning the patient completely to one side, a maneuver that could result in injuring a hip or other body part. Tympanic membrane thermometers are generally preferred in older adults and other populations because they are accurate, easy to use, and able to record temperatures within seconds.

Regardless of the method used, it is important to establish a norm for each patient and assess for trends. Once the norm is established, an increase in temperature alerts the health care professional to the possibility of infection. A 95-year-old patient with a temperature of 101°F (whose normal body temperature is 96°F) is in trouble. This patient's temperature is equivalent to 103.6°F in a person whose normal temperature is 98.6°F.

The thermoregulatory mechanism in older adults is blunted, and environmental temperatures may be more influential. During room temperature extremes (hot or cold), monitor the patient's body temperature on a regular basis.

### Pulse

The heart rate at rest is regulated by sympathetic and to a greater degree parasympathetic tone. In healthy men, the supine resting heart rate does not change with age. In a sitting position, the heart rate in the same individual will drop slightly from the rate exhibited when supine. In an inactive older adult, the pulse rate may decrease to 50 to 55 beats/min. In active older adults, although heart rates vary, a normal pulse may range between 60 and 100 beats/min. Arrhythmias that produce a rapid heart rate are not tolerated well by elderly patients, who may already have a decreased level of daily functioning. If there are any new (not previously noted) irregularities in pulse volume or rhythm, consult a nurse or physician about a follow-up assessment. To most accurately assess pulse in an older patient, use a stethoscope and count beats at the apex.

### Blood Pressure

The measurement of blood pressure is essential. Hypertension is an important cardiovascular risk factor in elderly people. Blood pressure and pulse pressure increase progressively with age. In most populations, average diastolic blood pressure increases with age until the sixth decade and then stabilizes, whereas systolic blood pressure continues to rise. As a result, the pulse pressure (the difference between systolic and diastolic pressures) may widen. A normal pulse pressure is anywhere between 50 and 100 mm Hg in older adults. If when documenting blood pressure you note a narrowing of the pulse pressure, it might be wise to monitor the patient. A narrowing pulse pressure can be an early sign of a slow leak tamponade.

Systolic blood pressure rises with aging as a consequence of the loss of elasticity in the peripheral vessels. It is estimated that 60% of older adults have either elevated systolic or diastolic blood pressures or both. Elevation of only the systolic pressure is termed isolated systolic hypertension (ISH). The American Heart Association (AHA) defines blood pressure using five categories: normal (less than 120/less than 80), prehypertension (120 to 139/80 to 89), hypertension stage one (140 to 159/90 to 99), hypertension stage two (160 or higher/100 or higher), and hypertensive crisis (higher than 180/ higher than 110).

High blood pressure is a common and dangerous condition. Approximately 70 million people have high blood pressure; however, only about half have their blood pressure under control. High blood pressure increases the risk for heart disease and stroke, two of the leading causes of death for Americans. It is very important for people to have their blood pressure checked regularly, especially because there often are no symptoms or warning signs of high blood pressure. There are many ways to prevent the onset of high blood pressure (e.g., maintaining a healthy weight and avoiding smoking), and if a person already has high blood pressure there are ways to control it.

Blood pressure may be falsely high in older adults because of arterial stiffness. An overestimated blood pressure (pseudohypertension) should be suspected in patients with elevated systolic and diastolic pressures but no end-organ damage.

Blood pressure must be measured accurately. Ask the patient to sit quietly for 3 to 5 minutes before taking a measurement, and use a cuff large enough to cover at least one third of the patient's upper arm. Measure pressure in both arms, and note any significant difference. Both supine and standing (or sitting) blood pressures, taken 1 to 3 minutes after the positional change, may reveal the presence of orthostatic hypotension/postural hypotension (i.e., a form of low blood pressure that happens when a person stands up from sitting or lying down). (Exercise caution, however, when testing volume-depleted patients.) A drop of 20 mm Hg systolic or 10 mm Hg diastolic or an increased heart rate of 20 beats/min is abnormal. Orthostatic hypotension in older adults is often associated with syncope and falls. Failure to check both supine and standing blood pressure is an oversight in potentially diagnosing an important and often correctable problem. Remember that emergency department blood pressures are not baseline data. They are measured under less than optimal conditions. Check blood pressure again before acting on a single measurement. Also, document any blood pressure trends. Safe drug therapy may depend on accurate daily blood pressure measurement.

As indicated in Chapter 4, a systolic blood pressure of 150 mm Hg or more and/or a diastolic pressure of 90 mm Hg or more are major causes of morbidity and mortality, especially in those 60 years old or older. As a result, if an assessment reveals a blood pressure of 150/90 mm Hg or more in this patient population, pharmacologic treatment is generally recommended as part of the management plan.

### SIMPLY STATED

Emergency department blood pressure measurements are generally not considered reliable baseline data because the setting can cause significant variability.

## Respiratory Rate

Residual volume (RV) increases almost 50% by age 70. The total lung capacity remains relatively stable, and the increase in RV comes at the expense of the vital capacity. In older adults, the respiratory rate may increase as a result of a decreased depth of ventilation. Normal respiratory rates in elderly patients range from 16 to 25 breaths/min.

Tachypnea or hyperpnea may be the result of exercise, for example, in a patient who just ambulated in the hallway or returned from therapy. Other factors that could result in an increased rate or depth of breathing are anxiety, fever, pneumonia, hypoxemia, acidemia, or lesions in the pons and medulla. Bradypnea might be secondary to pharmacologic respiratory depressants, or the patient may just be sleeping. When an abnormally slow rate of breathing is noted, other causes could be alkalosis, hypothermia, or hypoglycemia. Older adults are more susceptible to hypothermia. Additionally, older patients with diabetes have a greater risk for hypothermia, most likely a result of vascular disease that alters the body's thermoregulatory mechanism particularly among those with polyneuropathy. In patients being treated with oral antidiabetic agents (e.g., sulfonylureas), the incidence of hypoglycemia increases with age or with concomitant use of aspirin or sulfonamide antibiotics. Accurate respiratory rates, documented in a timely manner, can assist caregivers in looking for trends and can lead to additional diagnoses. If shallow breathing is noted, respiration may be easier to count by watching the rise and fall of the abdomen instead of the chest. If both the respiratory rate and pulse are elevated (>25 breaths/min and >100 beats/min) in an elderly patient for no apparent reason and the patient has other respiratory symptoms, pneumonia should be suspected. Dyspnea in older adults is abnormal. If a patient with airway disease exhibits significant shortness of breath at rest, the forced expiratory volume in 1 second ($FEV_1$) is likely less than 50% of predicted. Next to pain, dyspnea is the symptom most feared by patients and clinicians alike. An increased respiratory rate may signal a lower respiratory tract infection, CHF, or another disorder before the appearance of other clinical signs.

## Inspection and Palpation

Generally defined as a visual examination of the patient, inspection can be done while taking a patient history, checking vital signs, or auscultating lung sounds. Palpation is the process of using the hands to feel for body movement, lumps, masses, and skin characteristics.

### Inspection

**Breathing Patterns.** Note the pattern of breathing. Is Cheyne-Stokes or periodic breathing perceptible? If so, document the length of the apnea episodes. Older adults with heart disease may demonstrate this pattern of irregular breathing while sleeping. The more common etiologic factors of Cheyne-Stokes breathing include CHF, uremia, decreased blood flow to the respiratory center of the brain, drug-induced respiratory depression, or brain damage. Biot breathing, an irregular breathing pattern, also has characteristic periods of apnea. Again, document the length of apnea episodes in seconds. Biot breathing occurs most often in patients with brain damage and increased intracranial pressure (see Chapter 6).

*Cyanosis.* If the extremities (i.e., fingers, toes, tip of nose, lips, and earlobes) are bluish in color, the patient has peripheral cyanosis. Peripheral cyanosis is often related to inadequate circulation but can also be seen in patients who are cold, anxious, or have some measure of venous obstruction.

Central cyanosis results from a decreased concentration of oxygen in arterial blood and may be a result of advanced lung disease or CHF.

In older adults, two other manifestations of cyanosis may be noted. Small vessel syndrome can present as local areas of cyanosis or necrosis in a hand or foot that generally has adequate circulation. A number of predisposing conditions, such as disseminated intravascular coagulation, essential thrombocytosis, polycythemia, scleroderma, or emboli from arterial aneurysms, can result in small vessel syndrome. Raynaud phenomenon is another syndrome that can present with intermittent cutaneous pallor or cyanosis. It is typically caused by exposure to cold or emotional stimuli and related to peripheral vasospasm. However, older adults may experience the pallor and cyanosis at room temperature.

*Skin turgor.* Diminished skin turgor or fullness of the skin is a normal age-related integumentary change. The loss of subcutaneous fat and water, deterioration of elastin, and decreased vascularity can result in wrinkling and loose skin. Pinching the skin to check for tenting used to be a quick check for the presence of dehydration; however, because of structural changes tenting is not a valid indicator of dehydration among older adults. Other signs of dehydration among older adults should be assessed (e.g., dry tongue, dizziness, decreased urine output). If dehydration in an elderly patient is suspected, appropriate members of the patient care team should be consulted.

---

**SIMPLY STATED**

Dehydration should be treated as a potentially life-threatening situation.

---

*Clubbing.* The abnormal enlargement of the distal phalanges, most easily noted in the fingers, is not age related. However, the conditions that lead to clubbing are chronic, and older adults have a higher incidence of chronic disease. COPD alone, even in the presence of hypoxemia, does not lead to clubbing. If older adult patients with COPD have clubbing, something other than obstructive lung disease is occurring, such as pulmonary manifestations of connective tissue disease.

*Edema.* The visible signs of fluid accumulation can signal the presence of a variety of diseases. Check the patient's lower extremities for the presence of edema or swelling. Ask about or check the chart for any recent sudden weight gain. A gain of more than 2 pounds in a day or more than 5 pounds in a week may be fluid retention and could signal CHF. A rapid onset of unilateral leg swelling and dependent edema suggests a diagnosis of deep vein thrombosis.

Unfortunately, because they more commonly exhibit atypical presentations, peripheral edema is not always a reliable indicator of heart failure in elderly people.

*Jugular venous distention.* Peripheral edema may not be a reliable indicator of heart failure, but jugular venous distention in older adults is highly suggestive of right heart failure. Chapter 5 contains a detailed description of estimating jugular venous pressure. Hepatojugular reflux, or distention of the jugular vein induced by manual pressure over the liver, is also a reliable indicator of right heart failure in elderly patients. When performing the inspection portion of the physical examination, be sure to make a neck vein assessment.

## Palpation

Touching the patient to evaluate for the presence of pathology can assist in the process of assessment. Normally, palpation includes an evaluation for fremitus, including an estimation of thoracic expansion and feeling for crepitus. In older patients, palpation may initially be a scouting maneuver for skin condition, scars, signs of infection, and the presence of bumps or bruises.

When assessing patients whose respiration is being aided with mechanical ventilators, patients who have had thoracic surgery, or patients who have sustained trauma, palpate first for subcutaneous emphysema. Start assessing at the neck, and using the fingertips, gently "walk" down the sides of the neck from the jaw to the clavicle. Crepitus feels like crackling under the skin. Crepitus associated with subcutaneous emphysema is more common in patients who have sustained intrathoracic trauma or barotrauma.

Fremitus consists of palpable vibrations felt on the chest wall when the patient is repeating a sound. The vibrations caused by sound increase over areas of consolidation. Evaluating for fremitus requires a cooperative patient. Likewise, estimating thoracic expansion by palpation requires deep inspiratory and expiratory maneuvers. These maneuvers may be physically difficult for elderly patients to perform. Palpate for chest excursion on a case-by-case basis.

## Pulmonary Auscultation

Assessing lung sounds can generate very useful diagnostic information. Abnormal or added lung sounds are referred to as adventitious and can be classified as crackles or wheezes. A few simple questions can be used to classify lung sounds and guide the diagnosis.

---

**QUESTIONS TO ASK**

**Lung Sounds**
*When assessing lung sounds, ask yourself the following questions:*
- Is the sound continuous or discontinuous?
- Is the sound on one side or both?
- Is the sound on inspiration or expiration?
- Does the sound clear with coughing?

---

Older adult patients may not always be able to take several consecutive good-quality, deep breaths. They may only be able to give you three to four good, deep breaths before they tire. In a quiet environment, with the patient leaning forward, assess posterior lobes first. Position your stethoscope (on skin) midway between the patient's waist and scapula, and get four good bilateral breaths. Listen for a full inspiratory-to-expiratory (I/E) cycle. Moving the stethoscope from side to side, compare sounds, and then proceed with anterior and lateral chest assessment. The patient will be taking deeper breaths during the examination, so caution must be exercised to prevent hyperventilation. Ask the patient to report any feelings of dizziness.

Auscultation may reveal diminished breath sounds even in older patients with healthy lungs. An increased anteroposterior (AP) diameter and shallow breathing are common in elderly people and add to the difficulty of hearing normal vesicular breath sounds. However, pathologic conditions still produce characteristic wheezes and crackles. Fine, inspiratory crackles are more likely to represent atelectasis, pulmonary fibrosis, CHF, or an acute inflammatory process in elderly patients. When present, coarse crackles heard on both inspiration and expiration that do not clear with a cough may indicate an upper respiratory infection or severe pulmonary edema. Although very different disease processes, both CHF and asthma may cause wheezing due to the airway edema that generally accompanies these conditions.

## SIMPLY STATED

During auscultation, start on the back and at the lung bases, place the stethoscope on the patient's skin, and listen for a full I/E cycle.

## Cardiac Auscultation

The growing population of older patients is presenting a unique challenge for health care providers. Care of adult patients requires at least a working knowledge of cardiac assessment. Cardiac conduction defects, disease, and valvular incompetence can all result in altered heart sounds and murmurs.

### Heart Sounds

In about 30% to 40% of elderly patients, you may note an audible splitting of the second heart sound ($S_2$). Significant splitting of the $S_2$ that increases with inspiration suggests the presence of right bundle branch block. An $S_3$ is indicative of ventricular disease in elderly patients and can be auscultated in the same vertical line as $S_2$ but about 2 inches lower at the fourth intercostal space. It may be one of the earliest markers of CHF. $S_4$ sounds, when present, can be heard best on the left side, at the fifth intercostal space, midclavicular line. An $S_4$ is a sign of ventricular disease, as in the patient with CHF or recent MI.

### Heart Murmurs

Heart murmurs are a swooshing sound also described as sustained noises (e.g., blowing, harsh, rough, or rumbling sounds). Heart murmurs are most often the result of valvular heart disease and can be caused by stenosis, regurgitation, or valvular incompetence. Murmurs can be further classified as systolic or diastolic. Some murmurs indicate life-threatening illness. Trauma, infective endocarditis, aortic dissection, papillary muscle, or septal rupture are all acute, severe heart problems and may cause harsh regurgitant murmurs. Urgent attention is indicated.

Infective endocarditis has become more prevalent in older adults despite advances in antibiotic therapy. The increased numbers of older adults account for some of the statistical increases. Also factoring into the picture are an increase in the number of older adults with prosthetic valves, a higher prevalence of hospital-acquired bacteremia, and longer survival of persons with a history of rheumatic heart disease. Cardiac murmurs are found in more than 90% of patients with infective endocarditis.

Heart sounds are usually softer in older adults. This may be the result of weakened myocardial function or an increased AP diameter. An increased AP diameter increases the distance between the heart and chest wall and will make detection of the heart sounds more difficult. Take time to listen to heart sounds. The more you listen, the more skilled you will become at distinguishing subtle abnormalities.

## SIMPLY STATED

Chest auscultation of an elderly patient can provide a quick and accurate assessment of both the heart and lungs.

## DIAGNOSTIC TESTS

Physiologic and structural changes in the pulmonary system will be manifested as alterations in common diagnostic tests. Arterial blood gases, pulse oximetry, and pulmonary function studies reveal age-associated changes. Age-appropriate norms should be taken into consideration when interpreting diagnostic tests.

### Gas Exchange

The effects of pulmonary aging result in a reduced vital capacity and expiratory flow rates, as well as reduced partial pressure of arterial oxygenation ($Pao_2$). To a certain degree, gas exchange is altered even in healthy older adults.

As stated earlier, there is an age-associated loss of alveolar surface area. The alveolar-arterial oxygen partial pressure gradient ($P[A-a]o_2$) is also increased in older adults; this could be a consequence of either intrapulmonary shunting, diffusion limitation of oxygen and carbon dioxide gas exchange, or ventilation-perfusion (V/Q) abnormalities. A study was conducted on normal subjects (lifetime nonsmokers with normal spirometry) ages 18 to 71 years. The age-related increase in V/Q mismatching was confirmed, but it was not as great as expected. The amount of intrapulmonary shunting was almost negligible (<1% of cardiac output in 90% of cases), and the $PaO_2$ was reduced but only slightly.

## Arterial Blood Gases

$PaO_2$ (arterial oxygen) declines at a relatively predictable rate with age. A normal $PaO_2$ for a 30-year-old is approximately 95 mm Hg, compared with about 83 mm Hg for an 80-year-old. This equates to a decline in arterial oxygen tension associated with aging of about −0.245 mm Hg per year (Table 13.1).

Given that arterial oxygenation values are used to determine therapeutic interventions and eligibility for home oxygen therapy, it is important for therapists to understand the effect of age, body position, and gender on $PaO_2$. A blood gas drawn from an older patient in the supine position on average will produce a $PaO_2$ about 5 mm Hg less than that produced in the seated position. Interestingly, after age 75 years, $PaO_2$ also tends to be higher in men than in women.

Even though the $PaO_2$ is reduced as a result of aging, in the absence of disease, the $PaO_2$ is adequate to provide for tissue oxygenation. Oxygen consumption declines with age in both men and women as a result of reduced metabolism and the replacement of lean tissue with fat.

Some hypercapnia is occasionally noted in elderly patients, but there does not seem to be a consistent age-related alteration in partial pressure of arterial carbon dioxide ($PaCO_2$). Mild hypercapnia in elderly patients could be the result of numerous physiologic changes in the lung seen with age.

## Pulse Oximetry

The mild reduction in $PaO_2$ common among older adults will be consistent with lower oxygen saturation as measured by pulse oximetry ($SpO_2$), but in a healthy older adult saturations should be above 93% to 94%. A $PaO_2$ of 60 mm Hg corresponds to an $SpO_2$ of about 90%. As long as the patient's $PaO_2$ values remain on the flat portion of the oxyhemoglobin dissociation curve, the aging process does not significantly decrease the $SpO_2$.

Some factors that may cause pulse oximeters to inaccurately record $SpO_2$ are severe or rapid desaturation, hypotension, hypothermia, abnormal hemoglobin, and low perfusion. The presence of a good, measurable pulse is essential to the measurement of $SpO_2$. Unfortunately, in some older patients with poor perfusion or circulation, obtaining a reading can be a problem.

### SIMPLY STATED

Both $PaO_2$ and $SpO_2$ decline slightly with age.

## Pulmonary Function Studies

After age 25 years, pulmonary function in adults starts to decline gradually. The loss of elastic recoil and stiffening of the chest wall shift the balance of lung volumes and capacities. The total lung capacity and tidal volume remain relatively stable throughout the adult life span.

The effect of senescence on pulmonary function measurements has been well documented. When trying to diagnose functional impairment of airflow by performing pulmonary function studies in older adults, it is important that age-appropriate norms be used as a standard (Box 13.2).

The effects of changes in lung and chest wall mechanics cause forced vital capacity (FVC) and $FEV_1$ to diminish as early as age 20 years. The mean rate of decline is approximately 30 mL per year for men and 23 mL per year for women.

Diffusing capacity of the lung for carbon monoxide ($D_{LCO}$) peaks in persons in their early twenties and then gradually decreases. The reduction is estimated to be 2.03 mL/min/mm Hg per year in men. Women normally have a 10% lower diffusing capacity than men of equal height and weight. As a result of age-related changes in V/Q and loss of alveolar surface area, the age-related decline in $D_{LCO}$ is not linear. Decremental changes in total pulmonary diffusing capacity become more prominent after 40 years of age.

Standard pulmonary function testing in elderly people requires significant coordination and cooperation on the part of the therapist and patient. Explaining the procedure to the patient may take additional time and require more demonstration. Frequent maneuvers such as repeated breath holding and timed effort-dependent exhalations are required. The extra exertion may be difficult for some patients. After

## TABLE 13.1   Estimated Age-Associated Change in $PaO_2$ by Decade

| Age (yr) | Estimated $PaO_2$ (mm Hg) |
|---|---|
| 10 | 100 |
| 20 | 97.55 |
| 30 | 95.1 |
| 40 | 92.65 |
| 50 | 90.2 |
| 60 | 87.75 |
| 70 | 85.30 |
| 80 | 82.85 |
| 90 | 80.4 |
| 100 | 77.95 |

*$PaO_2$,* Partial pressure of arterial oxygenation.

## BOX 13.2   Age-Associated Pulmonary Function Test Changes

- Reduced vital capacity, both slow and forced
- Reduced peak expiratory flows
- Reduced inspiratory capacity
- Reduced $FEF_{25\%-75\%}$
- Reduced $FEV_1$
- Decreased diffusing capacity
- Increased RV
- Increased FRC

*FEF,* Forced expiratory flow; *$FEV_1$,* forced expiratory volume in 1 second; *FRC,* functional residual capacity; *RV,* residual volume.

obtaining the best data possible, a consultation with the pulmonologist concerning the patient's level of comprehension and performance may assist in the interpretation of results.

Prediction regression formulas for pulmonary function tests and prediction nomograms for spirometric values are available. The formulas are both age variable and gender specific. The nomograms can accommodate persons 20 to 90 years of age and are also gender specific.

It is important to remember that the predicted values are derived from a statistical analysis of "normal" subjects. These test subjects are classified as normal based on the absence of history or symptoms of lung disease in themselves or their families. Minimal exposure to environmental risk factors (e.g., smoking or pollution) would also be a criterion in selecting these subjects.

Older adults being seen by pulmonary specialists rarely are without a component of lung disease or environmental risk factors. When interpreting pulmonary function studies as part of a geriatric assessment, the age-related deviation from normal must be taken into consideration.

## Laboratory Values

Many factors are responsible for the alteration in laboratory values of older adults. Diet, exercise, multisystem disease, and physiologic and structural age-related changes are all variables that make determination of normal a challenge. The normal value for a laboratory test is its mean value ±2 standard deviations in a population of healthy persons. An abnormal result does not necessarily confirm the presence of disease or disorder. The likelihood of disease is estimated by knowing the test's specificity and sensitivity. Clinicians do not always have precise information on the specificity and sensitivity of tests in elderly patients, and the prevalence of disease often differs in older populations. Chapter 7 outlines clinical laboratory studies, and Box 13.3 shows some laboratory values and the increases and decreases that can result from the aging process.

### Hematology

Total hemoglobin in both males and females may remain in the normal range or decrease slightly with age. The decrease is related to the reduced formation and development of blood cells in the bone marrow. In men, reduced hemoglobin may also be a factor of a drop in androgen. Hematocrit may also decrease slightly, which is related to reduced hematopoiesis (see Chapter 7). Aging is not associated with significant changes in the white blood cell count; however, leukopenia, most frequently neutropenia, occurs in conjunction with a broad spectrum of medical problems. In older adults, leukopenia is likely the result of acquired or secondary disorders, either reactive (e.g., medications, nutritional deficits, infections, or diminished T and B lymphocytes) or malignant.

### Blood Chemistry

Age-related albumin reduction is related to a reduced liver size, blood flow, and enzyme production. Low serum albumin can also be a factor of malnutrition. Blood urea nitrogen may

---

### BOX 13.3    Effect of Aging on Laboratory Values

**Increased Values**
- Sedimentation rate (mild elevation)
- Glucose
- Cholesterol
- Triglycerides
- Uric acid
- Fibrinogen
- Copper
- Norepinephrine
- Prostate-specific antigen
- Serum potassium (slight increase)

**Decreased Values**
- Creatinine clearance
- Albumin
- Calcium
- Iron
- Phosphorus
- Zinc
- Vitamins $B_6$, $B_{12}$, and C

**Unchanged Values**
- Hemoglobin
- Red blood cell count
- White blood cell count
- Blood urea nitrogen
- Serum creatinine
- Serum electrolytes (sodium, chloride, and bicarbonate)

Data from Abrams WB, Beers MH, Berkow R, editors: *The Merck manual of health and aging*, Whitehouse Station, NJ, 2004, Merck; and Lamy PP: *Prescribing for the elderly*, New York, NY, 1980, PSG.

---

remain unchanged or may increase when related to compromised renal function. Creatinine (Cr) clearance declines, but serum Cr levels remain stable because elderly persons have less muscle mass. Cr clearance as a measure of kidney function is useful information in prescribing drugs for elderly people. Formulas and nomograms are available for determining age-adjusted normal values for clearance of creatinine. In patients with a reduced Cr clearance, some drugs need to be modified as to dosage to prevent the development of a drug toxicity.

Serum calcium levels will be slightly decreased, whereas potassium will be slightly increased. Fasting glucose increases with age, but values usually remain within the normal range. Glucose tolerance decreases gradually with age. The lack of exercise, obesity, and some medications, however, can exert more influence on glucose tolerance than age alone.

Variability is a hallmark of aging, so it is difficult to extrapolate norms with confidence in elderly people. The establishment of norms for each individual when healthy would be useful to compare with laboratory values when diagnosing a new condition or disease. This, of course, is not feasible with anything except routine tests performed at the time of annual physical examinations. The value of doing an occasional blood screening test in healthy elderly adults is appreciated when facing a challenging disease or diagnosis.

In older adults, do not assume that variations from the norm are always abnormal or that normal values are always an indicator of health.

**FIG. 13.2** Ensuring that patients understand their medication regimens is very important.

## COMPREHENSIVE GERIATRIC ASSESSMENT

Performing a comprehensive geriatric assessment has become an established component of medical practice, given the growing population of older adults. The needs of many elderly patients are too broad to be met by an assessment based only on diagnosis. The symptoms that cause the patient to seek medical attention are not always directly related to the disease, and a more thorough investigation is warranted. For example, a patient may seek help because of an unstable gait and an inability to walk. The underlying diagnosis may be CHF that has produced peripheral edema, causing problems with physical movement before the obvious shortness of breath is noticeable.

Comprehensive geriatric assessment is considered by most geriatricians to be an important and effective form of secondary and tertiary care for elderly patients. The Affordable Care Act (ACA), which was signed into law on March 23, 2010, provides seniors with greater access to comprehensive health care and provides seniors with greater control over their own health care. In addition, the ACA aims to improve the quality of services delivered and to reduce the rate of increase in health care spending. Specifically, the ACA lowers health care costs for seniors. For example, the ACA reduces or eliminates deductibles, copayments, and other cost-sharing for preventive care in Medicare and provides free yearly checkups. Additionally, the ACA increases access to quality, affordable health care for seniors by promoting better care after a hospital discharge, better control of chronic disease, and overall improvement of the quality of care by all providers and in long-term care facilities. Better access to preventive care and improved health care may help seniors to maintain or improve their functional ability and independence. An improvement in functional ability, rather than a cure, is often the most important goal of geriatric assessment. Geriatric assessment is time consuming. It involves not only physical health but also upper and lower extremity function, nutrition, and mental status. Screening for depression, urinary incontinence, a social support network, the adequacy and safety of the home environment, and functional ability are all components of the comprehensive geriatric assessment (Fig. 13.2).

### Functional Ability

Although not usually assessed by RTs, the functional ability of older adults is closely related to a perceived index of health. As a general rule, health in older adults is usually not defined as staying out of the hospital so much as it is retaining the ability to perform ADLs.

Knowing that "health" is so closely correlated with "ability" in older patients, perhaps a brief review of a patient's abilities would be beneficial. How often, as clinicians, do we deal with older patients suffering from hospital psychosis? When patients are out of their familiar environment, away from their usual caregivers, and sick, depression often becomes a problem. Individuals with depression can present with physical symptoms—for example, dyspnea and fatigue. Asking simple questions about their abilities may put a more positive focus on what the patients can do versus the temporary losses they are suffering. A positive attitude can have a large impact on a patient's outlook for recovery.

### Activities of Daily Living

A number of instruments have been developed for measuring the older adult's ability to complete Activities of Daily Living (ADL). The basic ADLs usually assessed are mobility and the ability to participate in personal hygiene and grooming, feeding, toileting, and dressing. To carry out these ADLs, patients must have sufficient range of motion, strength, and endurance.

### Instrumental Activities of Daily Living

Some measurement tools, known as instrumental activities of daily living (IADLs), have been designed to evaluate more complex skills. Household management skills, money management, ability to use the telephone, writing skills, and the ability to shop are categorized as IADLs. Only about 5% of adults older than 65 years in the United States live in nursing homes, so the hospitalized patient population includes a large percentage of noninstitutionalized older adults with a relatively high degree of functional ability.

Deterioration of functional ability in a previously unimpaired elderly person is an early, subtle sign of illness and is often not accompanied by typical disease signs and symptoms. As soon as functional impairment develops, a thorough clinical evaluation will best serve the patient in maintaining quality of life.

## KEY POINTS

- Effective communication with patients will improve the assessment and enhance any therapeutic intervention.
- Age-related sensory change (decreased vision and hearing) may necessitate subtle adaptations when delivering therapy to the older patient.
- Age-associated changes in organ systems (cardiac, pulmonary, or immune system) may affect how your patients respond to therapy and how quickly they recover from illness.
- Signs and symptoms of disease in the elderly patient may be atypical. New onset of mental status changes, fatigue, confusion, and syncope should be investigated.
- Vital signs may be altered as a result of age-related decremental change. It is important to accurately assess and record heart rate, respiratory rate, blood pressure, temperature, and other clinical indicators. Subtle changes may indicate worsening of a patient's condition.

- Fine inspiratory crackles in the bases are likely associated with atelectasis. Wheezes and crackles in other areas of the lungs may indicate pathology.
- The $Pao_2$ in an older adult is slightly reduced as a consequence of aging but not as much as was previously thought. The $Pao_2$ in a healthy 75-year-old adult should be about 83 mm Hg. The $Spo_2$ should be above 94%. The $Pao_2$ is about 5 mm Hg lower when drawn on a patient in a supine position.
- Laboratory values are altered a little with aging. Changes in trending or shifting of values, up or down, should be investigated.
- A comprehensive geriatric assessment by a geriatrician is considered to be a very important and effective form of secondary and tertiary care for elderly patients.
- Preventive interventions to keep older patients healthy, functional, and at home are the best medical care.

## CASE STUDY

A breathing treatment with albuterol has been ordered for an 86-year-old female patient with asthma. She also has macular degeneration, and her vision is very poor. She lives in an assisted living facility and is otherwise fairly functional.

1. What are some of the issues related to medication delivery for this patient that need to be addressed? Will she be able to actuate a metered-dose inhaler (MDI)? Will her inspiratory flow be great enough to use a dry powder inhaler (DPI)? Will she see well enough to manipulate these medication delivery devices? If she is given more than one MDI/DPI, how will she tell them apart? Will a small volume nebulizer (SVN) or handheld nebulizer be the best choice? If an SVN is selected, will she be able to see to dispense the medication into the nebulizer cup?

2. How common is asthma in older adults? Why is asthma underdiagnosed in older adults? When should an asthma diagnosis be considered among older adults?

3. What are some adaptations to the selected medication delivery device that would this patient once she is discharged from the hospital?

This patient is visually impaired, so careful consideration must be given to what method of aerosol delivery is best. If an MDI or more than one MDI is used, some type of tactile adaptation (e.g., puff paint, 1 dot vs. 2 dots on the outside of the inhaler) is needed. Slipping a short length of large-bore flex tubing over the inhaler also gives it a different feel than the smooth inhalers. Therapists can be creative in helping visually impaired patients distinguish among MDIs. If an SVN is ordered, the patient needs to have a supply of unit dose medications and the ability to open the vials and place the medicine in the cup. DPIs might be too much of a challenge for a visually impaired older adult.

## CASE STUDY

A 78-year-old retired male executive presents to the clinic with complaints of fatigue and shortness of breath that have worsened over the past weeks to months.

1. What are some possible diagnoses based only on this information?

Physical examination reveals the following: temperature, 98.4°F; blood pressure, 200/110 mm Hg; pulse, 100 beats/min;

respiratory rate, 28 breaths/min; height, 6 feet, 1 inch; weight, 66 kg. The patient is alert and in no obvious distress, but on further questioning he admits to having a lot of heartburn, the inability to walk as far as he used to, and sleeping at night with two or three pillows or in his recliner.

2. Based on this information, what abnormalities are noted, and what diagnosis should be considered?

## ASSESSMENT QUESTIONS

1. Which of the following is true about communicating with older adult patients?
   a. It is waste of time if they cannot respond
   b. It is unnecessary; just check their ID band
   c. It is a time-consuming task if done appropriately
   d. It is impossible when they cannot see or hear well

2. Which of the following statements reflects an ageist attitude?
   a. Many older adults have poor vision
   b. Most older adults are sick and debilitated
   c. Many older adults have some measure of hearing loss
   d. Most older adults have some degree of cardiac hypertrophy

3. The major risk factor associated with the development of diabetic retinopathy is which of the following?
   a. Chronically high blood sugar
   b. Smoking
   c. Alcohol consumption
   d. Overexposure to bright light

4. Normal age-related restructuring of the heart results in an enlargement of what structure?
   a. Left ventricle
   b. Right ventricle
   c. Left atrial
   d. Right atrial

5. Typical symptoms of right-sided heart failure include all of the following *except:*
   a. Jugular venous distention
   b. Cheyne-Stokes breathing
   c. Cyanosis
   d. Hepatomegaly

6. Which of the following is *not* an age-related pulmonary change?
   a. Loss of elastic recoil
   b. Increase in FRC
   c. Increase in total lung compliance
   d. Decrease in vital capacity

7. Blunted cell-mediated immunity in older adults is one factor in the increased incidence of:
   a. Pneumonia
   b. Leukemia
   c. Emphysema
   d. Tuberculosis

8. A 90-year-old patient is admitted to the hospital with a diagnosis of pneumonia. Based on your knowledge of pneumonia in older adults, the clinical presentation would most likely include:
   a. An increased respiratory rate
   b. A productive cough
   c. An elevated body temperature
   d. Radiating chest pain

9. Which of the following is the definition of pulse pressure?
   a. A palpable apical pulse
   b. A pulse felt over the point of maximal impulse
   c. The sum of systolic and diastolic pressures
   d. The difference between systolic and diastolic pressures

10. Syncope associated with standing up quickly may be the result of which of the following?
    a. Hyperthermia
    b. Orthostatic hypertension
    c. Orthostatic hypotension
    d. Pulmonary hypertension

11. Which of the following is an abnormal heart sound in older adults that may be an early sign of CHF?
    a. $S_1$
    b. $S_2$
    c. $S_3$
    d. $S_4$

12. Which serum value may decrease as a result of the normal aging process?
    a. Glucose
    b. Calcium
    c. Creatinine clearance
    d. Cholesterol

13. Which of the following activities is classified as an IADL?
    a. Combing one's hair
    b. Walking from the bedroom to the kitchen
    c. Calling the neighbor on the telephone
    d. Getting dressed by oneself

14. Based on current data, which of the following is the projected $Pao_2$ of a healthy 74-year-old person?
    a. 74.4 mm Hg
    b. 80.8 mm Hg
    c. 84.2 mm Hg
    d. 87.2 mm Hg

15. Approximately what percentage of adults older than 65 years of age in the United States live in a nursing home?
    a. 5%
    b. 10%
    c. 15%
    d. 20%

16. A normal $Spo_2$ percent for a healthy active older adult should be no lower than which of the following?
    a. 98
    b. 96
    c. 94
    d. 92

17. True/False: The number of older adults both living with HIV and being diagnosed with the disease is increasing significantly.
    a. True
    b. False

18. Ageism is defined as which of the following?
    a. A study of the effects of aging on older adults
    b. Sociologic consequences of aging and how they affect individuals
    c. A discriminatory attitude against older adults
    d. The realization that all older adults are sick and debilitated

## BIBLIOGRAPHY

Administration for Community Living. *Profile of older Americans*; 2015. Available at http://www.aoa.acl.gov/aging_statistics/profile/index.aspx.

Administration for Community Living. *A statistical profile of black older Americans aged 65+*; 2015. Available at http://www.aoa.gov/Aging_Statistics/minority_aging/Facts-on-Black-Elderly-plain_format.aspx.

Alzheimer's Association. *Communication and Alzheimer's*; 2016. Available at http://www.alz.org/care/dementia-communication-tips.asp. 2016.

American Heart Association. *Diagnosing heart failure*; 2015. Available at http://www.heart.org/HEARTORG/Conditions/Heart-Failure/DiagnosingHeartFailure/Diagnosing-Heart-Failure_UCM_002047_Article.jsp.

American Heart Association. *Older Americans and cardiovascular diseases: statistical fact sheet*; 2013. Available at http://www.heart.org/idc/groups/heart-public/@wcm/@sop/@smd/documents/downloadable/ucm_319574.pdf.

American Heart Association. *Prevention and treatment of high blood pressure*; 2015. Available at http://www.heart.org/HEARTORG/Conditions/HighBloodPressure/PreventionTreatmentofHighBloodPressure/Prevention-Treatment-of-High-Blood-Pressure_UCM_002054_Article.jsp#.V2sew6KGPm0.

American Heart Association. *Problem: aortic valve stenosis*; 2016. Available at http://www.heart.org/HEARTORG/Conditions/More/HeartValveProblemsandDisease/Problem-Aortic-Valve-Stenosis_UCM_450437_Article.jsp#.V2skh6KGPm0.

American Heart Association. *Understanding blood pressure readings*; 2015. Available at http://www.heart.org/HEARTORG/Conditions/HighBloodPressure/AboutHighBloodPressure/Understanding-Blood-Pressure-Readings_UCM_301764_Article.jsp#.V2sfXKKGPm0.

American Heart Association. *What is atrial fibrillation (AFib or AF)?* 2016. Available at http://www.heart.org/HEARTORG/Conditions/Arrhythmia/AboutArrhythmia/What-is-Atrial-Fibrillation-AFib-or-AF_UCM_423748_Article.jsp.

American Tinnitus Association: Understanding the facts. Available at http://www.ata.org/understanding-facts.

Asthma and Allergy Foundation of America. *Asthma facts and figures*; 2015. Available at http://www.aafa.org/page/asthma-facts.aspx.

Asthma and Allergy Foundation of America. *Asthma information for patients*; 2015. Available at http://www.aafa.org/page/asthma.aspx.

Beers MH. *The Merck manual of health and aging*. Whitehouse Station, NJ: Merck; 1991.

Bickeley L, Szilagyi P. *Bate's guide to physical examination and history taking*. 11th ed. Philadelphia: Lippincott Williams & Wilkins; 2009.

Cardus J, Burgose F, Diaz O, et al. Increase in pulmonary ventilation-perfusion inequality with age in healthy individuals. *Am J Resp Crit Care*. 1997;156:648.

Centers for Disease Control and Prevention. *High blood pressure*; 2016. Available at http://www.cdc.gov/bloodpressure/index/htm.

Centers for Disease Control and Prevention. *HIV among people aged 50 and over*; 2016. Available at http://www.cdc.gov/hiv/group/age/olderamericans/index.html.

Centers for Disease Control and Prevention. *Most recent asthma data*; 2016. Available at http://www.cdc.gov/asthma/most_recent_data.htm.

Cerveri I, Zoia MC, Fanfulla F, et al. Reference values of arterial oxygen tension in the middle-aged and elderly. *Am J Resp Crit Care*. 1995;152:934.

Ciorba A, Bianchini C, Pelucchi S, et al. The impact of hearing loss on the quality of life of elderly adults. *Clin Interv Aging*. 2012;7:159.

Cleveland Clinic: Presbycusis. Available at http://my.clevelandclinic.org/health/diseases_conditions/hic_What_is_Presbycusis.

Cone B, Dorn P, Konrad-Martin D. *Ototoxic medication (medication effects)*; 2016. Available at http://www.asha.org/public/hearing/Ototoxic-Medications/.

Connolly MJ. *Respiratory disease in the elderly*. London: Chapman & Hall; 2003.

Crapo RO, Jensen RL, Hegewald M, et al. Arterial blood gas reference values for sea level and an altitude of 1,400 meters. *Am J Resp Crit Care*. 1999;160:1525.

Genther DJ, Betz J, Pratt S, et al. Association of hearing impairment and mortality in older adults. *J Gerontol A Biol Sci Med Sci*. 2015;70:85.

Gerontological Society of America. *Communicating with older adults: an-evidenced-based review of what really works*; 2012. Available at http://www.lasell.edu/Documents/talk-of-ages/GSA_Communicating-with-Older-Adults-low-Final.pdf.

Halter J. *Hazzard's principles of geriatric medicine and gerontology*. 6th ed. New York, NY: McGraw-Hill; 2009.

Hardie JA, Vollmer WM, Buist AS, et al. Reference values for arterial blood gases in the elderly. *Chest*. 2004;125:2053.

National Eye Institute. *Facts about age-related macular degeneration*; 2015. Available at https://nei.nih.gov/health/maculardegen/armd_facts.

National Eye Institute. *Facts about diabetic eye disease*; 2015. Available at https://nei.nih.gov/health/diabetic/retinopathy.

Rutkove SB, Veves A, Mitsa T, et al. Impaired distal thermoregulation in diabetes and diabetic polyneuropathy. *Diabetes Care*. 2009;32:671.

Strait JB, Lakatta EG. Aging-associated cardiovascular changes and their relationship to heart failure. *Heart Failure Clin*. 2012;8:143.

Taverner T. The evidence on perception of pain in older people. *Nurs Times*. 2005;101:36–38.

Tomioka K, Ikeda H, Hanaie K, et al. The Hearing Handicap Inventory for Elderly–Screening (HHIE-S) versus a single question: reliability, validity, and relations with quality of life measures in the elderly community, Japan. *Qual Life Res*. 2013;22:1151.

U.S. Census Bureau. *An aging nation: the older population in the United States: population estimates and projections*; 2014. Available at http://www.census.gov/prod/2014pubs/p25-1140.pdf.

U.S. Census Bureau. *FFF: older Americans month*; May 2015. Available at http://www.census.gov/newsroom/fact-for-features/2015/cb15-ff09.html.

White House: The Affordable Care Act gives America's seniors greater control over their own health care. Available at https://www.whitehouse.gov/files/documents/health_reform_seniors.pdf.

# 14

# Respiratory Monitoring in Critical Care

*David L. Vines*

## LEARNING OBJECTIVES

*After reading this chapter, you will be able to:*

1. Identify the methods, normal values, and significance of measuring the following lung volumes in the intensive care unit:
   a. Tidal volume
   b. Rapid-shallow breathing index
   c. Integrated weaning index
   d. Vital capacity
   e. Functional residual capacity
2. Identify the methods, normal values, and significance of measuring the following airway pressures or related indices in the intensive care unit:
   a. Peak pressure
   b. Plateau pressure
   c. Compliance
   d. Airway resistance
   e. Mean airway pressure
   f. Maximum inspiratory pressure
3. List the definition, methods of detection, and methods of minimizing auto-PEEP.
4. Describe the value of monitoring pressure, volume and flow waveforms, and pressure-volume curves in mechanically ventilated patients.
5. Describe the methods and significance of measuring the fraction of inspired oxygen and exhaled carbon dioxide in the intensive care unit.
6. List the components of oxygen transport and their significance.
7. List the components involved in the clinical evaluation of oxygenation and their significance.
8. Explain how the following parameters can be used to evaluate tissue oxygen delivery and utilization:
   a. Oxygen delivery and availability
   b. Oxygen consumption
   c. Mixed venous oxygen tension
   d. Venous saturation
   e. Arterial-to-mixed venous oxygen content difference
   f. Oxygen extraction ratio
   g. Blood lactate
   h. Regional tissue oxygenation
9. Describe the value and limitations of pulse oximetry in monitoring oxygenation and oxygen delivery.
10. Identify the techniques for monitoring tissue oxygenation and utilization.

## OUTLINE

## KEY TERMS

airway resistance
alveolar dead space
anatomic dead space
arterial-to-alveolar tension ratio
arterial-to-mixed venous oxygen content difference ($C[a - \bar{v}]o_2$)
auto–positive end-expiratory pressure (auto-PEEP)
barotrauma
capnography
capnometry
carbon dioxide production
compliance
dead space–to–tidal volume ratio ($V_D/V_T$)
dynamic compliance

dynamic hyperinflation
end-tidal $P_{CO_2}$
Fick principle
functional residual capacity (FRC)
iatrogenic
integrated weaning index (IWI)
intrapulmonary shunt ($\dot{Q}_s/\dot{Q}_t$)
lower inflection point
maximum inspiratory pressure ($P_Imax$)
mean airway pressure ($P_{\overline{aw}}$)
mixed venous oxygen saturation ($S\bar{v}o_2$)
mixed venous oxygen tension ($P\bar{v}o_2$)
monitoring
near-infrared spectroscopy (NIRS)

oxygen consumption
oxygen content
oxygen delivery ($Do_2$)
oxygen extraction ratio ($C[a - \bar{v}]o_2/Cao_2$)
oxygen transport
oxygen utilization
oxyhemoglobin dissociation curve
peak inspiratory pressure (PIP)
physiologic dead space
plateau pressure
pressure-volume loop
rapid-shallow breathing index (RSBI)
static compliance
upper inflection point
volutrauma

Monitoring refers to the repeated or continuous measuring and/or observations of physiologic functions, life support equipment, and patient responses to guide management decisions and therapeutic interventions. Respiratory monitoring, specifically, is the process of continuously evaluating the cardiopulmonary status of patients for the purpose of improving clinical outcomes. The goals of monitoring include alerting clinicians to changes in the patient's condition and determining the underlying pathophysiology and cost-effective clinical management. These goals are accomplished through the use of physical examination, monitoring equipment, measurements, calculations, and alarms.

The goals of this chapter are to introduce the most common forms of respiratory monitoring in the intensive care unit (ICU), describe the information they provide, and discuss their application. Some of the information that normally would be included under respiratory monitoring, such as physical assessment, blood gas interpretation, and hemodynamic monitoring, is reviewed in other chapters of this book.

## VENTILATORY ASSESSMENT

Arterial pressure of carbon dioxide ($Paco_2$) is commonly thought of as the standard for assessing ventilation (see Chapter 8). However, changes in the patient's metabolism, lung mechanics, ventilatory efficiency, and equipment function will occur before changes are seen in the patient's blood gases. Table 14.1 provides a list of frequently used ventilatory parameters that are important to monitor. This table includes their commonly cited reference ranges and critical values, with the critical value representing the threshold for *insufficiency*. In general, the patient's status should not be based on a single critical value but instead should assess these parameters in combination with each other.

Ventilatory measurements that can be monitored at the bedside in the ICU include the following:
- Lung volumes and flows
- Airway pressures
- Fractional gas concentrations

### Lung Volumes and Flows

Ventilation is the process of moving gas mixtures in and out of the lung. These gases occupy spaces commonly called *lung volumes*. Although lung volumes have been described and their measurement discussed in Chapter 9, their importance to the critical care clinician is emphasized here.

### Why Monitor Lung Volumes?

The reasons that lung volumes are important to the clinician are as follows:
- They affect gas exchange in the lung.
- They reflect changes in the patient's clinical status (improvement or deterioration).
- They indicate response to therapy.
- They signal problems with the patient-ventilator interface (i.e., circuitry or ventilator settings).
- They help ascertain the patient's ability to breathe spontaneously or be weaned from mechanical ventilation.

### Who Should Be Monitored for Lung Volumes?

Following is a list of the most common circumstances in which patients will benefit from the monitoring of lung volumes:
- Intubated patients
  - Patients being considered for mechanical ventilation
  - Patients receiving and being weaned from mechanical ventilation
  - Patients with an abnormal breathing pattern

**TABLE 14.1   Common Parameters Used for Ventilatory Assessment**

| Parameter | Common Reference Range | Critical Value |
|---|---|---|
| Tidal volume ($V_T$) | 5-8 mL/kg PBW | <4-5 mL/kg or <300 mL |
| Frequency (fb) | 12-20 breaths/min | >30-35 breaths/min |
| Rapid-shallow breathing index (RSBI) | | >105 without PS or CPAP |
| Integrated weaning index (IWI) | | < 25 mL/cm $H_2O$ breaths/min/L |
| Dead space–to–tidal volume ratio ($V_D/V_T$) | 0.25-0.40 | >0.60 |
| Minute volume ($\dot{V}_E$) | 5-6 L/min | >10 L/min |
| Vital capacity (VC) | 65-75 mL/kg | <10-15 mL/kg |
| Maximum inspiratory pressure ($P_Imax$) | −80 to −100 cm $H_2O$ | 0 to −20 cm $H_2O$ |

*CPAP,* Continuous positive airway pressure; *PBW,* predicted body weight; *PS,* pressure control.

- Nonintubated patients
  - Preoperative evaluation (especially upper abdominal and thoracic surgery)
  - Adult patients with respiratory rates greater than 30 breaths/min
  - Patients with neuromuscular disease
  - Patients with central nervous system (CNS) depression
  - Patients with deteriorating blood gases
  - Patients receiving noninvasive positive-pressure ventilation

**What Do We Measure?**

Tidal volume ($V_T$) is defined as the volume of air inspired or passively exhaled in a normal respiratory cycle. $V_T$ for a healthy person varies with each breath but usually ranges from 5 to 8 mL/kg of predicted body weight.

$V_T$ has two components: alveolar volume ($V_A$), or the portion of $V_T$ that effectively exchanges with alveolar-capillary blood, and dead space volume ($V_D$), or the portion of $V_T$ that does not exchange with capillary blood. The common reference range cited for $V_D$ is 25% to 40% of the $V_T$. The Conducting airways and alveolar units that are ventilated but not perfused create the true or physiologic dead space. If the dead space exceeds 60% of the $V_T$, the patient may need ventilator support to help with the associated increase in the work of breathing.

**SIMPLY STATED**

Patients with increased dead space must increase their respiratory rate and/or tidal volume to maintain an acceptable $Paco_2$.

In healthy, spontaneously breathing people, the $V_T$ occasionally increases to 3 or 4 times normal levels. These larger tidal breaths are known as *sighs* and normally occur about 6 to 10 times each hour. In acutely ill patients, there is often a loss of the sigh, and the size of the patient's $V_T$ tends to diminish. A $V_T$ less than 5 mL/kg may indicate the onset of a respiratory problem. Impending respiratory failure causes $V_T$ to become more irregular. If shallow breathing without occasional sighing is maintained for prolonged periods, atelectasis may result, especially in patients breathing high oxygen concentrations or having compromised mucociliary clearance.

**SIMPLY STATED**

Rapid and shallow breathing in a critically ill patient at rest may indicate impending respiratory failure.

Conditions that may cause the $V_T$ to be reduced include pneumonia, atelectasis, chest or abdominal surgery, chest trauma, acute exacerbation of chronic obstructive pulmonary disease (COPD), congestive heart failure (CHF), pulmonary edema, acute restrictive diseases such as acute respiratory distress syndrome (ARDS), neuromuscular diseases, and CNS depression (especially of the respiratory centers). Patients with metabolic acidosis, sepsis, or severe neurologic injury usually have a larger than normal $V_T$.

Critically ill patients without an artificial airway may not tolerate the measurement of $V_T$. To accurately measure $V_T$, a facemask or mouthpiece is required. Patients often change their breathing patterns when a mask or mouthpiece is applied, which alters their $V_T$.

Patients receiving continuous mechanical ventilation (CMV) are routinely ventilated with $V_T$ of 6 to 8 mL/kg which are slightly larger than normal spontaneous $V_T$. When 4 or 5 mL/kg $V_T$ is set during CMV without positive end-expiratory pressure (PEEP), there is a reduction in functional residual capacity (FRC), an increase in intrapulmonary shunt, and a fall in partial pressure of arterial oxygen ($Pao_2$). These potentially harmful conditions can be reversed in part or totally by applying PEEP.

The use of higher $V_T$ ventilation can cause complications, particularly in patients with severe respiratory failure or ARDS. A high $V_T$ that increases alveolar pressures (plateau pressure) beyond approximately 30 cm $H_2O$ may result in lung injury. The use of high-$V_T$ ventilation may predispose patients to volutrauma, a lung injury that occurs from overdistention of the alveolar units. This risk of lung injury increases in severe ARDS because of the small amount of available lung participating in gas exchange, which is known as the "baby lung concept." To avoid this lung injury, patients at risk for developing ARDS should be ventilated with mechanical $V_T$ of 6 mL/kg or less at a higher frequency (breaths per minute) to maintain an acceptable acid-base balance (pH >7.30). Unfortunately, patients receiving low $V_T$ (4 mL/kg) and who have a strong respiratory drive may experience breath "stacking." The stacking results from a patient trying to inhale a

$V_T$ greater than set, which can decrease airway pressure to a point that an additional breath is triggered on top of the previous one. If plateau pressures are less than 30 cm $H_2O$, tidal volume can be increased by 1-mL increments until 7 or 8 mL/kg is reached in an effort to stop the breath stacking.

When using a smaller $V_T$, the application of PEEP maintains FRC and prevents the fall in $Pao_2$. Although no single approach to setting PEEP has been adopted, a review recommends setting the PEEP level to that which results in the best compliance and lowest driving pressure. Others suggest that PEEP be adjusted to achieve an end-expiratory transpulmonary pressure (difference between alveolar and pleural pressures) of 0 to 10 cm $H_2O$ using an esophageal balloon, which is needed to accurately obtain such values.

Monitoring $V_T$ during mechanical ventilation of a critically ill patient is crucial. Discrepancies between set and measured $V_T$ are often seen in these patients. Most of the time the differences are not clinically significant, and the clinician can make small adjustments in the $V_T$ settings to meet the patient's delivered $V_T$ needs. The differences are often caused by the compressible volume of the ventilator circuit or environmental factors at the different locations of the inspiratory and expiratory flow sensors (i.e., heated, humidified gases or differing flow profiles). Compressible volume is an important consideration in neonatal and pediatric patients and in patients with higher peak airway pressures and lower $V_T$. Most of today's ventilators will correct for volume loss to the ventilator circuit and humidifier if circuit compliance correction is selected and performed before the ventilator and circuitry are connected to the patient. Other sources that may cause a difference between set and measured $V_T$ include leaks in the ventilator circuit, partially deflated endotracheal (ET) tube cuff, and bronchopleural fistula.

A low measured $V_T$ also can be caused by severe air trapping or dynamic hyperinflation, which is a problem seen with severe airway obstruction. If not enough time is allowed for exhalation before the next breath is initiated by the ventilator, the subsequent $V_T$ will stack on top of the previous breath. This problem creates higher peak airway pressure, and pressure injury to the lung, called barotrauma, may result. Increasing expiratory time, administering bronchodilators, or decreasing the $V_T$ may help resolve the problem. Expiratory time is increased by reducing ventilator rate (if inspiratory time remains constant), increasing inspiratory flow rate, or decreasing inspiratory time.

If the circuit compliance feature is not used, the corrected tidal volume will need to be calculated. The corrected or delivered $V_T$ is determined by calculating the compressible volume of the ventilator circuit and subtracting it from the exhaled $V_T$. To calculate the compressible volume of the ventilator circuit, the clinician needs to know the compliance of the ventilator circuit being used. If the circuit's compliance is unknown, it can be determined by increasing the high pressure limit to 120 cm $H_2O$, setting PEEP to 0 cm $H_2O$, and setting a $V_T$ of 100 mL. Then divide the 100 mL by the resulting peak inspiratory pressure to obtain circuit compliance. The compliance of the adult ventilator circuit varies with

the structure and diameter of the tubing but is generally 1 to 3 mL/cm $H_2O$. If the patient is being ventilated with high airway pressures, a significant portion of the $V_T$ is lost to tubing expansion, and erroneous respiratory system compliance measurements would be computed if this loss were not considered.

$$Corr \ V_T = (V_T - [(PIP - EEP) \times CF])$$

where
Corr $V_T$ = corrected or delivered tidal volume
$V_T$ = exhaled tidal volume
PIP = peak inspiratory pressure
EEP = total end-expiratory pressure (defined later)
CF = circuit compliance factor (mL/cm $H_2O$)

Where $V_T$ is monitored often plays an important role in data interpretation. Monitoring volume before the circuit's wye or proximally eliminates the loss of compressible volume to the circuit and may reflect a more accurately delivered $V_T$ than does expiratory limb monitoring. This is particularly true during conditions of low $V_T$, low lung compliance, and high airway resistance ($R_{aw}$). Proximal monitoring is not without drawbacks. Proximal sensing makes the measuring device more susceptible to condensate and secretions, potentially reducing reliability and accuracy. It also may increase circuit resistance and dead space, increasing the patient's imposed work of breathing.

Air trapping and dynamic hyperinflation often occur in mechanically ventilated patients with severe airway obstruction. One technique that can measure the degree of hyperinflation is to measure the volume of gas exhaled during an expiratory hold on the ventilator. This maneuver measures the additional trapped gas above the patient's normal FRC. Ventilatory adjustments that reduce minute ventilation ($\dot{V}_E$), reduce $V_T$, and lengthen expiratory time should reduce the degree of air trapping.

---

### SIMPLY STATED

$V_T$ for mechanically ventilated patients should be adjusted for clinical conditions. Some patients, including those at risk for air trapping and dynamic hyperinflation or ARDS, should be ventilated with a lower $V_T$ of 6 mL/kg and adjusted down to 4 mL/kg to keep plateau pressure less than 30 cm $H_2O$ or eliminate dynamic hyperinflation.

---

Patients receiving synchronous intermittent mandatory ventilation (SIMV) are allowed to breathe spontaneously through the ventilator circuit between mechanical breaths. As a result, their spontaneous $V_T$ may differ in size from the mechanical $V_T$ being delivered by the ventilator. It is important for the clinician to distinguish between spontaneous and mechanical $V_T$ during weaning so that a true assessment of the patient's ventilatory status can be made.

When a patient is ready to be weaned from mechanical ventilation, a spontaneous breathing trial (SBT) should be attempted. The patient should be monitored for gas

## BOX 14.1 Criteria Indicating Failure of a Spontaneous Breathing Trial (SBT)

- Twenty percent increase or decrease in blood pressure or heart rate
- Oxygen saturation via pulse oximetry ($SpO_2$) ≤85% to 90%
- Respiratory rate greater than 35 breaths/min
- Change in patient's mental status, accessory muscle use, or the onset of diaphoresis

exchange, respiratory distress, and hemodynamic stability during this trial. Box 14.1 outlines the criteria used to define SBT failure. $V_T$ also may decrease if the patient fatigues during the SBT, as indicated by breath volumes below 300 mL or less than 4 mL/kg. Usually more than one of these signs is present when a patient fails an SBT.

The **rapid-shallow breathing index (RSBI)** incorporates this spontaneous breathing rate change and measures the ratio of respiratory frequency (fb) to $V_T$:

$$RSBI = f \, (breaths/min)/V_T \, (L)$$

RSBI values greater than 105 have been reported to be strong prognostic indicators of weaning failure. Patients who demonstrate a significant increase in their RSBI on ventilator removal are very likely to fail weaning. Repeated measurements of the RSBI during a period of spontaneous breathing may more accurately predict the ability to be successfully weaned or discontinued from mechanical ventilator support. However, early measures of RSBI during a spontaneous breathing trial appear to be of little value in predicting weaning outcomes in COPD patients.

Perhaps a better predictor of successful discontinuing of mechanical ventilation is the **integrated weaning index (IWI)**. IWI has been reported as the best predictor of weaning outcome. IWI is calculated by multiplying respiratory system compliance by arterial oxygen saturation and then dividing by RSBI. An IWI of 25 mL/cm $H_2O$ breaths/min/L or more is associated with successful weaning from mechanical ventilation.

$\dot{V}_E$ is the product of $V_T$ and respiratory rate or frequency and represents the total volume of gas inspired or exhaled by the patient in 1 minute. The average $\dot{V}_E$ for a normal healthy adult is 5 to 6 L/min. As with $V_T$, approximately 25% to 40% of $\dot{V}_E$ is dead space ventilation. $\dot{V}_E$ is often increased in the early stages of respiratory failure; it is not until later stages of failure that $\dot{V}_E$ begins to fall.

$Paco_2$ is considered an indicator of the adequacy of ventilation. The relationship of $\dot{V}_E$ to $Paco_2$ indicates the efficiency of ventilation. A $\dot{V}_E$ of 6 L/min is usually associated with a $Paco_2$ of approximately 40 mm Hg in a healthy person with a normal metabolic rate. If a higher than normal $\dot{V}_E$ occurs with a normal $Paco_2$ in a patient with a normal metabolic rate, there must be an increase in dead space ventilation. This is usually result of hypovolemia, pulmonary embolism, or obstructive disease.

An increase in carbon dioxide production caused by an increased metabolism (as occurs with trauma or fever) or high carbohydrate loading accompanying parenteral feedings may result in an increase in $\dot{V}_E$ with a normal $Paco_2$ (see Chapter 18). The elevated production of $CO_2$ requires an increase in ventilation to maintain a normal $Paco_2$.

A resting spontaneous $\dot{V}_E$ of 10 L/min or less during an SBT is often considered an acceptable weaning criterion. $\dot{V}_E$ may fluctuate both during traditional T-piece weaning and during pressure support ventilation (PSV). Many therapeutic activities also can alter $\dot{V}_E$. A good example is the postoperative administration of opiates to control pain. Opiates such as morphine can blunt the respiratory drive sufficiently to cause a sudden onset of hypoventilation.

For these reasons, $\dot{V}_E$ should be monitored frequently before and during weaning. A sudden rise or drop in $\dot{V}_E$ should be investigated because both may signal ventilatory failure. If a $\dot{V}_E$ greater than 10 L/min is needed for a mechanically ventilated patient to maintain a normal $Paco_2$, weaning is not likely to be successful. The elevated $\dot{V}_E$ indicates that the patient's respiratory muscles will probably fatigue when the mechanical ventilation is discontinued. Compared with the RSBI or IWI, a patient's spontaneous $\dot{V}_E$, $V_T$, or frequency is a much less reliable predictor of weaning success.

Vital capacity (VC) is the maximum volume of gas that can be expired from the lungs following a maximal inspiration. The typical reference range for healthy subjects is 65 to 75 mL/kg of predicted body weight. The VC maneuver depends on the patient's effort and position; the largest values usually are recorded with the patient in the upright position.

The VC is an excellent measurement of ventilatory reserve in the cooperative patient. It reflects the respiratory muscle strength and volume capacity of the lung while the patient is performing a maximal inspiratory and expiratory maneuver. Adequate inspiratory reserve is needed to clear secretions from the airway and periodically sigh to help prevent alveolar collapse.

As described in Chapter 9, VC can be measured as either a forced maneuver (FVC) or a slow maneuver (SVC). The SVC maneuver is usually collected in the ICU because patients may be medicated, be experiencing pain, or have obstructive airway disease. The patient must to able to follow commands to accurately perform the SVC.

The accuracy and repeatability of the values depend on the patient's effort and the coaching abilities of the clinician. It is important that the patient understand how to perform the maneuver correctly. A tightly sealed mouthpiece or mask is crucial. Observing a tracing generated by their effort or receiving some similar visual feedback may improve patient performance.

During preoperative evaluation of a patient's lung function, an $FEV_1$% (ratio of FEV in 1 second to the FVC) less than 50% of normal or an FVC of less than 20 mL/kg indicates that the patient may be at high risk for developing pulmonary complications in the postoperative period. Factors that influence the degree of decrease in VC during the postoperative period and the incidence of postoperative pulmonary complications include the surgical site, smoking history, age, nutritional status, obesity, pain, type of anesthesia, and types of narcotics used for pain control.

Although many factors can contribute to a reduction in VC postoperatively, one of the most important is the incision site. Thoracic and abdominal surgeries produce a significant fall in VC postoperatively, and this reduction may persist for a week or more. Operative procedures below the umbilicus are associated with fewer pulmonary complications.

A VC of 10 to 15 mL/kg is usually needed for effective deep breathing and coughing. Values below this range are usually associated with impending respiratory failure. Values greater than 15 mL/kg usually indicate adequate ventilatory reserve and the possibility of discontinuing mechanical ventilation.

VC also is measured to follow the responsiveness of the patient to various respiratory therapies such as incentive spirometry or intermittent positive-pressure breathing (IPPB). A common goal of both these maneuvers is to promote lung expansion.

---

### SIMPLY STATED

Multiple, not individual, measurements of weaning indices (RSBI, VC, and $V_T$) are most likely to predict success or failure.

---

FRC is the volume of gas remaining in the lungs at the end of a normal passive exhalation. It is rarely measured in the ICU. The FRC is continuously in contact with pulmonary capillary blood and undergoing gas exchange. It is composed of a combination of residual volume (RV) and expiratory reserve volume (ERV). Normally, FRC is about 40 mL/kg of predicted body weight, or about 35% to 40% of total lung capacity (TLC). FRC can vary from breath to breath by as much as 300 mL in healthy people. Changes in body position affect FRC, with the greatest values being recorded in the upright position. These changes in FRC between 30-degree Fowler and supine positions may not occur in overweight or obese patients. When alveolar volume falls, as with atelectasis, FRC is reduced, and there are regional changes in alveolar pressure-volume curves. Initially, as FRC decreases, dependent alveoli collapse and require higher distending pressures to inflate. Because the apical alveoli remain at least partially open, they are more compliant. Thus subsequent positive-pressure breaths are preferentially distributed to the apices. This distribution of inspired volumes to nondependent, poorly perfused alveoli increases dead space and contributes to the abnormal gas exchange seen in patients with decreased FRC. Dependent atelectatic alveoli may open during inspiration as alveolar pressure increases and collapse during expiration. Research evidence now demonstrates that repeated collapse and reinflation of alveoli leads to alveolar damage, capillary rupture, and considerable lung injury. The application of PEEP prevents alveolar collapse and may reduce the extent of acute lung injury. Therapeutic modalities, such as PEEP or continuous positive airway pressure (CPAP), increase FRC. This is the primary benefit to patients with atelectasis and refractory hypoxemia.

## Airway Pressures

It is important to monitor airway pressures for the following reasons:

- To help determine the need for mechanical ventilation and the patient's readiness for weaning
- To help determine the site and thereby the cause of impedance to mechanical ventilation
- To evaluate the progression or resolution of the underlying lung pathophysiology
- To evaluate the airway resistance and response to bronchodilator therapy
- To evaluate elastic recoil and compliance of the intact thorax
- To help estimate the amount of positive airway pressure being transmitted to the heart and major vessels
- To help assess the patient's respiratory muscle strength

Ideally airway pressures should be measured as closely as possible to the ET tube. This prevents resistance caused by the ventilator circuit from influencing the peak pressure measurement. Most modern critical ventilators measure these pressures internally, so it is the serial pressure measurements documented over the course of the patient's need for mechanical ventilation that is most important.

### Peak Pressure

Peak inspiratory pressure (PIP) is the maximum pressure attained during the inspiratory phase of mechanical ventilation (Fig. 14.1). It reflects the amount of force needed to overcome opposition to airflow into the lungs. Factors that affect PIP include resistance associated with the ventilator circuit, artificial airway (ET tube), and patient's airways and the compliance of the thoracic cage and the lungs. Sudden increases in PIP or peak airway pressure should alert the clinician to the possible presence of a patient-ventilator interface problem. Potential causes of an increase in peak pressure are listed in Box 14.2.

An increase in PIP while the plateau pressure (explained below) remains unchanged suggests an increase in $R_{aw}$. Common causes include bronchospasm, airway secretions, and mucous plugging. As a result of the relationship between PIP and $R_{aw}$, monitoring the PIP provides valuable information about the bronchodilator-induced changes in airway resistance in mechanically ventilated patients. It is important to note that whenever changes in the PIP are used for evaluating $R_{aw}$, no changes in the inspiratory flow, flow pattern, or $V_T$ should be made.

High PIP may cause barotrauma. However, evidence suggests that high peak alveolar pressures from overdistention lead to alveolar rupture, or volutrauma. Some conditions that raise the PIP may not affect alveolar pressure such as increases in airway resistance. Static pressure (plateau pressure) more accurately reflects alveolar pressure compared to peak pressure and should be used as the primary indicator to evaluate the risk for alveolar rupture.

### Plateau Pressure

To determine the cause of an elevated peak pressure, it is beneficial to separate the resistance component from the elastic recoil of the combined lung and chest wall. This can be accomplished by measuring the plateau pressure. The plateau pressure (also referred to as *static pressure*) is the pressure required to maintain a delivered $V_T$ in a patient's lungs during a period of no gas flow (see Fig. 14.1). Plateau pressure is measured by occluding the ventilator's valves immediately after the set $V_T$ has been delivered and holding the exhalation valve closed until a plateau pressure is observed. In normal patients this may take a few tenths of a second. In patients with airway obstruction, achievement of a stable plateau pressure may take several seconds. Any patient effort to inhale or exhale during this inspiratory hold can invalidate the measurement (Fig. 14.2).

During the period of no gas flow, the $R_{aw}$ component of ventilation is eliminated, leaving the elastic recoil component as the force required to maintain inflation. If the delivered volume to the lungs is known during this plateau period, the static or respiratory system compliance can be determined.

### Mean Airway Pressure

Mean airway pressure ($P_{\overline{aw}}$) is the average pressure recorded during the positive-pressure and spontaneous phases of a respiratory cycle. $P_{\overline{aw}}$ is calculated to determine the average airway pressure being applied to the lungs. Ventilator measurements affecting $P_{\overline{aw}}$ include CPAP and PEEP levels, inspiratory time (flow rate and flow patterns), peak pressure, and rate. A simple method of estimating $P_{\overline{aw}}$ is as follows:

$$P_{\overline{aw}} = [1/2\,(PIP - PEEP) \times (\text{inspiratory time/total cycle time})] + PEEP$$

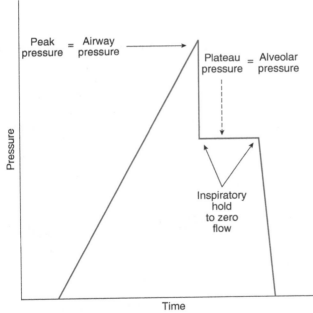

**FIG. 14.1** Theoretical pressure-time scalar during constant flow-volume control ventilation. The *solid-lined arrow* indicates peak airway pressure; the *dotted-lined arrow* indicates theoretical alveolar pressure. The difference between the dotted and solid line is the resistive component of the ventilator circuit, endotracheal tube, and airways. Notice that alveolar pressure equates to airway pressure only during the static, no-flow period.

Increases in $P_{\overline{aw}}$ are usually associated with an improvement in $PaO_2$ but can cause barotrauma and a reduction in cardiac output. When examining the aforementioned formula, it is easier to understand the greater impact that increasing PEEP and CPAP levels have on $P_{\overline{aw}}$ and thus oxygenation compared with increases in inspiratory time or inspiratory-to-expiratory (I/E) ratio. $P_{\overline{aw}}$ is often considered to be equivalent to mean alveolar pressure, but these values are not always equal. Discrepancies between the two values may be caused by imbalances in inspiratory and expiratory resistance, variable flow resistance, leakage of gas volume, and measurement error. Currently, no studies have shown a correlation between specific levels of $P_{\overline{aw}}$ and barotrauma in the adult population, but caution should be used when applying greater than 20 cm $H_2O$. Clinicians may need to adjust $P_{\overline{aw}}$ levels when switching from one ventilator modality to another. This is particularly important when switching to high-frequency oscillatory (HFO) ventilation. Typically, a $P_{\overline{aw}}$ 3 to 5 cm $H_2O$ higher is used when switching to HFO compared to the conventional ventilator.

---

**BOX 14.2 Potential Causes of Increased Peak Pressure**

**Resistance Factors**
*Patient Airways*
- Bronchospasm
- Peribronchiolar edema
- Retained secretions
- Airway obstruction caused by foreign body

*Artificial Airway*
- Internal diameter of tube too small
- Kinking of endotracheal tube
- Mucous plugging
- Cuff herniation
- Tube impinging on tracheal wall

*Ventilator Circuit*
- Water in tubing
- Kinking of circuit tubing
- High inspiratory flow rates (mechanical)

**Elastic Recoil**
*Thoracic Cage*
- Chest wall deformity
- Obesity
- Abdominal distention, compression, or herniation
- Diaphragmatic and intercostal muscle dyscoordination
- Active expiration, restlessness, pain
- Patient placement in lateral or prone position
- Chest wraps or casts

*Lung Involvement*
- Acute respiratory failure
- Pneumonia
- Acute respiratory distress syndrome
- Atelectasis
- Pneumothorax
- Fibrosis

**FIG. 14.2** Plateau pressure measurement during decelerating flow-volume control ventilation. The *dashed lines* indicate the point at which the inspiratory hold begins. **A**, Notice that the pressure-time waveform flattens and then squares as expiration begins, providing an accurate measure of plateau pressure. **B** and **C**, The pressure-time waveform dips, indicating patient effort during the inspiratory hold. Breathing efforts during the hold will cause inaccurate plateau pressure measurements. These inaccuracies are more common when low tidal volume strategies are used.

## Maximum Inspiratory Pressure

Maximum inspiratory pressure ($P_I$max), sometimes called the *negative inspiratory force (NIF)*, is the maximum inspiratory pressure the patient's ventilatory pump is capable of generating against a closed airway. The following factors influence the patient's ability to produce a normal $P_I$max:

- Respiratory muscle strength
- Patient effort
- Ventilatory drive
- Lung volume
- Phrenic nerve function
- Nutritional status
- Oxygenation status
- Acid-base status

Because $P_I$max is intended to be a measure of respiratory muscle strength, these variables must be considered when interpreting $P_I$max.

$P_I$max can be measured even if an artificial airway is not in place by using a mask or mouthpiece and an external pressure manometer. The alert patient should be asked to exhale to a volume between FRC and RV because this will improve the mechanical advantage of the inspiratory muscles. At the end of exhalation, the airway is occluded while the patient makes a maximal inspiratory effort.

There is a standardized approach to measuring $P_I$max in uncooperative critically ill patients. In this procedure, the patient is prepared for the maneuver by careful explanation of the procedure, proper positioning, and thorough suctioning with hyperoxygenation. Next, a one-way valve is placed in the expiratory path of a rigid T tube to allow exhalation but

not inhalation. This technique reduces lung volume to a level between FRC and RV. $P_I$max is usually generated within 20 seconds of occlusion. Careful explanation of the procedure is important because occlusion of the airway can be frightening.

A normal individual can generate a $P_I$max between $-80$ and $-100$ cm $H_2O$. Values more negative than $-30$ cm $H_2O$ have been used to predict successful weaning; however, there is limited agreement on this criterion. Although $P_I$max is useful in measuring the patient's respiratory muscle strength, it provides little information about muscle endurance. Most important, $P_I$max should never be used as the sole respiratory factor for predicting a patient's ability to wean. In combination with increasing respiratory rate and decreasing $V_T$, however, a low $P_I$max (0 to $-20$ cm $H_2O$) may indicate impending respiratory failure.

> ### SIMPLY STATED
>
> Mechanical ventilation is usually indicated in patients with neuromuscular disease (Guillain-Barré syndrome or myasthenia gravis) when multiple measurements of VC decrease to less than 10 mL/kg or less than 1 L, and the $P_I$max/NIF has dropped into the threshold range of 0 to $-20$ cm $H_2O$.

## Auto–Positive End-Expiratory Pressure

If mechanically ventilated patients do not complete exhalation before inspiration begins, they will develop auto–positive end-expiratory pressure (auto-PEEP). This can result from airway obstruction that increases during exhalation and causes insufficient time for exhalation. Therefore exhalation of each successive $V_T$ is incomplete, and a positive alveolar pressure occurs. The rise in alveolar pressure results in a PEEP-like effect, hence the term *auto-PEEP*. Auto-PEEP is not detected by the ventilator pressure indicator unless the expiratory valve is occluded at the end of expiration. When the flow is stopped at end-exhalation, pressure equilibrates throughout the closed system and registers on the pressure indicator.

Auto-PEEP is defined as the difference between the total PEEP (obtained by expiratory hold maneuver) and the ventilator's set PEEP value. All patients receiving mechanical ventilation should be assessed for the presence of auto-PEEP. It can be detected through observation, palpation, and auscultation of the patient's chest during exhalation to determine whether flow ends before the onset of the next inhalation. More accurately, the flow-time waveform can be examined to determine whether expiratory flow returns to baseline before the subsequent inhalation.

If auto-PEEP is detected, measurement of total PEEP should be attempted. It is not always possible to make accurate measurements of total PEEP because the patient must not inhale or exhale during the expiratory hold maneuver and the circuit cannot have any leaks. Many modern ventilators incorporate the ability to impose an expiratory pause that allows the measurement of total PEEP.

When auto-PEEP is caused by dynamic airway compression, the patient may be unable to trigger ventilator breaths despite spontaneous efforts. Forceful inspiratory efforts or the inability to trigger the ventilator will be seen. Increasing PEEP to approximately 80% of the measured total PEEP will reduce the inspiratory efforts needed to trigger the breaths. PIP will increase if the set PEEP level exceeds the resulting auto-PEEP. If this occurs, the set PEEP level should be lowered until PIP returns to its previous value.

Auto-PEEP varies with the time allowed for exhalation, the elastic recoil of the lung, and the resistance to flow of the airways, ET tube, and expiratory limb (exhalation valve) of the ventilator circuit. Bronchodilator therapy, clearing secretions, and increasing expiratory time by decreasing inspiratory time or the mandatory breath rate have been shown to reduce the amount of auto-PEEP. The most effective method to reduce auto-PEEP during conventional ventilation is through the reduction of $\dot{V}_E$. Strategies that alter $V_T$, ventilator rate, or inspiratory time without reducing $\dot{V}_E$ do little to reduce auto-PEEP.

### Compliance

Compliance is defined as volume change per unit of pressure change, or the amount of lung volume achieved per unit of pressure. This is further simplified by thinking of compliance as the willingness of the lungs to expand. Two forms of compliance are commonly reported: dynamic compliance and static compliance. Dynamic compliance represents the total impedance to gas flow into the lungs, and it is determined by dividing delivered or corrected $V_T$ by the peak airway pressure minus the positive end-expiratory pressure (PEEP):

$$\text{Dynamic compliance} = \text{Corr } V_T/\text{PIP} - \text{PEEP}$$

where Corr $V_T$ = corrected or delivered tidal volume.

Dynamic compliance incorporates both the flow-resistive characteristics of the airways and the elastic components of the lung and chest wall. Dynamic compliance curves are seen most commonly on ventilator graphic screens through the pressure-volume loops.

Static compliance, also called *respiratory system compliance,* is the lung volume change per unit of pressure during a period of no gas flow. Static compliance reflects the combination of chest wall and lung compliance. It is calculated clinically by dividing delivered $V_T$ by the plateau pressure minus PEEP:

$$\text{Static compliance} = \text{Corr } V_T/P_{\text{plateau}} - \text{PEEP}$$

where Corr $V_T$ = corrected or delivered tidal volume, and $P_{\text{plateau}}$ = plateau pressure.

In practice, static calculations should be based on at least three breaths. It is important to use the corrected or delivered $V_T$ (discussed earlier) to more accurately reflect the compliance of the lung-thorax unit.

Effective static compliance measurements can be useful in monitoring patients receiving mechanical ventilation. Lung diseases such as pulmonary edema, pneumothorax, pneumonia, and ARDS increase lung recoil and the observed static pressure. As a result, the static compliance is reduced in these situations.

The typically reported normal values for static compliance of 100 mL/cm $H_2O$ are rarely seen in mechanically ventilated patients because even patients with normal lungs usually develop a decrease in lung volume and compliance after receiving positive-pressure ventilation for a few hours. Thus normal static compliance values in patients receiving mechanical ventilation range from 40 to 80 mL/cm $H_2O$. Patients with static compliance values less than 20 to 25 mL/cm $H_2O$ may be hard to remove from ventilatory support and difficult to withdraw from PEEP.

### Airway Resistance

Airway resistance ($R_{aw}$) is the opposition to airflow by the inelastic forces of the lung. True $R_{aw}$ is not measured routinely in the ICU. A reliable estimate of the flow-restrictive components of $R_{aw}$ can be made by subtracting the static or plateau pressure from the PIP and dividing by flow in liters per second:

$$R_{aw} = \text{PIP (cm } H_2O) - P_{\text{plateau}} \text{ (cm } H_2O)/\text{Flow (L/sec)}$$

For this measure to be accurate a square flow waveform should be used and the patient should not be actively inhaling during the maneuver. For serial measure comparisons the same flow pattern and flow rate should be used.

The typical reference range cited for $R_{aw}$ is 1 to 3 cm $H_2O$/L/s. $R_{aw}$ can be elevated by numerous factors (discussed earlier). Increased $R_{aw}$ can cause problems not only during positive-pressure breathing but also during spontaneous breathing. A small-diameter ET tube will significantly increase the work of breathing for a spontaneously breathing patient. High flow rates from a continuous-flow SIMV system or high base flow through a demand valve system can increase expiratory work by forcing the patient to exhale against the high continuous flow through the patient's circuit and expiratory valve.

## Integrating Pressure, Flow, and Volume
### Evaluating the Patient-Ventilator Interface

Clinicians are often called on to evaluate the integration of the ventilator to the patient. Most often this consists of a sequential evaluation starting with the patient (use of accessory muscles, color, diaphoresis, heart rate, and respiratory rate) and airway (type, size, integrity, and stability), progressing down both limbs of the ventilator circuit (leaks, temperature, and condensate), and terminating with the ventilator settings and patient-monitoring panel. The RT also can observe the synchrony of the patient's breathing pattern and respiratory effort. This approach is beneficial at the beginning of the shift, after any ventilator-related event, and before and after adjustment of ventilator settings. The RT should then focus on the patient, ventilator settings, measured parameters, and, when available, ventilator graphics.

### Monitoring Pressure, Flow, and Volume in the Intensive Care Unit

Most ventilators manufactured today are equipped with a graphic display screen. This screen allows clinicians to review large amounts of patient ventilation data. Three of the most important parameters to follow are the pressure, flow, and volume tracings. The data can be displayed as a single parameter in a continuous tracing over time, called a *scalar*, or in combination with other parameters, called a *loop*. The individual parameters may be indexed to each other in a pressure-volume loop or a *flow-volume loop*. The integration of these three parameters provides a wealth of information important for proper ventilator management.

*Pressure-time waveforms.* The continuous display of the airway pressure waveform provides the opportunity to visually evaluate the following (Fig. 14.3):
- Airway pressure levels
- Characteristics of the airway pressure curve during all breath cycles
- Mode of ventilation
- Estimated respiratory work
- Adequacy of inspiratory flow pattern and peak flow
- Inspiratory resistive load (peak-plateau pressures)
- Gross estimates of patient inspiratory effort
- Estimations of the level of synchrony between the patient and ventilator

The pressure display on a ventilator graphic screen traces the rise and fall in airway pressure as measured within the ventilator circuit or at the airway opening. The clinician must remember that this tracing is a reflection of airway circuit pressure, ET tube resistance, airway resistance, and lung and chest wall compliance. If the ET tube is small or airway resistance is high, the tracings will not reflect alveolar pressures (intrapulmonary). In fact, only during a period of zero airflow (inspiratory or expiratory hold) does the ventilator airway pressure waveform reflect the actual intrapulmonary or alveolar pressure (see Fig. 14.1).

> ### SIMPLY STATED
>
> Increasing PIP while the plateau pressure remains unchanged is associated with an increased airway resistance. Patients should be assessed for bronchospasms, airway secretions, mucous plugging, and changes in set inspiratory flow.

The airway pressure waveform is helpful in setting rise time during pressure-limited modes. In adjusting rise time, the clinician is setting how fast the airway pressure rises to the set pressure limit. If airway pressure rises too rapidly, overshoot of the airway pressure curve may occur. This overshoot appears as a dog ear on the *right side* of the pressure-time curve (Fig. 14.4) or *left side* of the clinician assessing it. This problem is corrected by decreasing the rise time until this left-sided dog ear disappears. If airway pressure rises too slowly, the patient will feel air hungry, and patient comfort and synchrony will be compromised. This situation may increase the patient's work of breathing. Using a rise time that is slow can increase work of breathing. If possible, asking the patient if the breath feels comfortable can help the clinician achieve the optimal setting.

> ### SIMPLY STATED
>
> In spontaneously breathing patients on a pressure-limited mode, rise time should be adjusted to achieve the fastest raise to pressure without resulting in pressure overshoot.

Airway pressure tracings also are beneficial in adjusting the percentage of peak flow that cycles a pressure-supported breath (PS cycle %) into expiration. The lower this percentage is set, the greater the exhaled $V_T$ delivered for a given pressure-support level. Patients with high $R_{aw}$ typically need a higher PS cycle % setting to prevent active expiratory muscle effort to force expiration. If this occurs, the RT will likely see the abdominal muscles contract to push against the delivered pressure support and force the breath into exhalation. On the pressure-time waveform, this extra expiratory effort will appear as a dog ear on the *left side* of the pressure-time curve (Fig. 14.5) or *right side* of the clinician. If these conditions are occurring, the RT should increase the PS cycle % setting until the left-sided dog ear disappears or the patient is no longer using accessory muscles to force exhalation. If a targeted $V_T$ is desired during pressure-support ventilation, an increase in pressure-support level may be required after this setting is increased.

**FIG. 14.3** Pressure-time scalars. **A,** The patient is receiving assist/control ventilation, and the ventilator fails to sense the patient's inspiratory effort on the second attempt—missed effort. The trigger method and sensitivity should be adjusted to avoid missed efforts. **B,** Delayed onset of flow resulting from lack of sensitivity results in excessive trigger work. **C,** Scooping of the inspiratory pressure curve from inadequate flow relative to the patient's inspiratory flow demand. The *dotted line* represents the expected path of rise in inspiratory pressure.

**FIG. 14.4** Pressure-time curves can be used to set rise time during pressure-support and pressure-control ventilation. **A,** The rise time is too fast and results in pressure overshoot that appears as a left dog ear on the curve *(arrow)*. **B,** The rise time is set more appropriately, and the overshoot is no longer occurring.

**FIG. 14.5** In this patient with an obstructive disease process, the pressure-time curves can be used to set the percentage of peak flow that cycles a pressure support breath (PS cycle %). **A,** The patient is exhaling against the pressure support breath to cycle it into expiration. This expiratory effort by the patient creates the dog ear on the right side of the pressure-time curve *(arrow)*. **B,** The inspiration has been shortened by increasing the PS cycle %, and the patient is more synchronous.

### SIMPLY STATED

A lower flow cycle percentage or PS cycle percentage such as 10% should be used in patients with normal airway resistance and decreased compliance, whereas a higher PS cycle percentage such as 35% or 40% should be used in patients with airway obstructions.

During pressure-limited modes that are time cycled, such as pressure control (PC) and pressure-regulated volume control (PRVC), pressure-time waveforms are useful in determining if inspiratory time is too long. Prolonged inspiratory time can result in the patient breathing against or fighting the sustained inspiratory pressure (Fig. 14.6). Reducing the inspiratory time until the patient no longer opposes the sustained pressure should improve patient-ventilator synchrony. If shortening of inspiratory time causes inspiratory flow to no longer reach zero, the delivered $V_T$ may be reduced (discussed later).

*Volume-time waveforms.* The volume-time waveform is most often used to compare the inspiratory and expiratory delivered volumes. This can be particularly useful in checking for leaks within the ventilator circuit system or in determining the amount of leak around the ET tube or through a chest tube (Fig. 14.7).

**FIG. 14.6** In these flow-time and pressure-time waveforms, the patient is breathing against or fighting *(arrows)* the sustained inspiratory pressure during pressure-control ventilation. To correct this problem, the inspiratory time should be shortened.

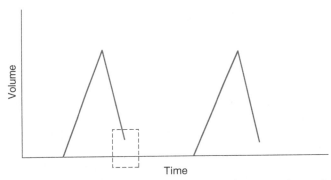

**FIG. 14.7** Volume-time scalar. The inspiratory volume is greater than the expiratory volume because of a leak in the patient-ventilator system, possibly from a bronchopleural fistula, endotracheal tube leak, or ventilator circuit leak.

## Flow-Time Waveforms

The flow-time waveform allows the clinician to evaluate the following:

- Both inspiratory and expiratory flow rates
- Characteristics of the flow profile during all breath cycles
- Presence of air trapping (i.e., auto-PEEP)
- Estimations of inspiratory effort
- Estimations of the level of synchrony between the patient and ventilator

The inspiratory flow profile provides information about how the ventilator breath is entering the patient. This profile is influenced by the flow pattern selected, mode of ventilation being used, and level of patient effort. During pressure-limited ventilation, airway resistance and respiratory system compliance also affect this profile, but the flow pattern usually assumes a decelerating appearance as set ventilator pressure equilibrates with alveolar pressure. The inspiratory flow rate and pattern should match the patient's efforts and breathing demands, demonstrating patient-ventilator synchrony. During volume ventilation, the set inspiratory flow and pattern chosen should create a smooth, consistent rise in airway pressure. If the set flow rate is too slow, the pressure-time waveform will show a dip or become concave (see Fig. 14.3C). Excessive flow rate creates a sharp, sudden rise in airway pressure. Some patients, particularly those with significant dyspnea, may require a higher inspiratory flow rate. Flow rate and flow profiles are particularly important to monitor during volume-limited modes of ventilation because the clinician sets the pattern and determines a finite flow rate. The inspiratory flow profile should be evaluated periodically and necessary adjustments made when using volume-limited modes of ventilation.

> **SIMPLY STATED**
>
> Scooping of the pressure-time waveform and a figure-of-eight pattern of the pressure-volume loop during volume-controlled ventilation indicate the need for higher peak inspiratory flows.

**FIG. 14.8** During pressure control ventilation, the flow-time waveform can be used to set inspiratory time. A, Inspiratory time is not long enough for inspiratory flow to reach zero (see *arrow*), which indicates that the set inspiratory pressure has not equilibrated in the lung. B, Inspiratory time has been increased, and inspiratory flow has reached zero (see *arrow*), which indicates that the set inspiratory pressure has equilibrated in the lung. In this pediatric patient, the increase in inspiratory time has resulted in a slightly larger tidal volume caused by the equilibration of set and alveolar pressures.

During pressure-limited ventilation, such as pressure support (PS), PC, PRVC, and volume support (VS), the inspiratory flow rate is determined by the resistive and elastic forces of the lungs and patient inspiratory effort. This flow pattern shows a rapid rise to a maximum flow rate, followed by a gradual tapering to a point of flow termination. This pattern is usually well matched to any changes in patient effort and allows the patient to determine the flow rate of the inspiratory phase of the breath. Adjusting rise time setting (previously discussed) also affects the peak flow rate and flow pattern created during pressure-limited ventilation.

During pressure-control ventilation, flow-time waveforms can be used to estimate inspiratory time needed for the set inspiratory pressure to equilibrate in the lung. When the inspiratory flow profile decreases to zero before expiration begins, the inspiratory pressure equilibrates throughout the lung, and maximum delivery $V_T$ for set pressure will have been achieved. Using an inspiratory time that does not allow inspiratory flow to reach zero will result in a lowered delivered $V_T$ (Fig. 14.8). If inspiratory flow is reaching baseline, further increases in inspiratory time will only result in a pause or inspiratory hold that increases $P_{aw}$. Unless the ventilator has an active exhalation valve that allows spontaneous breathing during the inspiratory phase, prolonged inspiratory time can result in severe patient dyssynchrony with the ventilator (see Fig. 14.6).

The expiratory flow profile displays how gas is leaving the lung and indicates the level of expiratory resistance and the expiratory time required to return to zero flow. The expiratory flow profile is used routinely to determine the presence of air trapping. When air trapping or auto-PEEP occurs, flow continues throughout expiration, and the onset of inspiration occurs before exhalation is complete (Fig. 14.9). However, a quantitative calculation of auto-PEEP cannot be made from an examination of the expiratory flow profile unless accompanied by a pressure-time tracing with an expiratory hold to zero flow.

**SIMPLY STATED**

If the expiratory flow of a flow-time waveform does not return to zero before inspiration begins, air trapping and auto-PEEP are occurring.

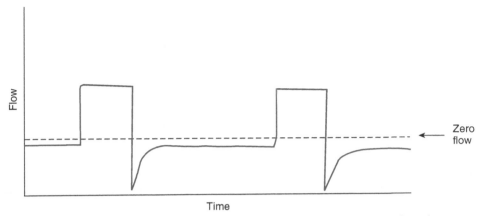

**FIG. 14.9** Flow-time scalar. The expiratory flow fails to return to baseline before the onset of the next inhalation. This demonstrates the presence of air trapping and auto-PEEP. The shape of the expiratory tracing demonstrates a prolonged expiratory time with low expiratory flow consistent with significant expiratory resistance in either the patient or the ventilator circuit.

*Pressure/volume curves.* The integration of pressure and volume data produces a useful tool: the pressure-volume loop. Pressure is most often displayed on the X-axis and volume on the Y-axis. The angle of the inspiratory and expiratory curves is known as the *slope* of the tracings. At normal inspiratory flows, the pressure-volume curve is a display of the dynamic compliance. It reflects both the resistive and elastic components of the circuit-patient interface. A typical tracing during constant inspiratory flow reveals a slightly concave inspiratory tracing, with the expiratory curve being slightly convex. The flatter the slope of the tracing, the less compliant the respiratory system is. Lower compliance tracings are most often seen with restrictive conditions such as ARDS and lung consolidation (Fig. 14.10). The wider the curve or the greater the difference between its inspiratory and expiratory limbs, the greater the airway resistance is (Fig. 14.11). However, proper interpretation of pressure-volume loop width must take into account the ventilator flow pattern. For example, as depicted in Fig. 14.12, a decelerating inspiratory flow pattern typically causes the inspiratory limb of the loop to bulge downward because of the higher initial flow.

The pressure-volume loop also can be helpful in setting inspiratory flow during volume-limited ventilation. The inspiratory limb should be slightly curved outward, as mentioned earlier. The tracings should move in a counterclockwise fashion. If the patient's effort exceeds the set inspiratory flow rate, the width of the curve will narrow and in some cases create a figure-of-eight appearance (Fig. 14.13). In such cases, the inspiratory flow should be increased until the curve resumes its normal shape. When using low-$V_T$ strategies to prevent lung injury in patients with an increased drive to breathe, the pressure-volume curve can be inverted and move in the clockwise instead of counterclockwise motion. If this happens, the patient's work of breathing would be significantly elevated. An increase in both $V_T$ and flow may be needed to

correct this problem. Remember that plateau pressure should remain below 28 to 30 cm $H_2O$ in patients receiving mechanical ventilation.

**SIMPLY STATED**

Graphic displays of ventilator pressure, volume, and flow waveforms are invaluable in the titration of ventilator settings and the assessment of patient-ventilator synchrony.

*Titrating PEEP and tidal volume with the pressure-volume curve.* Some investigators have advocated using a static pressure-volume curve to titrate PEEP and $V_T$. It is not routinely used in the ICU, mainly because it is time consuming and cumbersome, but it can be valuable for some patients, particularly those with acute lung injury. This technique, which incorporates a super-syringe filled with 100% oxygen and a pressure manometer, requires the sequential delivery of specific volumes to the airway. The volumes are delivered to the lung and held for a few seconds to allow equilibration and a static condition to occur. Sometimes the lung is inflated to a maximal level and then emptied in the same stepwise fashion. The corresponding pressures and volumes are recorded and plotted to form a curve. The initial points of the curve are fairly flat, indicating increasing pressure with minimal alveolar recruitment. As one moves up the curve, the compliance points change the slope of the curve. An upward change in slope is seen as a greater change in lung volume per unit of pressure or increase in compliance. The point on the curve at which a significant upslope first occurs is known as the lower inflection point. This point's corresponding pressure plus 2 cm $H_2O$ is considered to be the minimum PEEP that should be applied to the lung. As the remainder of the volume is delivered into the lungs,

FIG. 14.10 Dynamic pressure-volume loops. The slope of the curve represents the dynamic compliance of the system (*dashed lines*).

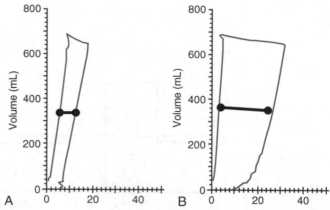

**FIG. 14.11** The difference in the width of the pressure-volume loop between A and B is due to airway resistance.

**FIG. 14.12** Dynamic pressure-volume loops. Nonconstant flow (decelerating ramp) changes the appearance of the pressure-volume loop. The decelerating inspiratory flow seen with pressure-limited ventilation will cause the inspiratory curve to bulge downward.

the corresponding line increases at the same slope unless compliance changes. Eventually, the slope flattens again, indicating that more pressure is being required to deliver the given volume or compliance has significantly decreased. This upper flattening characteristic identifies the **upper inflection point** and is referred to as *beaking*. Its presence in an apneic mechanically ventilated patient indicates a significant

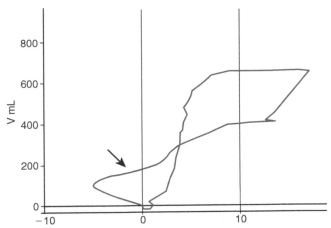

**FIG. 14.13** Pressure-volume loop indicating inadequate flow during volume control ventilation. The inward curve of the inspiratory limb of the loop, and especially a figure-of-eight appearance, indicates that the patient's inspiratory flow is exceeding the set flow rate.

**FIG. 14.14** Static and quasi-static pressure loops. The static pressure-volume loop is constructed by serial injection of aliquots of volume with a pause to zero flow and recording the resultant pressure. The volume and pressure data points are plotted through both inhalation and exhalation. The lower and upper inflection points (LIP, UIP) can often be determined by this method. It can be difficult to accomplish in the unstable, critically ill patient. The quasi-static method uses a constant, low-flow (<10 L/min) inhalation with continuous recording of the volume and pressure data points. Although there is a small error related to the pressure being recorded during flow, the error is fairly constant, and the inflection points can be approximated with this method. For both methods, the patient must remain completely passive, and attention to detail is critical in obtaining reliable results.

decrease in compliance caused by overdistention of the lung. The static pressure-volume curve can be used to adjust the minimum PEEP required to recruit and maintain open alveoli (lower inflection point) and to determine the maximal pressure level to limit the possibility of overdistention (upper inflection point) (Fig. 14.14).

---

### SIMPLY STATED

PEEP and tidal volume settings in mechanically ventilated patients should maintain lung volume between the lower and upper inflection points on the steepest part of the static pressure-volume curve.

---

The dynamic pressure-volume curves commonly displayed on ventilators in the ICU are different from the static curves just described. Because the pressure-volume points are being taken while the ventilator is delivering the breath, the ventilator tracings are incorporating the resistive and elastic characteristics of the ventilator circuit and the lungs. Consequently, the lower inflection point is typically higher than the minimal level of PEEP.

Quasi-static pressure-volume curves using specific settings have been advocated as a simple and reliable technique to determine the lower and upper inflection points. Inflation of the lungs is accomplished with a constant, low flow (<10 L/min) from FRC through the set $V_T$ range. The pressure-volume curve for this inflation is frozen on the screen for assessment. Patients must be sedated and paralyzed to obtain accurate lower and upper inflection points. It is thought that maintaining breath delivery above the lower inflection point and below the upper inflection point protects the lungs against ventilator-associated lung injury. Some ventilator manufacturers have incorporated this as an executable maneuver in their software.

## Fractional Gas Concentrations

The ability to monitor inspired oxygen concentrations is crucial for many respiratory procedures. Monitoring of exhaled gas concentrations also can be useful in patient management. These measurements can provide information about changes in gas exchange, tissue perfusion, ventilation/perfusion ($\dot{V}/\dot{Q}$) relationships, metabolic rate, and equipment function.

This section discusses oxygen concentration and carbon dioxide analysis and their use in the ICU.

## Fraction of Inspired Oxygen Concentration

Measurement of the fraction of inspired oxygen ($F_iO_2$) is essential to the modern ICU. Various oxygen delivery devices require at least intermittent analysis of $F_iO_2$ to ensure that the appropriate oxygen concentration is being delivered and to interpret blood gases. If the $F_iO_2$ is inappropriately low, hypoxia may result; an inappropriate elevation of $F_iO_2$ may lead to oxygen toxicity. Moreover, accurate measurement of both the inspired and expired $O_2$ concentration is required to conduct metabolic evaluations.

## Exhaled Carbon Dioxide

Carbon dioxide is one of the byproducts of tissue metabolism, and its elimination is a prime function of ventilation. Monitoring of exhaled carbon dioxide with either capnometry (simple measurement) or capnography (graphing the measurement against time) can detect changes in the following:

- Metabolic rate as a result of cardiac output and body temperature changes, shivering, seizures, trauma, and high carbohydrate infusion
- Ventilator function such as a patient disconnection or apnea
- Efficiency of ventilation (by looking at the increase and decrease in dead space)
- Transport of carbon dioxide as a result of changes in perfusion

Exhaled $CO_2$ analysis may be done on a breath-by-breath basis or by sampling mean concentration. The most common systems in current use employ infrared analysis (absorption of a specific wavelength of infrared radiation). Sampling can be done either by aspiration through a sample line or by placement of the sensor between the ventilator circuit wye and ET tube. Typically expired $CO_2$ is plotted against time. However, $CO_2$ levels also can be plotted against volume by incorporating a flow transducer. The latter technique allows the clinician to estimate dead space.

A single breath capnograph tracing for $CO_2$ concentration against volume is illustrated in Fig. 14.15. The tracing has three phases. Phase I contains no $CO_2$ and represents gas coming exclusively from dead space. Phase II shows a rapid increase in $CO_2$ concentration because alveolar gas begins mixing with the remaining dead space gas. In phase III, the $CO_2$ concentration begins to plateau with gas now coming mainly from the ventilated alveolar region.

The peak $CO_2$ concentration in phase III normally occurs at end-exhalation and is referred to as the end-tidal $P_{CO_2}$ ($P_{ET}CO_2$). The commonly cited reference range for $P_{ET}CO_2$ in normal subjects is 30 to 43 mm Hg, or about 2 to 5 mm Hg less than the $Pa_{CO_2}$. In individuals with healthy lungs, the difference between the arterial and end-tidal $P_{CO_2}$ (the arterial-$P_{ET}CO_2$ gradient) ranges between 2 and 5 mm Hg, and the $P_{ET}CO_2$ provides a good estimate of $Pa_{CO_2}$.

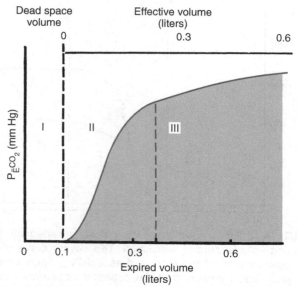

**FIG. 14.15** Single-breath tracing for exhaled carbon dioxide.

However, $CO_2$ elimination depends on many factors, including cardiac output, regional $\dot{V}/\dot{Q}$ ratios, and the emptying times of different areas of the lung. These factors commonly are seen among critically ill patients (e.g., mechanical ventilation, pulmonary disease, poor perfusion) and typically have the effect of altering $\dot{V}/\dot{Q}$ relationships and increasing the arterial-$P_{ET}CO_2$ gradient. For this reason, among critically ill patients, the $P_{ET}CO_2$ should never be used as a substitute for direct measurement of the $Pa_{CO_2}$.

Even among the critically ill, capnometry and capnography can be used to assess both equipment function and effectiveness of therapy. Current guidelines recommend that some form of $P_{ET}CO_2$ measurement be used to confirm proper placement of both ET tubes and supraglottic airway devices such as laryngeal mask airways. In terms of detecting equipment malfunction, Fig. 14.16 depicts several good examples of abnormal capnography waveforms indicating specific equipment-related problems. Furthermore, capnography is now considered a standard of care during moderate sedation to monitor the adequacy of ventilation and during cardiopulmonary resuscitation, both to confirm proper airway placement and to assess circulatory function. Specifically, during cardiopulmonary resuscitation, $P_{ET}CO_2$ levels below 10 mm Hg indicate poor circulation and the need to improve the quality of compressions. Moreover, an abrupt and sustained increase in $P_{ET}CO_2$ is a good indicator of return of spontaneous circulation.

## SIMPLY STATED

During cardiopulmonary resuscitation, capnography should be used both to confirm proper airway placement and assess circulatory function.

**Carbon dioxide production** ($\dot{V}CO_2$) is the carbon dioxide produced and excreted over 1 minute. The $\dot{V}CO_2$ values provide information about changes in metabolic rate and

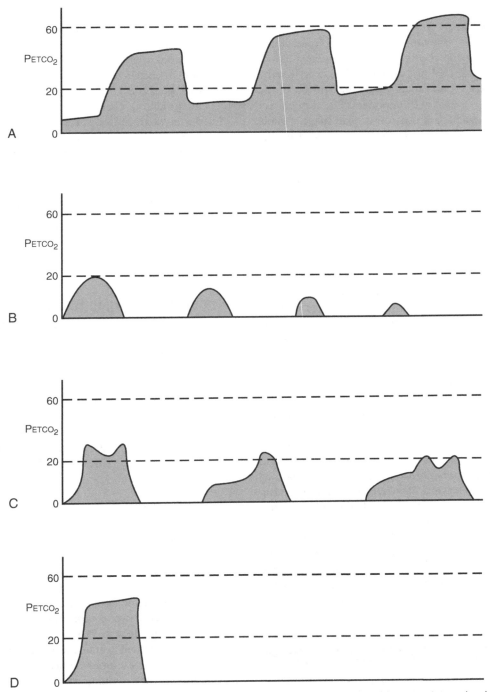

**FIG. 14.16** Examples of abnormal capnograms. **A,** Progressive rebreathing causing a rise in baseline $P_{ETCO_2}$. **B,** Placement of endotracheal (ET) tube in esophagus, causing a drop in $P_{ETCO_2}$ to 0. **C,** Leak in sample line or around ET tube cuff, resulting in low and variable $P_{ETCO_2}$ levels. **D,** Ventilator disconnect, causing an abrupt drop in $P_{ETCO_2}$ to 0.

transport of carbon dioxide. The formula for calculating $\dot{V}CO_2$ is as follows:

$$\dot{V}CO_2 = F_{\bar{E}}CO_2 \times \dot{V}_E$$

where $F_{\bar{E}}CO_2$ = mean fraction of expired carbon dioxide and $\dot{V}_E$ = minute volume exhaled at standard temperature and pressure dry (STPD).

The formula assumes that there is no carbon dioxide in inspired air. $\dot{V}CO_2$ is often increased in fever (10% increase per 1°C body temperature increase), trauma, peritonitis (25% to 50% increase), head trauma, rewarming after hypothermia, and high carbohydrate loading with total parenteral nutrition. A rapid decrease in $\dot{V}CO_2$ or carbon dioxide elimination accompanies a low cardiac output and a fall in tissue perfusion, decreased right ventricular output, decreased venous return, or pulmonary embolism.

*Dead space/tidal volume ratio.* $V_D$ is the inspired volume that does not come in contact with pulmonary capillary blood. The dead space–to–tidal volume ratio ($V_D/V_T$) expresses the relationship between $V_D$ and total $V_T$, or the portion of the $V_T$ that is "wasted." $V_D$ has two components: anatomic dead space and alveolar dead space. Anatomic dead space is made up of the conducting airways and is normally about 1 mL/kg of predicted body weight. Alveolar dead space is classically defined as alveoli that are ventilated but not perfused. The combination of anatomic and alveolar dead space is called physiologic dead space. $V_D/V_T$ is traditionally calculated by the Enghoff modification of the Bohr equation, as follows:

$$V_D/V_T = Paco_2 - P_{\overline{E}}co_2/Paco_2$$

where $Paco_2$ = arterial $Pco_2$ and $P_{\overline{E}}co_2$ = $Pco_2$ of mixed exhaled gas.

The patient is stabilized for 20 minutes, and arterial blood and exhaled gases are sampled simultaneously. $P_{\overline{E}}co_2$ should be provided by a capnometer as one of its measures, or the exhaled gases may be collected in a Douglas bag. Factors that may contaminate or dilute the $P_{\overline{E}}co_2$, such as compressible gas volume from the patient ventilator circuit or gases from a continuous-flow SIMV system, should be eliminated by double exhalation valves.

The common normal reference range for $V_D/V_T$ in healthy subjects is 25% to 40% and is position dependent. Patients receiving positive-pressure ventilation usually have a higher $V_D/V_T$ while they are upright or in the lateral position than when they are in the supine position. During anesthesia, $V_D/V_T$ is usually increased because of an overall reduction in lung volume. In patients receiving mechanical ventilation, higher inspiratory flow rates or small $V_T$s usually are associated with an increase in $V_D/V_T$. Variations in the inspiratory waveforms have less of an impact on $V_D/V_T$. Shortening inspiratory time from 33% to 15% and increasing pause time from 10% to 28% augmented $CO_2$ elimination by 14%. Changes in the pulmonary perfusion caused by emboli, hypoperfusion, and precapillary constriction may result in an increased $V_D/V_T$.

---

**SIMPLY STATED**

Increasing difference between $Paco_2$ and mean exhaled $CO_2$ indicates a worsening of dead space, which may result from inadequate perfusion.

---

## EVALUATION OF OXYGENATION

Inappropriate oxygenation is a common occurrence in critically ill patients. Recognition and correction of this problem are crucial to the patient's well-being. Respiratory care maneuvers, pharmacologic and fluid therapy, and diagnostic procedures often affect tissue oxygenation. The bedside clinician must be able to monitor and determine the effect of these activities.

This section describes the concepts and techniques used in the assessment of oxygenation. It includes the components of oxygen transport and the measurements used to monitor oxygenation. This section also discusses the indices of pulmonary gas exchange and indicators of systemic and regional tissue oxygenation.

The potential causes of hypoxemia and hypoxia are diverse. Hypoxic episodes can be iatrogenic (complication due to a procedure) in origin, as with suctioning or equipment failure. Worsening of lung pathophysiology, shock, or a new problem can make oxygenation more difficult. Therefore the bedside clinician must be able to identify the causes of these problems, select the appropriate therapy or therapies, and monitor the outcome. Causes of impaired oxygenation in critically ill patients are listed in Box 14.3. Haldane, the physiologist, said it best almost a century ago: "Anoxia not only stops the machine but wrecks the machinery."

## Evaluation of Oxygen Transport

Oxygen transport is the essential mechanism by which oxygen is carried from the lungs to the capillary bed. Equally important is how oxygen is used by the tissues, a process known as oxygen consumption or oxygen utilization. The majority of cellular oxygen is used for the production of adenosine triphosphate (ATP). Recent evidence shows that other activities, such as cell wall stabilization and chemical synthesis, are extremely oxygen dependent and sensitive to minor fluctuations in oxygen tension. Box 14.4 lists some of the crucial factors that determine oxygen delivery ($Do_2$) and oxygen utilization.

### Oxygen Reserves

In the critically ill patient, an increase in oxygen consumption or decrease in $Do_2$ to the tissues must be compensated for by an increase in one or more of the reserve systems:

- Cardiac output and distribution
- $Pao_2$ and oxygen saturation ($Sao_2$) values
- Functional hemoglobin levels

Patients with two compromised reserve systems are at high risk for inadequate $Do_2$ and subsequent tissue hypoxia. Critically ill patients often have compromised reserve systems. Low cardiac output (shock), blood flow maldistribution, anemia, and ventilatory failure do not allow adequate compensation to occur. As the abnormal situation persists, it becomes more difficult to correct and the more profoundly the "machinery" is damaged.

Oxygen content is defined as the total amount of oxygen carried in the blood as described in Chapter 8 and is calculated by summing its component parts:

$$O_2 \text{ content} = O_2 \text{ chemically bound to Hb} + O_2 \text{ dissolved in plasma}$$

$$O_2 \text{ content} = (\text{Hb content} \times 1.34 \times \% \text{ HbO}_2) + (Pao_2 \times 0.003)$$

## BOX 14.3  Causes of Impaired Oxygenation in Critically Ill Patients

**Equipment-Related Problems, Low- or High-Flow Oxygen Delivery Devices**
- Loose tubing connection, cannula
- Loose humidifier, nipple connector
- Inadequate flow to meet patient peak inspiratory flow, air entrainment
- Blender malfunction

**Ventilator-Related Problems**
- Endotracheal: tracheostomy tube malfunctions
- Ventilator and circuit malfunctions
- Improper settings, modes of ventilation

**Progression of Underlying Disease Process**
- Acute respiratory distress syndrome
- Cardiogenic pulmonary edema
- Pneumonia
- Airway obstruction, asthma, chronic obstructive pulmonary disease

**Onset of a New Clinical Problem**
- Pneumothoraces: simple, tension, loculated
- Lobar atelectasis
- Gastric aspiration
- Artificial airway problems: stenosis, fistula, malacia
- Nosocomial pneumonia
- Fluid overload
- Microatelectasis
- Bronchospasm
- Retained secretions
- Shock
- Sepsis
- Additional organ failure

**Interventions and Procedures**
- Endotracheal tube suctioning
- Position changes
- Chest physiotherapy
- Bronchoscopy
- Thoracentesis
- Peritoneal dialysis
- Hemodialysis
- Transport
- Diagnostic procedures
- Line or tube placement

**Medications**
- Bronchodilators
- Vasodilators
- Inotropic agents

**Miscellaneous**
- Leukocytopenia
- Intralipids

Data from Glauser FL, Polatty RC, Sessler CN: Worsening oxygenation in the mechanically ventilated patient. *Am Rev Respir Dis* 138:458-465, 1988.

## BOX 14.4  Factors That Determine Oxygen Delivery and Utilization

**Oxygen Transport**
Oxygen content of the blood
Cardiac output
Distribution of cardiac output
Oxyhemoglobin dissociation curve

**Oxygen Utilization**
Metabolic rate (disease, trauma, sepsis, nutrition)
Cell integrity (organ injury, sepsis)
Oxygen availability
Level of cellular toxins, byproducts (organ injury, sepsis)

Under normal conditions, Hb is responsible for carrying 99% or more of the $O_2$ in the blood, with the remainder (<1%) dissolved in plasma, and is measured as the $Pao_2$. $Pao_2$ reflects the degree of saturation of Hb and the driving pressure of oxygen between systemic capillary blood and the tissues.

Traditional respiratory care has focused on the physiologic mechanisms causing inadequate oxygenation of the pulmonary capillary blood (hypoxemia). Causes of hypoxemia include the following:
- $\dot{V}/\dot{Q}$ mismatch (most common cause)
- Diffusion defect (rare cause)
- Hypoventilation
- Shunt (extreme $\dot{V}/\dot{Q}$ mismatch)

Details on the differential assessment of these causes of hypoxemia are provided in Chapter 8.

### SIMPLY STATED

Oxygen transport depends primarily on the following three components:
   Cardiac output
   $Sao_2$ values
   Sufficient levels of functional hemoglobin
   A compromise in any of the three parameters must be compensated for by the other components. Patients with two compromised components are at high risk for inadequate $Do_2$ and subsequent tissue hypoxia.

### Cardiac Output

The techniques used to assess cardiac output are described in Chapter 16. $Do_2$ is extremely dependent on cardiac output and systemic distribution of blood flow. The major determinant of cardiac output is metabolic activity, whereas peripheral distribution of blood flow depends on regional oxygen consumption, temperature, humoral agents, and other factors. Cardiac output is not sensitive to moderate changes in oxygen tension ($Po_2$) and usually does not increase until the $Pao_2$ drops below 50 mm Hg. In the patient with shock, blood flow is redirected away from the low-oxygen-consuming regions of the body, such as the skin, to the vital organs, such as the heart and brain, in response to an increase in sympathetic tone.

## Oxyhemoglobin Dissociation Curve

Another factor influencing $Do_2$ is the oxyhemoglobin dissociation curve. This curve graphically depicts the relationship between $Pao_2$ and Hb saturation. The clinical significance of the curve is that large changes in $Pao_2$ may have little effect on the oxygen content or Hb saturation of arterial blood on the upper, flat portion of the curve ($Pao_2$ >70 mm Hg), but dramatic changes occur in oxygen content or Hb saturation on the steep portion of the curve ($Pao_2$ <70 mm Hg). At $Po_2$ below 70 mm Hg, large volumes of oxygen can be unloaded at the cellular level with relatively small changes in $Po_2$.

$O_2$ loading and unloading also are affected by the position of the curve. The position of the curve is measured by the $P_{50}$, which equals the $Po_2$ at which Hb is 50% saturated with $O_2$. A normal $P_{50}$ is approximately 27 mm Hg. A shift of the curve to the left decreases the $P_{50}$, whereas a shift to the right increases the $P_{50}$. Shifts of the curve to the left cause $O_2$ to bind more tightly to Hb and can impair unloading at the tissues. A left shift can be caused by massive transfusion of stored blood, rapid correction of acidosis that has been present for hours or days, or severe hyperventilation resulting in respiratory alkalosis. Other less commonly seen causes of a left-shifted curve are hypothermia and hypophosphatemia. Conversely, shifts of the curve to the right decrease Hb affinity for $O_2$ and improve $O_2$ delivery to the tissues. Acidosis, hypercapnia, and fever all shift the curve to the right.

The normal compensatory mechanism for a left-shifted curve is an increase in the cardiac output. Patients with compromised reserve systems who are not capable of increasing cardiac output or who cannot tolerate a further reduction in tissue oxygenation are at great risk for hypoxia if they have a significantly left-shifted curve.

To show how efficient the position of the curve is in improving $Do_2$, consider the following theoretical clinical situation. A patient with a normal fixed oxygen consumption of 250 mL/min, a cardiac output of 5.4 L/min, a mixed venous oxygen tension ($P\bar{v}o_2$) of 36 mm Hg, and a $P_{50}$ of 27 mm Hg develops a clinical condition in which the curve shifts to the left and reduces the $P_{50}$ to 20 mm Hg. This patient would need to increase cardiac output by 50% to deliver the equivalent volume of $O_2$ to the tissues. However, if $P_{50}$ were increased from 27 mm Hg to 30 mm Hg, the patient would require 20% less cardiac output. If such a patient had heart damage and was unable to increase cardiac output, the significant shift to the left of curve could result in tissue hypoxia.

## Monitoring the Adequacy of Arterial Oxygenation
### Partial Pressure of Arterial Oxygen

$Pao_2$ is used universally in the ICU as a measure of pulmonary gas exchange, but it is not specific or sensitive enough to be used exclusively in the estimation of oxygen transport.

Practitioners must keep this in mind when treating the critically ill patient who is hemodynamically unstable.

$Pao_2$ is an excellent value to follow to identify which therapies are effective to manage a pulmonary gas exchange problem (e.g., asthma) that is not associated with other complications. However, it should not be relied on in assessing systemic oxygen transport for the following reasons. First, it is a gas tension and does not directly reflect delivered oxygen. Second, $Pao_2$ reflects partial pressure available at the systemic bed, not what is used. Third, factors that may improve oxygen transport by improving cardiac output may cause $Pao_2$ to fall because of an increase in intrapulmonary shunt. It is not uncommon for multiple deficiencies to exist that adversely affect the oxygen transport system but are not directly related to pulmonary gas exchange.

Under most clinical conditions, $Pao_2$ should be kept within a range of 60 to 80 mm Hg. This usually ensures an arterial saturation of at least 90%. $Pao_2$ values greater than 80 mm Hg are usually unnecessary except in situations such as carbon monoxide poisoning and during periods of severe anemia or cardiogenic shock. A higher than normal $Pao_2$ does not necessarily improve oxygen transport. A $Pao_2$ greater than 125 mm Hg has been shown to cause a reduction of blood flow to both the kidneys and the brain, probably as a result of vasoconstriction.

### Alveolar-to-Arterial Oxygen Tension Difference

The alveolar-to-arterial oxygen tension difference ($P[A-a]o_2$) has commonly been used as an indication of gas exchange efficiency. Its major limitation is that it changes with alterations in $F_io_2$. See Chapter 8 for guidance on interpreting the $P(A-a)o_2$.

### Ratio of $Pao_2$ to $P_Ao_2$ (a/A Ratio)

The arterial-to-alveolar tension ratio ($Pao_2/P_Ao_2$, or a/A ratio) is a more useful index of pulmonary gas exchange than the $P(A-a)o_2$ because it remains relatively stable with changes in $F_io_2$. The a/A ratio is most stable when $F_io_2$ is greater than 0.30 and $Pao_2$ is less than 100 mm Hg.

An example computation is as follows. Given a $Pao_2$ of 50 mm Hg and a $Paco_2$ of 40 mm Hg while breathing an $F_io_2$ of 0.6, you would first compute the $P_Ao_2$:

$$P_Ao_2 = [0.6 \times (760 - 47)] - (1.25 \times 40) = 378 \text{ mm Hg}$$

Then divide the $P_Ao_2$ into the $Pao_2$:

$$Pao_2/P_Ao_2 = 50/378 = 0.13$$

The lower limit of normal of the a/A ratio is 0.77 to 0.82, with values below 0.20 to 0.25 (as above) indicating the presence of significant intrapulmonary shunting and acute lung injury.

The a/A ratio also can be used to predict the $F_io_2$ required for a desired $Pao_2$. In the above example, were we to increase the $F_io_2$ to 0.7, we could estimate the new $Pao_2$ as follows:

$$\text{New } P_Ao_2 (70\% \text{ } O_2) = [0.7 \times (760 - 47)] - (1.25 \times 40)$$
$$= 449 \text{ mm Hg}$$

$$\text{a/A ratio} = 0.13 \text{ (given)}$$

$$\text{a/A ratio} \times \text{new } P_{A}O_2 = \text{estimated new } Pao_2$$
$$0.13 \times 449 = 58 \text{ mm Hg}$$

Because the a/A ratio requires calculation of the alveolar $Po_2$, many clinicians prefer one of two other simpler measures of oxygenation, the P/F ratio or the oxygenation index (OI).

### Ratio of $Pao_2$ to $F_IO_2$ (P/F Ratio)

The $Pao_2/F_iO_2$ or P/F ratio is computed simply by dividing the arterial $Po_2$ by the decimal value of the $F_IO_2$. Using the same patient example above, the P/F ratio would be calculated as follows:

$$Pao_2/F_IO_2 = 50/0.6 = 83$$

A "normal" P/F ratio breathing room air would be 95/0.21, or about 450. The 1994 American-European Consensus Conference on ARDS used the P/F ratio as one of the criteria to define and distinguish between acute lung injury (ALI) and ARDS. A P/F ratio between 200 and 300 mm Hg is associated with ALI, whereas a P/F ratio of less than 200 is associated with ARDS. The other criteria required by both were acute onset, bilateral infiltrates, and a pulmonary artery wedge pressure of 18 mm Hg or less.

Note that although simpler to compute, the P/F ratio does not take into account changes in $Paco_2$. Moreover, unlike the a/A ratio, it cannot be used to predict the $Pao_2$ resulting from changes in $F_IO_2$.

### Oxygenation Index

The OI was initially developed as an index of ventilatory oxygenation support for a neonatal surfactant trial and then adapted as a prognostic index for morbidity and mortality for infants requiring extracorporeal membrane oxygenation (ECMO). The OI is defined as the reciprocal of P/F ratio multiplied by the mean airway pressure ($P_{\overline{aw}}$) times 100:

$$OI = F_IO_2/Pao_2 \times P_{\overline{aw}} \times 100$$

Again using our prior patient as an example ($Pao_2$ of 50 mm Hg with $F_IO_2 = 0.6$) and assuming $P_{\overline{aw}} = 15$ cm $H_2O$, the patient's OI would be computed as follows:

$$OI = F_IO_2/Pao_2 \times P_{\overline{aw}} \times 100$$
$$OI = 0.60/50 \times 15 \times 100$$
$$OI = 18$$

In general, OI values less than 5 are considered acceptable. Values in the 10 to 20 range indicate impaired oxygenation, with an OI above 25 associated with a severe oxygenation disturbance and poor clinical outcomes.

### SIMPLY STATED

Parameters that incorporate ventilator settings (oxygenation index) are helpful in determining severity of illness and can guide the initiation of other forms of care (i.e., if OI is ≥25 for 4 hours, consider other strategies).

### Intrapulmonary Shunt

Intrapulmonary shunting ($\dot{Q}_s/\dot{Q}_T$) is a major contributor to hypoxemia in critically ill patients. An **intrapulmonary shunt** occurs when there is perfusion to alveolar regions that lack ventilation. Clinical states that increase $\dot{Q}_s\dot{Q}_T$ include atelectasis, pneumonia, ARDS, pulmonary edema, and, rarely, congenital heart anomalies or arteriovenous anastomosis. The $\dot{Q}_s\dot{Q}_T$ and $\dot{V}/\dot{Q}$ relation may be measured by tracer gas techniques or radioactive gas and microsphere techniques, but the calculation most often used in the ICU is the following classic shunt equation:

$$\dot{Q}_s\dot{Q}_t = \frac{Cc'o_2 - Cao_2}{Cc'o_2 - C\overline{v}o_2}$$

where $Cc'o_2$ = end-capillary oxygen content (an idealized value computed using the $P_AO_2$), $Cao_2$ = arterial oxygen content, and $C\overline{V}O_2$ = mixed venous oxygen content.

Note that this measurement requires simultaneous collection of both arterial and mixed venous blood samples and thus necessitates having a pulmonary artery catheter in place (see Chapter 15).

$\dot{Q}_s/\dot{Q}_T$ is often measured while the patient is breathing 100% oxygen. However, breathing 100% oxygen for 30 minutes can lead to nitrogen washout and collapse of low $\dot{V}/\dot{Q}$ units. This phenomenon of alveolar collapse appears to be caused by poor ventilation of low $\dot{V}/\dot{Q}$ units so that oxygen uptake by the blood exceeds oxygen delivered to the alveoli by means of ventilation. The resulting microatelectasis increases the shunt fraction. Regional blood flow is usually reduced to areas of the lung with low $\dot{V}/\dot{Q}$ as a protective mechanism. Breathing 100% oxygen alters this natural autoregulation, causing increased shunt.

Pulmonary vasodilation and inotropic agents (e.g., dopamine) increase cardiac output but also can increase $\dot{Q}_s/\dot{Q}_T$. If oxygen transport is improved with this pharmacologic support, its use may be indicated regardless of the increased shunt.

In patients without pulmonary artery catheters, an estimation of $\dot{Q}_s/\dot{Q}_T$ can be made by substituting the value of 3.5 mL/dL for the actual measured arteriovenous difference in the denominator (a typical value in critically ill patients). Compared with the other previously described oxygenation indices, this method for estimating the shunt fraction correlates best with the actual measured $\dot{Q}_s/\dot{Q}_T$. This is because all the other oxygenation indices fail to account for the mixed venous $O_2$ content and, except for the a/A ratio, ignore the effects of alveolar ventilation.

### Pulse Oximetry

The principles of measurement, clinical use, interpretation, and limitations of $HbO_2$ saturation measured by pulse oximetry are detailed in Chapter 8. Because pulse oximetry is quick and noninvasive and can be used for continuous monitoring, it has become a standard of care in critical care units, in operating rooms and emergency departments, and during transport and special procedures such as bronchoscopy, computed tomography, sleep studies, exercise testing, and weaning from supplemental oxygen and mechanical ventilation. Oximetry also can be helpful in the ambulatory care setting to support pulmonary rehabilitation and justify and monitor home oxygen therapy.

Many studies have been performed to compare the accuracy and responsiveness of pulse oximeters to direct measures of $HbO_2$ saturation. Studies of healthy and critically ill patients with adequate cardiac output generally show a high degree of accuracy and correlation compared with direct arterial saturation, as long as saturation exceeds 65%. However, as described in Chapter 8, numerous factors can cause erroneous $SpO_2$ readings and must be taken into account when interpreting this measurement.

Selecting the monitoring site can be crucial to obtaining accurate measurement of $SpO_2$. Pulse oximetry sensors are primarily applied to the thumb or a finger of the hand if available. Unfortunately, use of the digits increases the likelihood of motion artifact that can interfere with good signal acquisition. Secondarily, the great toe of the foot, an earlobe, or the forehead can be used with the appropriate equipment. Earlobe and forehead sensors are specifically designed for those sites and less prone to motion artifact. Forehead and ear sensors also may be less affected than the extremities by poor perfusion. Fortunately, ongoing improvements in pulse oximetry technology have resulted in better artifact filtration and pulse signal recognition. These changes enable pulse oximeters to more accurately provide $SpO_2$ readings during periods of movement and during low perfusion states.

Pulse oximetry can be a useful tool in the ICU but also is prone to overuse and misinterpretation. Normal pulse oximetry values do not guarantee adequate $DO_2$ to the tissues. The anemic patient may be adequately saturated, but hypoxia may be present because of the low arterial oxygen concentration ($CaO_2$). In addition, the pulse oximeter does not measure $PcO_2$ or acid-base status. Abnormalities in these variables can be just as life threatening as hypoxia yet may go undetected when the $SpO_2$ reads normal.

## MONITORING TISSUE OXYGEN DELIVERY AND UTILIZATION

### Oxygen Delivery and Availability

Oxygen delivery ($DO_2$) is calculated as follows:

$$DO_2 \, (mL/min) = CO \, (L/min) \times CaO_2 \, (mL/dL) \times 10$$

The delivered oxygen value reflects the total amount of oxygen carried in the blood per unit of time. Adjusted for body surface area, the reference range for $DO_2$ for normal subjects is 550 to 650 $mL/m^2$ per minute. The delivered oxygen often is elevated with hyperdynamic states such as septic shock. Reduced values indicate low cardiac output or decreased $CaO_2$. Measuring $DO_2$ is one way to see whether the overall effect of a specific therapy is positive or negative. For example, increasing the PEEP level of a patient with ALI may well increase the $PaO_2$, $SaO_2$, and $CaO_2$, but this improvement

may be offset by a fall in cardiac output due to higher $P_{\overline{aw}}$ and resulting impaired venous return.

## Oxygen Consumption

Oxygen consumption ($\dot{V}O_2$) is defined as the oxygen consumed by the entire body in milliliters per minute. The reference range is 2.86 to 4.29 mL/kg per minute at STPD or 100 to 140 $mL/m^2$ per minute of body surface area. If one thinks of $DO_2$ as the supply, the $\dot{V}O_2$ is the utilization. Adequate supply does not always ensure proper utilization.

Many factors determine tissue $\dot{V}O_2$. $\dot{V}O_2$ can be limited by decreased oxygen availability because of a reduction in regional perfusion or a decrease in oxygen content. Demand may exceed supply, as in a hypermetabolic state, or cellular metabolism may be impaired, as in cyanide poisoning.

$\dot{V}O_2$ can be measured directly, through the analysis of inspired and exhaled gas volumes and concentrations, or indirectly, by multiplying the cardiac output by the arteriovenous oxygen content difference (Fick calculation). The formula for calculating $\dot{V}O_2$ using the direct method is as follows:

$$\dot{V}O_2 = \left( \left[ \left( 1 - F_{\overline{E}}O_2 / 1 - F_IO_2 \right) \times F_IO_2 \right] - F_{\overline{E}}O_2 \right) \times \dot{V}_E$$

All volumes are converted to STPD conditions. Fraction of exhaled gas that is oxygen ($F_EO_2$) is measured directly. The formula assumes that nitrogen is an inert (nonreactive) gas and that no other gases are present. The presence of nitrous oxide (a gas used in surgery by anesthesiologists) may introduce a considerable error if the patient's $\dot{V}O_2$ is measured immediately after anesthesia.

Direct $\dot{V}O_2$ measurement techniques are extremely demanding. The circuit must be completely free of leaks. Gas volumes and concentrations must be accurately collected and measured. The $F_IO_2$ must remain stable with minimal fluctuation. Technologic advances allow $\dot{V}O_2$ to be monitored continuously in critically ill patients during continuous mechanical ventilation.

The indirect calculation of $\dot{V}O_2$ is based on the Fick principle:

$$\dot{V}O_2 \, (mL/min) = CO \, (L/min) \times C \, (a - \overline{v})O_2 \, (mL/dL) \times 10$$

The Fick principle is used often in the ICU because of its convenience more than its accuracy. Variations between Fick calculations and direct measurement of $\dot{V}O_2$ may be clinically significant, primarily because of errors in venous gas sampling and cardiac output analysis. This error is greatest in patients with high cardiac output.

When $DO_2$ is adequate, $\dot{V}O_2$ is determined by the metabolic demands of the patient. $\dot{V}O_2$ will stay constant as long as the delivered oxygen is greater than a critical threshold of approximately 8 to 10 mL/kg per minute in anesthetized humans. This critical threshold is significantly elevated in ARDS and sepsis (Fig. 14.17). In patients with ARDS, $\dot{V}O_2$ is linearly related to $DO_2$ up to 21 mL/kg per minute. ICU patients often exhibit alterations in $\dot{V}O_2$ caused by trauma, sepsis, shock, changes in body temperature, anesthesia, therapeutic modalities such

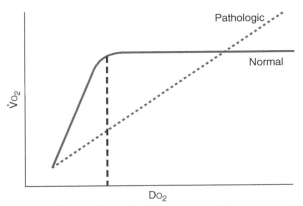

**FIG. 14.17** Supply dependence of oxygen consumption ($\dot{V}o_2$). Under normal conditions *(solid line)*, $\dot{V}o_2$ will increase until a critical threshold *(dashed line)* of delivered oxygen ($Do_2$) is reached. Beyond this critical threshold, $\dot{V}o_2$ remains stable, despite the increase in $Do_2$. In pathologic conditions *(dotted line)*, such as acute respiratory distress syndrome (ARDS), $\dot{V}o_2$ may not plateau but will continue to rise, as $Do_2$ increases, until well past the normal critical threshold.

as chest physiotherapy, and ventilator settings. $\dot{V}o_2$ has been shown to be an excellent predictor of survival in patients with trauma and shock and is helpful in determining the adequacy of resuscitation. It also has been advocated as an index of the cost of breathing in terms of oxygen use and therefore is useful in predicting the patient's ability to be weaned from mechanical ventilation.

$\dot{V}o_2$ values of 100% to 150% of normal after trauma or shock are associated with a better prognosis and have been identified as appropriate therapeutic goals for the high-risk surgical patient. Values less than 100% may be the result of decreased oxygen availability, as with low cardiac output or oxygen content, or with decreased use, as in hypothermia. In patients with severe injury, values greater than 150% may indicate a poor prognosis. If $Do_2$ is increased for any reason, increased availability may lead to increased consumption. This phenomenon has been observed in patients with ARDS, cardiogenic pulmonary edema, COPD, and pneumonia.

### SIMPLY STATED

Oxygen consumption is partially influenced by oxygen availability. In many critically ill patients, as $Do_2$ goes, so goes oxygen consumption.

### Mixed Venous Oxygen Tension

Mixed venous oxygen tension ($P\bar{v}o_2$) is a measure of the partial pressure of oxygen in mixed venous blood and is an indication of oxygen use by the entire body. Factors that influence oxygen transport and consumption invariably affect $P\bar{v}o_2$. The normal reference range is 38 to 42 mm Hg. Low $P\bar{v}o_2$ may result from the following:

- Inadequate cardiac output
- Anemia

- Significant hypoxia
- "Affinity" hypoxia (low $P\bar{v}o_2$ with increased $S\bar{v}o_2$)

A $P\bar{v}o_2$ of less than 27 mm Hg is usually associated with lactic acidosis. Increased $P\bar{v}o_2$ (>45 mm Hg) may result from the following:

- Poor sampling technique (pulmonary artery catheter in wedge position)
- Left-to-right shunt
- Septic shock
- Increased cardiac output
- Cyanide poisoning

Because $P\bar{v}o_2$ reflects the components of the supply-and-demand balance in perfused tissues, it is possible to have normal values of $P\bar{v}o_2$ and still have inadequate $Do_2$ to certain organs (e.g., kidneys). Organs with poor perfusion make a minimal contribution to venous return; therefore $P\bar{v}o_2$ may remain in the normal range even though an oxygen deficit exists, as in the vasodilated, septic patient with normal cardiac output.

$P\bar{v}o_2$ may not reflect changes in $Do_2$ and cardiac output. Because variations in $\dot{V}o_2$ also affect the balance between supply and demand, elevated $P\bar{v}o_2$ may indicate inadequate tissue oxygen utilization and marked maldistribution in systemic blood flow. This is common in septic shock. A low $P\bar{v}o_2$ is expected when the tissues are using the available oxygen effectively but the supply is insufficient.

$\dot{V}o_2$ is particularly high for the heart and the brain, so the $P\bar{v}o_2$ of these organs is extremely critical. A fall in perfusion would require a compensatory mechanism to maintain blood flow and oxygen to these organs.

The mixed venous sample is obtained by slowly aspirating, over about 1 minute, 3 to 5 mL of blood from the distal port of a pulmonary artery catheter. Central venous blood samples may trend well if the catheter is properly positioned, but generally there is a difference of 2 to 3 mm Hg between the $Po_2$ of central venous and pulmonary artery samples. The technique used for mixed venous gas analysis is important because errors in sampling may result in erroneous readings. The pressure waveform should be inspected before the sample is aspirated to ensure that the catheter is not wedged. Wedging may result in aspirating postcapillary blood resulting in an erroneously high measurement of $P\bar{v}o_2$. Air bubbles in the sample are also a possible cause of falsely elevated values.

### Mixed Venous Oxygen Saturation

Mixed venous oxygen saturation ($S\bar{v}o_2$) is measured from a mixed venous blood sample. Small changes in $P\bar{v}o_2$ lead to large changes in $S\bar{v}o_2$ and therefore large changes in mixed venous oxygen content ($C\bar{v}o_2$). As a result, the measurement is a sensitive index of cardiac output and tissue perfusion if $\dot{V}o_2$ is stable (Table 14.2). Like $P\bar{v}o_2$, $S\bar{v}o_2$ is a means of monitoring the general supply-and-demand differences in $Do_2$, not the use of oxygen at a specific site.

$S\bar{v}o_2$ can be monitored continuously through a fiberoptic system incorporated in a five-lumen pulmonary artery catheter. The system incorporates the principle of *reflection*

**TABLE 14.2 Interpretation of Venous Oxygen Saturation ($S\bar{v}o_2$)**

| $S\bar{v}o_2$ | Interpretation |
|---|---|
| 68%–77% | Normal |
| >77% | Sepsis, left-to-right shunt, excessive cardiac output, hypothermia, cell poisoning, wedged catheter |
| <60% | Cardiac decompensation |
| <50% | Lactic acidosis |
| <30% | Unconsciousness |
| <20% | Permanent damage |

*spectrophotometry* (traditional oximetry uses transmission spectrophotometry). An optical module transmits light through the blood by means of a fiberoptic monofilament. Reflected light is transmitted by a separate monofilament to a photodetector in the module. Because reduced Hb and oxygenated Hb absorb different wavelengths of light, a microprocessor can quantify the reflected wavelengths and calculate $S\bar{v}o_2$ (Fig. 14.18). When the catheter is properly positioned and calibrated, values correlate well with benchmark saturation measurements. Continuous monitoring has the advantage of providing immediate feedback for purposes of evaluating therapy. The continuous measurement of central venous oxygen saturation ($Scvo_2$) has been shown to be comparable to $S\bar{v}o_2$ monitoring, although others question its reliability.

Various factors, such as suctioning, shivering, pharmacologic intervention, extubation, weaning, and positive-pressure therapy, can decrease the $S\bar{v}o_2$ measurement, signifying a deterioration in pulmonary gas exchange, an increase in $\dot{V}o_2$, or a reduction in cardiac output.

## Arterial-to-Mixed Venous Oxygen Content Difference

The arterial-to-mixed venous oxygen content difference ($C[a-\bar{v}]o_2$) reflects the difference in oxygen content between arterial and venous blood. It is derived after simultaneous arterial and mixed venous blood gases are drawn. The normal reference range is 4 to 6 vol%.

Values greater than 6 vol% may be the result of the following:
- Low cardiac output
- Increasing $\dot{V}o_2$

Values less than 4 vol% may be the result of the following:
- Septic shock
- Increased cardiac output
- Anemia
- Increased oxygen affinity caused by a left-shifted oxyhemoglobin dissociation curve

The $C(a-\bar{v})o_2$ is useful in determining the effects of mechanical ventilation and PEEP on cardiac output and evaluating the need for additional circulatory support. It has a slight advantage over the $P\bar{v}o_2$ measurement in that it reflects content differences instead of partial pressure.

## Oxygen Extraction Ratio

The oxygen extraction ratio ($C[a-\bar{v}]o_2/Cao_2$) expresses the relationship between available oxygen ($Cao_2$) and oxygen extracted ($C[a-\bar{v}]o_2$). The normal reference range is 25% to 30%. Values greater than 30% indicate one of the following:
- Increased extraction caused by low cardiac output
- Increased $\dot{V}o_2$
- Decreased oxygen availability caused by decreased $Cao_2$

Values less than 25% indicate that supply is out of proportion to demand, which may be a result of the following:
- High cardiac output
- Sepsis with systemic shunts

The $C(a-\bar{v})o_2/Cao_2$ ratio identifies the portion of the delivered oxygen actually consumed and is therefore an index of the efficiency of circulation.

## Blood Lactate

If oxygen transport or its use by the tissues is insufficient for metabolic demands, anaerobic metabolism occurs and lactic acid is produced. Clinically this is seen as a metabolic acidosis with an elevation in blood lactate concentrations. The degree of lactic acidosis corresponds to the severity of oxygen deficit and is therefore a good indicator of prognostic outcome in patients with shock and multisystem organ dysfunction syndrome. The reference range for normal blood lactate is less than 1.7 to 2.0 mM/L. In patients with shock, lactate levels greater than 3.83 mM/L are associated with a 67% mortality rate, and values greater than 8 mM/L are associated with a greater than 90% mortality rate. β-Adrenergic stimulator drugs increase lactate levels because of glycolysis, and β-blockers decrease blood lactate levels. Patients with lactic acidosis are often treated with alkaline solutions such as sodium bicarbonate. This alkalinization may increase blood lactate levels because of a redistribution of extracellular and intracellular lactate but does not indicate a worsening metabolic acidosis.

Patients with cirrhosis have a reduced ability to clear peak lactate concentrations after periods of increased production. As a result, lactate is useful in confirming the presence of tissue hypoxia in these patients, but it is not a useful prognostic index.

## Regional Tissue Oxygenation (Near-Infrared Spectroscopy)

Recent advances in technology now provide the means to monitor regional tissue oxygenation noninvasively. The principle is basically the same as that used for estimating arterial $O_2$ saturation by pulse oximetry (see Chapter 8). Instead of using visible light, however, tissue oxygenation monitors use near-infrared light, a technique called near-infrared

Narrow waveband light source

Flowing blood

Microprocessor

$S\overline{v}O_2$

Photodetector

Fiberoptic bundles

A

B

**FIG. 14.18** **A,** Principles of reflection spectrophotometry. **B,** Fiberoptic catheter system used for continuous monitoring of venous oxygen saturation ($S\overline{v}O_2$). (A, From Mottram C: *Ruppel's manual of pulmonary function testing,* ed 10, St. Louis, 2013, Mosby. B, Courtesy ICU Medical, San Clemente, CA.)

**spectroscopy (NIRS).** Light in the near-infrared spectrum (700 to 1100 nm) can penetrate tissues and bone to a depth of several centimeters. As with pulse oximetry, using different wavelengths of light allows quantification of the relative differences in the amount of oxygenated and deoxygenated hemoglobin present and thus provides a measure of $HbO_2$ saturation in the tissues. This measure is commonly abbreviated as either $StO_2$ or $SrO_2$ (regional $O_2$ saturation). In addition to $StO_2$, some tissue oxygenation monitors also can provide an estimate of the Hb concentration that correlates well with in vitro blood Hb measurement.

The most common application of NIRS has been to assess cerebral oxygenation during surgery. NIRS monitors and sensors designed to assess peripheral tissue oxygenation are now being used in critical care. Sampling sites include the thenar eminence (group of muscles on the palm of the hand at the base of the thumb) or the inner surface of the forearm (Fig. 14.19). As a measure of regional oxygenation, the $StO_2$ reflects not only the $HbO_2$ saturation but also the matching of $O_2$ delivery to $O_2$ utilization of the underlying tissues, including the extent of peripheral vasoconstriction and regional ischemia that occurs in shocklike states. Often not detectable using central venous blood measures, regional ischemia is associated with poor outcomes among critically ill patients. Because $StO_2$ levels fall well before standard markers of tissue

**FIG. 14.19** Tissue oxygenation monitor (InSpectra $StO_2$ Monitor) used to measure regional $HbO_2$ saturation, in this case using a probe placed over the thenar eminence. (Photograph courtesy Hutchison Technology, Inc., BioMeasurement Division, Hutchison, MN.)

**FIG. 14.20** Example of trend monitoring of $StO_2$. Goal-directed therapy (e.g., fluid resuscitation, pharmacologic therapy) aims to maintain the $StO_2$ at or above the threshold value of 75%. Note that higher than normal $StO_2$ values can occur in hyperdynamic states such as septic shock.

hypoxia such as blood lactate, tissue oxygenation monitors can provide an early warning of potential perfusion deficits. In addition to providing early detection of regional ischemia or hypoxia, tissue oxygenation monitors can help guide therapy to treat it.

Among patients suffering from trauma or sepsis, keeping $StO_2$ levels above 75% decreases the likelihood of organ dysfunction. Indeed, the mortality rate has been shown to increase as much as twofold to threefold when the $StO_2$ remains significantly below this level and cannot be restored. For this reason, an $StO_2$ of 75% has been recommended as the threshold for intervention (Fig. 14.20). The addition of a vascular occlusion test (VOT) improves the ability of $StO_2$ to identify tissue hypoperfusion. To perform a VOT, blood flow to the arm is rapidly stopped by inflating a sphygmomanometer cuff to 30 mm Hg above systolic pressure either for 3 minutes or until the forearm or thenar $StO_2$ drops to a defined minimal value (usually 40%), followed by rapid release of the cuff and restoration of perfusion. The slope of the fall in $StO_2$ with arterial occlusion is termed the *deoxygenation rate* ($DeO_2$), which reflects the metabolic rate of the underlying tissues. The slope of the rise in $StO_2$ with restoration of blood is termed the *reoxygenation rate* ($ReO_2$), which is a measure of local cardiovascular reserve and microcirculatory flow.

Because maintenance of adequate tissue oxygenation is a primary goal, clinicians must be more involved in both the collection and interpretation of relevant data and incorporate the information provided by this new technology into their clinical decision making.

## KEY POINTS

- The ventilatory measurements that can be monitored at the bedside in the ICU routinely include lung volumes and flows, airway pressures, and fractional gas concentrations.
- $V_T$ for a healthy person varies with each breath but typically ranges from 5 to 8 mL/kg of predicted body weight.
- If shallow breathing without occasional sighing is maintained for prolonged periods, atelectasis and pneumonia may result, especially in patients breathing high oxygen concentrations or having compromised mucociliary clearance.
- Conditions that may cause the $V_T$ to be reduced include pneumonia, atelectasis, the postoperative period after chest and abdominal surgeries, chest trauma, acute exacerbation of COPD, CHF, acute restrictive diseases such as ARDS, neuromuscular diseases, and CNS depression (especially of the respiratory centers).
- The use of high $V_T$ ventilation may predispose patients to volutrauma, a lung injury that occurs from overdistention of the terminal respiratory units.
- A low measured $V_T$ also can be caused by "stacking" or dynamic hyperinflation, a problem seen with severe airway obstruction. If not enough time is allowed for exhalation before the next breath is initiated by the ventilator, the subsequent $V_T$ will "stack" on top of the previous breath.

- When a patient is ready to be weaned from mechanical ventilation, a spontaneous breathing trial (SBT) should be attempted. The patient should be monitored for gas exchange, respiratory distress, and hemodynamic stability during this trial.
- If a higher than normal $\dot{V}_E$ is associated with a normal $PaCO_2$ in a patient with a normal metabolic rate, there must be an increase in wasted or dead space ventilation.
- If a spontaneous $\dot{V}_E$ greater than 10 L/min is needed for a mechanically ventilated patient to maintain a normal $PaCO_2$, weaning is not likely to be successful.
- VC is the maximal volume of gas that can be expired from the lungs following a maximal inspiration. The normal reference range for healthy persons is 65 to 75 mL/kg of predicted body weight.
- A VC of 10 to 15 mL/kg is usually needed for effective deep breathing and coughing.
- PIP is the maximal pressure attained during the inspiratory phase of mechanical ventilation. It reflects the amount of force needed to overcome opposition to airflow into the lungs.
- If the PIP increases while the plateau pressure is unchanged, an increase in $R_{aw}$ is probably occurring. Common causes include bronchospasm, airway secretions, and mucous plugging.

- The plateau pressure (also referred to as static pressure) is the pressure required to maintain a delivered $V_T$ in a patient's lungs during a period of no gas flow.
- $P_I$max, sometimes called the NIF, is the maximal inspiratory pressure the patient's ventilatory pump is capable of generating against a closed airway.
- A normal $P_I$max or NIF is approximately −80 to −100 cm $H_2O$. A $P_I$max of −30 cm $H_2O$ may be useful when considered in conjunction with other parameters in predicting successful weaning.
- If mechanically ventilated patients do not complete exhalation before inspiration begins, they will develop auto-PEEP. This can result from airway obstruction that increases during exhalation and causes insufficient time for exhalation.
- Auto-PEEP varies with the time allowed for exhalation, the elastic recoil of the lung, and the resistance to flow of the airways, ET tube, and expiratory limb (exhalation valve) of the ventilator circuit. Bronchodilator therapy, decreased inspiratory time, and a reduction in the mechanical frequency have been shown to reduce the amount of auto-PEEP.
- Static (or respiratory system) compliance is the lung volume change per unit of pressure during a period of no gas flow. Static compliance reflects a combination of chest wall and lung compliance.
- Most ventilators manufactured today are equipped with a graphic display screen. Three of the most important parameters to follow are the pressure, flow, and volume tracings of mechanically ventilated patients. The individual parameters may be indexed to each other, as in a pressure-volume loop or a flow-volume loop.
- $V_D$ is the inspired volume that does not come in contact with pulmonary capillary blood. The $V_D/V_T$ ratio expresses the relationship between $V_D$ and total $V_T$, or the portion of the $V_T$ that is "wasted." $V_D$ has two components: anatomic dead space and alveolar dead space.
- The normal $V_D/V_T$ ratio for healthy persons is between 25% and 40% and is position dependent.
- Oxygen delivery to the tissues is a function of $Cao_2$ and cardiac output. If either component fails, tissue hypoxia may occur.
- Intrapulmonary shunt ($\dot{Q}_s/\dot{Q}_T$) is a major contributor to hypoxemia in most critically ill patients and represents the proportion of blood flow perfusing the lungs that does not pass by ventilated alveoli.
- Pulse oximetry is a noninvasive technique for measuring $HbO_2$ saturation in the arterial blood.
- $\dot{V}o_2$ is defined as the oxygen consumed by the entire body in milliliters per minute. The normal reference range is 2.86 to 4.29 mL/min/kg at STPD or 100 to 140 mL/min/m² of body surface area.
- $P\bar{v}o_2$ is a measure of the $O_2$ partial pressure in mixed venous blood and is an indication of oxygen use by the entire body; the normal reference range of $P\bar{v}o_2$ is 38 to 42 mm Hg, with low values associated with low cardiac

output or reduced $Cao_2$ in a patient with limited cardiac reserve.
- Keeping noninvasively monitored tissue $O_2$ saturation ($Sto_2$) levels above 75% decreases the likelihood of organ dysfunction and mortality among shock and trauma patients.

## CASE STUDY

Lucy is a 30-year-old woman with asthma who presented to the emergency room with shortness of breath, respiratory distress, and wheezing. She has been given steroids and bronchodilators for the past 3 hours. The following data were recently collected: arterial blood gas (ABG) values (pH, 7.36; $Paco_2$, 44 mm Hg; $Pao_2$, 65 mm Hg; $Sao_2$, 91%; $F_Io_2$, 0.40); respiratory rate, 30; and $V_T$, 220 mL. Lucy is using abdominal muscles to force exhalations and is wheezing and appears severely dyspneic. She was unable to perform bedside spirometry and weighs 60 kg.

### Interpretation

Even though the pH and $Paco_2$ are normal, we would expect this patient with an asthma exacerbation and mild hypoxemia to be hyperventilating (see Chapter 8). The fact that this patient's $Paco_2$ is 44 mm Hg is a sign of fatigue and impending respiratory failure. The high respiratory rate and $V_T$ of less than 4 mL/kg are also signs of fatigue and impending respiratory failure. When these factors are combined with the patient's severe respiratory distress, the need for mechanical ventilation and admission to the ICU is apparent.

## CASE STUDY

When assessing a patient with COPD who requires mechanical ventilation, the RT notices that the patient is using his abdominal muscles when exhaling and that he appears to be in some respiratory distress. When assessing the ventilator, she found the following parameters and graphics: PS, 15 cm $H_2O$; PEEP, 0 cm $H_2O$; $F_Io_2$, 0.40; PS cycle %, 10%; flow trigger, 2 L/min; PIP, 18 cm $H_2O$; spontaneous respiratory rate, 20; and spontaneous $V_T$, 420 mL. The pressure-time waveform is as follows:

### Interpretation

When assessing this pressure-time waveform, the inspiratory time during PS is too long on the first breath, and the second breath ends earlier because of the patient exhaling against the set PS level. The clinician's observation of the patient confirms that the patient has some expiratory dyssynchrony and the patient's work of breathing is elevated.

This type of dyssynchrony is most likely to occur in patients with obstructive lung disease with high PS levels and low set PS cycle %. To correct this patient's dyssynchrony, the PS cycle % of 10% would need to be increased until the dog ear on the right side of the pressure-time waveform disappears. A PS cycle % of 30% to 40% will usually correct the problem.

## ASSESSMENT QUESTIONS

1. Which of the following patients is *least* likely to benefit from having his or her lung volumes monitored?
   a. A patient receiving mechanical ventilation through an ET tube
   b. A patient with neuromuscular disease
   c. A patient with mild to moderate hypoxemia
   d. A patient with CNS depression

2. Which of the following is true regarding the measurement of $V_T$ as a means of ventilatory assessment in intensive care?
   a. It is normally 3 to 4 mL/kg of predicted body weight
   b. It should be at least 450 mL before weaning from mechanical ventilation
   c. It may decrease after abdominal or thoracic surgery
   d. It should be increased to keep plateau pressures above 30 cm $H_2O$

3. Which of the following conditions is most likely to cause an increase in a patient's $V_T$?
   a. Metabolic acidosis
   b. Pneumonia
   c. Atelectasis
   d. CHF

4. What is the primary concern with ventilating patients using larger $V_T$?
   a. Heart failure
   b. Volutrauma
   c. Atelectasis
   d. Aortic rupture

5. What diagnosis is most likely to lead to dynamic hyperinflation during mechanical ventilation?
   a. ARDS
   b. CHF
   c. COPD
   d. Pneumonia

6. Determine the corrected or delivered $V_T$ using the following data: set $V_T$, 600 mL; exhaled $V_T$, 590 mL; frequency, 10 breaths/min; PIP, 25 cm $H_2O$; plateau, 20 cm $H_2O$; PEEP, 5 cm $H_2O$; spontaneous $V_T$, 400 mL; spontaneous frequency, 6 breaths/min; and circuit compliance, 2 mL/cm $H_2O$.
   a. 550 mL
   b. 560 mL
   c. 570 mL
   d. 590 mL

7. You are attending to a 45-year-old man weighing 80 kg who has been mechanically ventilated for 3 days as a result of bilateral pneumonia. The physician asks you to check his spontaneous breathing parameters, and you find the spontaneous $V_T$ to be 250 mL with a respiratory rate of 30 breaths/min. What is your advice about proceeding with weaning?
   a. The patient is ready
   b. The patient is not ready
   c. The patient needs a higher $F_{IO_2}$
   d. The patient needs a PEEP level

8. Which of the following would reduce air trapping or auto-PEEP during mechanical ventilation?
   a. Increasing the inspiratory flow
   b. Increasing the machine rate
   c. Increasing the set $V_T$
   d. Increasing the I/E ratio

9. An increased $\dot{V}_E$ with a normal $Paco_2$ indicates which of the following?
   a. Shunt
   b. Decreased metabolic rate
   c. Increased dead space
   d. Atelectasis

10. Which of the following is true regarding the measurement of vital capacity in the ICU?
    1. The measured value depends on patient position and effort
    2. It reflects the ventilatory reserve of the patient
    3. A value less than 10 to 15 mL/kg suggests respiratory failure
    a. 1 and 2
    b. 2 and 3
    c. 3 only
    d. 1, 2, and 3

11. Which of the following increases FRC?
    a. Long expiratory times
    b. High tidal volumes
    c. Air trapping and auto-PEEP
    d. High inspiratory flows

12. Which of the following would cause peak airway pressures to decrease on a mechanical ventilator?
    a. Partial airway obstruction
    b. Tension pneumothorax
    c. High inspiratory flow setting
    d. Leak in the ventilator circuit

13. Given a peak pressure of 50 cm $H_2O$, a static pressure of 35 cm $H_2O$, a PEEP of 5 cm $H_2O$, and a delivered $V_T$ of 850 mL, what is the effective static compliance?
    a. 2 mL/cm $H_2O$
    b. 18 mL/cm $H_2O$
    c. 24 mL/cm $H_2O$
    d. 28 mL/cm $H_2O$

14. Which of the following is true regarding auto-PEEP?
    a. It normally is not detected by airway pressure monitoring
    b. It can be reduced by decreasing the inspiratory flow
    c. Administration of bronchodilators worsens the condition
    d. It decreases the patient's work of breathing

15. Given a peak airway pressure of 40 cm $H_2O$, a static pressure of 32 cm $H_2O$, a PEEP of 7 cm $H_2O$, a $V_T$ of 675 mL, and an inspiratory flow of 60 L/min, what is the $R_{aw}$?
    a. 2 cm $H_2O$/L/s
    b. 5 cm $H_2O$/L/s
    c. 8 cm $H_2O$/L/s
    d. 12 cm $H_2O$/L/s

16. Which of the following ventilator graphic displays would be most useful in adjusting the level of PEEP applied to a patient with acute lung injury?
    a. Flow-pressure loop
    b. Volume-time scalar
    c. Pressure-volume loop
    d. Pressure-time scalar

17. The pressure-time ventilator graphic display can be used to assess all of the following *except:*
    a. Mode of ventilation
    b. Estimate of patient effort
    c. Adequacy of inspiratory flow
    d. Presence of circuit leaks

18. Which of the following is true regarding the measurement of $V_D/V_T$ in the ICU?
    a. It is calculated using the $Pao_2$ and $Paco_2$
    b. It is often increased during mechanical ventilation
    c. It is normally ranges between 50% and 60%
    d. It requires that the patient be fully preoxygenated

19. What is the normal range for $V_D/V_T$?
    a. 10% to 25%
    b. 15% to 30%
    c. 25% to 40%
    d. 30% to 60%

20. Which of the following would most likely result in a significant decrease in oxygen transport to the tissues?
    a. Cardiac output of 6 L/min
    b. Arterial saturation of 75%
    c. Hb level of 15 g/dL
    d. Arterial $Po_2$ of 60 mm Hg

21. Which of the following clinical indices denotes poor oxygenation?
    a. $Pao_2$ of 80 mm Hg
    b. $Pao_2/F_Io_2$ ratio of 400
    c. $P(A-a)o_2$ of 55 mm Hg on room air
    d. Oxygen index of 10

22. Which of the following would cause a low $P\overline{v}o_2$?
    a. Left-to-right shunt
    b. Increased cardiac output
    c. Septic shock
    d. Hypoxia

23. Which of the following is true regarding the measurement of blood lactate?
    1. It corresponds to the level of oxygen deficit
    2. It is usually a result of anaerobic metabolism
    3. It can be increased by the administration of β-adrenergic drugs
       a. 2 only
       b. 1 and 2
       c. 2 and 3
       d. 1, 2, and 3

24. Which of the following oxygen delivery values falls within the normal reference range?
    a. 200 mL/min/m²
    b. 300 mL/min/m²
    c. 500 mL/min/m²
    d. 600 mL/min/m²

25. What is the effect of cyanide poisoning on the body?
    a. Reduced oxygen consumption
    b. Reduced oxygen content
    c. Increased oxygen delivery
    d. Decreased $P\overline{v}o_2$

26. What is the normal reference range for $P\overline{v}o_2$?
    a. 26 to 30 mm Hg
    b. 38 to 42 mm Hg
    c. 44 to 58 mm Hg
    d. 56 to 60 mm Hg

27. Your patient has a $P\overline{v}o_2$ of 55 mm Hg. Which of the following may explain the finding?
    a. Low cardiac output
    b. Septic shock
    c. Lung disease
    d. Renal failure

28. At what level of regional tissue $HbO_2$ saturation ($Sto_2$) should intervention to improve $O_2$ delivery be recommended?
    a. <95%
    b. <85%
    c. <75%
    d. <65%

## BIBLIOGRAPHY

AARC Clinical Practice Guideline. Capnography/capnometry during mechanical ventilation, 2011 revision and update. *Respir Care*. 2011;56(4):503–509.

Aboussouan LS. Respiratory failure and the need for ventilatory support. In: Kacmarek RM, Stoller JK, Heuer AL, eds. *Egan's fundamentals of respiratory care*. 11th ed. St. Louis: Mosby; 2017.

Bakker J, Nijsten MWN, Jansen TC. Clinical use of lactate monitoring in critically ill patients. *Ann Intensive Care*. 2013;3(12).

Bouton AK, Abatzidou F, Tryfon S, et al. Diagnostic accuracy of the rapid shallow breathing index to predict a successful spontaneous breathing trial outcome in mechanically ventilated patients with chronic obstructive pulmonary disease. *Heart Lung*. 2011;40(2):105–110.

Cairo JM. Final considerations in ventilator setup. In: Cairo JM, ed. *Pilbeam's mechanical ventilation: physiological and clinical applications*. 6th ed. St. Louis: Mosby; 2016.

Cairo JM. Improving oxygenation and management of ARDS. In: Cairo JM, ed. *Pilbeam's mechanical ventilation: physiological and clinical applications*. 6th ed. St. Louis: Mosby; 2016.

Curley GF, Laffey JG, Zhang H. Biotrauma and ventilator induced lung injury: clinical implications. *Chest*. 2016 Nov; 150(5):1109–1117. http://dx.doi.org/10.1016/j.chest.2016.07.019.

Edmark L, Auner U, Enlund M, et al. Oxygen concentration and characteristics of progressive atelectasis formation during anaesthesia. *Acta Anaesthesiol Scand*. 2010;55:75–81.

Feiner JR, Severinghaus JW, Bickler PE. Dark skin decreases the accuracy of pulse oximeters at low oxygen saturation: the effects of oximeter probe type and gender. *Anesth Analg*. 2007;105:S18–S23.

Hess DR. Approaches to conventional mechanical ventilation of the patient with acute respiratory distress syndrome. *Respir Care*. 2011;56(10):1555–1572.

Kacmarek RM. Initiating and adjusing invasive ventilator support. In: Kacmarek RM, Stoller JK, Heuer AL, eds. *Egan's fundamentals of respiratory care*. 11th ed. St. Louis: Mosby; 2017.

Kodali BS, Urman RD. Capnography during cardiopulmonary resuscitation: current evidence and future directions. *J Emerg Trauma Shock*. 2014;7(4):332–340.

Lipcsey M, Woinarski NC, Bellomo R. Near infrared spectroscopy (NIRS) of the thenar eminence in anesthesia and intensive care. *Ann Intensive Care*. 2012;2(1):11.

MacIntyre NR, Cook DJ, Ely EW, et al. Evidence-based guidelines for weaning and discontinuing ventilatory support: a collective task force facilitated by the American College of Chest Physicians; the American Association for Respiratory Care; and the American College of Critical Care Medicine. *Chest*. 2001;120(6):S375–S395.

Milner QJW, Mathews GR. An assessment of the accuracy of pulse oximeters. *Anesthesia*. 2012;67:396–401.

Murata S, Yokoyama K, Sakamoto Y. Effects of inspiratory rise time on triggering work load during pressure-support ventilation: a lung model study. *Respir Care*. 2010;55(7):878–884.

Neto AS, Pereira VG, Manetta JA. Association between static and dynamic thenar near-infrared spectroscopy and mortality in patients with sepsis: a systematic review and meta-analysis. *J Trauma Acute Care Surg*. 2014;76:226–233.

Petrucci N, De Feo C. Lung protective strategy for the acute respiratory distress syndrome. *Cochrane Database of Systematic Reviews*; 2013. http://dx.doi.org/10.1002/146551858. CD003844.pub4.

Pinsky MR, Payen D. Probing the limits of regional tissue oxygenation measures. *Crit Care*. 2009;13(Suppl 5):S1.

Pohlman MC, McCallister KE, Schweickert WD, et al. Excessive tidal volume from breath stacking during lung-protective ventilation for acute lung injury. *Crit Care Med*. 2008;36(11):3019–3029.

Sabatini S, Kurtzman NA. Bicarbonate therapy in severe metabolic acidosis. *J Am Soc Nephrol*. 2009;20(4):692–695.

Scheeren TW, Schober P, Schwarte LA. Monitoring tissue oxygenation by near infrared spectroscopy (NIRS): background and current applications. *J Clin Monit Comput*. 2012;26(4):279–287.

Segal LN, Oei E, Oppenheimer BW, et al. Evolution of pattern of breathing during a spontaneous breathing trial predicts successful extubation. *Intensive Care Med*. 2010;36:487–495.

Sturesson LW, Malmkvist G, Allvin S, et al. An appropriate inspiratory flow pattern can enhance CO2 exchange, facilitating protective ventilation of healthy lungs. *Br J Anaesth*. 2016;117(2):243–249.

Vorwerk C, Coats TJ. The prognostic value of tissue oxygen saturation in emergency department patients with severe sepsis or septic shock. *Emerg Med J*. 2012;29(9):699–703.

Wysocki M, Cracco C, Teixeira A, et al. Approximate entropy of respiratory rate and tidal volume during weaning from mechanical ventilation. *Crit Care Med*. 2006;34(8):2076–2083.

# 15

# Vascular Pressure Monitoring

*Ruben Restrepo and Craig L. Scanlan*

## LEARNING OBJECTIVES

*After reading this chapter, you will be able to:*

1. Describe the indications for placing an arterial line, a central venous line, and a pulmonary artery catheter.
2. List the most common insertion sites for hemodynamic monitoring lines.
3. Identify the monitoring equipment setup used for hemodynamic monitoring.
4. Describe the steps required for placement of the catheters.
5. Interpret the pressure waveforms and the values derived from all hemodynamic monitoring equipment.
6. Identify potential complications associated with placement of hemodynamic monitoring lines.
7. Describe the relationship of central venous pressure to left and right ventricular function.
8. Describe how to obtain an accurate pulmonary artery wedge pressure (PAWP) reading.
9. Explain the relationship between pulmonary artery diastolic pressure, transmural pressure, and PAWP.
10. Explain the effect of positive end-expiratory pressure on PAWP measurements.
11. Outline the key interventions recommended to minimize central line–associated bloodstream infections (the central line bundle).

## OUTLINE

## KEY TERMS

central venous pressure (CVP)
dicrotic notch
inotropic agent
mean arterial pressure (MAP)
phlebostatic axis

pulmonary artery occlusion pressure (PAOP)
pulmonary artery wedge pressure (PAWP)
pulmonary capillary wedge pressure (PCWP)

pulse pressure
transmural pressure

Hemodynamic monitoring plays an important role in the assessment and treatment of critically ill patients. It evaluates intravascular fluid volume by measuring central venous pressure (CVP); cardiac function by measuring arterial blood pressure, pulmonary artery wedge pressure (PAWP), and cardiac output (CO); and vascular function by measuring systemic and pulmonary vascular resistance (PVR).

Invasive hemodynamic monitoring is needed because basic clinical assessments such as evaluating jugular venous distention or heart sounds alone may not accurately reflect patients' hemodynamic status. Before a catheter is placed in a patient, however, clinicians must consider the risk-to-benefit ratio of invasive monitoring. The risk for invasive hemodynamic monitoring is minimized when properly trained clinicians insert and maintain the system. The complications associated with placing a catheter in a major blood vessel are detailed throughout this chapter.

Bedside monitors acquire and calculate physiologic data in real time and often transfer the data automatically to computers for trend analysis. However, optimal invasive monitoring requires not only knowledge of the procedural complications and use of the information but also understanding and control of the factors affecting the validity of the data.

This chapter provides an introduction to the hemodynamic pressures most often monitored invasively in critically ill patients: arterial pressure, CVP, and pulmonary artery pressures (Box 15.1). Indications and complications of invasive monitoring, normal and abnormal pressure waveforms, and clinical applications are discussed. It should be noted that as a result of the risks and complications, as well as technologic advancements, newer, less invasive techniques are emerging for monitoring hemodynamics both within and outside of an acute care setting. However, the main focus of this chapter is the more traditional techniques that respiratory therapists (RTs) are likely to encounter in practice and in the credentialing examinations.

Table 15.1 summarizes the common reference ranges and the abbreviations for the pressures discussed in this chapter. Although intracardiac pressures are essentially the same in adults and children, heart rate and blood pressure vary significantly by age. Table 15.2 lists the common reference ranges for heart rate and blood pressure for children from infancy through 16 years of age. Although knowledge of these reference ranges is essential in the interpretation and application of hemodynamic data, reference ranges are obtained from studies on healthy people and may be neither normal nor desirable for a specific patient.

## ARTERIAL PRESSURE MONITORING

### Indications for Arterial Pressure Monitoring

Patients with significant hemodynamic instability (hypotension, hypertension), receiving medications that affect blood pressure (e.g., vasodilators or inotropic agents), or requiring

---

**BOX 15.1    The Heart as Two Pumps: An Overview of Hemodynamic Pressure Relationships**

When discussing hemodynamic parameters, it is necessary to think of the heart as two separate pumps. The right side of the heart receives blood from the venous system (venous return) and pumps blood to the pulmonary system. The left side of the heart receives blood from the pulmonary system and pumps blood to the systemic circulation. In normal states, both sides of the heart pump at the same time and move the same amount of blood.

Both atria are filling chambers for the ventricles. Their pressures are about equal, and they have the same waveform. When the atrioventricular valves open (tricuspid and mitral), the pressures in the atrium and ventricle are equal; therefore atrial pressure usually reflects the ventricle's filling pressure (end-diastolic pressure).

Both ventricles pump blood into arterial systems and create two waveforms: ventricular and arterial. Their waveforms have the same shape characteristics, but their pressures are significantly different. The right side of the heart pumps to a low-resistance circuit, the lungs, and thus produces a lower pressure. The left side of the heart pumps to a high-pressure circuit, the body, so it has to produce a high pressure.

Alterations in blood flow and resistance to flow are reflected backward through the cardiopulmonary circuit as pressure changes. Pulmonary hypertension causes pressure to increase in the right side of the heart and eventually the venous system.

$$\uparrow \text{Lung pressure} \rightarrow \uparrow PAP \rightarrow \uparrow CVP \rightarrow \uparrow \text{Venous congestion}$$

A failing left ventricle will cause blood to "dam up" in the left side of the heart, then the lungs, and eventually alters the entire circuit.

$$\rightarrow \uparrow LAP \rightarrow \uparrow PAWP \rightarrow \uparrow PAP \rightarrow \uparrow CVP \rightarrow \uparrow \text{Venous congestion}$$

The following simple diagram illustrates the dynamic relationship between the two sides of the heart and shows where pressures are measured. Marking a patient's pressure changes helps clarify where there is and is not a problem (e.g., increased PAWP with normal PAP and CVP indicates a left-sided heart problem that has not altered the lungs or right side of the heart).

| Pressures: | CVP | | | PAP | PAWP | LAP | | | Arterial BP | |
|---|---|---|---|---|---|---|---|---|---|---|
| Venous system | | RA | RV | Lungs | | LA | | LV | Aorta | Arterial circulation |

Blood flow →        ← Alterations in resistance and flow are reflected backward

---

*AV,* Arteriovenous; *BP,* blood pressure; *CVP,* central venous pressure; *LA,* left atrium; *LAP,* left atrial pressure; *LV,* left ventricle; *PAP,* pulmonary artery pressure; *PAWP,* pulmonary artery wedge pressure; *RA,* right atrium; *RV,* right ventricle; vertical bars indicate heart valves.

frequent arterial blood sampling (unstable respiratory failure) may benefit from placement of an arterial catheter and continuous pressure monitoring.

## Arterial Catheter Insertion Sites

Arterial catheters may be placed in the radial, ulnar, brachial, axillary, or femoral arteries. The radial site is preferred because it is readily accessible, is easy to monitor, provides a stable location for blood sampling, and usually has adequate collateral circulation through the ulnar artery. The femoral artery provides pressure measurements that are less affected by peripheral vasoconstriction, but significant leakage of blood into the surrounding tissue can occur without

detection. The femoral site also is more prone to contamination than the other locations.

## Equipment Setup

Fig. 15.1 shows the basic equipment used for an indwelling vascular line in the brachial artery. Once inserted, the catheter connects to a disposable continuous flush device by low-compliance tubing. The flush device keeps the line open by providing a continuous low flow of fluid (2 to 4 mL/h) through the system. To maintain continuous flow, the intravenous bag supplying these systems must be pressurized, usually by a hand bulb pump. A pressure transducer, connected to the flush device, provides an electrical signal to an amplifier or monitor, which displays the corresponding pressure waveform. A sampling port (not shown) typically is included to allow blood withdrawal. CVP and pulmonary artery monitoring systems use the same basic setup.

## Procedure for Inserting an Arterial Line

Box 15.2 outlines the key procedural steps for inserting a radial artery line. Note that if the Allen test for collateral

### TABLE 15.1  Reference Ranges for Hemodynamic Pressures

| Pressure | Abbreviation | Normal Value (mm Hg) |
|---|---|---|
| Arterial pressure (i.e., blood pressure) | BP | Systolic 100-140 Diastolic 60-90 120/80 (90/60 in teenage girls) |
| Mean arterial pressure | MAP | 70-105 |
| Central venous pressure | CVP | 2-6 (mean) |
| Right atrial pressure | RAP | 2-6 (mean) |
| Right ventricular pressure | RVP | Systolic 15-30 Diastolic 2-8 |
| Right ventricular end-diastolic pressure | RVEDP | 2-6 |
| Pulmonary artery pressure | PAP | Systolic 15-30 Diastolic 8-15 |
| Mean pulmonary artery pressure | MPAP or PAP | 9-18 |
| Pulmonary artery wedge pressure | PAWP, PCWP, PAOP | 6-12 |
| Left atrial pressure | LAP | 4-12 |
| Left ventricular pressure | LVP | Systolic 100-140 Diastolic 0-5 |
| Left ventricular end-diastolic pressure | LVEDP | 5-12 |

### TABLE 15.2  Reference Ranges for Heart Rate and Blood Pressure in Children

| Age | Blood Pressure Average for Males (Females 5% Lower) | HEART RATE[a] Average | Range |
|---|---|---|---|
| Neonate | 75/50 | 140 | 100-190 |
| 1-6 mo | 80/50 | 145 | 110-190 |
| 6-12 mo | 90/65 | 140 | 110-180 |
| 1-2 yr | 95/65 | 125 | 100-160 |
| 2-6 yr | 100/60 | 100 | 65-130 |
| 6-12 yr | 110/60 | 80 | 55-110 |
| 12-16 yr | 110/65 | 75 | 55-100 |
|  | Range: ±20% |  |  |

[a]Heart rates rounded to nearest 5.
Data from Rubenstein JS, Hageman JR: Monitoring of critically ill infants and children, *Crit Care Clin* 4:621, 1988.

**FIG. 15.1** An indwelling vascular line system (brachial artery catheter) used to monitor blood pressures and obtain blood samples. See text for description. (From Kacmarek R, Stoller J, Heuer A: *Egan's fundamentals of respiratory care*, ed 11, St. Louis, 2017, Mosby-Elsevier.)

**FIG. 15.2** Arterial pressure waveform. Increase of circulating catecholamines can cause the inotropic phase to become steeper and form a point that may be higher than in the volume displacement phase. The *circle* marks the dicrotic notch that results from closure of the aortic valve. If the dicrotic notch cannot be visualized and the patient's systolic pressure is greater than 50 mm Hg, the measuring system likely is dampened.

circulation is negative, the opposite wrist should be assessed. If collateral circulation cannot be confirmed on either side, the brachial site typically is used.

There are two common arterial line insertion methods: direct cannulation and the guidewire (Seldinger) technique. The direct cannulation method uses a puncture needle sheathed with the catheter. Using this approach, once a flash of blood is observed in the needle hub, the catheter sheath is advanced over the needle into the artery, and the needle is then removed.

With the Seldinger technique, a needle is used to penetrate the artery, with a soft-tipped guidewire then threaded through the needle into the vessel. Next, the needle is removed, leaving the guidewire in place. Finally, the indwelling catheter is advanced over the guidewire into position, and the guidewire is removed.

## Arterial Pressure Waveforms

An arterial pressure waveform should have a clear upstroke on the left, with a **dicrotic notch** representing aortic valve closure on the downstroke to the right (Fig. 15.2). If the dicrotic notch is not visible, the pressure tracing is dampened and probably inaccurate, and the measured pressures likely are lower than the patient's actual values. The dicrotic notch

disappears in some patients when the systolic pressure drops below 50 or 60 mm Hg.

Arterial pressure waves take on many different configurations (Fig. 15.3). The left side of the pressure wave may become straight and even pointed on the top when there is an increase in circulating catecholamines that increase cardiac contractility (a positive inotropic response). A tall, narrow pressure wave is also seen in patients with a stiff aorta caused by arteriosclerotic vascular disease. In these patients the diastolic pressure may also fall, producing an exaggerated tall and narrow complex. Increases in heart rate and vascular resistance increase diastolic pressure. On the other hand, vasodilation decreases vascular resistance and can cause a fall in diastolic pressures. Because approximately 70% of coronary artery perfusion occurs during diastole, coronary artery perfusion may be compromised if the diastolic pressure falls below 50 mm Hg.

### Respiratory Variations

Respiratory variations in the arterial pressure waveform normally go unnoticed because arterial pressures are substantially higher than intrathoracic pressure changes during breathing. Also, the monitor scale usually is set to a pressure range of 0 to 300 mm Hg, making changes of 10 mm Hg barely visible. When respiratory variations in the arterial pressure waveform are seen, the possibility of cardiac tamponade or other causes of paradoxic pulse must be considered (see Chapter 4). Increases in arterial pressure during inspiration (reverse pulsus paradoxus) are seen after heart surgery and in patients with left ventricular failure who are mechanically ventilated with techniques that produce high mean airway pressures, such as positive end-expiratory pressure (PEEP). Dysrhythmias and *pulsus alternans* also cause variations in the height and shapes of the arterial pressure waveform.

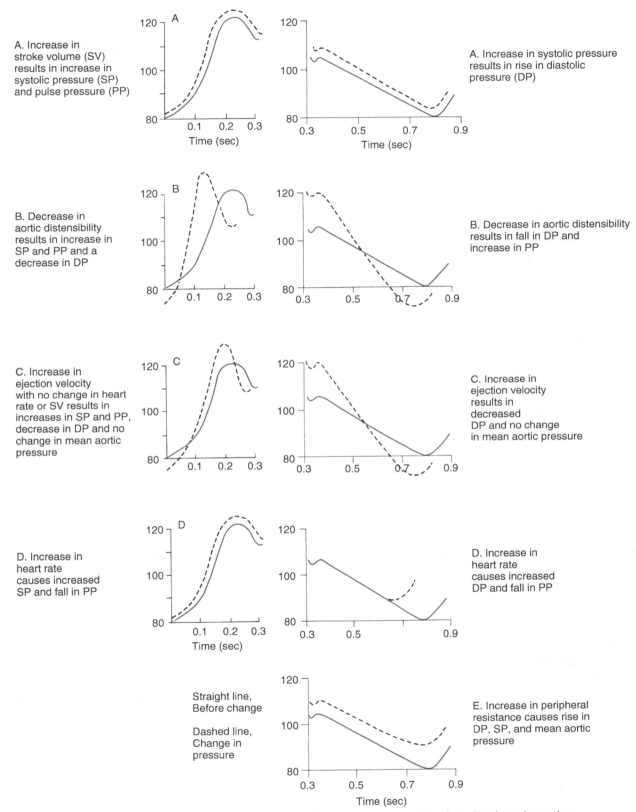

A. Increase in stroke volume (SV) results in increase in systolic pressure (SP) and pulse pressure (PP)

A. Increase in systolic pressure results in rise in diastolic pressure (DP)

B. Decrease in aortic distensibility results in increase in SP and PP and a decrease in DP

B. Decrease in aortic distensibility results in fall in DP and increase in PP

C. Increase in ejection velocity with no change in heart rate or SV results in increases in SP and PP, decrease in DP and no change in mean aortic pressure

C. Increase in ejection velocity results in decreased DP and no change in mean aortic pressure

D. Increase in heart rate causes increased SP and fall in PP

D. Increase in heart rate causes increased DP and fall in PP

Straight line, Before change

Dashed line, Change in pressure

E. Increase in peripheral resistance causes rise in DP, SP, and mean aortic pressure

**FIG. 15.3** Determinants of aortic pressures. Diagrams indicate general tendencies when other factors are held constant. (Modified from Smith JJ, Kampine JP: *Circulatory physiology: the essentials*, Baltimore, 1980, Williams & Wilkins.)

### Use of Arterial Pressure Waveform to Estimate Cardiac Output

Recently, monitors have been developed that use sophisticated software algorithms to calculate and display continuous beat-to-beat stroke volume and CO based on the shape and area of the arterial pressure waveform. This method is called *arterial pulse contour analysis* and is among the most commonly used minimally invasive methods to measure CO in critically ill patients. Chapter 16 provides details on the use of these systems.

### Interpretation of Arterial Pressure Measurements

The normal average arterial pressure in the adult is slightly less than 120/80 mm Hg and increases gradually with age. Systolic pressures greater than 140 and diastolic pressures greater than 90 are considered hypertensive (see Chapter 4 for the current classification of hypertension). A blood pressure significantly below 120/80 mm Hg (particularly if it is below 90/60 mm Hg) in adults is termed *hypotension*.

Although arterial pressure is one of the most frequently monitored vital signs, it reflects only the general circulatory status. Pressure is the product of flow and resistance. Because neurovascular compensatory mechanisms can maintain blood pressure by vasoconstriction while flow is decreasing, low blood pressure is a late sign of hypovolemia or impaired cardiac function. Earlier evidence of decreased blood volume or CO includes cold, clammy extremities caused by catecholamine-mediated peripheral vasoconstriction.

Arterial pressure decreases in the following circumstances:
- With hypovolemia from fluid or blood loss (most commonly, bleeding)
- During cardiac failure and shock (most commonly, heart attack)
- With vasodilation (most commonly, sepsis or anesthetic agents)

Diastolic pressure must be watched carefully during the administration of vasodilators such as sodium nitroprusside, which may reduce diastolic pressure more rapidly than systolic or mean pressure. Diastolic pressure less than 50 mm Hg and mean pressure less than 60 mm Hg in an adult may result in compromised coronary perfusion.

Arterial pressure increases with the following:
- Improvement in circulatory volume and function
- Sympathetic stimulation (e.g., fear or medications)
- Vasoconstriction
- Administration of vasopressors

Administration of inotropic agents may or may not increase blood pressure. If a positive inotropic drug stimulates the heart under conditions of inadequate myocardial oxygenation or hypovolemia, the pressure may fall. Additionally, if the inotropic agent also causes vasodilation, the pressure may stay the same or fall as the medication is increased. In addition to systolic and diastolic blood pressure, arterial pressure monitoring allows assessment of pulse and mean arterial pressure.

The **pulse pressure** is the difference between the systolic and diastolic pressure. Normal pulse pressure is 30 to 40 mm Hg and is a reflection of left ventricular stroke volume (SV) and arterial system compliance. A decreasing pulse pressure

is a sign of low SV. An increasing SV in a patient receiving fluid therapy is consistent with improved preload.

**SIMPLY STATED**

A pulse pressure lower than 30 mm Hg indicates low left ventricular SV. If the pulse pressure increases with fluid therapy, the patient was probably hypovolemic.

**Mean arterial pressure (MAP)** is an average of pressures in the systemic circulation and thus the pressure best associated with the adequacy of tissue perfusion. The normal reference range for MAP is 70 to 105 mm Hg. MAP is not an arithmetic average of systolic and diastolic pressures because the cardiac cycle spends about twice as long in diastole as in systole when the heart rate is normal. Most monitors compute MAP and display it digitally. MAP can be estimated mathematically by either of the following formulas:

$$MAP = 1/3 \text{ Pulse Pressure} + \text{Diastolic Pressure}$$

or

$$MAP = \frac{\text{Systolic Pressure} + (\text{Diastolic Pressure} \times 2)}{3}$$

Circulation to the vital organs (i.e., kidneys, coronary arteries, and brain) may be compromised when MAP falls below 60 mm Hg. In such cases, the patient may need fluid therapy or medications to increase left ventricular contractility (inotropics) or to increase vascular resistance. Elevated MAP is associated with increased risk for stroke and heart failure. Pharmacologic treatment of elevated MAP may include vasodilators or negative inotropic agents. MAP is used in calculating derived hemodynamic variables such as systemic vascular resistance (SVR), left ventricular stroke work, and cardiac work (see Chapter 16).

### Complications Associated with Arterial Lines
#### Ischemia

Ischemia resulting from embolism, thrombus, or arterial spasm is the major complication of direct arterial monitoring. It is evidenced by pallor distal to the insertion site and usually is accompanied by pain and paresthesia (numbness and tingling). Ischemia can proceed to tissue necrosis if the catheter is not repositioned or removed. Thrombosis is prevented by irrigation with diluted heparinized solution. Bolus irrigation is done in very small amounts because flushing the line can result in retrograde flow and cerebral embolization.

#### Hemorrhage

Hemorrhage is possible if the line becomes disconnected or a stopcock is left open; therefore the tubing should be kept on top of the bed sheets, where it can be observed. Blood flow through an 18-gauge catheter is sufficient to allow a 500-mL blood loss per minute, and exsanguination (whereby the patient "bleeds out") can occur. Bleeding and hematoma at the insertion site can also occur, especially if the catheter was placed through a needle. Sites should be assessed regularly while the catheter is in place and after its removal.

## Infection

As with all invasive lines, the presence of an arterial catheter increases the risk for infection. The incidence of infection increases over time and is directly related to the care of the lines and transducers; frequency of dressing, tubing, and solution change; to-and-fro motion of the catheter; and altered host defenses. Fever in any patient with invasive lines must trigger questions about the necessity of the lines and their role as a cause of the infection process. This risk partially explains why invasive lines are used less frequently now than in the past. More detail on preventing catheter-associated infections is provided later in this chapter.

> ### SIMPLY STATED
>
> All invasive hemodynamic monitoring lines are a potential source of infection, bleeding, hematoma, embolus, thrombus, and impaired circulation. Fever in any patient with invasive lines must trigger questions about the necessity of the lines and their role in an infectious process.

## CENTRAL VENOUS PRESSURE MONITORING

Central venous pressure (CVP) is the pressure of the blood in the right atrium or vena cava. Because the tricuspid valve is opened between the right atrium and ventricle during diastole (ventricular filling), CVP also represents the end-diastolic pressure in the right ventricle and reflects right ventricular preload (filling volume). To obtain a CVP measurement, a venous catheter is placed in a major vein (see the later section on insertion).

### Indications for Central Venous Pressure Monitoring

CVP monitoring is indicated to assess the circulating blood volume (adequacy of cardiac filling), adequacy of venous return, or right ventricular function. Patients who have had major surgery or blood loss caused by trauma and those suspected of severe dehydration may benefit from placement of a CVP catheter to guide fluid replacement therapy. Patients with either cardiogenic or noncardiogenic pulmonary edema also need CVP monitoring to guide fluid therapy. In addition, CVP measurements are useful in evaluating patients suspected of having right ventricular damage due to myocardial infarction. Once the catheter is in place, the line can be used for rapid infusion of fluids or medications and to obtain blood samples for measurement of routine laboratory studies (e.g., complete blood counts and electrolytes).

### Central Venous Pressure Catheters and Insertion Sites

The most common central venous catheters are 7-French, triple-lumen catheters with one distal port and two ports 3 to 4 cm from the distal end of the catheter (Fig. 15.4). The multiple-lumen catheter allows infusion of blood and various medications and solutions through different ports as well as permits aspiration of blood samples and continuous

**FIG. 15.4** Triple-lumen central venous pressure catheter designed for placement through the internal or external jugular vein. The tip ends in the right atrium. The catheter does not have a balloon; air is never injected into ports.

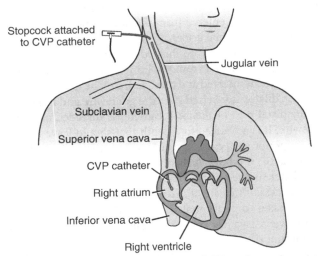

**FIG. 15.5** Central venous pressure (CVP) catheter inserted through the jugular vein with the tip positioned in the right atrium.

monitoring of CVP. Catheters with walls that are impregnated with antibiotics are more effective in preventing infection than standard catheters.

Common sites for the introduction of central venous catheters include the subclavian and internal jugular veins (Fig. 15.5). An advantage of the subclavian vein approach is that it results in a much more stable catheter after placement. Disadvantages of the subclavian vein approach are that it is technically more difficult because the vein is harder to find and the catheter guidewire does not follow the subclavian vein as easily as it turns to form the superior vena cava. The subclavian vein is close to the subclavian artery, which is easily punctured, and the mediastinum can hold a fair amount of blood without external evidence of blood loss. The pleural surface is not far below the vein, so pneumothorax is a potential complication of the procedure.

The internal jugular vein approach is easier because there is nearly a straight shot for the guidewire to reach the superior vena cava and less risk for pneumothorax, and hematomas are easier to see and control. Disadvantages of the internal jugular vein approach are that the catheter is much less stable after placement and is subject to kinking, breakage, and accidental removal.

## Procedure for Inserting a Central Venous Pressure Catheter

Central venous line kits commonly include a needle for venous penetration, a stiff plastic dilator, and a guidewire coiled in a plastic sheath with a "J" tip to prevent venous wall penetration. The J tip is held straight by a small separate sheath to accommodate entry into the hub of the insertion needle.

The technique is nearly identical for subclavian and internal jugular line insertions. Normally, the head of the patient's bed is lowered, which increases venous pressure and causes the vein to swell, making it easier to penetrate and thread the guidewire. This also decreases the risk for inadvertent air embolism. The subclavian vein is entered from an insertion site at the edge of the distal third of the clavicle. The internal jugular vein can be entered from the head of the clavicle or a site behind the brachial artery.

The catheter lumens are flushed with heparinized saline, and the cap is removed from the lumen with the distal port. The guidewire is inserted and threaded, and the needle is withdrawn. A dilator is inserted over the guidewire and removed, and the distal port of the CVP catheter is threaded onto the guidewire. It is advanced to a depth that should leave the tip in the superior vena cava. The guidewire is then removed, the hub replaced, the port flushed with heparinized saline, and the catheter secured in position.

Regardless of the site of insertion, a chest radiograph typically is taken to verify that the tip of the catheter is in the superior vena cava just above the right atrium and to rule out pneumothorax.

Once inserted and secured, the CVP catheter is attached to a flushed and calibrated monitoring system like that used for pressure measurement through an arterial line (see Fig. 15.1). However, because CVP typically is much lower than arterial pressures, two key differences in the procedure are required. First, the monitor scale for CVP measurement should be set to the low range, typically 0 to 30 mm Hg. Second, to ensure accuracy in measurement and interpretation, the pressure transducer must be placed level with the patient's right atrium, identified externally at the phlebostatic axis. As indicated in Fig. 15.6, the phlebostatic axis

**FIG. 15.6** The phlebostatic axis at the intersection of the fourth intercostal space (ICS) and midaxillary line corresponds with the location of the right atrium. Central venous pressure and pulmonary artery transducers need to be level with this point. *AP*, Anteroposterior. (From Sole ML, Klein D, Moseley M: *Introduction to critical care nursing*, ed 5, St. Louis, 2008, Saunders-Elsevier.)

is located at the intersection of the fourth intercostal space and midaxillary line. Positioning of the transducer below the phlebostatic axis will result in erroneously high CVP readings, whereas positioning the transducer above this level will cause the reading to be lower than the patient's actual value.

## Central Venous and Atrial Pressure Waveforms

The CVP waveform reflects pressure changes in the right atrium and normally consists of three waves for each cardiac cycle: a, c, and v (Fig. 15.7).

The a-wave results from atrial contraction and occurs during ventricular diastole. When there is no atrial contraction (atrial fibrillation), there is no a-wave. Conversely, when the atrium contracts against a closed valve, as occurs during atrioventricular (AV) dissociation or with some junctional or ventricular pacemaker rhythms, large a-wave called *cannon waves* occur. The downslope of the a-wave (X descent) results from the decrease in atrial pressure as the blood moves into the ventricle and ends with the closure of the tricuspid valve (tricuspid on right, mitral on left).

The c-wave occurs at the completion of AV valve closure. It represents the movement or bulging of the AV valve back toward the atrium during ventricular contraction.

The v-wave results from atrial filling while the AV valve is closed during ventricular systole. The downslope of the v-wave (Y descent) occurs when the tricuspid and mitral valves open and the ventricle begins to fill with blood. When an AV valve does not close all the way (incompetent or leaky valve), some of the blood is ejected backward into the atrium during systole (tricuspid regurgitation), creating exaggerated v-wave and an elevated CVP measurement.

### Respiratory Variations

Respiratory-induced pressure changes are normal on CVP waveforms. In fact, the absence of respiratory oscillations on a CVP tracing indicates a measurement error that requires

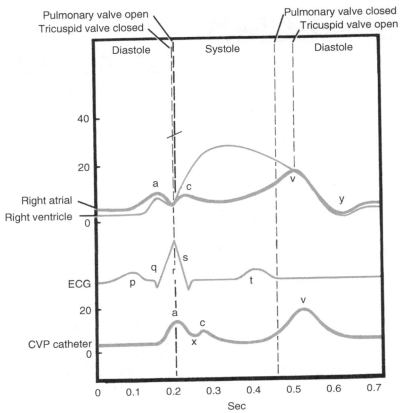

**FIG. 15.7** Central venous pressure (CVP) and right atrial pressure traces with a, c, and v waves shown in relation to the electrocardiogram (ECG) and ventricular pressure waves. When traces are recorded from long catheters, especially pulmonary artery catheters, there is usually a time delay in visualizing the pressure waveform so that the a wave coincides with the QRS complex rather than preceding it slightly, as occurs with the right atrial pressure trace. *a*, Atrial contraction; *b*, closure of the AV valve; *v*, ventricular contraction.

troubleshooting. The most likely cause of absent respiratory oscillations is a kink or air in the tubing, a stopcock turned in the wrong direction, or a small clot or kink in the catheter. Rarely, when a hypovolemic patient is breathing spontaneously at small tidal volumes, respiratory oscillations may not be apparent and the typical a, c, and v wave pattern may not be seen. If the patient is asked to take a deep breath, the waveform should fall below baseline as intrathoracic pressure falls with inspiration. The catheter and tubing should still be checked carefully for air and other causes of dampened pressure traces.

Because the CVP decreases with spontaneous inspiration and increases with delivery of positive pressure breaths, accurate determination of this parameter can be problematic. For spontaneously breathing patients who are awake and cooperative, having them briefly suspend their breathing for a few cardiac cycles can yield an accurate CVP measurement. For patients receiving positive-pressure ventilation, it is best to view a simultaneous tracing of CVP with the airway pressure and record the CVP value that most closely corresponds to the average end-expiratory pressure over several respiratory cycles. Patients should not be removed from the ventilator to measure the CVP, especially if PEEP is in use.

**SIMPLY STATED**

To avoid errors due to respiratory artifact, the CVP and all pulmonary artery pressures should be measured at end-expiration.

## Interpretation of Central Venous Pressure Measurements

CVP is regulated by a balance between the volume of blood being returned to the heart (venous return) and the ability of the right side of the heart to pump this blood out into the pulmonary circulation. In general, any peripheral factor that decreases the amount of blood returning to the heart decreases CVP, and any factor that increases venous return increases CVP. When the pumping capacity of the right heart is increased, more blood is moved out of the right ventricle, and CVP decreases. Conversely, any impairment to the pumping ability of the right side of the heart tends to increase CVP. Box 15.3 summarizes the common causes of increased and decreased CVP.

In patients with poor perfusion and a low CVP, a fluid challenge may be given to determine whether the cause is hypovolemia. A fluid challenge involves the rapid administration of

## BOX 15.3    Causes of Changes in Central Venous Pressure

**Increased Pressure**
- Volume overload or fluids being given more rapidly than the heart can tolerate
- Increased intrathoracic pressure (central venous pressure [CVP] increases with positive-pressure breath or tension pneumothorax)
- Compression around the heart: constrictive pericarditis or cardiac tamponade
- Pulmonary hypertension (primary or secondary)
- Right ventricular failure (e.g., myocardial infarction or cardiomyopathy)
- Left-sided heart failure severe enough to cause right-sided heart failure
- Pulmonary valvular stenosis
- Tricuspid valvular stenosis or regurgitation
- Pulmonary embolism
- Increased large vessel tone throughout the body, resulting in venoconstriction
- Arteriolar vasodilation that increases the blood supply to the venous system
- Infusion of solution into the CVP line (especially by infusion pumps)
- Placement of the transducer below the patient's right atrium and phlebostatic axis

**Decreased Pressure**
- Vasodilation (drugs, hyperpyrexia, sepsis)
- Inadequate circulating blood volume (hypovolemia) caused by dehydration, blood loss, gastrointestinal loss, wound drainage, perspiration, urine output (diuresis), insensible losses (high temperature, low humidity), and losses to the interstitial space (edema, third spacing)
- Spontaneous inspiration
- Placement of the transducer above the patient's right atrium and phlebostatic axis
- Air bubbles or leaks in the pressure line

200 to 500 mL of intravenous fluid over a short time period, such as 10 minutes. If the CVP does not change after a fluid challenge, this indicates that the poor perfusion is due to hypovolemia, with the administration of additional fluid warranted. However, if the CVP increases by 2 mm Hg or more during the challenge, hypovolemia is unlikely, and additional fluid should be administered with caution. It is important to note that with more and better ways to monitor cardiac function, the CVP fluid challenge has fallen out of favor. Real-time measures of stroke volume and CO in response to a fluid challenge are now considered the best predictor of hemodynamic response to changes in circulating blood volume. Details on these methods are provided in Chapter 16.

Note also that a normal CVP does not necessarily indicate normal circulating volume or cardiac function. For example, if a patient is hypovolemic but has pulmonary hypertension with decreased right ventricular function, the balance of these opposing factors may result in a normal CVP. This is most commonly seen in patients with cor pulmonale who become dehydrated and hypovolemic. In such cases, correcting the hypovolemia will cause an abnormal elevation in the CVP.

### SIMPLY STATED

CVP rises as the efficiency of the right side of the heart to move blood through the lungs decreases. When the CVP is elevated and accurately measured while pulmonary artery pressures are normal or low, the cause of the problem resides in the right side of the heart (e.g., right ventricular infarction or tricuspid stenosis and regurgitation). If both CVP and pulmonary artery pressures are elevated while the left-sided filling pressures are normal, the problem probably resides in the lung.

### Central Venous Pressure as a Reflection of Left Ventricular Function

In patients with an ejection fraction greater than 0.50 (50% of the left ventricular end-diastolic volume [LVEDV]) and no cardiopulmonary disease, excellent correlation has been found between central venous, left atrial, and pulmonary artery wedge pressures.

CVP is an acceptable option for management of intraoperative fluid levels, postoperative fluid levels, or volume replacement in young patients with no history of heart disease or hypertension. However, in patients with valvular heart disease or coronary artery disease and in critically ill patients, CVP may not correlate well with left-sided heart filling pressures.

In a patient with pulmonary disease, the left-sided heart pressures remain normal or may even be decreased, whereas the pulmonary artery pressure and therefore right-sided heart pressures are significantly elevated. Therefore a patient with pulmonary hypertension may benefit from monitoring of both the left- and right-sided heart pressures.

### SIMPLY STATED

Patients with pulmonary hypertension have increased pulmonary vascular pressures and CVP resulting from the pulmonary disease process; therefore CVP is not a good reflection of volume status. It is necessary to look more directly at left-sided heart filling pressure to determine whether the patient's volume status is adequate.

## Complications of Central Venous Pressure Monitoring

Complications of using a CVP catheter can occur during placement or during its use over time. Placement of the catheter can cause problems such as bleeding or pneumothorax. Bleeding is often minimal because of the low pressures characterizing the venous system. Bleeding is more likely if the patient is taking heparin or has low platelet counts. Bleeding also can be severe if the subclavian artery is accidentally penetrated. Pneumothorax is uncommon but can occur if the catheter punctures the pleural lining. The most common complication associated with use of the catheter over time is infection (see Central Line Bundle later in this chapter). A less common complication is development of thrombus around the catheter. Accidental opening of the central venous line stopcock could allow air to enter the vein and result in an air embolus.

The development of the pulmonary artery catheter (PAC) by Drs. Swan and Ganz in the late 1960s began a new era in assessment of left ventricular function and hemodynamic performance. Placement of a flow-directed PAC into the patient's pulmonary artery allows assessment of the filling pressures of the left side of the heart. Before the PAC was developed, measurement of left-sided filling pressures required cardiac catheterization, with bedside care estimates based on the CVP measurement. However, as previously mentioned, many critically ill patients have factors present that make CVP a poor estimate of left heart filling pressures. Thus, the PAC provides better assessment of left-sided heart function. In addition, a PAC provides the means to assess CO and tissue oxygenation.

These values allow assessment of the following (Box 15.4):

- Left ventricular preload through measurement of the pulmonary artery wedge pressure (PAWP)
- Cardiac output and its related computations (stroke volume and cardiac index)
- Pulmonary vascular resistance (PVR) through measurement of pulmonary artery pressure, wedge pressure, and CO
- Mixed venous $O_2$ content (reflecting tissue oxygenation) and the AV oxygen content difference
- Proportion of left-to-right shunted pulmonary blood flow
- Patient's response to therapy with vasoactive agents, fluid, and positive-pressure ventilation

## INDICATIONS FOR PULMONARY ARTERY PRESSURE MONITORING

Significant improvements in the diagnostic ability and availability of less invasive and noninvasive cardiac imaging techniques, in addition to evidence of potential harm associated with PAC compared with CVP catheter in patients in critical care, have led to a decline in right-sided heart catheterization over recent years. The additional risk is present because the catheter must pass through the right side of the heart and into the pulmonary artery. The procedure may cause dysrhythmias or other serious complications (see later discussion). However, it can provide direct hemodynamic data that can be used to determine CO, as well as evaluate intracardiac shunts and valve dysfunction. It is also considered the gold standard method for diagnosing pulmonary hypertension and an essential component in the evaluation of patients before heart and/or lung transplantation. Evidence exists to suggest that use of the PAC in patients with respiratory failure often results in a change in diagnosis and therapy. However, the research results are inconclusive with regard to accurately determining benefit or harm from PAC use in patients with respiratory failure.

As a result, the PAC must be inserted only in those patients in whom the anticipated benefit outweighs the potential risks. Unfortunately, there is no specific diagnosis or group of patients in which PAC placement is an absolute indication.

---

**BOX 15.4   Interpreting Pulmonary Artery Pressure**

Pulmonary artery pressure is the product of the volume ejected by the right ventricle and resistance of flow through the pulmonary vasculature.

Pulmonary artery pressure measures right-sided heart function and reflects the following:
- Preload and end-diastolic filling pressure
- Ability of the right side of the heart to move blood through the lungs and left side of the heart

Pulmonary artery pressure can reflect left-sided heart filling pressure in young patients with no hypertension, cardiac disease, or pulmonary disease.

Pulmonary artery pressure increases with the following:
- Increased venous return (volume)
- Increased intrathoracic pressure
- Increased PVR

Pulmonary artery pressure decreases with the following:
- Decreased venous return (volume)
- Decreased intrathoracic pressure
- Decreased PVR

Normal pulmonary artery pressure is as follows:
- Systolic: 15 to 30 mm Hg
- Diastolic: 8 to 15 mm Hg[a]
- Mean: 9 to 18 mm Hg

If pressure is abnormally low or falling, think of the following:
- Inadequate volume, volume loss
- Vasodilation (could be fever or medications)
- Plumbing or measurement problem

If pressure is abnormally high or climbing, think of the following:
- Increased PVR
- Constriction, obstruction, compression of pulmonary vasculature (e.g., ↑ intrathoracic pressure, pulmonary hypertension, or cardiac tamponade)
- Backpressure from high left-sided heart pressures
- Volume overload
- Technical problem or not reading at end-expiration

Pulmonary diastolic pressure can be used instead of wedge pressure if the diastolic is higher than the wedge and if none of the following is present:
- Tachyarrhythmia
- Vasoconstriction, increased pulmonary resistance
- Pulmonary emboli
- Fluctuating PVR

*PVR,* Pulmonary vascular resistance.
[a]Normal pulmonary artery diastolic pressure is 2 mm Hg higher than wedge pressure.

---

Rather, the decision to place a PAC is individualized on a case-by-case basis.

The common situations in which PAC monitoring is considered include the diagnosis and treatment of patients with severe cardiogenic pulmonary edema, diagnosis and treatment of patients with severe ARDS who are hemodynamically unstable, monitoring of patients who have had major thoracic surgery, and diagnosis and treatment of patients in cardiogenic or septic shock.

## Pulmonary Artery Catheters and Insertion Sites

PACs, also called *Swan-Ganz catheters*, are made of radiopaque polyvinylchloride, with the adult version being about 110 cm long (marked in 10-cm increments) and tipped with a small inflatable balloon. The balloon is used both to float the catheter into position and to obtain wedge pressure measurements. A 5-French catheter typically is used with children up

to 20 kg, with 7- and 8-French versions selected respectively for large children/small adults and average-sized adults.

Typically, the catheter has at least three lumens connecting to three external ports:

- Proximal CVP/atrial lumen: use for aspirating blood samples, measuring CVP, injecting drugs, and injecting the thermal bolus used for thermodilution CO measurements (see Chapter 16)
- Distal pulmonary artery lumen: used for measuring pulmonary artery pressures, aspirating mixed venous blood samples, and injecting medications
- Balloon lumen (Fig. 15.8): used for inflating/deflating the balloon

**FIG. 15.8** Idealized pulmonary artery (PA) catheter showing many of the features available; no catheters have all the features shown. Distal lumen opens into the PA. Fiberoptic filaments used for Svo$_2$ monitoring (see Fig. 14.18) and the balloon are also located at the tip. The thermistor bead is located 1.5 inches from the tip and is connected by a wire through the catheter to the connector for the thermodilution cardiac output computer. The proximal lumen located 30 cm back from the tip opens into the right atrium. Catheters are available for ventricular, atrial, or atrioventricular sequential pacing using either pacemaker bands positioned on the catheter or pacing leads, which are passed through the lumen. Ventricular bands or lumens are located 20 cm from the tip; atrial, 30 cm from the tip. *CVP*, Central venous pressure.

Other connectors may include those for a CO computer, atrial and ventricular pacemakers, and a mixed venous $O_2$ sensor (not shown).

Most balloons hold approximately 1.5 mL of air when fully inflated. To help the catheter float through the right side of the heart and into the pulmonary artery, the balloon is fully inflated during insertion. Once the catheter is properly positioned, the balloon is deflated and maintained in that state except when obtaining wedge pressure measurements.

PACs are available with bands for atrial, ventricular, or AV sequential cardiac pacing. The pacemaker bands must stay in contact with the wall of the atrium or ventricle to work effectively.

The insertion sites for the PAC are the same as those for the CVP catheter, with the subclavian route being the most common site used in the intensive care unit (ICU).

## Placement of the Pulmonary Artery Catheter

The PAC can be positioned using fluoroscopy but is more often floated into place using pressure waveforms to indicate the catheter's position. The distal lumen of the catheter is connected to the same basic transducer-monitoring system depicted in Fig. 15.1. Before insertion, both the proximal and distal lumens are flushed with sterile saline to make sure they are free of air bubbles, and then the catheter is placed through an introducer. The clinician placing the catheter usually inflates the balloon on the tip of the catheter when it reaches the superior vena cava or the right atrium. The clinician observes the pressure waves transmitted through the distal lumen as displayed on the bedside monitor. As the catheter passes through the various anatomic structures (e.g., right atrium, right ventricle, and pulmonary artery), distinct

waveforms are observed (Fig. 15.9). Based on these waveforms, the clinician placing the catheter can know when the tip passes into the pulmonary artery and is near the wedge position. The wedge position is reached when the balloon arrives at an artery that is too small to allow further advancement of the catheter. The waveforms generated by the catheter as it is inserted are briefly discussed in the next sections according to anatomic site.

In most adults, insertion of the catheter through the subclavian or jugular vein to the 50-cm marker is sufficient to reach the pulmonary artery. If the insertion depth exceeds 50 cm and no pulmonary artery waveform is observed, it is generally assumed that the catheter is curling in the atrium or ventricle or is going down the inferior vena cava. In these cases, the clinician deflates the balloon and withdraws the catheter until the tip is in the atrium. The balloon is then reinflated and the catheter repositioned.

When the catheter wedges in a smaller branch of the pulmonary artery, the forward flow of the pulmonary arterial blood is occluded. With pulsatile arterial blood flow stopped, the tip of the catheter "reflects" the back pressure from the pulmonary venous system and left atrium, and the waveform takes on the appearance of an atrial/CVP pressure waveform with its typical a, c, and v waves (Fig. 15.10). The pulmonary artery waveform should return when the balloon is deflated. Adjustments in catheter placement are often needed to keep the catheter tip in position to easily wedge but to avoid a permanently wedged position. Care should be taken to inflate the balloon only enough to provide a wedge reading because overdistention of the pulmonary artery could cause rupture of the artery, which could be fatal.

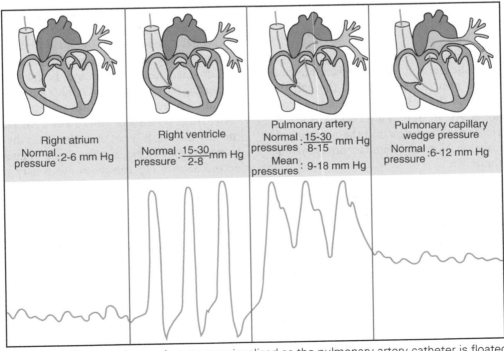

| Right atrium | Right ventricle | Pulmonary artery | Pulmonary capillary wedge pressure |
|---|---|---|---|
| Normal pressure: 2-6 mm Hg | Normal pressure: 15-30 / 2-8 mm Hg | Normal pressures: 15-30 / 8-15 mm Hg  Mean pressures: 9-18 mm Hg | Normal pressure: 6-12 mm Hg |

**FIG. 15.9** Schematic of waveforms and normal pressures visualized as the pulmonary artery catheter is floated into position.

**FIG. 15.10** Pulmonary artery pressure (PAP) trace converting to wedge pressure. A, Patient is on intermittent mandatory ventilation of 12 and positive end-expiratory pressure (PEEP) of 5 cm $H_2O$. Note respiratory swing in pressure wave. Heart rate: 98/min, normal sinus rhythm; PAP, 27/15 mm Hg; wedge pressure (PAWP), 13 mm Hg. B, Note difference in appearance of waveforms in patient with atrial fibrillation. Heart rate: 87 to 102/min; PAP: 23/14 mm Hg; PAWP: 13 mm Hg. *I*, Spontaneous inspiration; *V*, intermittent ventilator breath.

## Interpretation of Pulmonary Artery Pressures

As seen in the previous discussion, the PAC provides numerous measurements, including pulmonary artery systolic and diastolic pressures and the wedge pressure. Interpretation of each is discussed in the following sections.

### Pulmonary Artery Systolic Pressure

Pulmonary artery systolic pressure is the highest pressure created when the right ventricle ejects blood through the pulmonary valve and into the lungs. Like systemic arterial pressure, pulmonary artery pressure is a product of the volume of blood ejected by the ventricle and the resistance of the pulmonary circulation. Normal pulmonary artery systolic pressure is 15 to 30 mm Hg.

Pulmonary artery pressures decrease when the volume of blood ejected by the right ventricle decreases or when the pulmonary vasculature relaxes or dilates (decreased PVR).

Pulmonary artery pressures increase when pulmonary blood flow increases or when PVR increases. The right ventricle pumps increased amounts of blood into the lungs with volume overload or when it receives excess blood from left-to-right intracardiac shunts (e.g., atrial or ventricular septal defects or patent ductus arteriosus).

Resistance to pulmonary flow (increased PVR) can be caused by constriction, obstruction, or compression of the pulmonary vasculature or by back pressure from the left heart. Examples of conditions that can cause increased PVR include the following:

- Pulmonary emboli
- Acute or chronic lung disease that causes pulmonary vasoconstriction in response to hypoxia
- Cardiac tamponade or increased intrathoracic pressure compressing the vasculature and impeding forward flow
- Left-sided heart failure and mitral valve regurgitation causing back pressure from the left heart into the lungs

Pulmonary arterial pressures average about 25/12 mm Hg, with a mean pressure of about 16 mm Hg. However, with pulmonary disease, it is not uncommon for the systolic pressure to exceed 45 mm Hg and the mean pulmonary pressure to exceed 35 mm Hg. Advanced pulmonary hypertension can result in pressures approaching systemic artery pressures. Such severe pulmonary hypertension can impair right ventricular function, which in turn decreases right ventricular output. With less blood moving forward, left ventricular preload is decreased, and subsequently left ventricular SV and systemic oxygen transport may also decrease.

### Pulmonary Artery Diastolic Pressure

Pulmonary artery diastolic pressure (PADP) normally ranges between 8 and 15 mm Hg and under normal conditions reflects pulmonary venous, left atrial, and left ventricular end-diastolic pressure (the mitral valve is open during diastole). In the absence of severe pulmonary vascular changes, marked tachycardia, pulmonary embolism, and mitral valve stenosis or regurgitation, PADP can be used to monitor left ventricular filling pressure. Unfortunately, such ideal conditions are uncommon in the ICU, and PADP is often unreliable as a measure of left ventricular filling pressure.

Normally, PADP is approximately 2 mm Hg higher than wedge pressure, but elevated PVR increases the gradient. In fact, a PADP-PAWP gradient that is greater than 5 mm Hg is characteristic of ARDS, sepsis, excessive PEEP, or other conditions that increase PVR. In contrast, pulmonary hypertension caused by left ventricular failure is characterized by a normal PADP-PAWP gradient (<5 mm Hg). With heart rates greater than 120 beats per minute, the time for diastolic runoff is shortened, and diastolic pressure and the gradient increase.

## SIMPLY STATED

Pulmonary artery diastolic pressure may reflect filling pressures of the left ventricle if the mitral valve of the patient is normal and the PVR is normal. In most ICU patients, however, these conditions are not present.

### Wedge Pressure

Normal PAWP is 6 to 12 mm Hg. Wedge pressure is lower than mean pulmonary artery pressure and is usually about 2 mm Hg lower than PADP. These normal pressure relationships are easier to remember by keeping in mind that blood flows from higher pressure to lower pressure. Wedge pressure is also called pulmonary capillary wedge pressure (PCWP) or pulmonary artery occlusion pressure (PAOP).

The PAWP reading is used to monitor left ventricular filling during diastole. Under normal conditions (e.g., healthy heart) the filling pressure correlates well with the volume of blood filling the ventricle (preload). However, when the heart is damaged, healthy myocardium often is replaced with scar tissue, resulting in the ventricles becoming stiffer than normal. When the ventricle is stiff or noncompliant, the same filling volume results in a higher filling pressure. As a result, the PAWP reading must be interpreted in light of the patient's medical history.

Optimal PAWP values for any one patient depend on the condition of the left ventricle. In the normal heart, an optimal SV is obtained with a PAWP of 10 to 12 mm Hg. In the patient with left ventricular hypertrophy, a PAWP of 18 mm Hg or higher may be needed to optimize SV. Thus optimal PAWP varies from patient to patient and is identified by construction of left ventricular function curves for each patient. The function curves are created by measuring the SV at various PAWP readings. This allows determination of the pressure readings that result in the best CO. PAWP readings above or below this range cause the SV to decrease.

PAWP increases for a variety of reasons. Left ventricular failure is a common cause. The lack of forward flow out of the left ventricle causes the left ventricle to dilate and blood to back up into the pulmonary circulation, resulting in an

---

**BOX 15.5  Conditions in Which PAWP Overestimates Left Ventricular Filling Volume**

**Physiologic Conditions**
- Pulmonary venous obstruction and compression (e.g., lung or mediastinal tumors, left atrial myxoma)
- Mitral valve stenosis or occlusion
- Mitral valve insufficiency: large v waves
- Decreased left ventricular compliance
- Inotropic drugs, hypertension
- Acute cardiac dilation
- Myocardial ischemia, hypertrophy, injury, infarction, infiltrate
- Pericardial disease or tamponade
- Increased intrathoracic pressure
- High mean airway pressures (e.g., PEEP >10 cm $H_2O$ or APRV)

**Technical Problems**
- Overinflation of balloon
- Incomplete wedging
- Catheter fling
- Underdampened trace
- Occluded catheter tip (e.g., clot, vessel wall, embolism)
- Transducer below left atrial level and phlebostatic axis
- Reading not made at end-expiration
- Tubing or patient movement
- Cough or Valsalva maneuver during measurement

*APRV,* Airway pressure release ventilation; *PEEP,* positive end-expiratory pressure.

---

elevated PAWP. In some cases, the PAWP is markedly elevated, indicating overstretching of the left ventricle. This overstretching of the left ventricle causes the SV to decrease and adds to the problem. In these cases, diuretics usually are needed, along with other therapy to reduce the PAWP and optimize left ventricular function. PAWP also increases with mitral valve regurgitation and when the pulmonary venous circulation is obstructed with a tumor. In these cases, the elevated PAWP tends to overestimate the filling volume of the left ventricle. Additional physiologic conditions and technical problems in which the wedge pressure tends to overestimate left ventricular filling volume are outlined in Box 15.5.

The most common cause for a reduction in PAWP is hypovolemia. This is common after major surgery or trauma in which blood loss is significant. Severe dehydration can also lead to a reduction in PAWP.

## SIMPLY STATED

The most common cause of an elevated PAWP is left ventricular failure.

*Obtaining an accurate wedge pressure.* The accuracy of the wedge pressure reading is related to numerous factors, including technical issues and position of the catheter within the chest. Table 15.3 summarizes the criteria used to ensure that the pressure measured is really wedge pressure.

**TABLE 15.3    Criteria for Wedge Pressure That Represents Left-Sided Heart Filling Pressure**

| Criteria | Characteristics |
| --- | --- |
| Distinct and valid pulmonary artery pressure trace before inflation | Frequency response not overdampened or underdampened |
| | Transducer calibrated at left atrial level (phlebostatic axis) |
| | Patient supine, head of bed ≤45 degrees |
| Catheter tip in zone III | At or below left atrial level with lateral radiograph |
| PADP > PAWP | If PADP < PAWP, consider non–zone III, tachycardia >120/min, and increased PVR |
| Distinct PAWP trace immediately on wedge | Clearly visible a and c waves |
| | Elevated v waves suggest mitral regurgitation; may also be seen with MI and mitral stenosis |
| Free flow with catheter wedged | No overinflation (climbing wave) |
| | Easy withdrawal of blood |
| | Nondampened tracing |
| Change in PAWP <½ change in airway pressure | Applies to both increase and decrease of PEEP or CPAP |
| Aspiration of "arterialized" blood from distal port while catheter is wedged | $P_wO_2 - PaO_2 \geq 19$ mm Hg |
| | $PaCO_2 - P_wCO_2 \geq 11$ mm Hg |
| | $pH_w - pH_a \geq 0.08$ |
| Pressure reading using the a wave at end-expiration | Obtain from paper recording to ensure accuracy |
| | If monitor has algorithm to find end-expiration and if digital and paper recording agrees: |
| | • Use systolic pressure for spontaneous breathing |
| | • Use diastolic pressure for positive-pressure breathing |

*CPAP*, Continuous positive airway pressure; *MI*, myocardial infarction; *PaCO₂*, arterial carbon dioxide tension; *PADP*, pulmonary artery diastolic pressure; *PaO₂*, arterial oxygen tension; *PAWP*, pulmonary artery wedge pressure; *PEEP*, positive end-expiratory pressure; *pHₐ*, arterial pH; *pHᵥᵥ*, wedge pH; *PᵥᵥCO₂*, wedge pressure, carbon dioxide; *PᵥᵥO₂*, wedge pressure, oxygen.

**FIG. 15.11** Pulmonary artery catheter wedged in zone III, where both pulmonary arterial pressures are greater than alveolar pressure, resulting in uninterrupted blood flow to the left side of the heart and a wedge pressure that reflects pulmonary venous and left heart pressures. Relationship of pressures is shown at the right. *LA,* Left atrium; *LV,* left ventricle; *PA,* alveolar pressure; *Pa,* pulmonary arterial pressure; *Pv,* pulmonary venous pressure; *RA,* right atrium; *RV,* right ventricle.

The technical aspects of setting up a pressure monitoring system include calibrating the monitor and transducer, positioning the transducer and patient, verifying and maximizing frequency response and dampening characteristics, and recording the pressures at end-expiration. Attention to proper management of the technical steps is vital to obtaining accurate pulmonary artery and wedge pressure measurements.

Another key point related to obtaining an accurate PAWP reading is the position of the catheter tip in relation to the heart (Fig. 15.11). For wedge pressure to reflect pulmonary venous and therefore left atrial pressure, blood flow must be uninterrupted between the catheter tip and the left heart.

This condition exists only in what is termed *zone III*, an area of the lung where both pulmonary arterial and venous pressures exceed alveolar pressure. When intravascular volume decreases (diuresis, hypovolemia, hemorrhage) or alveolar pressure increases (PEEP), zone III areas can convert to zone I or II.

The following observations indicate inappropriate catheter positioning in zones I or II:
- PADP < PAWP
- Smooth trace: no a or v waves
- With changes in PEEP
  - PAWP increase >50% of PEEP increase
  - PAWP decrease >50% of PEEP reduction

- With catheter wedged
  - Inability to withdraw blood
  - Mixed venous blood rather than "arterialized" blood
  - Catheter tip above left atrial level on lateral chest film

Alterations in ventilatory patterns cause fluctuations in intrapleural pressure. End-expiration minimizes the influence of the pressure swings for both spontaneous and mechanical ventilation, provided the patient is not exhaling against positive pressure. Ideally, the pressure will be recorded from a calibrated paper trace that also records the ventilatory pattern so that the end-expiratory pressures are clearly identified over several respiratory cycles.

*Wedging the balloon.* The balloon should be inflated with the minimum amount of air needed to obtain a clear wedge reading and waveform (systolic, dicrotic notch, and diastolic segments). Placing too much air in the balloon (hyperinflation) results in a pressure waveform without clearly distinguishable a and v waves that gradually climbs upward across the screen. Rarely, hyperinflation may produce a waveform that gradually declines, without clearly distinguishable a and v waves.

Normally, a period of 5 to 20 seconds is required for equilibration of the left-sided heart and pulmonary pressures. Once equilibration is achieved, the waveform should convert to an atrial pressure trace resembling a CVP pressure pattern. On balloon deflation, the waveform should convert back to a crisp pulmonary artery pattern. To avoid damage to the balloon (which would require catheter reinsertion), it should deflate passively rather than by aspiration.

*Relationship between transmural pressure and wedge pressure.* Transmural pressure is the net distending pressure within the ventricle. It provides a true estimation of LVEDV filling because the effect of pressure around the heart is considered. Transmural pressure cannot be measured directly but is calculated by subtracting the pressure around the heart from the measured filling pressure in the heart.

Wedge pressure is used to estimate left ventricular filling pressure inside the heart. Intrapleural or esophageal pressure is used to approximate the pressure pushing on the heart from the outside.

During spontaneous breathing, intrapleural pressure is nearly zero at end-expiration. Therefore as shown in the example that follows, end-diastolic pressure and transmural pressure are approximately equal, and wedge pressure is a good estimator of left ventricular filling pressure in the patient during normal spontaneous breathing. However, positive-pressure ventilation, labored respiratory effort, coughing, and the Valsalva maneuver cause large swings in intrapleural pressure. These pressure fluctuations can cause wedge pressure to overestimate or underestimate left ventricular filling pressure. The following example shows how a PAWP of 12 mm Hg can occur with very different transmural pressures. Remember that left ventricular filling pressure (PAWP) minus pressure around the heart (pleural pressure) equals pressure distending the left ventricle (transmural pressure).

| PAWP | (minus) | Pleural | Pressure (equals) | Transmural Pressure |
|---|---|---|---|---|
| Spontaneous breathing | 12 | − | 0 | = | 12 mm Hg |
| 20 cm PEEP | 12 | − | 10 | = | 2 mm Hg |
| Partial airway obstruction | 12 | − | −10 | = | 22 mm Hg |

The relationship between wedge and transmural pressures must be kept in mind in interpreting the numbers. The example "20 cm PEEP" shows how transmission of positive pleural pressure can cause the wedge pressure reading on the monitor or on paper to appear normal (12 mm Hg) while, in fact, the patient is really hypovolemic, with a transmural pressure of 2 mm Hg. The example "partial airway obstruction" shows how filling pressure can appear to be normal (12 mm Hg) when the true filling pressure would be high (22 mm Hg).

Clinically, PEEP levels less than 10 cm $H_2O$ tend to have little effect on intrapleural pressure. However, when PEEP exceeds 15 cm $H_2O$, the effect of PEEP on transmural pressure is uncertain and is altered by lung compliance and changing venous return. As lung compliance decreases, the lung gets stiffer, and a smaller amount of the positive pressure is passed to the pleural space. This has led to the practice of estimating the effect of PEEP on wedge pressure by converting PEEP to millimeters of mercury (1.36 cm $H_2O$ = 1 mm Hg) and subtracting part of PEEP from wedge pressure as follows:

- Compliant lungs: subtract one-half of PEEP from PAWP
- Noncompliant lungs: subtract one-fourth of PEEP from PAWP

The effects of PEEP on transmural pressure also can be assessed by measuring pleural pressure. In practice, esophageal pressure is measured with a fluid-filled tube while the patient is in the lateral decubitus position. The esophageal pressure, which is essentially the same as pleural pressure, is then subtracted from the wedge pressure.

Removing the patient from PEEP while the wedge pressures are obtained has been suggested. However, this maneuver alters the pressure gradient for venous return to the thorax and may result in sudden "autotransfusion." In addition, sudden removal of PEEP has been reported to cause deterioration in gas exchange that is not readily corrected. In patients with left ventricular dysfunction, removal from mechanical ventilation with PEEP may be associated with increased pulmonary artery pressure, hypoxemia, and deterioration in cardiac function. For these reasons, removal of patients from mechanical ventilation with PEEP to obtain pressure readings is not recommended.

## Complications of Pulmonary Artery Catheters

PAC has been associated with multiple complications. During cannulation of a central vein, it is possible for pneumothorax, hydrothorax, hemothorax, air embolism, and damage to the vein, nearby arteries, or nerves to occur. Movement of the catheter inside the heart can trigger bundle branch block and supraventricular or ventricular dysrhythmia. Hypoxemia, acidosis, hypokalemia, hypocalcemia, and hypomagnesemia increase the likelihood of a dysrhythmia. In addition, perforation of the heart or pulmonary artery is possible.

The PAC, like all other invasive lines, is a source of embolus, thrombus, bleeding, hematoma, site infection, and sepsis. The constant movement of the catheter with heartbeat, breathing, and patient movement can result in catheter migration. It should be remembered that a balloon left inflated or a catheter that migrates into wedge position acts like a pulmonary embolus.

Pulmonary infarction and even pulmonary artery rupture can result from overfilling the balloon while obtaining a wedge pressure, as well as from catheter migration. Pulmonary infarction should be suspected and assessed whenever a patient with a PAC coughs up blood-tinged sputum. An overfilled balloon can rupture, causing possible fragment or air embolism.

Catheter movement and catheter removal can trigger dysrhythmia, as well as looping of the catheter in the ventricle, with possible knotting and valve damage. Lidocaine and emergency resuscitation equipment should be immediately available at both insertion and removal. Blood gases and serum electrolytes should be optimized to decrease the risk for dysrhythmia. Catheter resistance during removal is not normal and is an indication for obtaining a chest radiograph to assess the cause.

## CENTRAL LINE BUNDLE

As discussed throughout this chapter, a common complication associated with all intravascular lines is infection. Indeed, it is estimated that each year more than 80,000 catheter-related bloodstream infections occur in the nation's ICUs, with as many as 28,000 deaths associated with this serious complication of medical management. In addition to mortality, catheter-related bloodstream infections increase morbidity, length of stay, and hospital costs.

Reducing the incidence of these infections requires a multidisciplinary approach among all those caring for patients with intravascular lines. Because RTs are part of the multidisciplinary critical care team, they must be active contributors to this effort.

As with ventilator-associated pneumonia, a "bundle" of evidence-based interventions for patients with intravascular catheters has been established that, when implemented together, can reduce the incidence of catheter-related infections. Although the bundle focuses on central lines (i.e., those with the tip terminating in a great vessel), it applies equally to arterial line insertion and maintenance. The five key components in a bundle are as follows:

1. Hand hygiene
2. Maximal barrier precautions
3. Chlorhexidine skin antisepsis
4. Optimal catheter site selection
5. Daily review of line status

Box 15.6 outlines the specific actions involved in applying each of the bundle's components. Given their active participation in the use of intravascular lines among the critically ill patients they care for, RTs must assume major responsibility for implementing and assuring application of these important infection-control strategies.

---

### BOX 15.6   Central Line Bundle

**Hand Hygiene**
Hand hygiene involves washing hands or using an alcohol-based waterless hand cleaner.
- When caring for central lines, appropriate times for hand hygiene include the following:
  - Before and after palpating catheter insertion sites
  - Before and after inserting, replacing, accessing, repairing, or dressing an intravascular catheter
- When hands are obviously soiled or if contamination is suspected:
  - Before and after invasive procedures
  - Between patients
  - Before donning and after removing gloves
  - After using the bathroom

**Maximal Barrier Precautions**
- Strict compliance with hand hygiene (above)
- Wear a cap, mask, sterile gown, and sterile gloves; consider protective eyewear for arterial line insertion
- Cover the insertion area with a sterile fenestrated drape
- Use a sterile sleeve to protect pulmonary artery catheters during insertion

- Wear either clean or sterile gloves when changing the dressing on intravascular catheters
- Use either sterile gauze or sterile, transparent, semipermeable dressing to cover the catheter site
- Replace catheter site dressing if the dressing becomes damp, loosened, or visibly soiled
- Avoid using topical antibiotic ointment or creams on insertion sites (can promote fungal infections)
- Replace gauze dressings every 2 days and transparent dressings at least every 7 days
- Scrub access port and diaphragm with antiseptic (e.g., chlorhexidine, povidone iodine, 70% alcohol), and access only with sterile devices

**Chlorhexidine Skin Antisepsis**
The technique, for most kits, is as follows:
- Prepare skin with antiseptic-detergent chlorhexidine 2% in 70% isopropyl alcohol
- Pinch wings on the chlorhexidine applicator to break open the ampule (when ampule is included)
- Hold the applicator down to allow the solution to saturate the pad

## BOX 15.6    Central Line Bundle—cont'd

- Press sponge against skin, using a back-and-forth friction scrub for at least 30 seconds
- Let solution dry completely before puncturing the site (about 2 minutes)
- If chlorhexidine is contraindicated, use tincture of iodine, an iodophor, or 70% alcohol
  
  *Note:* Palpation of the insertion site should not be performed after antiseptic application.

**Optimal Catheter Site Selection**
- Whenever possible, avoid the femoral site in adults
- For central venous pressure and pulmonary artery catheters, prioritize the subclavian site over the jugular
- Avoid brachial site for arterial lines in children

**Daily Review of Central Line Status**
- Remove the arterial catheter as soon as it is no longer needed
- Evaluate the catheter insertion site daily by palpation and inspection
- Monitor the catheter sites visually when changing the dressing
- If the patient has local tenderness or other signs of infection, remove dressing and visually inspect the site
- Do not routinely replace catheters to prevent catheter-related infections; replace only when there is a specific indication
- Encourage patients to report any changes in their catheter site or any new discomfort to their provider
- Replace tubing assembly, continuous flow device, and transducers every 96 hours

## KEY POINTS

- Patients with severe hypotension (shock), severe hypertension, or unstable respiratory failure are likely candidates for continuous arterial pressure monitoring.
- An arterial waveform should have a clear upstroke on the left, with a dicrotic notch representing aortic valve closure on the downstroke to the right.
- Normal arterial pressure in the adult is approximately 120/80 mm Hg and increases gradually with age. Systolic pressures greater than 140 mm Hg and diastolic pressures greater than 90 mm Hg are considered hypertensive. A pressure below 90/60 mm Hg in adults is known as hypotension.
- Arterial pressure decreases with hypovolemia from fluid or blood loss (most commonly, bleeding), during cardiac failure and shock (most commonly, heart attack), and with vasodilation (most commonly, sepsis).
- Normal MAP is considered to be 70 to 105 mm Hg.
- Ischemia resulting from embolism, thrombus, or arterial spasm is the major complication of direct arterial monitoring.
- As with all invasive lines, the presence of an arterial catheter increases the risk for infection.
- CVP is the pressure of the blood in the right atrium or vena cava, in which the blood is returned to the heart from the venous system.
- CVP monitoring is indicated to assess the circulating blood volume (adequacy of cardiac filling) or the degree of venous return or to evaluate right ventricular function.
- Patients who have had major surgery or blood loss caused by trauma and those suspected of severe dehydration may benefit from placement of a CVP catheter to guide fluid replacement therapy.
- CVP is regulated by a balance between the ability of the heart to pump blood out of the right atrium and ventricle and the amount of blood being returned to the heart by the venous system (venous return).
- Elevations of CVP occur under the following conditions:
  - Volume overload or fluids being given more rapidly than the heart can tolerate
  - Increased intrathoracic pressure (CVP increases with positive-pressure breath or tension pneumothorax)

- Compression around the heart: constrictive pericarditis or cardiac tamponade
- Pulmonary hypertension (primary or secondary)
- Right ventricular failure (e.g., myocardial infarction or cardiomyopathy)
- Left-sided heart failure severe enough to cause right-sided heart failure
- Pulmonary valvular stenosis
- Tricuspid valvular stenosis or regurgitation
- Pulmonary embolism
- Causes of decreased CVP include vasodilation and inadequate circulating blood volume (hypovolemia).
- Complications of using a CVP catheter can occur during placement or during its use over time. Placement of the catheter can cause problems such as bleeding or pneumothorax. Infection is the most common side effect over time.
- Insertion of the PAC represents increased risk compared with the CVP catheter. The additional risk is present because of the need for the catheter to pass through the right side of the heart and into the pulmonary artery.
- The PAC may be helpful in monitoring selected patients with cardiogenic or septic shock and ARDS.
- Normal PAWP is 6 to 12 mm Hg.
- The lack of forward flow out of the left ventricle causes the left ventricle to dilate and blood to back up into the pulmonary circulation, resulting in an elevated PAWP.
- The most common cause of a decreased PAWP is hypovolemia.
- Pulmonary artery catheterization has been associated with multiple complications. During cannulation of a central vein, it is possible for pneumothorax, hydrothorax, hemothorax, air embolism, and damage to the vein, nearby arteries, or nerves to occur.
- To help prevent catheter-related bloodstream infections, RTs must work together with the critical care team to implement the components of the central line bundle, including hand hygiene, barrier precautions, chlorhexidine skin antisepsis, optimal catheter site selection, and daily review of line status.

## CASE STUDY

A 32-year-old man is brought to the emergency department (ED) after a motor vehicle accident in which he suffered a broken femur, multiple lacerations, and a possible ruptured spleen. The paramedics state that the patient lost several units of blood at the scene, but the bleeding was stopped before he was transported to the ED. On entering the ED, he is semiconscious and has the following vital signs: pulse, weak and 122/min; respirations, 34/min; blood pressure, 80/60 mm Hg; body temperature, normal. A CVP catheter is placed, and the initial reading is 0 mm Hg.

1. What is your assessment of the patient at this point?
   The CVP reading of 0 mm Hg and the blood pressure of 80/60 mm Hg indicate significant hypovolemia. The narrow pulse pressure is consistent with a low stroke volume, probably the result of poor preload of the heart. The patient is suffering from hypovolemic shock.
2. Should a PAC be placed?
   A PAC is not needed at this time. The patient can be managed with volume replacement using the CVP readings before taking him to the operating room to repair the ruptured spleen.

## CASE STUDY

A 55-year-old woman was admitted to the cardiac unit for chest pain and dyspnea. Her hospital stay has been complicated by severe pulmonary edema and a poor response to initial therapy with inotropic agent. The attending physician decided to place a PAC to assist with treatment. Initial findings after placement of the PAC are as follows:

Pulse: 98/min
Respirations: 28/min
Blood pressure: 90/60 mm Hg
$SpO_2$: 92% on $FiO_2$ of 0.40
CO: 2.3 L/min
CI: 1.5 $L/min/m^2$
PVR: 310 $dynes/s/cm^5$
SVR: 1700 $dynes/s/cm^5$
PAWP: 22 mm Hg
CVP: 8 mm Hg
PAP: 38/28 mm Hg

1. What is your interpretation of the PVR and the SVR? What could cause these findings?
   The PVR and SVR are both elevated. The increase in PVR is probably related to the pulmonary edema and hypoxemia. The increase in SVR is caused by the peripheral vasoconstriction in response to a reduced CO.
2. What is the patient's SV? How do you interpret it?
   The SV is determined by dividing the CO by the heart rate. In this case, it is 23.5 mL, which is markedly reduced.
3. What is your interpretation of the PAWP and CO? What is probably causing the overall hemodynamic picture?
   The PAWP is increased, and the CO is reduced; these indicate that the left ventricle is not pumping blood forward effectively, causing a backup of blood into the pulmonary circulation and increasing the hydrostatic pressure in the pulmonary capillaries. The high hydrostatic pressure in the pulmonary capillaries is the cause of her pulmonary edema. The overall clinical picture is one of cardiogenic shock.

## ASSESSMENT QUESTIONS

1. What is the preferred site for insertion of an arterial catheter for continuous pressure monitoring?
   a. Femoral artery
   b. Brachial artery
   c. Radial artery
   d. Ulnar artery
2. A patient with which of the following conditions is least likely to need placement of an indwelling arterial catheter?
   a. Septic shock
   b. Cardiogenic shock
   c. ARDS
   d. Pneumonia
3. Just after insertion of a radial arterial catheter, you note that the pressure waveform appears dampened. All connecting tubing is secure and free of air. Which of the following actions is appropriate at this time?
   a. Remove the catheter and cannulate the other wrist
   b. Increase the sensitivity setting on the monitor
   c. Withdraw and then reinject 5 mL of blood
   d. Reposition the catheter while observing the waveform

4. The dicrotic notch on the arterial pressure waveform represents closure of which of the following heart valves?
   a. Pulmonic
   b. Aortic
   c. Tricuspid
   d. Mitral
5. Which of the following will cause a tall, narrow arterial pressure waveform?
   a. A stiff aorta
   b. Vasodilation
   c. Mitral valve stenosis
   d. Ventricular hypertrophy
6. What change in the arterial pressure waveform is normally seen with respiration?
   a. A large decrease with inspiration
   b. A large increase with inspiration
   c. A large increase with expiration
   d. Minimal changes with inspiration and expiration

7. Which of the following will cause the arterial pressure to decrease?
   1. Vasodilators
   2. Cardiac failure
   3. Hypovolemia
      a. 1 and 2
      b. 2 and 3
      c. 2 only
      d. 1, 2, and 3

8. Which of the following is true about MAP?
   1. It normally ranges between 70 and 105 mm Hg.
   2. It is the arithmetic average of the systolic and diastolic pressures.
   3. Organ perfusion is reduced if MAP is less than 60 mm Hg.
      a. 1 and 3
      b. 2 and 3
      c. 1 only
      d. 1, 2, and 3

9. Which of the following are possible complications of arterial cannulation?
   1. Infection
   2. Arterial spasm
   3. Thromboembolism
      a. 1 and 2
      b. 2 and 3
      c. 1 only
      d. 1, 2, and 3

10. CVP is a reflection of which of the following?
    a. Right atrial pressure
    b. Left ventricular filling volume
    c. Left atrial pressure
    d. Pulmonary artery diastolic pressure

11. A patient with which of the following conditions is least likely to need placement of a CVP catheter?
    a. Cardiogenic pulmonary edema
    b. Noncardiogenic pulmonary edema
    c. Large pleural effusion
    d. Major trauma

12. Which of the following is true about the CVP catheter?
    1. It is commonly inserted by way of the subclavian vein.
    2. The catheter can have multiple lumens.
    3. A balloon is located on the distal end.
       a. 1 and 2
       b. 2 and 3
       c. 1 only
       d. 1, 2, and 3

13. The c wave of a CVP waveform represents which of the following?
    a. Atrial contraction
    b. Ventricular contraction
    c. Atrial filling
    d. Ventricular filling

14. In which of the following conditions would an elevated CVP be expected?
    a. Pneumonia
    b. Hypovolemia

c. Cor pulmonale
d. Pleural effusion

15. Which of the following is the correct method of measuring CVP in a patient receiving mechanical ventilation with PEEP?
    a. At end-inspiration on the ventilator
    b. At end-inspiration off the ventilator
    c. At end-expiration on the ventilator
    d. At end-expiration off the ventilator

16. What is the normal value for CVP?
    a. 2 to 6 mm Hg
    b. 6 to 8 mm Hg
    c. 8 to 12 mm Hg
    d. 12 to 18 mm Hg

17. Which of the following causes the CVP to increase?
    a. Vasodilator therapy
    b. Spontaneous inspiration
    c. Fluid overload
    d. Air in the pressure-sensing line

18. The proximal port of a pulmonary artery catheter can be used for all of the following *except*:
    a. Measuring the CVP
    b. Withdrawing blood samples
    c. Injecting medications
    d. Measuring stroke volume

19. What is the approximate amount of air required to fill the balloon on a pulmonary artery catheter?
    a. 0.5 mL
    b. 1.5 mL
    c. 2.5 mL
    d. 3.5 mL

20. During insertion of a pulmonary artery catheter, when is the balloon inflated?
    a. Immediately after insertion into the venous site
    b. When the catheter enters the superior vena cava and right atrium
    c. When the catheter passes through the tricuspid valve and enters the right ventricle
    d. When the catheter passes through the pulmonic valve and enters the pulmonary artery

21. What would be considered a normal value for pulmonary artery pressure?
    a. 15/4 mm Hg
    b. 18/10 mm Hg
    c. 25/12 mm Hg
    d. 36/22 mm Hg

22. Which of the following would increase pulmonary artery pressure?
    1. Severe hypoxemia
    2. Thromboembolism
    3. Acidosis
       a. 1 and 2
       b. 2 and 3
       c. 1 and 3
       d. 1, 2, and 3

23. Which of the following statements is true about pulmonary artery wedge pressure?
    1. It is normally 6 to 12 mm Hg
    2. It is normally higher than PADP
    3. It reflects left ventricular preload
       a. 1 only
       b. 1 and 3
       c. 2 and 3
       d. 1, 2, and 3

24. What clinical condition is most likely to cause the PAWP to be elevated?
    a. ARDS
    b. Left-sided heart failure
    c. Cor pulmonale
    d. Pneumonia

25. Which of the following could cause PAWP to be overestimated?
    1. PEEP or CPAP greater than 10 cm $H_2O$
    2. Mitral valve stenosis
    3. Reduced left ventricular compliance
       a. 1 only
       b. 2 only
       c. 1 and 3
       d. 1, 2, and 3

26. Your patient has a pulmonary artery catheter in place and suddenly starts coughing up bloody sputum. What is the most likely cause of this?
    a. Pneumothorax
    b. Pulmonary infarction
    c. Mitral valve stenosis
    d. Myocardial infarction

27. What complication is most likely to occur during removal of a pulmonary artery catheter?
    a. Pneumothorax
    b. Pulmonary infarction
    c. Pulmonary embolism
    d. Dysrhythmias

28. When obtaining an arterial blood sample from an arterial line, you note that the patient complains of significant tenderness at the insertion site. You should recommend which of the following to the patient's nurse?
    a. Removal of the dressing and inspection of the site
    b. Immediate removal of the catheter
    c. Replacement of the catheter with a new one
    d. Application of an antibiotic cream to the insertion site

## BIBLIOGRAPHY

Augusto JF, Teboul JL, Radermacher P, et al. Interpretation of blood pressure signal: physiological bases, clinical relevance, and objectives during shock states. *Intensive Care Med.* 2011;37(3):411–419.

Burchell PL, Powers KA. Focus on central venous pressure monitoring in an acute care setting. *Nursing.* 2011;41(12):38–43.

Callan P, Clark AL. Right heart catheterization: indications and interpretation. *Heart.* 2016;102(2):147–157.

Cole E. Measuring central venous pressure. *Nurs Stand.* 2007;22(7):40–42.

Cooper LB, Mentz RJ, Stevens SR, et al. Hemodynamic predictors of heart failure morbidity and mortality: fluid or flow? *J Card Fail.* 2016;22(3):182–189.

Cruz K, Franklin C. The pulmonary artery catheter: uses and controversies. *Crit Care Clin.* 2001;17:271–291.

Frazier SK, Skinner GJ. Pulmonary artery catheters: state of the controversy. *J Cardiovasc Nurs.* 2008;23(2):113–121.

Hakata S, Ota C, Kato Y, et al. An analysis of the factors influencing pulmonary artery catheter placement in anesthetized patients. *Ann Card Anaesth.* 2015;18(4):474–478.

Healthcare Infection Control Practices Advisory Committee. *Guidelines for the prevention of intravascular catheter-related infections.* Atlanta, GA: Centers for Disease Control and Prevention; 2011.

Hofer CK, Cecconi M, Marx G, et al. Minimally invasive haemodynamic monitoring. *Eur J Anaesthesiol.* 2009;26(12):996–1002.

Husain S, Pamboukian SV, Tallaj JA, et al. Invasive monitoring in patients with heart failure. *Curr Cardiol Rep.* 2009;11(3):159–166.

Marik PE, Baram M, Vahid B. Does central venous pressure predict fluid responsiveness? A systematic review of the literature and the tale of seven mares. *Chest.* 2008;134(1):172–178.

Montenij LJ, de Waal EE, Buhre WF. Arterial waveform analysis in anesthesia and critical care. *Curr Opin Anaesthesiol.* 2011;24(6):651–656.

Mooney DM, Fung E, Doshi RN, et al. Evolution from electrophysiologic to hemodynamic monitoring: the story of left atrial and pulmonary artery pressure monitors. *Front Physiol.* 2015;6:271.

Polanco PM, Pinsky MR. Practical issues of hemodynamic monitoring at the bedside. *Surg Clin North Am.* 2006;86(6):1431–1456.

Richard C, Monnet X, Teboul JL. Pulmonary artery catheter monitoring in 2011. *Curr Opin Crit Care.* 2011;17(3):296–302.

Teboul JL, Saugel B, Cecconi M, et al. Less invasive hemodynamic monitoring in critically ill patients. *Intensive Care Med.* 2016;42(9):1350–1359.

Wiener B, Chacko S, Cron SG, et al. Guideline development and education to insure accurate and consistent pulmonary artery wedge pressure measurement by nurses in intensive care units. *Dimens Crit Care Nurs.* 2007;26(6):263–268.

Wong FW. Where is end expiration? Measuring PAWP when the patient is on pressure support ventilation. *Dynamics.* 2010;21(1):11–16.

# 16

# Cardiac Output Measurement

*Ruben D. Restrepo and Richard B. Wettstein*

## LEARNING OBJECTIVES

*After reading this chapter, you will be able to:*

1. Define cardiac output, cardiac index, stroke volume, and venous return.
2. Describe the method of calculation, common reference range, and effect of sympathetic nervous stimulation on cardiac output.
3. Describe the effects of metabolism and reduced oxygen availability on the regulation of blood flow through organs.
4. Explain the effect of blood loss (hypovolemia) on circulatory function.
5. Describe the effect of mechanical ventilation on cardiac output and blood flow.
6. Explain the significance of the following indicators of cardiac output:
   a. Cardiac index
   b. Ejection fraction
   c. Stroke volume
   d. End-diastolic volume

e. Cardiac work
f. Ventricular stroke work

7. List the most important factors that regulate cardiac preload, afterload, and contractility.
8. Calculate systemic and pulmonary vascular resistance.
9. Describe the technique for obtaining cardiac output through the following invasive methods:
   a. Fick
   b. Thermodilution (pulmonary artery and transpulmonary)
   c. Pulse contour analysis
   d. Doppler ultrasound
10. Describe the noninvasive methods for evaluating cardiac performance:
    a. Transthoracic electrical bioimpedance
    b. Echocardiography
    c. Radionuclide cardiac imaging
    d. Partial carbon dioxide rebreathing

## OUTLINE

## KEY TERMS

afterload
cardiac index
cardiac output
cardiac work
cardiac work index
central venous pressure
contractility
ejection fraction

end-diastolic pressure
end-diastolic volume
negative inotropic effect
positive inotropic effect
preload
pulmonary capillary wedge pressure
pulmonary vascular resistance
pulse pressure

rate-pressure product
stroke volume
systemic vascular resistance
venous return
ventricular compliance
ventricular function curves
ventricular stroke work

Cardiac output monitoring provides essential information regarding the adequacy of perfusion and helps guide patient management. Adequacy of perfusion is the most important factor in the assessment of the cardiovascular system's ability to meet the body's metabolic demands. Early detection of circulatory problems allows for early proactive interventions. This is important because most patients do not succumb to their disease but to vital organ failure.

The aim of this chapter is to describe the physiologic principles and common techniques used to measure cardiac output. Chapter 15 on the other hand describes the specific vascular pressure parameters used in the intensive care unit (ICU) to monitor patients with circulatory problems.

## CARDIAC OUTPUT

The amount of blood the heart pumps in a minute is known as cardiac output (CO). It is the product of heart rate (HR) and stroke volume (SV), which is the volume of blood ejected by a single ventricular contraction (Box 16.1). Normal SV for adults is 60 to 130 mL/beat and is roughly equal for both the left and right ventricles. The average CO for men and women of all ages is approximately 5 L/min at rest (normal range is 4 to 8 L/min); however, the normal CO for an individual varies with age, sex (10% higher in men), body size, blood viscosity (hematocrit), and the tissue demand for oxygen.

When stimulated by the sympathetic nervous system the heart is capable of pumping approximately 20 to 25 L/min. A well-trained athlete's heart enlarges sometimes as much as 50% and is capable of pumping up to 35 L/min. Under normal conditions, the heart serves as a demand pump, pushing forward all the blood that returns to it. Congestive heart failure occurs when the diseased or damaged heart can no longer pump all the blood returned to it.

## VENOUS RETURN

The volume of blood returning to the right atrium is known as the venous return. The blood flow through an organ is determined by its metabolic needs. As the organ's demand for oxygen increases, perfusion to the organ increases. The muscles, liver, and kidneys receive the greatest amount of blood flow in the resting state because of their high metabolic needs. When the metabolic activity of the tissues increases (as during exercise) or when the availability of oxygen to the tissues decreases (as occurs at high altitudes or with carbon monoxide or cyanide poisoning), vasodilation allows more blood to flow to the tissues.

The concentrations of oxygen, carbon dioxide ($CO_2$), hydrogen ions, electrolytes, and other humoral substances regulate capillary blood flow. The presence of low oxygen concentration and increased levels of hydrogen ions and $CO_2$ at the tissue level causes vasodilation and increases blood flow to the affected area.

In addition to providing tissue regulatory control of CO, the venous system acts as a reservoir of blood. Normally about two-thirds of the total blood volume resides in the venous

---

### BOX 16.1 Cardiac Output: An Overview

**Cardiac Output (CO)**
Amount of blood pumped by the heart per minute:
  CO = HR × SV
Varies with age, gender, body size, blood viscosity, and tissue demand for oxygen
Adult reference range for cardiac output: 4-8 L/min

**Cardiac Index (CI)**
Ratio of cardiac output to body surface area (m²): CO/BSA
Reference range for cardiac index: 2.5-4.0 L/min/m²

**Stroke Volume (SV)**
Volume of blood ejected with each beat, determined by the following:
  Preload: stretch on ventricle at filling before contraction volume, venous return, compliance
  Afterload: resistance to ventricular emptying, vasoconstriction versus vasodilation, blood viscosity, ventricular wall tension, negative intrathoracic pressure
  Contractility: strength of ventricular contraction sympathetic stimulation, inotropes, depressants, coronary flow, heart muscle damage

**Frank-Starling Mechanism (Ventricular Function Curve)**
Defines a characteristic relationship between the following:
  Volume filling the ventricle (end-diastolic volume/preload) and volume ejected per contraction (ventricular stroke volume): ↑ filling volume → ↑ muscle stretch → ↑ energy → ↑ output
  If the ventricle becomes too large, overdistention: → ↓ SV

**Ventricular Filling Volume and Filling Pressure Are Closely Related**
Filling pressure is used to evaluate ventricular filling volume.
Atrial pressures approximate ventricular end-diastolic pressure.
Right atrial pressure (RAP or CVP) for right-sided heart filling
Left atrial pressure (LAP) for left-sided heart filling
Pulmonary artery wedge pressure (PAWP), also known as pulmonary capillary wedge pressure (PCWP), approximates LAP and left-sided heart filling pressure in most patients (see, Chapter 15). For consistency throughout the chapter, the acronym PAWP is used.

**Cardiac Output Can Be Used to Determine Vascular Resistance**
Resistance = pressure/flow
↑ Vascular resistance → ↑ heart work
↓ Vascular resistance (vasodilation) → ↓ heart work
Right side of the heart: pulmonary vascular resistance (PVR)
Left side of the heart: systemic vascular resistance (SVR)
Ventricular filling pressure, volume, vascular resistance, and blood pressure can be manipulated by fluids and drugs to optimize CO and perfusion of oxygen and nutrients to the tissues.

*CVP*, Central venous pressure; *HR*, heart rate.

system. When blood volume to vital organs decreases, the veins and the spleen constrict and redistribute volume to maintain venous return and cardiac pressures. In fact, 20% to 25% of the total blood volume can be lost without altering circulatory function and pressures. In cases of severely reduced CO such as heart failure, the central nervous system causes a sympathetic stimulation that increases vasoconstriction. As the heart fails, this compensatory mechanism reduces blood flow to the liver, kidneys, and other body areas to maintain perfusion to the most vital organs (heart and brain).

### SIMPLY STATED

- The adequacy of perfusion is the most important factor in the assessment of the cardiovascular system's ability to meet the body's metabolic demands.
- Blood flow to tissues can be inadequate when blood pressure is too low, but a normal blood pressure does not always indicate optimal blood flow to the tissues.
- The venous system serves as a reservoir for the entire circulatory system and through vasoconstriction can compensate for loss of up to one-fourth of the total blood volume.

## MEASURES OF CARDIAC OUTPUT AND PUMP FUNCTION

### Cardiac Index

Because CO, like most other hemodynamic measurements, varies with body size, cardiac index (CI) is often used to describe flow output. CI is obtained by dividing CO by body surface area (BSA) and is reported as liters per minute per square meter (L/min/m²). BSA is calculated using the patient's weight and height and the DuBois nomogram (Fig. 16.1). The advantage of using an index is that values are standardized, and comparisons can be made among patients of different heights and weights.

A commonly cited resting CI reference range for patients of all ages is 2.5 to 4.0 L/min/m², with the average for adults being about 3.0 L/min/m² (Table 16.1). The CI is highest at 10 years of age and decreases with age to approximately 2.4 L/min/m² at age 80 years.

### SIMPLY STATED

The advantage of using a cardiac index is that comparisons of CO can be made among patients of different sizes.

### Cardiac Work

Cardiac work is a measure of the energy the ventricles use to eject blood against the aortic or pulmonary pressures (resistance). It increases as the end-diastolic ventricular size increases and correlates well with the oxygen requirements of the heart. Although the left and right ventricles eject the same volume of blood, the work performed by the left

**FIG. 16.1** DuBois body surface area (BSA) nomogram. BSA is found by locating the patient's height on scale I and weight on scale III and placing a straightedge between the two points. The line intersects scale II at the patient's BSA. (From DuBois EF: *Basal metabolism in health and disease*, Philadelphia, 1936, Lea & Febiger.)

ventricle is much greater since it must eject against the mean aortic pressure (MAP), which is about 6 times greater than the mean pulmonary artery pressure (MPAP). The cardiac work index (CWI) measures the work per minute per square meter for each ventricle and is calculated using the following formulas:

$$LCWI = CI \times MAP \times 0.0136 = 3.4 - 4.2 \text{ kg/min/m}^2$$
$$RCWI = CI \times MPAP \times 0.0136 = 0.4 - 0.66 \text{ kg/min/m}^2$$

where 0.0136 is a conversion factor for changing pressure to work.

### Ventricular Stroke Work

Ventricular stroke work is a measure of myocardial work per contraction. It is the product of the stroke volume index (SVI) times the pressure across the vascular bed. Normal left

**TABLE 16.1  Hemodynamic Variables, Example Reference Ranges, and Formulas**

| Variable | Example Reference Range[a] | Formula |
|---|---|---|
| Cardiac output (CO) | 4-8 L/min | CO = direct measurement |
| Cardiac index (CI) | 2.5-4.0 L/min/m² | CI = CO/BSA |
| Stroke volume (SV) | 60-130 mL/beat | SV = CO/HR or EDV − ESV |
| Stroke volume index (SVI) | 30-50 mL/m² | SVI = CI/HR or SV/BSA |
| Ejection fraction (EF) | 65%-75% | EF = SV/EDV or direct measurement |
| End-diastolic volume (EDV) | 120-180 mL/beat | EDV = direct measurement |
| End-systolic volume (ESV) | 50-60 mL | ESV = direct measurement |
| Rate-pressure product (RPP) | <12,000 mm Hg | RPP = systolic BP × HR |
| Coronary perfusion pressure (CPP) | 60-80 mm Hg | CPP = diastolic BP − PAWP |
| Left cardiac work index (LCWI) | 3.4-4.2 kg/min/m² | LCWI = CI × MAP × 0.0136[b] |
| Right cardiac work index (RCWI) | 0.4-0.66 kg/min/m² | RCWI = CI × MPAP × 0.0136[b] |
| Left ventricular stroke work index (LVSWI) | 50-60 g/min/m²/beat | LVSWI = SI × MAP × 0.0136[b] |
| Right ventricular stroke work index (RVSWI) | 7.9-9.7 g/min/m²/beat | RVSWI = SI × MPAP × 0.0136[c] |
| Pulmonary vascular resistance (PVR) | <2 units | PVR = (MPAP − PAWP)/CO |
|  | 110-250 dynes-s/cm⁵ | PVR = (MPAP − PAWP)/CO × 80[d] |
| Pulmonary vascular resistance index (PVRI) | 225-315 dynes-s/cm⁵/m² | PVRI = (MPAP − PAWP)/CI × 80[d] |
| Systemic vascular resistance (SVR) | 15-20 units | SVR = (MAP − CVP)/CO × 80 |
|  | 900-1400 dynes-s/cm⁵ |  |
| Systemic vascular resistance index (SVRI) | 1970-2400 dynes-s/cm⁵/m² | SVRI = (MAP − CVP)/CI × 80[d] |

*BP*, Blood pressure; *BSA*, body surface area; *CVP*, central venous pressure (mm Hg); *HR*, heart rate; *MAP*, mean arterial pressure (mm Hg); *MPAP*, mean pulmonary artery pressure (mm Hg); *PAWP*, pulmonary artery occlusion pressure (mm Hg).
[a]Commonly cited references ranges for adults. Sources vary somewhat in the ranges reported.
[b]Conversion factor to convert L/mm Hg to kg/min/m²; 0.0144 is used by some sources.
[c]Conversion factor to convert mL/mm Hg to g/min/m²; 0.144 is used by some sources. An alternative version of the formula includes subtraction of the filling pressures: LVSWI = SV × (MAP − PAWP) × 0.0136; RVSWI = SV × (MPAP − CVP) × 0.0136.
[d]Conversion factors of 79.92 and 79.96 may also be used.

ventricular stroke work index (LVSWI) and right ventricular stroke work index (RVSWI) values are as follows:

$$LVSWI = SVI \times MAP \times 0.0136 = 50 - 60 \text{ g/min/m}^2/\text{beat}$$
$$RVSWI = SVI \times MPAP \times 0.0136 = 7.9 - 9.7 \text{ g/min/m}^2/\text{beat}$$

## Ventricular Volume

The end-diastolic volume (EDV), defined as the amount of blood in the ventricle at the end of filling (diastole), and the end-diastolic pressure (EDP), can help estimate the ventricular size. Further discussion of the EDV and EDP relationship is found in the Ventricular Function Curves section of this chapter.

## Ejection Fraction

Ejection fraction (EF) represents the percentage of the EDV that is ejected with each heartbeat. EF is either measured directly or calculated from the following formula:

$$EF = SV/EDV$$

Normal EF is 65% to 70%. When the EF falls to the 30% range, a patient's exercise tolerance is severely limited because of the heart's inability to maintain an adequate CO.

## DETERMINANTS OF PUMP FUNCTION

CO is determined by HR and SV, and SV is determined by three factors: preload, afterload, and contractility (Fig. 16.2).

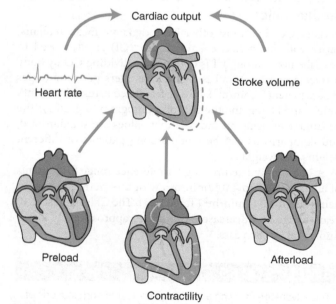

**FIG. 16.2** Cardiac output is determined by stroke volume and heart rate. Stroke volume is determined by preload, afterload, and contractility.

## Heart Rate

HR normally does not play a large role in control of CO in the adult except when it is outside the normal range or when a dysrhythmia is present.

Bradycardia (HR <60 beats/min in an adult) does not drop CO as long as the heart can compensate with increased SV.

A well-trained athlete may have a resting pulse rate below 50 beats/min but still maintain normal blood pressure. However, a failing heart cannot alter SV to compensate for bradycardia, and thus CO falls.

Tachycardia (adult HR >100 beats/min) is the body's way of maintaining CO when compensatory mechanisms to increase SV are inadequate. In the resting patient, CO may begin to decline at rates of 120 to 130 beats/min. In the presence of tachycardia, premature ventricular contractions, and premature atrial contractions, the time for ventricular filling is decreased, leading to decreased CO. Maintaining a higher HR requires an increased oxygen consumption that may not be available in the patient with coronary artery disease. In subjects with a healthy heart the CO does not decline until the HR reaches about 180 beats/min.

## Preload

Preload is the stretch on the ventricular muscle fibers before contraction. Preload is created by the EDV. In 1914 Starling found that up to a critical limit, the force of a muscle contraction was directly related to the initial length of the muscle before contraction. His theory is known as *Starling's law of the heart*. Simply put, the greater the stretch on the resting ventricle, the greater the strength of contraction within physiologic limits. When the physiologic limits are exceeded, greater stretching of the muscles does not result in an increased force of contraction.

### Ventricular Function Curves

Fig. 16.3 shows ventricular function curves (often called *Starling curves*) for the right and left ventricles. The horizontal axis represents the volume (preload), and the vertical axis is a measure of the heart's output: CO, CI, SV, stroke index, or ventricular SWI. Increasing the volume increases output. However, when the pump becomes overstretched, it can no longer eject all of its blood efficiently, and CO begins to fall.

Continuously measured EDV is an ideal but time-consuming way to assess preload. Most critical care units only measure ventricular volumes on a periodic basis using echocardiography or radionuclide imaging. Therefore atrial pressures, which can be measured continuously, are used to reflect EDV. During diastole, the atrioventricular valves (tricuspid and mitral) are open. If the valves are not dysfunctional, the pressures in the atrium and ventricle should be the same at end-diastole. The filling pressure for the right side of the heart is right atrial pressure, commonly measured as the central venous pressure (CVP). The filling pressure for the left side of the heart is left atrial pressure, commonly measured as pulmonary artery wedge pressure (PAWP). Measuring these pressures is discussed in Chapter 15. Because a nonlinear relationship exists between the EDV and EDP, filling pressure does not always reflect ventricular volume when ventricular compliance is altered. An example in which EDP does not accurately reflect EDV is in patients with increased ventricle chamber stiffness (e.g., myocardial infarction). In these cases, EDP may remain constant as EDV decreases.

A

B

FIG. 16.3 Ventricular function curves for right and left ventricles. Note that filling pressures are used to represent end-diastolic volume. **A,** Ventricular function curves for the right ventricle. Upstroke of curve shows rapid change in cardiac output for small change in end-diastolic volume initially, but the curve then plateaus, with little change in output for large changes in right atrial pressure. *Dashed curves* show change in output for given pressure occurring with altered contractility from sympathetic stimulation (as occurs with exercise or fear) and heart failure. **B,** Ventricular function curves for left ventricle. End-diastolic volume can be used for plotting horizontal axis. Cardiac index, stroke volume, or left ventricular stroke work index can be graphed on the vertical axis rather than cardiac output. Output begins to decline after pulmonary capillary wedge pressure reaches 20 mm Hg unless ventricular compliance is abnormal.

### Ventricular Compliance

Pressure is the result of the volume, space, and compliance of the chamber the volume is entering. Forcing 100 mL of water into a small, rigid chamber takes more pressure than filling a compliant balloon with 100 mL of water. Fig. 16.4 shows how ventricular pressure is affected by changes in volume and ventricular compliance (distensibility). When compliance is reduced, a much higher pressure is generated for a given volume. Pressure also increases more rapidly as the ventricle fills; thus the ends of the curves rise more abruptly as the ventricle becomes full and tension is developed in the ventricular walls.

Factors that decrease ventricular compliance and therefore cause the pressure to increase out of proportion to the volume include the following:
- Myocardial ischemia and infarction
- Hemorrhagic and septic shock
- Pericardial effusions

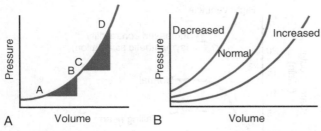

**FIG. 16.4** Compliance can be altered along a single pressure-volume relationship or by a change in the rate of increase in diastolic pressure. **A,** Small rise in pressure (point A to point B) for given change in end-diastolic volume is in contrast to large increase in pressure seen from point C to point D with the same (or smaller) change in end-diastolic volume. Therefore the ventricle described by A to B is more compliant than the ventricle described by C to D. **B,** Ventricular compliance curves. Not only may compliance fall along the ascending curve, but disease and drugs may also effect a change in the compliance curve up and to the left (reduced compliance) or down and to the right (increased compliance). (From Sibbald WJ, Driedger AA: Right and left ventricular preload and diastolic ventricular compliance: implications for therapy in critically ill patients. In Shoemaker WC, Thompson WL, editors: *Critical care: state of the art,* vol 3, Fullerton, CA, 1982, Society for Critical Care Medicine.)

- Right ventricular dilation and overload (causing the septum to shift to the left and impinge on the left ventricle)
- Positive end-expiratory pressure (PEEP) or continuous positive airway pressure (CPAP)
- Inotropic drugs (increase the strength of myocardial contraction)

Factors that increase ventricular compliance include the following:
- Relief of ischemia
- Vasodilator drugs (nitroprusside or nitroglycerin)
- Cardiomyopathies

### Factors That Affect Venous Return, Preload, and Cardiac Output

The three main factors affecting the amount of blood returned to the heart are the following:
1. Changes in circulating blood volume
2. Changes in the distribution of the blood volume
3. Atrial contraction

*Circulating blood volume.* Although bleeding directly impacts circulating blood volume, excessive urine output (as occurs with diuretics), wound drainage, diarrhea, perspiration, and gastric secretions can result in a large decrease in blood volume (hypovolemia). Clinical conditions such as sepsis, burns, and shock may result in tremendous amounts of fluid being moved into the interstitial space, or the so-called third space. On the other hand, fluids ingested or given intravenously increase the circulating blood volume. Administration of colloids (large-molecular-weight solutions) pulls water from the interstitial space to "dilute out" the large molecules, resulting in an increase in blood volume. Use of continuous bland aerosols or even heated humidification to overcome a patient's humidity deficit can also cause a net fluid gain, especially in small children.

*Distribution of the blood volume.* Distribution of the blood volume is altered not only by third spacing but also by changes in body position, venous tone, intrathoracic pressure, and, rarely, obstruction of the large veins returning to the heart. As the body changes position, blood tends to move to dependent areas. Standing decreases venous return; conversely, raising the legs of a patient who is lying down increases venous return.

Venous tone also alters the distribution of blood in the body. Venous tone may increase (vasoconstriction) as a compensatory mechanism and shift more blood to the vital organs (heart, lungs, and brain). Vasodilation therapy relaxes vascular tone and may decrease venous return.

The presence of conditions such as tension pneumothorax, Valsalva maneuver, breath holding in children, prolonged bouts of coughing, and positive-pressure ventilation increases intrathoracic pressure and thereby decreases venous return.

*Atrial contraction.* Atrial contraction, so-called atrial kick, contributes approximately 30% of the SV and total CO by loading the ventricle at the end of diastole. When a patient develops atrial fibrillation, atrioventricular dissociation, or third-degree heart block, or is being paced by a ventricular pacemaker, the CO may fall.

### Clinical Applications of Ventricular Function Curves

Preload is the major determinant of contractility, but ideal filling pressures vary greatly with cardiac compliance and the patient's condition. Ventricular function curves may be constructed to find a patient's ideal filling pressure at a given time and provide information about ventricular compliance. Most commonly, they are used when large amounts of fluid are administered; however, they may also be used to monitor CO response to changes in filling pressure resulting from volume unloading (diuresis) and administration of intravenous cardiopulmonary drugs such as inotropes and vasodilators.

To construct a ventricular function curve, CI, CO, SV, or another measure of heart output is plotted on the vertical axis. Filling pressure (usually pulmonary artery diastolic or PAWP) is plotted on the horizontal axis. A baseline CO measurement is obtained, and the point corresponding to the CO reading and simultaneous pressure reading is plotted (Fig. 16.5A). A fluid challenge is administered, and another set of output and pressure measurements is obtained. Pressure is again plotted against output. When satisfactory CO is achieved or when CO begins to decline as the filling pressure increases, the fluid challenge is stopped. The pressure that corresponds to the highest CO reading obtained is used to indicate optimal preload. Volume can then be administered as needed to maintain this optimal pressure. It is important to remember that the venous system will begin to "relax" and expand as the volume status is corrected, so it is necessary to follow the patient carefully and reassess the need for additional volume.

| # | PAWP (mm Hg) | CO (L/min) | IV Fluid Challenge in response to hemodynamics |
|---|---|---|---|
| a | 4 | 2.4 | 200 mL × 10 min |
| b | 7 | 2.8 | 200 mL × 10 min |
| c | 8 | 3.3 | 200 mL × 10 min |
| d | 10 | 3.8 | 200 mL × 10 min |
| e | 16 | 3.5 | stop challenge, monitor |
| f | 12 | 4.1 | monitor |

| # | PAWP (mm Hg) | CO (L/min) | Rx or Fluid Challenge in response to hemodynamics |
|---|---|---|---|
| a | 23 | 2.2 | furosemide 40 mg IV |
| b | 19 | 3.3 | furosemide 40 mg IV |
| c | 17 | 3.8 | monitor |
| d | 14 | 3.9 | monitor |
| e | 11 | 3.0 | 100 mL × 10 min |
| f | 14 | 3.9 | monitor |

**FIG. 16.5** Ventricular function curves constructed to determine optimal filling pressure using pulmonary artery wedge pressure (PAWP, mm Hg) as the filling pressure measurement and cardiac output (CO, L/min) as the heart output measurement. **A,** Fluid challenge curve for a patient with low output (CO 2.4 L/min) and low filling pressure (PAWP 4 mm Hg) treated with four intravenous (IV) fluid challenges. Administrations of the first three fluid challenges (a to c) were followed by increases in filling pressure and output (↑ PAWP to 8, ↑ CO to 3.3). After the fourth challenge (d), filling pressure continued to increase, but output began to fall (e) (↑ PAWP to 16, ↓ CO to 3.5), suggesting volume overload. The fluid challenge was stopped. Subsequent measurements confirmed that output increased as the filling pressure dropped back toward normal (f) (↓ PAWP to 12, ↑ CO to 4.1). An optimal filling pressure near 12 mm Hg using PAWP was suggested. **B,** Diuresis curve for a heart failure patient with low cardiac output (2.2 L/min) and high filling pressure (PAWP 23 mm Hg) treated with two doses of IV furosemide. Diuresis after the first dose of furosemide decreased the filling pressure with a corresponding improvement in heart output (b) (↓ PAWP to 19, ↑ CO to 3.3). A second dose of furosemide was given to further unload the ventricle and improve pulmonary congestion. Filling pressure decreased toward the normal range and output improved (c, d) (↓ PAWP to 14, ↑ CO to 3.9). However, continuing diuresis caused the filling pressure and the output to drop (e) (↓ PAWP to 11, ↓ CO to 3.0). A fluid challenge was given to increase filling pressure, and output improved (f) (↑ PAWP to 14, ↑ CO to 3.9). An optimal filling pressure near 14 mm Hg using PAWP was suggested.

## Effects of Mechanical Ventilation on Preload and Venous Return

***Normal spontaneous breathing.*** During normal spontaneous inspiration, contraction of the diaphragm and enlargement of the thoracic cage reduce the intrapleural pressure to approximately −6 cm $H_2O$. The drop in intrapleural pressure increases the negative gradient between the intrathoracic and extrathoracic vessels. This higher gradient favors the movement of blood into the chest and right atrium, thus increasing venous return (preload).

During spontaneous expiration, the reverse occurs. Recoil of the thoracic cage causes the intrathoracic pressure to rise, augmenting CO and creating the slight rise in arterial blood pressure that is normally seen with expiration. Thus spontaneous inspiration functions as a circulatory assist pump for the heart. During labored breathing, as often seen in the patient having a severe asthma attack, these pressure swings are exaggerated and may result in a *paradoxic pulse*, which is a drop in blood pressure of more than 10 mm Hg during inspiration.

*Increased intrapleural pressure.* Increased intrapleural pressure, as occurs during the Valsalva maneuver, decreases venous return and thereby may decrease CO. Increased intrapleural pressure also occurs with loss of spontaneous breathing, disruption of the chest wall, collection of fluid or air in the pleural space, or positive-pressure ventilation.

*Positive-pressure ventilation and compliance.* The effect of positive-pressure ventilation on venous return depends on how much airway pressure is transferred to the pleural space. When lung and thorax compliances are equal, only about half of the change in airway pressure is transmitted to the pleural space. If the lung compliance decreases, as occurs with certain types of respiratory failures, less positive pressure is transmitted to the pleural space; thus these patients can tolerate positive-pressure ventilation better and may experience little effect on cardiovascular function.

When chest wall compliance decreases, as commonly seen with abdominal distention or after thoracic or abdominal surgery, more airway pressure is transmitted to the pleural space. If chest wall compliance is decreased while lung compliance is increased (e.g., chronic obstructive pulmonary disease), even more of the elevated airway pressure is transmitted to the pleural space. These patients are more likely to develop problems of both decreased venous return and increased pulmonary vascular resistance during positive-pressure ventilation, with the potential result being a reduction in CO.

*Positive end-expiratory pressure and continuous positive airway pressure.* Positive expiratory pressures, including auto-PEEP (intrinsic PEEP), exaggerate the inspiratory effects of positive-pressure ventilation and maintain increased intrapleural pressure throughout expiration, thus having an even greater potential for decreasing venous return. It has been shown that venous return is affected most by continuous mechanical ventilation with PEEP. However, if intravascular volume is maintained or increased to offset the ventilator-induced reduction in venous return, CO may not be affected when positive airway pressure is used. The effect of mechanical ventilation on vascular pressure measurements is discussed in Chapter 15.

---

### SIMPLY STATED

Because the heart is inside the chest, it is subject to the pressure changes occurring in the chest:
- Positive pressures around the heart push on the heart, making it harder for blood to enter the heart (decrease venous return) but easier for blood to be ejected.
- Negative pressures around the heart pull blood toward the heart (increase venous return and preload) but make it more difficult for blood to leave the heart.

---

## Afterload

Afterload, the resistance or sum of the external factors that oppose ventricular ejection, has the following two components:
1. Ventricular wall stress
2. Peripheral vascular resistance

### Ventricular Wall Stress

Ventricular wall stress is directly related to the tension on the wall of the ventricle (ventricular pressure × radius) and inversely related to the wall thickness. Cardiac factors that decrease ventricular emptying include the following:
- Ventricular overdistention
- Abnormally high intraventricular pressure
- Thinning of the ventricular wall
- Negative intrathoracic pressure

*Increased afterload.* When the ventricle is distended from too much volume and pressure, tension in the muscle increases, and more oxygen and energy are required for contraction; thus afterload increases. Similarly, as intrathoracic pressure becomes more negative, the vacuum-like effect aids the opening and filling of the ventricle but increases resistance to ventricular emptying.

*Decreased afterload.* Positive intrathoracic pressure facilitates compression of the ventricle, decreases the pressure gradient across the ventricular wall, and decreases resistance to ventricular emptying but opposes right ventricular filling. Positive-pressure ventilation with PEEP may compress the heart during inspiration, reducing diastolic filling but at the same time enhancing systolic emptying. This combination may be beneficial for many patients in congestive heart failure.

### Peripheral Resistance

The peripheral component of afterload is determined by the following:
- Elasticity (compliance) of the vessels
- Size (radius) of the vessels
- Viscosity of the blood
- Driving pressure (changes in pressure from one end of the vessel to the other)

*Increased vascular resistance.* The radius of the vessels is the greatest determinant of peripheral resistance to blood flow. In the presence of vasoconstriction, the heart must exert more energy to eject the blood. As afterload increases, the myocardial oxygen demands on the heart also increase. When the heart is receiving an inadequate supply of oxygen (as occurs with coronary artery disease), it is not able to produce the amount of energy needed to eject efficiently against the afterload, and failure worsens. A downward cycle of cardiac failure ensues if afterload is not decreased. Inadequate CO causes vasoconstriction, which causes increased work for the heart, resulting in less CO and more vasoconstriction. The cycle is broken by maximizing cardiac oxygenation and performance and decreasing the afterload, either by vasodilator therapy or with a cardiac assist device such as an intraaortic balloon pump.

Afterload also increases as the viscosity of the blood increases. This is an important consideration in some patients with chronic pulmonary disease because the concentration of red blood cells often rises above normal in order to increase their oxygen-carrying capacity (see Chapter 7). When hematocrit levels exceed 60%, the viscosity or thickness of blood is very high and CO often decreases. Conversely, one of the causes of high CO (hyperdynamic state) is anemia (low hematocrit).

Blood flow is also dependent on a pressure gradient. When the backpressure in the venous system increases, as occurs when the right side of the heart is not able to pump blood efficiently, the pressure gradient across the capillary beds decreases. Blood flow from the arteries through the capillaries to the venous system slows. This damming effect causes the afterload to increase, which can lead to left-sided heart failure.

*Decreased vascular resistance.* Although vasodilator therapy decreases afterload and thus the energy demands on the heart, it also increases the ability of the blood vessels to hold blood and act as a "vascular reservoir." If the reservoir is made larger but the volume in the container stays the same, the amount of blood returning to the heart (venous return) decreases, and preload decreases. Conversely, when the volume in the ventricle is more than the ventricle can pump effectively, decreasing the preload will reduce the mechanical work of the ventricle and improve CO. However, if the venous return (preload) decreases too much, the stretch on the ventricle (preload) will be inadequate, and CO will fall. In addition, if vasodilation causes the arterial diastolic pressure to fall below 50 mm Hg or MAP to fall below 60 mm Hg, perfusion to the coronary arteries may decrease, and CO will be compromised even further.

### Calculating Systemic and Pulmonary Vascular Resistance

Calculated values for systemic vascular resistance (SVR) and pulmonary vascular resistance (PVR) are helpful in evaluating the vascular component of afterload for each of the ventricles. The values typically are reported as absolute resistance units (dynes-s/cm$^5$) or divided by CI and reported as an index.

Elevated SVR is associated with clinical conditions that cause vasoconstriction, such as cold, inadequate perfusion, hypertension, or administration of vasopressors such as norepinephrine (Levophed), methoxamine (Vasoxyl), or epinephrine (Adrenalin). Warming a hypothermic patient to normal temperature or administering vasodilators such as nitroprusside decreases SVR.

PVR is increased by conditions that decrease blood flow through the pulmonary artery, such as constriction, obstruction (e.g., emboli), or compression of the pulmonary vasculature. In addition, hypoxemia, acidosis, and release of histamine from an allergic response also cause vasoconstriction of the pulmonary vasculature, which results in an increase in PVR. Over time, increased PVR results in pulmonary hypertension and eventually right-sided heart failure or cor pulmonale (Table 16.2).

---

**SIMPLY STATED**

CO may decrease by one-third before a significant drop in arterial blood pressure occurs. Because systemic arterial pressure is the product of SVR and CO, reflex vasoconstriction may increase SVR and maintain a normal or increased blood pressure despite the decreasing CO. However, once compensatory vasoconstriction is maximized, the patient may suddenly "crash" because this mechanism may no longer be able to maintain an adequate blood pressure.

---

**TABLE 16.2   Causes of Pulmonary Hypertension and Cor Pulmonale**

| Mechanisms | Related Disorders |
|---|---|
| Loss of pulmonary vasculature and tissue (blockage, compression, destruction) | Primary pulmonary hypertension, multiple pulmonary emboli, pulmonary thrombosis |
| | Malignant metastasis, collagen vascular diseases |
| | Inflammatory and fibrotic disease of the lung (diffuse interstitial pneumonia, sarcoidosis, pneumoconiosis) |
| Pulmonary vasoconstriction resulting from hypoxemia and/or acidosis | COPD (emphysema, bronchitis, asthma) |
| | Neuromuscular disorders (e.g., myasthenia gravis, Guillain-Barré syndrome, poliomyelitis) |
| | Extreme obesity (pickwickian syndrome) |
| | Thoracic spine and chest wall deformities |
| Increased pulmonary venous pressure | Mitral valve stenosis, left atrial embolus or tumor, rheumatic heart disease |
| | Idiopathic venoocclusive disease |
| Increased pulmonary blood flow | Ventricular septal defect, patent ductus arteriosus |
| Increased blood viscosity | Polycythemia |

*COPD,* Chronic obstructive pulmonary disease.
Modified from Margulies DM, Thaler MS: *The physician's book of lists,* New York, 1983, Churchill Livingstone.

### Contractility

The third primary factor determining CO is contractility, which is a measure of myocardial contraction strength. The strength of a cardiac contraction is modified by the following two major influences:

1. Change in the initial muscle length caused by stretch of the cardiac muscle (preload)
2. Change in contractility or inotropic state of the heart at any given amount of muscle stretch

For all practical purposes, contractility represents the force generated when myocardial muscle fibers shorten during systole, independent of preload or afterload. In Fig. 16.3, an increase in contractility is shown to be associated with an increase in CO, despite no change in the preload. Conversely, heart failure is usually accompanied by decreased contractility (and a lower ejection fraction) with a downward shift of the ventricular function curve and a lowering of CO for a given preload.

### Factors Related to Contractility

Myocardial contractility is affected by the following factors:
- Sympathetic nerve stimulation
- Inotropic drugs

- Physiologic depressants
- Damage to the heart
- Coronary blood flow

***Sympathetic nerve stimulation.*** Sympathetic nerve stimulation with release of norepinephrine and other circulating catecholamines increases the strength and the rate of cardiac contraction (the fight-or-flight response). Conversely, inhibiting the sympathetic nervous system with a drug or by total spinal anesthesia depresses contractility. Parasympathetic stimulation (vagal stimulation) also decreases contractility.

***Inotropic drugs.*** Inotropic drugs are medications that affect the force or energy of muscular contraction. A drug with a positive inotropic effect increases the strength of contraction of the myocardial fibers, most often by increasing intracellular calcium levels. These drugs also increase myocardial oxygen consumption because cells are pushed beyond their metabolic rate to increase the force of contraction. Positive inotropic drugs include calcium, digitalis, epinephrine, norepinephrine, dopamine, dobutamine, amrinone, isoproterenol, and caffeine. If a positive inotropic drug is used to strengthen the heart when there is inadequate preload, myocardial oxygen supply and demand can become increasingly mismatched and even result in myocardial infarction. Therefore it is necessary to maximize preload before "driving" the heart with these drugs.

Drugs with a negative inotropic effect decrease the strength of contraction but may also decrease the myocardial oxygen demand. Negative inotropic drugs include β-blockers, barbiturates, and many antidysrhythmic agents such as procainamide and quinidine. In a patient with angina resulting from myocardial ischemia, negative inotropic agents, such as β-blockers, may be used to enhance the relationship of myocardial oxygen supply to demand.

***Physiologic depressants.*** Physiologic depressants of cardiac contractility include hypoxia, hypercapnia, and acidosis. Decreased extravascular calcium and elevated potassium and sodium levels can severely depress myocardial contractility. An excess of calcium ions has the opposite effect, causing the heart to go into spastic contraction. Low potassium and sodium levels are associated with conduction disturbances and dysrhythmia associated with decreased cardiac performance.

***Damage to the heart.*** Damage to the myocardium, valves, or conduction system reduces the pumping ability of the heart. Loss of ventricular tissue results in decreased contractility because of the reduced effectiveness of muscle contraction, as in cardiomyopathy, myocardial ischemia, and myocarditis. The muscle in the area of a myocardial infarction typically loses contractile ability or, over time, may even balloon out and develop into a ventricular aneurysm.

Chronic increase in myocardial work will result in enlargement of the chambers and hypertrophy of the muscle.

***Coronary blood flow.*** Although coronary blood flow continues throughout the cardiac cycle, it is significantly higher during diastole and is directly influenced by myocardial oxygen demand. When myocardial oxygen demand increases, coronary blood flow increases. This autoregulation of coronary blood occurs within an MAP range of 60 to 180 mm Hg. When MAP or diastolic pressure falls, coronary artery perfusion may be compromised, resulting in decreased myocardial oxygen delivery and a subsequent fall in contractility.

Normal coronary perfusion pressure (CPP) is 60 to 80 mm Hg and is calculated as follows:

$$CPP = Diastolic\ arterial\ blood\ pressure - PAWP$$

---

**SIMPLY STATED**

Decreased contractility generally is caused by loss of contractile muscle mass resulting from injury, disease, dysrhythmias, drugs, or poor perfusion. Increased contractility can be caused by sympathetic nerve stimulation or inotropic drugs.

---

### Variables Used to Assess Contractility

Unfortunately, it is not possible to directly conclude that the cause of low CO is decreased contractility. In addition, there is no definitive hemodynamic measure of contractility.

SV is a good indicator of ventricular performance and is directly related to the degree of myocardial fiber shortening and circumferential ventricular size. Other variables used to describe ventricular performance and pumping efficiency include EF, cardiac work, stroke work, and their indices, which were described earlier in this chapter. These calculations are used to describe the work the heart can do and thereby indicate its contractile ability.

Rate-pressure product is a simplified approach to evaluating cardiac work and reflects hemodynamic distress measured at rest and during various stages of exercise. It is obtained by multiplying HR and systolic blood pressure. Values greater than 12,000 are thought to indicate increased myocardial work and increased oxygen demand.

Echocardiography and radionuclide cardiac imaging can provide visual assessment of ventricular volumes and function. Transthoracic electrical bioimpedance (described later in this chapter) is a noninvasive method of measuring cardiac performance variables that can also can be used to assess the ventricular contractile state. These three methods for assessing contractility are discussed later in this chapter.

---

**SIMPLY STATED**

CO is determined by a complex set of interrelated physiologic variables, including the volume of blood in the heart (preload), the downstream resistance to ejecting blood from the heart (afterload), the contractility and compliance of the heart muscle, and the metabolic requirements of the body. A single measurement of CO represents the interaction of all the variables. CO reflects not only heart function but also the response of the circulatory system to acute and chronic disease and the effect of therapeutic interventions (Table 16.3).

**TABLE 16.3  Conditions Associated with Alteration in Hemodynamic Measurements Used to Evaluate Low Cardiac Output**

| Normal Hemodynamics | Altered Hemodynamics | Conditions | Corrective Therapy |
|---|---|---|---|
| **Preload** | | | |
| Right-sided heart CVP and RAP = 2-6 mm Hg or 4-12 cm $H_2O$ | Low pressure or EDV ↓ CVP, ↓ PAWP, and ↓ urine output | 1. Inadequate vascular volume | 1. Volume expansion: intravenous solutions, blood, albumin |
| Left-sided heart LAP, PAWP, PADP 8-15 mm Hg EDV = 120-180 mL/beat | ↓ PAWP | 2. ↓ SVR (vasodilation) from drugs, spinal anesthetic, fever, sepsis | 2. Stop vasodilators; volume expansion, vasoconstriction |
| | | 3. SVR may ↑ (vasoconstriction) to maintain MAP and CO if significant hypovolemia has developed | 3. Volume expansion; if SVR does not ↓, vasodilation and additional volume may be needed |
| Urine output 30 mL/h | High pressure or EDV poor pump/too much volume | | |
| | 1. ↑ CVP or PAWP | 1. a.  Cardiac failure | 1. a.  Inotropic drugs, diuretics |
| | | b.  Cardiac tamponade | b.  Volume expansion and isoproterenol until correction of tamponade |
| | 2. ↓ CVP and ↑ PAWP | 2. Left-sided heart failure, intraoperative myocardial infarction, left heart valve malfunction | 2. Inotropic drugs, vasodilate to ↓ SVR, surgical correction |
| | 3. ↑ CVP and ↓ PAWP | 3. a.  Right-sided heart failure/valve malfunction | 3. a.  Inotropic drugs, surgical correction |
| | | b.  Chronic pulmonary disease | b.  ↓ PVR, watch for hypovolemia with low PAWP |
| | | c.  Pulmonary embolism | c.  Heparin, inotropic drugs, vasopressors, surgical correction |
| **Afterload** | | | |
| SVR = <20 units or 900-1400 dyne-s/cm⁵ | 1. ↑ SVR, ↓ CVP, and PAWP | 1. Vasoconstriction: body's natural response to maintain perfusion to vital organs when BP drops; ↓ temperature | 1. Volume expansion; warm to normal temperature, watch for hypovolemia with vasodilation from warming |
| Urine output Adult = 30 mL/h Pediatric = ≥1 mL/kg/h | 2. ↑ SVR and ↑ PAWP | 2. ↑ SVR is compensation for failing pump; if uncorrected, will proceed to downward cycle of cardiac failure to cardiogenic shock | 2. Vasodilators, diuretics, inotropic drugs |
| Extremities warm Capillary refill = <3 sec | 3. ↓ SVR | 3. Vasodilation: spinal anesthetic, ↑ temperature, vasovagal response, sepsis | 3. Stop vasodilators/diuretics; consider volume expansion; inotropic drugs, possible vasoconstrictors |
| **Contractility** | | | |
| CI = 2.5-4.0 L/min/m² | Causes of decreased contractility: | | |
| SV = 60-130 mL SVI = 30-50 mL/m² RVSWI = 7.9-9.7 g/min/m² LVSWI= 50-60 g/min/m² | 1. ↓ Volume | 1. Dehydration | 1. Volume expansion; in some failing hearts, PAWP must be kept at 15 mm Hg or higher to maintain contractility |

*Continued*

**TABLE 16.3 Conditions Associated with Alteration in Hemodynamic Measurements Used to Evaluate Low Cardiac Output—cont'd**

| Normal Hemodynamics | Altered Hemodynamics Conditions | | Corrective Therapy |
|---|---|---|---|
| MAP = 70-105 mm Hg (see Table 16.2 for formulas) | 2. Inadequate coronary perfusion/heart muscle | 2. Inadequate diastolic pressure; coronary stenosis, occlusion; myocardial ischemia, infarction; ventricular aneurysm, congenital defects, surgery | 2. Maintain MAP >60 mm Hg, diastolic pressure >50 mm Hg (watch for drop in diastolic pressure with vasodilators)<br><br>Angioplasty, surgery<br>Inotropic drugs when volume is adequate (driving heart when volume is low could lead to myocardial infarction); low-dose inotropic support may be used continuously for 24-48 h after surgery to support a weak myocardium |
|  | 3. HR >100 beats/min<br>HR <60 beats/min |  | 3. ↓ HR: ensure adequate volume; β-blockers, calcium antagonists<br>↑ HR: atropine; rarely, isoproterenol<br>Pacemaker (CO may ↓ if loss of atrial kick) |
|  | 4. Dysrhythmia | 4. ↓ K+, Ca2, O2<br>Drug induced<br>Other | 4. Replace K+, Ca2, maintain adequate Pao2<br>Withdraw/change medication<br>Treat with antidysrhythmics, cardioversion, pacemaker |
|  | 5. Hypotension | 5. Negative inotropic drugs β-Blockers (propranolol), antiarrhythmics, barbiturates | 5. Decrease or discontinue medication; inotropic drugs as needed |
|  | 6. ↑ SVR (heart must work harder to pump against vasoconstriction) |  | 6. Vasodilators with volume expansion if necessary; inotropic drugs |
|  | 7. ↓ Po2, pH, K+, Na+, Ca2; ↑ Pco2, K+, Na+ | 7. ARDS, pulmonary edema | 7. Correct oxygenation electrolytes, acid-base balance |

*BP,* Blood pressure; *CPP,* cerebral perfusion pressure; *CVP,* central venous pressure; *LAP,* left atrial pressure; *PADP,* pulmonary artery diastolic pressure; *PAWP,* pulmonary artery wedge pressure; *RAP,* right atrial pressure; *SVR,* systemic vascular resistance. For other abbreviations, see text.

# METHODS OF MEASURING CARDIAC OUTPUT

Accurate clinical assessment of the circulatory status is particularly desirable in critically ill patients in the ICU and in patients undergoing cardiac, thoracic, or vascular interventions. Invasive techniques are still considered the gold standard for measuring CO. However, greater emphasis now is being placed on minimally invasive and noninvasive techniques. The ideal CO monitoring techniques should be accurate, reproducible or precise, fast responding, noninvasive, operator independent, easy to use, continuous, cost-effective, cheap, and safe. None of the methods currently used meet all these criteria.

## SIMPLY STATED

The ideal characteristics for CO monitoring techniques are accuracy, reproducibility or precision, fast response time, operator independence, ease of use, continuous use, noninvasive access, cost-effectiveness, and safety.

## Invasive Methods
### Fick Cardiac Output

Several invasive techniques have been introduced to measure CO in humans. The direct Fick method, described by Adolph Fick in 1870, became the accepted standard for the measurement of CO until the development of usable dye dilution techniques. The CO is calculated as the quotient of oxygen uptake ($\dot{V}O_2$) and the difference of the arterial and mixed venous oxygen content ($C\,[a-\bar{v}]O_2$). The direct Fick technique, however, is only rarely used in clinical practice, primarily because the bedside measurement of oxygen uptake is technically demanding.

The CO can be calculated as follows:

$$CO\,(mL/min) = \frac{\text{Whole body } O_2 \text{ consumption}\,(mL/min)}{\text{Arterial} - \text{mixed } O_2 \text{ content difference}\,(mL/dL) \times 10}$$

Or, symbolically:

$$CO \ (L/min) = \frac{\dot{V}O_2}{C(a-\bar{v})O_2 \times 10}$$

Using a normal or expected value of oxygen consumption and measuring the $C(a-\bar{v})O_2$, an estimated Fick CO reading can be obtained in the ICU setting. The following three steps are required:

1. Calculate the expected oxygen consumption $(\dot{V}O_2)$. The normal range of $\dot{V}O_2$ is 120 to 160 mL/min/m², with an average of 125 mL/min/m². $\dot{V}O_2$ for a patient with a body surface area of 2 m² would be calculated as follows:

$$\dot{V}O_2 = 125 \ mL/min/m^2 \times 2 \ m^2 = 250 \ mL/min$$

2. Calculate the arterial and mixed venous oxygen contents and $C(a-\bar{v})O_2$. For example, given a hemoglobin of 14 g/dL, an arterial oxygen saturation $(SaO_2)$ of 90%, and a mixed venous oxygen saturation $(S\bar{v}O_2)$ of 60%, the $C(a-\bar{v})O_2$ is computed as follows:

Arterial $O_2$ content = 14 g/dL × 1.34 mL/g × 0.90 = 16.9 mL/dL
Venous $O_2$ content = 14 g/dL × 1.34 mL/g × 0.60 = 11.3 mL/dL
$$C(a-\bar{v})O_2 = 5.6 \ mL/dL$$

The normal range for the $C(a-\bar{v})O_2$ is 3.0 to 5.5 mL/dL. The lower the $C(a-\bar{v})O_2$, the smaller the amount of oxygen removed per 100 mL of blood passing through the capillaries. Low values are seen when the following occurs:

- Well-oxygenated blood moves rapidly through the capillaries (high CO)
- Cells extract less oxygen (septic shock)
- Oxygen is not released from hemoglobin (left-sided shift in the oxyhemoglobin dissociation curve)

Higher values indicate more oxygen was removed, as when the following occurs:

- Blood flow is slow (low CO), *or*
- Tissue extraction of oxygen is high (increased oxygen consumption)
- Calculate the CO:

$$CO \ (L/min) = \frac{\dot{V}O_2}{C(a-\bar{v})O_2 \times 10}$$
$$CO \ (L/min) = 250 \ mL/min/5.6 \ mL/dL \times 10$$
$$CO \ (L/min) = 250 \ mL/min/56 \ mL/L$$
$$CO \ (L/min) = 4.46 \ L/min$$

To derive actual $O_2$ consumption, the expired gas volume over a known time and the difference in $O_2$ concentrations between this expired gas and inspired gas must be measured. Accurate collection of the gas is difficult unless the patient is intubated. Analysis of the gas is straightforward if the inspired gas is air, but if it is oxygen-enriched air, there are two problems: (1) potential fluctuations in the inspired $O_2$

concentration $(FiO_2)$, and (2) difficulty in measuring small changes in $O_2$ concentrations at high $FiO_2$. Moreover, measurement of mixed venous blood $O_2$ contents is required, which can only be obtained from the distal port of a pulmonary artery catheter. Clearly, if pulmonary artery catheter placement is needed, other simpler methods to compute CO are available and used.

## Pulmonary Artery Thermodilution Cardiac Output

The pulmonary artery (PA) catheter thermodilution method is considered the most accurate and reproducible method for CO determination and the one to which all other methods are compared. However, thermodilution CO measurement (TDCO) requires placement of a PA catheter and thus carries with it all the potential complications of central venous access. For this reason, PA catheter use has decreased substantially during the past two decades, mostly owing to the lack of evidence demonstrating improved patient outcomes, as well as concerns related to cost and hazards.

The indicator measured for TDCO is change in blood temperature. Sterile dextrose in water or normal saline solution at least 2°C colder than blood temperature is injected into the proximal port (right atrium) of the PA catheter. The resultant cooling is detected by a thermistor bead located just behind the balloon of the catheter, which is positioned in the pulmonary artery (Fig. 16.6). A temperature-time curve is recorded by the computer, with the CO inversely proportional to the area under the curve (Steward-Hamilton equation). As with all indicator-dilution methods, TDCO measurement makes three major assumptions: (1) complete mixing of blood and indicator, (2) no loss of indicator between place of injection and place of detection, and (3) constant blood flow. Errors in measurement are primarily related to the violation of these conditions.

*Acceptable variations in thermodilution injection technique.* Accurate TDCO results can be achieved using iced, refrigerated, or room-temperature injectant in most patients. Because SV can vary significantly with intrapleural pressures, an average of multiple determinations with injections equally spaced throughout the respiratory cycle has been shown to provide the best estimate of mean CO. Manual injection at end exhalation may not accurately reflect the average CO, especially in mechanically ventilated patients. Use of an injection gun and a connecting system that measures the injectant temperature as it enters the catheter produces more consistent TDCO readings.

Accuracy and reproducibility of results depend on extremely careful attention to detail and technique. Indicators must be measured precisely and injected as a bolus in less than 3 seconds. Computers must be calibrated, carefully maintained by biomedical engineers, and balanced before each measurement. Catheters must be properly located and patent, and tips must be away from the wall of the vessel. The cardiac monitor should be watched during CO measurements because dysrhythmias may alter the CO. When a significant dysrhythmia does occur, the CO should be recorded separately (not averaged into the set) and noted to occur with the

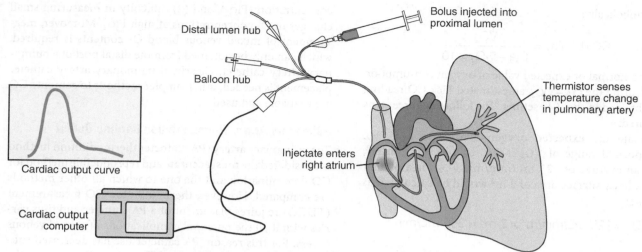

**FIG. 16.6** Thermodilution cardiac output measurement. See text for details.

identified dysrhythmia. Another output measurement is then obtained, averaged into the set, and recorded as CO without the presence of dysrhythmia.

### Transpulmonary Indicator Dilution Cardiac Output

As a result of the numerous complications associated with the placement and presence of a PA catheter, alternative less invasive ways to measure CO have been developed. One approach is to use the same indicator-dilution method as with a PA catheter, but instead inject the indicator into a central vein and measure the change through an arterial line placed in a large artery. This technique is referred to as the *transpulmonary indicator-dilution CO method*. CO determination by this method is reliable and agrees well with the results from pulmonary artery thermodilution. Because most critically ill patients already have CVP and arterial lines in place, this method is not only less risky than PA thermodilution but also more practical. As with PA thermodilution, repeated measurements are possible. Moreover, transpulmonary indicator dilution methods are less influenced by respiratory variations than CO measured by PA thermodilution.

Two methods are in current use: (1) transpulmonary thermodilution (PiCCO, Pulsion Medical Systems) and (2) transpulmonary lithium dilution (LiDCO, LiDCO Group). Both methods also are used to calibrate CO measurement through arterial pulse contour analysis, as discussed elsewhere in this chapter.

*PiCCO.* The PiCCO system is based on the injection of a cold fluid bolus into a central vein. A thermistor located in the tip of a catheter inserted into a large artery (usually femoral) is used to measure blood temperature changes. A thermodilution curve is created, and CO is computed using

the same basic Steward-Hamilton equation as applied with pulmonary artery thermodilution. The only major difference is that the transpulmonary curve appears later and has a lower peak temperature than that observed with pulmonary artery thermodilution. Research indicates that TDCO and PiCCO may be used interchangeably for CO measurement even under acute hemodynamic changes.

*LiDCO.* The LiDCO (lithium dilution cardiac output) method consists of injecting a small dose of lithium chloride (LiCl) through a peripheral venous line. The resulting lithium concentration-time curve is recorded by withdrawing blood past a lithium sensor attached to the patient's existing arterial line (Fig. 16.7). Primary and secondary indicator dilution curves for lithium dilution CO are obtained, and CO is calculated using a variation of the Steward-Hamilton formula that accounts for packed cell volume (needed because lithium is distributed only in the plasma). Research evidence indicates that this method correlates well with TDCO in a variety of clinical settings.

Although less risky and generally as accurate and repeatable as pulmonary artery thermodilution, transpulmonary indicator-dilution methods still provide only intermittent measures of CO.

### Continuous Cardiac Output Monitoring

Continuous cardiac output (CCO) monitoring is preferable to intermittent measurement, especially during rapid changes in hemodynamic function of critically ill patients. CCO is considered the ideal method for monitoring the response to a fluid challenge because it has been shown to reduce hospital stay and postoperative complications. Two CCO methods are in current use: (1) continuous PA thermal dilution and (2) arterial pulse contour analysis.

*Continuous pulmonary artery thermal dilution cardiac output monitoring.* PA-based continuous thermodilution methods use a modified PA catheter that includes a thermal filament located between 14 and 25 cm from the distal tip of the catheter. Every 30 to 60 seconds, the thermal filament heats the surface of the catheter to about 5°C above body temperature.

**FIG. 16.7** LiDCO system. The sensor consists of a disposable lithium-selective electrode in a flow-through cell. The sensor is connected to a three-way tap on the arterial line, and a small peristaltic pump restricts the flow through it to 4.5 mL/min.

$$CO = cal \cdot HR \cdot \int_{Systole} \left( \frac{P(t)}{SVR} + C(p) \cdot \frac{dP}{dt} \right) dt$$

Patient-specific calibration factor (determined with thermodilution) — Heart rate — Area under pressure curve — Compliance — Shape of pressure curve

**FIG. 16.8** Computation of cardiac output from arterial pulse contour (APC) analysis (PiCCO system as an example). The calibration factor is determined by intermittent transpulmonary indicator dilution measurement of CO (thermodilution for the PiCCO system). SV is computed as a complex integral that includes three factors: the area and shape of the pressure curve and the compliance of the arterial system. (From PULSION Medical Systems.)

As with intermittent bolus injections, the subsequent change in blood temperature (in this case warming) is measured by a thermistor near the PA catheter tip, with CO calculated using the same basic Steward-Hamilton equation.

*Invasive arterial pulse contour analysis.* In recent years, several techniques that estimate CO by analysis of the arterial line waveform have been developed and applied at the bedside. Collectively, these techniques, known as *arterial pulse contour (APC) analysis,* have become the most frequently described method for continuous CO monitoring in the literature. APC analysis is considered a minimally invasive and indirect method used to assess CO. CO is computed from a pressure pulsation on the basis of a criterion or a model. APC provides beat-to-beat CO measurement and permits preload assessment using volumetric parameters, an assessment tool critically important to guide fluid therapy. The origin of the APC method for estimation of beat-to-beat SV goes back

to the classic model described by Otto Frank in 1899. In its simplest conceptual formulation, SV is proportional to the area under the arterial pulse-pressure waveform.

As of this writing, four invasive APC methods are in common clinical use: (1) PulseCO (LiDCO, Cambridge, UK), (2) PiCCO (Pulsion, Munich, Germany), (3) FloTrac (Edwards Lifesciences, Irvine, CA), and (4) PRAM (MostCare System; Vyetrech Health, Padua, Italy). All methods use arterial blood pressure measured invasively through an arterial line (see Chapter 15). The PulseCO and PiCCO methods require calibration through one of the indicator-dilution methods previously described. The FloTrac system requires no external calibration, and the PRAM system does not require calibration or preloaded data.

The PulseCO and PiCCO systems both calculate continuous beat-to-beat SV and CO through complex analysis of the arterial blood pressure waveform (Fig. 16.8). The PulseCO system requires calibration by a transpulmonary lithium dilution CO measurement using the LiDCO technology previously described, and the PiCCO system calibration is by transpulmonary thermodilution. Both systems have proved accurate and reliable in the perioperative and ICU settings. In an evaluation of this method in patients undergoing off-pump coronary artery bypass grafting, calibrated PulseCO values were interchangeable with the those obtained by intermittent PA TDCO. However, other studies have indicated that the values of cardiac function measured by calibrated PulseCO may not always be consistent with those measured by the gold standard of PA TDCO. A check on the calibration is required only every 8 hours, and the software can track changes in CO even in the presence of moderately dampened arterial lines.

In combination with the Vigileo monitor, the FloTrac sensor only requires access to the radial or femoral artery using a standard arterial catheter and does not need an external calibration. This technique has been recently validated in critically ill patients and has been found to correlate well with values obtained by TDCO and PulseCO. CO measurement based on uncalibrated pulse contour analysis correlates well with CO measured with the continuous thermodilution method in patients undergoing uncomplicated coronary artery surgery. However, in situations in which the arterial pressure waveform is changed, agreement among techniques may be altered, and data obtained with uncalibrated pulse contour analysis may become less reliable.

The PRAM system automatically calibrates, does not require a recalibration indicator, and measures SV variations and pulse pressure variations. However, this technique has not been well studied.

---

**SIMPLY STATED**

CCO monitoring is preferable to intermittent cardiac output measurement, especially during the rapid changes in hemodynamic function that commonly occur in critically ill patients.

---

### Transesophageal, Transtracheal, and Intravascular Doppler Monitoring

Technologic advances have led to new miniature Doppler ultrasonic probes that can be positioned on tubes or catheters inserted into different body locations to obtain CO measurements. The technique measures the velocity of blood flow and vessel diameter in a nearby artery. With blood velocity and vessel diameter known, volumetric blood flow in liters per minute can be calculated.

The transesophageal probe is positioned in the esophagus at the level of the fifth and sixth vertebrae (approximately 35 to 45 cm from the nose) and pointed posteriorly to assess descending thoracic aortic blood flow. It can be used to derive CO from measurement of blood flow velocity by recording the Doppler shift of ultrasound reflected from the red blood cells. Signals can be obtained every 2 to 10 minutes.

Transesophageal probes have been left in place for up to 4 days without significant complications. Esophageal Doppler has been considered clinically acceptable and has shown good agreement with values obtained by CCO and PulseCO. The main disadvantages of the method are that a skilled operator is needed, the probe is large and therefore heavy, sedation or anesthesia is needed, the equipment is very expensive, and the probe cannot be fixed to give continuous CO readings without an expert user being present.

Transtracheal Doppler ultrasound is accomplished by a transducer attached to the end of an endotracheal tube so that it can be in continuous contact with the tracheal wall. Because these devices look at flow in the descending aorta, which does not reflect total CO, they cannot provide an actual CO measurement. However, they can provide measures of flow—including flow time, peak velocity, and stroke distance—that correlate with SV. One-time calibration using transcutaneous Doppler ultrasound CO measurements has been used to convert the descending aorta flow measurements to total CO measurement. This technique has not proven to be reliable. However, these devices may find more use in situations in which it is important to identify hemodynamic changes but not necessary to know the actual CO.

Continuous intravenous Doppler ultrasound CO measurements are obtained by a transducer mounted on the distal section of a PA catheter and positioned in the main pulmonary artery proximal to the bifurcation. CO measurements obtained by this method have a moderate correlation to the bolus PA thermodilution technique.

## Noninvasive Methods

Early assessment of SV or CO is important for the management of critically ill patients in the ICU or high-risk surgical patients in the operating room, as well as for assisting in the triage of patients with hemodynamic compromise in the emergency department. However, the invasiveness and complexity of the established CO monitoring techniques often discourage this early evaluation. To that end, newer, noninvasive methods are gaining acceptance among clinicians.

### Continuous Measurement of Cardiac Performance Using Transthoracic Electrical Bioimpedance

Transthoracic electrical bioimpedance was first described by Kubicek and associates in 1966 and reviewed by Critchley in 1998. It allows the intrabeat measurement of changes in transthoracic voltage amplitude in response to an injected high-frequency current. It provides continuous, real-time, noninvasive measurement of variables that describe global blood flow, left ventricular performance, pumping efficiency, and volume status. Because blood is the most electrically conductive substance in the body and because the thorax can act like a transducer, the electrical conductivity in the thorax can be translated into blood flow data. Eight electrocardiogram-type electrodes, two on each side of the neck and two on each side of the chest, form the interface between the patient and the computer terminal. Digitally displayed variables include CO, SV, HR, ejection velocity, ejection time, and thoracic fluid index. Additional variables include end-diastolic volume, peak flow, index of contractility, acceleration index, ejection ratio, and systolic time ratio.

This technique is promising because continuous real-time hemodynamic data can be obtained noninvasively at no risk to the patient. Changes in fluid content also induce changes in thoracic capacitive and inductive properties; thus bioimpedance is limited in some clinical settings such as sepsis, intracardiac shunts, cardiac dysrhythmias, and hypertension because of inherently low signal-to-noise ratio. Preclinical and clinical data demonstrate the feasibility of using transthoracic electric signals to perform noninvasive CCO monitoring that closely correlates with TDCO.

An endotracheally sourced impedance cardiography-based CO monitor (ECOM, ConMed Corporation) increases accuracy of SV measurement by placing the monitoring electrodes on an endotracheal tube, resulting in close proximity to the ascending aorta. Once the ECOM endotracheal tube is placed, two cables connect the endotracheal tube and arterial catheter transducer to the ECOM monitor. The system reports CO, CI, SV, and SVR. Although ECOM may show poor correlation with measurements obtained with the gold standard, TDCO, as well as other transesophageal echocardiographic monitoring, the method does provide clinically acceptable trending of CO, and it retains potential utility for monitoring changes in whole body perfusion of critically ill patients.

## Periodic Noninvasive Measurement of Cardiac Performance

*Transthoracic echocardiography.* Transthoracic echocardiography (TTE) provides a noninvasive method of obtaining periodic data on cardiac performance. The use of Doppler color-flow mapping with two-dimensional and M-mode echocardiography allows assessment of global ventricular function, including left ventricular volume, EF, fractional shortening, and circumferential fiber shortening. Additionally, echocardiography can be used to describe intracardiac blood flow and the origin of intracardiac shunts, diagnose pathologic lesions in and around the heart, evaluate regional wall motion and its relationship to coronary artery insufficiency, and suggest the possibility of rejection in the infant with a transplanted heart. Although echocardiography does not provide continuous assessment of cardiac function, the portability of the current machines allows quality studies to be performed at the patient's bedside in the ICU or ED. However, bandages, obesity, inability to turn or maintain a desired position, and air trapping (as occurs in patients with emphysema) may make it difficult to obtain an adequate study using transthoracic imaging. This technique has been shown to accurately predict fluid responsiveness in critically ill patients because it measures the dynamic markers of preload that affect SV or CO.

Real-time three-dimensional echocardiography, unlike two-dimensional echocardiography, can measure SV without inaccurate geometric assumptions, and it has a close correlation with TDCO under the same hemodynamic conditions.

When a quality image cannot be obtained using a chest transducer, transesophageal imaging can be performed. Esophageal imaging provides especially good images of the chambers and the mitral valve because the transducer is positioned immediately behind the left ventricle or left atrium.

Although TTE has the potential of becoming a valuable method for rapid assessment of CO, especially in the emergency setting, further studies are still warranted. Given the currently moderate level of evidence, the use of TTE should be restricted to well-defined clinical studies until more evidence has emerged.

*Radionuclide cardiac imaging.* Radionuclide cardiac imaging techniques can be used to provide periodic information about cardiac performance. Thallium-201 can be injected, and myocardial perfusion scanning can be done with a gamma camera or single-photon emission computed tomography. Areas of decreased perfusion or scars pick up reduced amounts of thallium, creating "cold" spots on the image. Radionuclide angiography can be done by two techniques: first-pass method and gated blood pool (multiple-gated acquisition) technique. Technetium-99m is the radioisotope injected in both cases. The images obtained permit visualization of wall motion and calculation of EF.

*Blood pressure.* Obtaining CO measurements noninvasively during routine blood pressure recording can improve management of hypertension. A method that estimates CO using pulse waveform analysis from a brachial cuff sphygmomanometer that correlates well with CO values derived by Doppler ultrasound during dobutamine stimulation has been developed.

*Pulse pressure* (the difference between the systolic and diastolic arterial pressure) can be used as a rough estimate of stroke index (1 mm Hg = 1 mL/m$^2$) because SV is the major determinant of pulse pressure. This estimate does not take into account the effects of peripheral vascular resistance on CO but may be useful for trending when perfusion parameters are changing rapidly and no other methods are available for measuring CO.

Elevation of the lower limbs or passive leg raising induces an autotransfusion hemodynamically equivalent to an exogenous fluid challenge. For this reason, changes in CO and pulse pressure in response to passive leg raising are considered good predictors of fluid responsiveness, even in patients receiving positive-pressure ventilation.

*Finger arterial pressure waveform.* Two technologies currently are used to provide cardiac performance data noninvasively by measurement of a finger arterial pressure waveform: (1) the Finometer (Finapres Medical Systems) and the (2) Nexfin monitor (BMEYE).

The Finometer measures arterial pressure using a finger cuff and an inflatable bladder in combination with an infrared plethysmograph. As with a pulse oximeter, the infrared light is absorbed by the blood, and the arterial pulsations are measured by a light detector. To correct for distortions in finger pressure relative to brachial artery pressure, electronic filtering and computer reconstruction techniques are applied. Then a proprietary algorithm (Modelflow) is used to model aortic flow from the reconstructed brachial artery waveform. Although the technology appears to provide useful beat-to-beat information on arterial pressure trends, marked variability in pressure and flow (CO) accuracy limits its utility in the critical care setting.

The Nexfin monitor also employs analysis of the blood pressure waveform produced by a finger cuff to measure blood pressure, HR, SV, and CO. Because of its ease of use, this method may be best suited for clinical areas where blood pressure measurement is necessary but blood sampling is not. Although this method has demonstrated a good correlation with thermodilution measurements of CO during and after cardiac surgery, it was determined to be less reliable than invasive blood pressure monitoring. Although an invasively derived calibration is still needed to obtain absolute data on CO, relative changes in CO can be accurately monitored using this method.

*Partial CO2 rebreathing.* Partial $CO_2$ rebreathing is a method of CO monitoring based on a modification of the Fick principle. This "indirect Fick" method uses the Fick method applied to $CO_2$ produced by the body and eliminated through gas exchange by the lungs. The equation for differential Fick partial rebreathing $CO_2$ is as follows:

$$CO = \frac{(V_{CO_2}N - V_{CO_2}R)}{(Ca_{CO_2}R - Ca_{CO_2}N)} = \frac{\Delta V_{CO_2}}{\Delta Ca_{CO_2}} = \frac{\Delta V_{CO_2}}{S\Delta etco_2}$$

where $V_{CO_2}N$ and $V_{CO_2}R$ are the arterial $CO_2$ concentrations during normal and rebreathing periods, respectively; $\Delta V_{CO_2}$ and $\Delta Ca_{CO_2}$ represent the changes in $CO_2$ and arterial content of $CO_2$ ($Ca_{CO_2}$) between normal and rebreathing periods, respectively; changes in arterial $CO_2$ concentration are reflected in end-tidal $CO_2$ ($etco_2$) value; and S represents the $CO_2$ dissociation curve.

The use of noninvasive methods, although attractive, has to be validated against the gold standard thermodilution method. A review of the literature related to the accuracy and precision invasive methods (transthoracic electric bioimpedance, pulse contour, esophageal Doppler, and partial $CO_2$ rebreathing) found that they did not achieve agreement with bolus thermodilution in patients during surgery and in the critical care setting. The correlations between these methods and the thermodilution were 0.79, 0.75, 0.69, and 0.57, respectively.

The literature further indicates that pulse wave analysis may be used reliably as an alternative to the PA catheter in a variety of clinical settings. The use of transesophageal echography and Doppler monitoring is limited because it requires high operator dependency; the partial $CO_2$ rebreathing technique should be applied in a precisely defined clinical setting to mechanically ventilated patients only; and pulsed dye densitometry and the bioimpedance technique are currently primarily applied in an investigational setting. Although minimally invasive and noninvasive CO monitoring may replace measures obtained from the PA catheter in some settings, the traditional invasive approach may still be recommended for CO measurement when PA pressure monitoring is needed.

## KEY POINTS

- The amount of blood pumped out of the left ventricle in 1 minute is known as CO. It is the product of HR and SV, which is the volume of blood ejected by the ventricle by a single heartbeat.
- CI is CO divided by BSA and is reported as liters per minute per square meter ($L/min/m^2$) so that comparisons can be made among patients of different heights and weights.
- Cardiac work is a measurement of the energy the heart uses to eject blood against the aortic or pulmonary pressures (resistance) and increases as the end-diastolic ventricular size increases. Cardiac work correlates well with the oxygen requirements of the heart.
- End-diastolic ventricular size can be assessed by the EDV, defined as the amount of blood in the ventricle at the end of filling (diastole). The most common indirect method of measuring the end-diastolic ventricular size is the measurement of the EDP.
- EF represents the percentage of the EDV ejected with each beat. Normal EF is 65% to 70%.
- The performance ability of the heart (CO) is determined by both HR and SV. SV is determined by three factors: preload, afterload, and contractility.
- Preload is the stretch on the ventricular muscle fibers before contraction. Preload is created by the end-diastolic volume.

- The filling pressure for the right side of the heart is right atrial pressure, commonly measured as CVP.
- The filling pressure for the left side of the heart is left atrial pressure, commonly measured as PAWP.
- Afterload, the resistance or sum of the external factors that oppose ventricular ejection, has two components: tension in the ventricular wall and peripheral resistance (sometimes called *impedance*).
- Contractility is a measure of myocardial contraction strength.
- Inotropic drugs are medications that affect the force or energy of muscular contraction, typically by increasing cellular levels of calcium. A drug with a positive inotropic effect increases the strength of contraction but also may increase myocardial oxygen consumption as cells are stimulated to work beyond their metabolic capacity.
- Drugs with a negative inotropic effect decrease the strength of contraction but may also decrease the myocardial oxygen demand.
- The ideal characteristics for CO monitoring techniques are accuracy, reproducibility or precision, fast response time, operator independence, ease of use, noninvasive access, continuous use, cost-effectiveness, and no increased mortality and morbidity.

- Despite the introduction of various less invasive concepts of CO measurement, pulmonary artery thermodilution is still considered the gold standard technique for measuring CO.
- APC analysis is an indirect method to assess CO. CO is computed from a pressure pulsation on the basis of a criterion or model.
- Continuous intravenous Doppler ultrasound CO measurements are obtained through a transducer mounted on the distal section of a PA catheter and positioned in the main pulmonary artery proximal to the bifurcation.

- Echocardiography provides a noninvasive method of obtaining periodic data on cardiac performance. Near-continuous invasive measurement of cardiac performance can be provided by a special thermodilution PA catheter that heats the blood, by arterial line pulse contour analysis, or Doppler ultrasound using an esophageal, tracheal, or PA transducer.
- True noninvasive methods for assessing cardiac performance include transthoracic electrical bioimpedance, transthoracic echocardiography, finger arterial pressure waveform analysis, and partial $CO_2$ rebreathing.

## ASSESSMENT QUESTIONS

1. Given a stroke volume of 62 mL and an HR of 88 beats/min, what is the CO?
   a. 5.5 L/min
   b. 6.2 L/min
   c. 7.0 L/min
   d. 11.0 L/min
2. What is the normal range for CO in an adult?
   a. 2 to 4 L/min
   b. 4 to 8 L/min
   c. 6 to 10 L/min
   d. 10 to 13 L/min
3. A 75-year-old man is admitted to the ICU after aortic valve surgery. A pulmonary artery catheter yields the following data: central venous pressure (CVP): 5 mm Hg; cardiac output (CO): 4.0 L/min; mean arterial pressure (MAP): 80 mm Hg; mean pulmonary artery pressure (MPAP): 26 mm Hg; pulmonary artery wedge pressure (PAWP): 10 mm Hg; and heart rate (HR): 80 beats/min. Calculate the patient's pulmonary vascular resistance (PVR):
   a. 40 dynes-s/cm$^5$
   b. 320 dynes-s/cm$^5$
   c. 160 dynes-s/cm$^5$
   d. 220 dynes-s/cm$^5$
4. What happens to CO in the presence of sympathetic nervous stimulation?
   a. Increases significantly
   b. Decreases significantly
   c. Remains unchanged
   d. Decreases by only 20%
5. Which of the following statements are true regarding the distribution of blood flow and venous return?
   1. 60% to 70% of the total blood volume is in the venous system
   2. Blood is shunted to vital organs during cardiac failure
   3. Circulatory function and pressures can be maintained with a loss of 20% of the blood volume
   4. 50% of the total blood volume is in the venous system
   a. 1, 2, and 3
   b. 2 and 3
   c. 1 and 2
   d. 2, 3, and 4

6. What is the normal range for CI?
   a. 0.2 to 1.3 L/min/m$^2$
   b. 1.5 to 2.6 L/min/m$^2$
   c. 2.5 to 4.0 L/min/m$^2$
   d. 4 to 8 L/min/m$^2$
7. Which of the following correlates best with the oxygen requirements of the heart?
   a. SV
   b. EF
   c. EDV
   d. Cardiac work
8. What is the normal range for ejection fraction?
   a. 25% to 40%
   b. 40% to 55%
   c. 65% to 75%
   d. 75% to 85%
9. The amount of precontraction stretch applied to the ventricles is called:
   a. Preload
   b. Afterload
   c. Contractility
   d. EF
10. Preload of the left ventricle is assessed by which of the following parameters?
   a. Arterial diastolic blood pressure
   b. MAP
   c. CVP
   d. PAWP
11. Which of the following conditions would cause a reduction in ventricular preload?
   a. Decreased ventricular compliance
   b. Increased venous return
   c. Cardiac tamponade
   d. Hypovolemia
12. Which of the following are possible hemodynamic effects of using mechanical ventilation?
   1. Reduced preload
   2. Reduced CO
   3. Increased PVR
   4. Increased preload
   a. 1, 2, and 3
   b. 2, 3, and 4
   c. 1 and 2
   d. 3 and 4

13. Which of the following conditions would increase left ventricular afterload?
    a. Pulmonic valve stenosis
    b. Decreased blood viscosity
    c. Positive end-expiratory pressure
    d. Systemic hypertension

14. Which of the following is most closely related to systemic vascular resistance?
    a. Right ventricular afterload
    b. Left ventricular afterload
    c. CO
    d. Left ventricular preload

15. Which of the following abnormalities would increase PVR?
    1. Hypoxemia
    2. Acidosis
    3. Pulmonary emboli
    4. Hypervolemia
        a. 1, 3, and 4
        b. 1, 2, and 3
        c. 2 and 4
        d. 1, 2, 3, and 4

16. Which of the following is TRUE regarding cardiac contractility?
    a. It cannot be measured directly
    b. It is increased by β-blocking drugs
    c. It is increased by hypercapnia
    d. It is increased by parasympathetic neural stimulation

17. Which of the following invasive CO techniques requires the measurement of inhaled and exhaled gas concentrations?
    a. Thermodilution
    b. Fick
    c. Pulse contour
    d. Transtracheal Doppler

18. Which of the following techniques can provide beat-by-beat measurement of stroke volume and cardiac output?
    a. Thermodilution
    b. Fick
    c. Pulse contour
    d. NM3

19. Which of the following are noninvasive techniques for determining cardiac performance?
    1. Echocardiography
    2. Transthoracic electrical bioimpedance
    3. Partial $CO_2$ rebreathing
    4. Thermodilution
        a. 1, 2, and 3
        b. 1, 2, and 4
        c. 2, 3, and 4
        d. 2 and 4

## BIBLIOGRAPHY

Broch O, Renner J, Gruenewald M, et al. A comparison of the nexfin and transcardiopulmonary thermodilution to estimate cardiac output during coronary artery surgery. *Anaesthesia.* 2012;67:377–383.

Cecconi M, Dawson D, Casaretti R, et al. A prospective study of the accuracy and precision of continuous cardiac output monitoring devices as compared to intermittent thermodilution. *Minerva Anestesiol.* 2010;76:1010–1017.

Cecconi M, Parsons AK, Rhodes A. What is a fluid challenge? *Curr Opin Crit Care.* 2011;17:290–295.

Chew MS, Aneman A. Haemodynamic monitoring using arterial waveform analysis. *Curr Opin Crit Care.* 2013;19:234–241.

Critchley LA, Lee A, Ho AM. A critical review of the ability of continuous cardiac output monitors to measure trends in cardiac output. *Anesth Analg.* 2010;111:1180–1192.

Davey R, Raina A. Hemodynamic monitoring in heart failure and pulmonary hypertension: from analog tracings to the digital age. *World J Transplant.* 2016;24:542–547.

Geerts BF, Aarts LP, Jansen JR. Methods in pharmacology: measurement of cardiac output. *Br J Clin Pharmacol.* 2011;71:316–330.

Hathaway R. The Swan-Ganz catheter: a review. *Nurs Clin North Am.* 1978;13:389–407.

Hattori K, Maeda T, Masubichi T, et al. Accuracy and trending ability of the fourth-generation FloTrac/Vigileo system in patients with low cardiac index. *J Cardiothorac Vasc Anesth.* 2016. epub ahead of print.

Mandeville JC, Colebourn CL. Can transthoracic echocardiography be used to predict fluid responsiveness in the critically ill patient? A systematic review. *Crit Care Res Pract.* 2012;2012:513480.

Marik PE. Noninvasive cardiac output monitors: a state-of the-art review. *J Cardiothor Vasc Anesth.* 2013;27:121–134.

Maus TM, Reber B, Banks DA, et al. Cardiac output determination from endotracheally measured impedance cardiography: clinical evaluation of endotracheal cardiac output monitor. *J Cardiothorac Vasc Anesth.* 2011;25:770–775.

Middleton PM, Davies SR. Noninvasive hemodynamic monitoring in the emergency department. *Curr Opin Crit Care.* 2011;17:342–350.

Møller-Sørensen H, Hansen KL, Ostergaard M, et al. Lack of agreement and trending ability of the endotracheal cardiac output monitor compared with thermodilution. *Acta Anaesthesiol Scand.* 2012;56:433–440.

Nusmeier A, van der Hoeven JG, Lemson J. Cardiac output monitoring in pediatric patients. *Expert Rev Med Devices.* 2010;7:503–517.

Peyton PJ. Continuous minimally invasive peri-operative monitoring of cardiac output by pulmonary capnotracking: comparison with thermodilution and transesophageal echocardiography. *J Clin Monit Comput.* 2012;26:121–132.

Phan TD, Kluger R, Wan C. Minimally invasive cardiac output monitoring: agreement of oesophageal Doppler, LiDCOrapid™ and Vigileo FloTrac™ monitors in non-cardiac surgery. *Anaesth Intensive Care.* 2016;44:382–390.

Proulx F, Lemson J, Choker G, et al. Hemodynamic monitoring by transpulmonary thermodilution and pulse contour analysis in critically ill children. *Pediatr Crit Care Med.* 2011;12:459–466.

Pugsley J, Lerner AB. Cardiac output monitoring: is there a gold standard and how do the newer technologies compare? *Semin Cardiothorac Vasc Anesth.* 2010;14:274–282.

Reuter DA, Huang C, Edrich T, et al. Cardiac output monitoring using indicator-dilution techniques: basics, limits, and perspectives. *Anesth Analg.* 2010;110:799–811.

Sangkum L, Liu GL, Yu L, et al. Minimally invasive or noninvasive cardiac output: an update. *J Anesth.* 2016;30:461–480.

Wagner JY, Grond J, Fortin J, et al. Continuous noninvasive cardiac output determination using the CNAP system: evaluation of a cardiac output algorithm for the analysis of volume clamp method–derived pulse contour. *J Clin Monit Comput.* 2016;30:487–493.

Wernly B, Lichtenauer M, Franz M, et al. Pulse contour cardiac output monitoring in acute heart failure patients: assessment of hemodynamic measurements. *Wien Klin Wochenstr.* 2016. epub ahead of print.

Wetthersley M, Sorensen H, Johansen RR, et al. Systematic review of cardiac output measurements by echocardiography vs. thermodilution: the techniques are not interchangeable. *Intensive Care Med.* 2016;42:1223–1233.

# 17

# Bronchoscopy

*Zaza Cohen*

## LEARNING OBJECTIVES

*After reading this chapter, you will be able to:*

1. Define the basic terms used with endoscopy.
2. Describe the characteristics and capabilities of the flexible bronchoscope.
3. Identify common indications for bronchoscopy.
4. Distinguish diagnostic and therapeutic indications for bronchoscopy.
5. Explain the uses of bronchoalveolar lavage, brushings (both sterile and nonsterile), and forceps and needle biopsies.
6. Discuss the major concepts of interventional bronchoscopy.
7. Discuss the complications of flexible bronchoscopy and the relative risks involved in the procedure.
8. Identify the contraindications to performing a bronchoscopy.
9. List the essential equipment needed to perform a bronchoscopy safely.
10. Review the role of the respiratory therapist in bronchoscopy.
11. Discuss step-by-step preparation of the patient and the equipment for the bronchoscopy.

## OUTLINE

## KEY TERMS

bronchoalveolar lavage (BAL)
bronchoscope
bronchoscopy
electromagnetic navigation
    bronchoscopy (ENB)

endoscopy
fiberoptic bronchoscope
fluoroscopy
informed consent
interventional bronchoscopy

moderate sedation
transbronchial biopsy (TBB)

---

The word **endoscopy** (from the Greek words *endo,* meaning "inside," and *skopeo,* "to examine") describes examination of the internal organs by means of a special instrument, such as an endoscope. Endoscopy is a somewhat general term that includes procedures, such as *laryngoscopy,* examination of the larynx; **bronchoscopy,** examination of the bronchi; *gastroscopy,* examination of the stomach; and *colonoscopy,* examination of the colon, among many others. Gustav Killian, widely regarded as the "father" of bronchoscopy, was the first person to visualize the bronchial tree through a

hollow tube (**bronchoscope**) inserted in the patient's larynx in 1897. Two major advances of the 20th century in the field of bronchoscopy were the addition of the suction channel by Chevalier Jackson and the use of fiberoptics for the light source by Shigeto Ikeda. The first application of flexible fiberoptics to the field of endoscopy was in 1957 and was initially applied to gastroscopy. As experience grew and the techniques improved, it was applied to the other disciplines within the field of endoscopy. In the 1960s Shigeto Ikeda of Japan designed the first **fiberoptic bronchoscope,** which incorporated fiberoptics into a flexible tube suitable in size and length to enter the trachea and visualize the lower airway. The first bronchoscopy in the United States using flexible fiberoptic technique was done in the Mayo Clinic in 1969.

Today's bronchoscopes are much more advanced and sophisticated instruments with a light source at the tip and valves to allow general anesthesia, oxygenation, suctioning, and biopsy. The new rigid bronchoscopes remain useful for a few problems, such as removal of difficult foreign bodies and management of severe bleeding, but well over 90% of bronchoscopy procedures now are done with flexible fiberoptic bronchoscopes. Given that the emphasis of this text is on patient assessment and that rigid bronchoscopy is relatively infrequently performed, the focus of this chapter is on flexible fiberoptic bronchoscopy.

The flexible fiberoptic bronchoscope has greatly expanded the practice of pulmonary medicine by allowing inspection of the airways, removal of many different foreign bodies, and biopsy of airway and peripheral lung tissue. Most of these activities can be performed in the outpatient setting with moderate sedation, whereby the patient is sedated but is generally arousable.

In most institutions, flexible bronchoscopy is performed by a properly trained and licensed physician (usually a pulmonologist but sometimes a surgeon or a critical care physician) and one or two assistants, usually a respiratory therapist (RT) and a registered nurse (RN). For the remainder of this chapter, we refer to the physician performing the procedure as "the bronchoscopist" and the RN or the RT assisting as "the assistant." In many teaching institutions, students, medical residents, or other trainees may also be present and participate in various parts of the procedure under the supervision of a licensed health care provider. Sometimes a radiology technician is available to perform fluoroscopy (see the discussions on fluoroscopy later in this chapter and in Chapter 10), as well as a histology technician to evaluate the quality of the specimen from biopsy or brushings. RTs are educated and trained about flexible fiberoptic bronchoscopes because they often maintain the equipment and the materials needed for the procedure. The RT has become indispensable in helping the physician perform the procedure both in hospitals and outpatient clinics.

### SIMPLY STATED

Endoscopy is a field of medicine that uses instruments to look into different parts of the body to diagnose various diseases and explain certain conditions. Bronchoscopy is the process of visualizing the airways below the larynx with a bronchoscope.

## CHARACTERISTICS AND CAPABILITIES OF THE BRONCHOSCOPE

The bronchoscopes available today serve a wide range of applications, from small-diameter scopes used for viewing the airways of infants and children to large-diameter scopes

with suction channels used to remove thick secretions from patients on ventilators in the intensive care unit (ICU), to scopes that incorporate ultrasound equipment for better visualization of the structures. Many bronchoscopes are now digital. Light is produced in an external light source and carried into the airways through a fiberoptic bundle. A digital video camera on the end of the bronchoscope acquires the images of the lighted airways, and the real-time images are displayed on a large video monitor. This allows easier and more hygienic manipulation of the bronchoscope and allows both still photographs and video recordings of the procedure for documenting and teaching purposes.

The standard flexible bronchoscope has an external diameter of 5.3 mm and a total length of 605 mm (Fig. 17.1). It can pass easily down the trachea (first-order bronchus) and into the right or left main stem bronchus (second-order bronchi). From there, it can be advanced through most fourth- and one-third of all fifth-order bronchi (Fig. 17.2). Ultrathin

FIG. 17.1 Flexible fiberoptic bronchoscope. (Courtesy Olympus America, Inc., Melville, NY.)

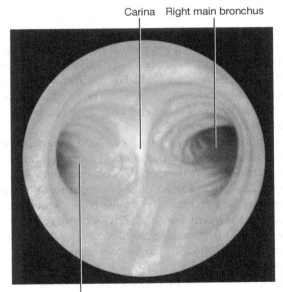

Carina    Right main bronchus

Left main bronchus

FIG. 17.2 Normal main carina showing left (L) and right (R) mainstem bronchi. (From Drake RL, Vogl RA, Mitchell A: *Gray's basic anatomy*, Philadelphia, 2012, Elsevier Health Sciences.)

scopes with a 2.7-mm external diameter and 0.8-mm biopsy channels will pass down 3.5-mm or larger endotracheal tubes, making it easier to study and perform biopsies on infants and children who are intubated. One must keep in mind that even with such depth of visualization, bronchoscopy still allows examination of only a small percentage of all airways. For comparison, colonoscopy allows the entire length of the colon to be examined during the procedure.

### SIMPLY STATED

The standard adult bronchoscope is an instrument about 60 cm long and 5 mm thick, with hand controls for directing the tip. There are two ports near the hand controls: one for suctioning and the other for inserting biopsy tools and flushing fluids or medications into distal airways.

The amount of tip angulation, which makes the scope directional, is crucial to the scope's utility and ability to visualize hard-to-reach but important airways. Most bronchoscope tips can bend from the axial plane at least 130 degrees in one direction and 160 degrees in the other. Bronchoscopes flex less with a brush, forceps, or needle in place, and all bronchoscopes lose flexibility at the tip over time and with use.

A light source is the foundation for fiberoptic bronchoscopy. Light sources range in size from 2-inch battery cases that attach to the head of the bronchoscope to large units that deliver light at varied intensities, in different wavelengths, in pulses for photography, or other special purposes.

In addition to visually inspecting the airways, various devices can be passed down the scope and greatly extend its use. The devices include biting and grasping forceps, brushes (shielded and unshielded), sheathed needles, baskets to remove foreign objects, and sampling catheters.

The biting forceps come in various types (biting cusps with smooth edges or serrated edges). Smooth-cusped flexible forceps can be used if the physician needs to obtain a piece of lung parenchyma during the procedure. If a large, dense (tough) lesion is seen in the larger airways, a serrated forceps capable of cutting tissue is preferred. Forceps are metallic, are easily visualized by radiographs, and can be directed to the desired area for biopsy of peripheral lung lesions using real-time radiography (fluoroscopy).

A hollow needle fixed to a long, small-lumen plastic tube can be passed down the scope to perform biopsy on lesions under the mucosa. Unlike the specimens obtained during forceps biopsy that contain a larger piece of actual tissue sample with preserved lung architecture, needle biopsy specimens usually contain a few cells. Positive yields (obtaining diagnostic tissue samples) from needle biopsies of the submucosal lesions are less than those for large cancers growing in the larger airways.

Unshielded brushes are used to harvest cells from tumor masses, located both centrally and in the periphery. The double-shielded sterile brush is used to gather microbiologically important material to diagnose infections in the lung. Because the bronchoscope is passed into the lung by way of the nose,

mouth, or artificial airway, the entire scope immediately becomes contaminated with the patient's upper-tract bacterial mix (normal flora) or the biofilm within the artificial airway. Thus unshielded sampling may misrepresent the specific infection-causing bacteria in the lung and result in a misdirected treatment plan. To prevent this, sterile double-shielded brushes are passed through the entire length of the scope until the bronchoscopist sees that the tip is well in view into the airway of concern. The inner sheath is then advanced, followed by the wire brush that comes out of the sterile inner sheath. The sampling is done by gently brushing the airway. The wire is then drawn back into its sheath and pulled from the bronchoscope. The wire tip is cut off with sterile scissors, placed in a sterile container with sterile normal saline, and sent for microbiologic studies.

During bronchoalveolar lavage (BAL), the bronchoscope is passed to the affected part of the lung, and the tip of the scope is positioned into a fourth-generation bronchus. A total of about 100 mL of normal saline is flushed through the scope's suction channel in four or five increments of 20 to 30 mL to distend the distal bronchioles and fill the alveoli, thereby washing out samples of any microorganisms or cells. The fluid is collected very carefully to avoid contamination from oral or upper airway secretions. In normal patients, the fluid is sterile and contains predominantly macrophages. A little more than half of the BAL fluid can usually be suctioned back into a collection chamber, and the rest is absorbed by the lymphatic system. The lavage is typically done for diagnostic purposes: to look for infection (smears and cultures), certain types of interstitial diseases (cell count and differential), or malignant cells (cytology). In rare situations, such as patients with pulmonary alveolar proteinosis and highly selected patients with severe asthma, the lavage can be done for therapeutic purposes.

### SIMPLY STATED

Because the mouth, nose, and artificial airways (through which a bronchoscope is passed) harbor bacteria, shielded brushes must be used to get uncontaminated material from the area of the lung where an infection is suspected. When the offending organism is identified, the appropriate antibiotic can be selected.

Patients accidentally inhale a remarkable variety of objects, including food, teeth (or other dental appliances), pills, hard candy, coins, beads, and toys. These objects, as well as mucous plugs or clots, can be retrieved with a bronchoscope. In some cases these items or conditions do not show up on the chest radiograph, and their discovery by bronchoscopy is based on the patient's history or is an unexpected discovery during an evaluation for chronic cough. Grasping forceps and snares can be used with the bronchoscope to retrieve foreign objects (Figs. 17.3 and 17.4) and come in various shapes and designs to accommodate the variety of aspirated objects.

Laser beams and other types of phototherapies, tissue coagulation, thermal manipulation (burning and freezing),

FIG. 17.3 Electrosurgical snare. (Courtesy Olympus America, Inc., Melville, NY.)

FIG. 17.4 Retrieval snare. (Courtesy Olympus America, Inc., Melville, NY.)

and various other types of tissue destruction have been used to remove the endobronchial tumors. Placement of airway stents allows the patency of airways that would otherwise collapse. Development of these and other advanced techniques in the past two decades of the 20th century led to the growth of a new discipline—interventional bronchoscopy—within the field of bronchoscopy. In a combined European Respiratory Society and American Thoracic Society (ERS/ATS) statement, interventional bronchoscopy was defined as "the art and science of medicine as related to the performance of diagnostic and invasive therapeutic procedures that require additional training and expertize beyond that required in a standard pulmonary medicine training program." The field of interventional bronchoscopy includes procedures such as autofluorescent bronchoscopy, endobronchial ultrasound (EBUS), laser bronchoscopy, endobronchial electrosurgery, electromagnetic navigation bronchoscopy (ENB), argon-plasma coagulation, bronchial thermoplasty, endobronchial cryotherapy, airway stent placement, endobronchial brachytherapy, photodynamic therapy, percutaneous tracheostomy placement, and endobronchial valve placement, and it is constantly expanding. A detailed description of these procedures is outside the scope of this chapter. A review of the aforementioned ERS/ATS statement is highly recommended for a better understanding of these procedures.

## BOX 17.1 Indications for Flexible Bronchoscopy

**Diagnostic**
- Radiographic finding suggestive of neoplasia
- Pneumonia
- Hemoptysis
- Persistent atelectasis
- Unexplained and persistent pleural effusion
- Unexplained and persistent paralysis of a hemidiaphragm
- Interstitial lung disease
- Unexplained hoarseness

**Therapeutic**
- Atelectasis (to remove mucous plugs and secretions)
- Removal of foreign bodies
- Tamponade of a bleeding source
- Advanced procedures (see section on interventional bronchoscopy)

**Miscellaneous**
- Difficult intubations
- Research

### SIMPLY STATED

The field of interventional bronchoscopy is rapidly expanding and permits many secondary therapeutic procedures to be performed during bronchoscopy.

## INDICATIONS FOR BRONCHOSCOPY

There are two basic categories of indications for flexible fiberoptic bronchoscopy: diagnostic and therapeutic (Box 17.1). The flexible fiberoptic bronchoscope is used most often for diagnostic purposes, with therapeutic indications being less common. The most common indication for flexible bronchoscopy is to diagnose the cause of an abnormality seen on a chest radiograph. These abnormalities include infiltrates of any size or location, atelectasis, or mass lesions. These lesions are of particular concern if they have appeared recently on the chest radiograph, or if the patient has risk factors for malignancy, such as history of previous cancer or history of smoking. Bronchoscopy may be indicated in the patient with a normal chest radiograph if the patient has symptoms of chronic cough, stridor, hoarseness, or history of choking.

### Nodules and Masses

Radiologists and pulmonologists often distinguish between pulmonary nodules and masses. An abnormal solid structure in the pulmonary parenchyma that is smaller than 3 cm on a chest radiograph or computed tomography (CT) scan is typically called a *nodule*. Structures larger than 3 cm are referred to as *masses*. Rounded small lesions are often called *coin lesions* because their shadows resemble coins. The malignant potential of these lesions depends on their size, location, shape, rate of growth, and the patient's history (smoking, weight loss, hemoptysis, history of cancer, or other risk factors for malignancy). Although most nodules and some masses turn out to be benign, a biopsy is often necessary for accurate diagnosis. The possibility of obtaining adequate tissue for diagnosis depends on the lesion size, its location (endobronchial or not, central vs. peripheral), and the expertise of the bronchoscopist.

Naturally, large lesions that are in the central airways are easy to find and excise for biopsy. However, coin lesions are often in the lung periphery and cannot be seen through a flexible bronchoscope. Fluoroscopy is used to aim the tip of the bronchoscope toward the lesion (see Chapter 10 on chest imaging for the utility and limitations of the fluoroscopy). Biopsy forceps can then be advanced into the appropriate subsegmental bronchus to reach the lesion and snip off pieces to be sent for analysis. New advanced bronchoscopy techniques such as ENB and EBUS increase the likelihood of obtaining adequate tissue sample. During ENB, the patient's lungs and the lesion are mapped out using conventional CT scan, and then the software guides the bronchoscope toward the lesion even when the lesion cannot be directly visualized. During EBUS, the ultrasound probe that is mounted on a special bronchoscope guides the biopsy needle into the submucosal lymph nodes that cannot otherwise be seen.

FIG. 17.5 Placement of a rigid bronchoscope in the trachea of an anesthetized patient. (From Stradling P: *Diagnostic bronchoscopy,* ed 6, New York, 1991, Churchill Livingstone.)

### SIMPLY STATED

The larger the lung tumor and the closer to the hilar area it is located, the easier it is to make a histologic diagnosis. If the cancer is outside an airway and in the periphery of the lung, it is less likely that flexible bronchoscopy will be able to get adequate tissue to make a diagnosis.

## Hemoptysis

Hemoptysis is commonly caused by infection of the lower respiratory tract, and milder cases frequently can be treated with antibiotics. Lung tumors can also cause moderate to severe hemoptysis. As a result, bronchoscopy is usually indicated for the evaluation of more severe cases of hemoptysis, particularly in patients with risk factors for lung cancer.

Usually, the patient with hemoptysis coughs up small amounts of blood and then stops. Occasionally, massive hemoptysis (>200 mL/24 hours) occurs, making intervention more urgent. Large-bore rigid bronchoscopes (Figs. 17.5 and 17.6) are often used in this setting because they allow more rapid removal of blood than do flexible fiberoptic bronchoscopes, but they generally require an operating room, which takes more preparation time than a flexible fiberoptic bronchoscopy performed at the bedside. Fiberoptic bronchoscopy also provides a more detailed and distal examination of the airways, making it a good alternative in most instances of hemoptysis. Sometimes, flexible bronchoscopy is performed at bedside urgently to localize the site of bleeding, without attempts to stop it. Once the site has been identified, the patient is then taken to a special suite in radiology, where a corresponding bronchial vessel is cannulated and then special material injected into it, leading to obstruction of the blood

FIG. 17.6 Lateral neck radiograph of a rigid bronchoscope in place. (From Stradling P: *Diagnostic bronchoscopy,* ed 6, New York, 1991, Churchill Livingstone.)

flow through the vessel (a procedure called *bronchial artery embolization*) in hope of stopping the bleeding.

## Pneumonia

Most patients with pneumonia do not require bronchoscopy. The diagnosis is usually made based on clinical information (history and physical examination), routine laboratory tests, and chest imaging. The treatment is often started empirically, without the knowledge of sputum or blood culture results. A more accurate microbiologic diagnosis—microorganism species and antibiotic sensitivity—may be necessary in certain situations, such as in a patient with persistent pneumonia, on mechanical ventilation, or with severe immunosuppression (human immunodeficiency virus infection or acquired immunodeficiency syndrome, chronic steroid use, organ transplantation, or cancer therapy). In such patients, BAL fluid and sometimes biopsy samples are obtained and sent to the laboratory for smears and cultures. If biopsy samples are obtained for culture purposes, the specimens must be placed in sterile saline solution, rather than formalin, to avoid suppression of bacterial growth by formalin.

For patients on ventilators who are receiving antibiotics, diagnosis of the organisms responsible for persistent and severe pneumonias is a serious issue. In these cases, the double-sheathed sterile brush is used to distinguish the pathogenic organism from organisms that have merely colonized the lower respiratory tract. It is assumed that some bacteria will grow from a respiratory sample of nearly every intubated patient, so the cultures are often done in a quantitative fashion, and a certain threshold of bacterial load must be reached for the cultures to be considered positive. This approach is the best available, but even with careful attention to technique, the results of sterile brushing directly into an infiltrate may not establish the identity of the offending pathogen. Biopsies are typically not performed while the patient is on a ventilator because positive-pressure ventilation increases the risk for pneumothorax.

## Interstitial Lung Diseases

*Interstitial lung disease* is a loosely defined term that encompasses about 200 clinical syndromes and diagnoses. Many of these diseases affect not only the lung interstitium but also the parenchyma, the airways, and the pleural space, leading to a certain degree of confusion. In addition, many other diseases that do not affect the interstitial space give a pattern of infiltrates on a chest radiograph that is often described as "interstitial infiltrates," leading to further confusion. Flexible bronchoscopy has a limited role in the evaluation of patients with interstitial lung disease or the interstitial pattern of infiltrates. With the exception of sarcoidosis, some cancers, and most infections, fiberoptic bronchoscopy provides insufficient material to make a definitive diagnosis of interstitial lung disease. The lavage analysis for cell count and differential is often nonspecific (Table 17.1). Transbronchial biopsy (TBB), or biopsy done with use of a bronchoscope, often gives a poor diagnostic specimen for one or more of several reasons, including the small amount of tissue sample often obtained, sampling error (excising an area with minimal involvement), or crushing artifact (distortion of the lung architecture from the shearing forces of the biopsy forceps). This usually creates a dilemma for the patient care team regarding whether to perform a bronchoscopy first (easy, safe, outpatient procedure but less likely to lead to a definitive diagnosis) or an open lung biopsy, which requires general anesthesia, opening the chest in an operating room, and allowing postoperative time in the hospital. Ultimately, the decision is based on a balance between the risks and the likelihood that

### TABLE 17.1   Interstitial Lung Diseases and Fiberoptic Bronchoscopy

| Disease | Technique | Findings |
|---|---|---|
| Sarcoidosis | TBB | Noncaseating granulomas |
|  | BAL | Altered T-lymphocyte helper-to-suppressor ratio |
| Pulmonary alveolar proteinosis | TBB | PAS stain and alveolar exudates |
| Lymphangitic spread of cancer | TBB | Tumor cells in interstitial areas |
| Alveolar cell cancer | TBB | Tumor cells in alveolar space |
| Idiopathic interstitial fibrosis | BAL | Increased PMNs |
| Collagen vascular diseases | BAL | Increased PMNs |
| Pneumoconiosis | BAL | Increased PMNs |
| Bronchiolitis obliterans | BAL | Increased PMNs |
| Amiodarone toxicity | BAL | Lipid-laden macrophages |
| Goodpasture syndrome | BAL | Hemosiderin-laden macrophages |
| Eosinophilic pneumonia | BAL | High eosinophil concentration |
| Hypersensitivity pneumonitis | BAL | Altered T-lymphocyte helper-to-suppressor ratio |

*BAL,* Bronchoalveolar lavage; *PAS,* periodic acid–Schiff; *PMN,* polymorphonuclear cells (neutrophils); *TBB,* transbronchial biopsy.

the patient has sarcoidosis, cancer, or infection—diseases that can be reliably diagnosed by the specimens obtained during bronchoscopy.

### SIMPLY STATED

Interstitial lung diseases may require several methods (transbronchial biopsy, bronchoalveolar lavage) to obtain diagnostic material through a flexible bronchoscope or an open lung biopsy.

## Foreign Bodies

As described earlier, various objects have been reported to have been aspirated and then retrieved from the airways. The bronchoscopy (rigid vs. flexible) method for retrieval often depends on the size of the object and the expertise of the bronchoscopist. If a large foreign body has been inhaled into the proximal airway, a large-bore rigid bronchoscope inserted during general anesthesia is most useful to remove the object. Sometimes the aspirated object is small and passes beyond the reach of a rigid scope. In these cases, the flexible fiberoptic bronchoscope is used. Regardless of the type of scope used, control of the airway is of the greatest concern. If the object is dislodged, it can move to a new location where obstruction of the airway can further endanger the patient.

## BOX 17.2   Complications of Flexible Bronchoscopy

1. Adverse effects of associated medications (e.g., lidocaine)
2. Hypoxemia
3. Hypercarbia
4. Bronchospasm
5. Hypotension
6. Laryngospasm, bradycardia, or other vagal responses
7. Mechanical complications such as epistaxis, pneumothorax, and hemoptysis
8. Increased airway resistance
9. Death
10. Cross-contamination of specimens or bronchoscopes
11. Nausea, vomiting, fever, and chills
12. Cardiac dysrhythmias

Adapted from AARC Clinical Practice Guidelines, bronchoscopy assisting—2007 revision and update, *Respir Care* 52:1, 2007.

## COMPLICATIONS OF BRONCHOSCOPY

Few complications are associated with fiberoptic bronchoscopy (Box 17.2). When they do occur, they are most often associated with transient hypoxemia or medications used in the procedure and not the procedure itself. The overall mortality rate from flexible bronchoscopy is less than 0.01%. A careful preprocedure history and physical will identify high-risk patients, and questions about previous bleeding problems to screen for clotting abnormalities will alert the bronchoscopist that biopsy may be risky.

Respiratory failure is more common in patients with advanced lung disease. There are typically multiple factors that lead to the development of respiratory failure in a given patient undergoing bronchoscopy.

Bleeding and pneumothorax are potentially serious complications associated with transbronchial biopsies. The risk for both problems can be reduced with careful attention to technique. In some studies, bronchial brushings were reported to cause rates of bleeding similar to those from TBB. Bilateral TBB is usually avoided because bilateral postprocedure pneumothorax could be life threatening.

Suction is frequently used to remove secretions, blood, or foreign material. Prolonged suctioning while performing bronchoscopy may significantly reduce the inspired oxygen, thereby creating a risk for intraoperative atelectasis and hypoxemia.

After bronchoscopy, patients may develop a transient low-grade fever. It occurs in about 5% of bronchoscopy patients, usually starting 6 to 8 hours after the procedure but lasting only 12 to 24 hours. The exact cause of the fever is unknown, but it is believed not to be a sign of a new infection. Similarly, small amounts of blood may be expectorated up to 24 hours after the procedure. This is considered an expected finding and does not require additional attention.

The longer the procedure duration, the greater is the risk for hypoxemia and hypercapnia. When these conditions occur, side effects of the anesthetic agents and arrhythmias become more likely.

## SIMPLY STATED

Flexible fiberoptic bronchoscopy is safe. Careful patient selection and attention to detail during and after the bronchoscopy make the risk-to-benefit ratio excellent for this procedure.

## PREPARATION

As previously described, bronchoscopies are typically performed by an experienced team consisting of the bronchoscopist (physician) and two assistants, often an RT and an RN; one monitors the patient's clinical status and records vital signs, and the other prepares the equipment and directly assists the bronchoscopist in performing the procedure. It is extremely important that the roles of each team member are clearly defined in advance and that all members of the team communicate clearly with one another before, during, and after the procedure. Appropriate preparation is crucial to the successful and efficient performance of the procedure.

### Personnel and Equipment Preparation

Bronchoscopy is an invasive procedure with hazards and side effects, so safety protocols for patients, as well as the health care workers, must be in place. Infection control protocols require that all personnel wear gowns, masks, goggles, and gloves. Additional protective equipment, such as lead aprons, may be necessary if fluoroscopy, which involves ionizing radiation, is performed. Another protocol commonly in place in many institutions is to take a preprocedure time-out to confirm that the right procedure is being performed on the right patient.

It is assumed that even patients with normal gas exchange before the procedure will require supplemental oxygen. The need for the oxygen comes from decreased alveolar ventilation due to anesthesia, loss of tidal volume due to suctioning, airway obstruction from the bronchoscope, additional airway edema from the mechanical trauma, local pulmonary edema after instillation of saline for the lavage, or a combination thereof. Almost all patients should receive supplemental oxygen during bronchoscopy. This is usually achieved by giving oxygen by nasal cannula at 2 to 6 L/min. Some patients will require higher flow that cannot be delivered by nasal cannula. In such situations, a small hole is cut out of the mask that is used for oxygen delivery to allow passage of the bronchoscope. Yet other patients will have such a degree of gas exchange compromise that the procedure may need to be performed in the ICU, or even after intubation, to ensure the availability of appropriate level of supportive care. The decision about the need for supplemental oxygen or the need for mechanical ventilation before bronchoscopy is often done in collaboration among the bronchoscopist, the RT, and other clinicians, including the patient's nurse. It is usually the RT's responsibility to have various oxygen delivery devices available and ready to use.

Suctioning through the bronchoscope is critical to keep the airway clear of mucus and blood and to help keep the bronchoscope lens clear. The suction is connected to a sterile

80-mL specimen trap, which must be secured so that it will not tip and thereby lose the sample from the patient's airway. Several of these traps are needed. Because the first one is usually contaminated with mouth flora, it is usually discarded, along with its contents. If heavy bleeding occurs during biopsy, the trap may become clogged with blood and thus inappropriate for cytologic analysis or cultures and may need to be discarded. A separate suction channel is set up for oropharyngeal suctioning to avoid cross-contamination with lower airway specimens.

Once the procedure starts, events occur at a fast pace so the assistant must have an organized working surface with easily accessible supplies. The exact list of supplies requested for bronchoscopy varies somewhat from hospital to hospital and bronchoscopist to bronchoscopist. Medications are placed in individual cups and are clearly labeled. A labeled syringe is placed with each labeled medication cup to match each medication. Commonly used materials include the following:

- Equipment to monitor vital signs and oxygen saturation
- Various oxygen delivery devices
- Artificial airways of various sizes and shapes
- Suction/specimen traps
- 2% topical lidocaine to be used if needed above the vocal cords
- 1% topical lidocaine to be used if needed below the vocal cords
- 0.9% sodium chloride (NaCl) for irrigation (a larger container may be necessary if BAL is needed)
- 1:20 solution of epinephrine (1 mL 1:1000 epinephrine diluted with 19 mL 0.9% NaCl)
- Syringes of various size, with the proper tip to adapt to the working channel of the bronchoscope
- Brushes, aspiration needles, and biopsy forceps of various sizes and shapes

It is important that when the syringes with lidocaine are handed to the bronchoscopist during the procedure, they contain a known amount of lidocaine, with plenty of air in the syringe barrel. This allows the bronchoscopist to push the lidocaine all the way down the approximately 2 feet of the scope's channel. Because it is possible to administer an overdose of lidocaine, having a small amount (1 to 2 mL) in each syringe helps limit the lidocaine given. It is impossible to know how much lidocaine the patient absorbs as a total dosage because suctioning during the procedure removes some of the lidocaine before it is absorbed. Nevertheless, it is important to keep the total dosage of instilled lidocaine below 300 mg. Seizures are the most common sign of acute lidocaine overdose.

## Patient Preparation

The patient preparation starts the night before so that when the patient arrives for the procedure, he or she has been fasting for a minimum of 6 hours. Taking essential medications with a small sip of water in the morning of the procedure is usually allowed. Before the procedure can be performed, an informed consent must be obtained from the patient (or a surrogate, such as close relative, if the patient is unable due to physical or mental disability). The patient must understand the reason for the bronchoscopy (diagnostic or therapeutic) and other alternatives available to obtain similar results. The patient also must understand the potential risks and complications of both the procedure and the anesthesia to be used, and be aware of what to expect after the procedure.

The patient is encouraged to ask questions about the bronchoscopy before signing the consent form. The bronchoscopist should already have explained the procedure in detail and should be available to answer any new questions. Risks and benefits are again discussed. Issues such as the patient's inability to speak during the procedure, the use of supplemental oxygen, and local anesthetic medicines are covered. The concept of intravenous (IV) moderate sedation is explained to the patient, and possible medication allergies are reviewed again. The effects and side effects of the anesthetic drugs must be explained. An adult must accompany the patient after the procedure because the sedative effects of the medications may linger long after the procedure. The patient is then informed of the process necessary for adequate preparation. It is explained to the patient that during the procedure the assistant will monitor and record the patient's vital signs.

After all issues are covered to the patient's satisfaction, the consent is signed and witnessed. It is important to steer clear of medical terminology and use simple language to avoid patient confusion.

It is also important that the assistant carefully review the chart to ensure that there is appropriate documentation for the procedure and that no contraindications exist (see Chapter 21). This involves ensuring that the informed consent has been properly signed, the time-out procedure has been completed, there is a valid physician's order, and there are no absolute contraindications.

### SIMPLY STATED

Patient preparation should include answering all the patient's questions. The RT usually has this responsibility and must understand all aspects of the procedure.

For the bronchoscopy to be successful, the patient will need moderate sedation with IV agents, as well as local anesthesia. There are numerous ways to achieve local anesthesia, and the chosen method for a given procedure usually depends on the clinician's experience and the patient's characteristics (e.g., anatomy, personal choices). The patient is usually positioned upright, and 10 to 20 mg of lidocaine is delivered topically to the nasopharynx and oropharynx. The delivery methods include instillation of liquid or viscous lidocaine, inhalation through nebulizer or atomizer, or combination thereof. Some bronchoscopists choose to administer recurrent laryngeal nerve block, which involves injection of 1 to 2 mg of lidocaine in the area of the recurrent laryngeal nerve bilaterally. Throughout the administration of the local anesthesia, it is common to track progress and repeat the steps until the desired level of anesthesia is achieved.

The final stage of preparation is to administer IV moderate sedation. Moderate sedation is a state of consciousness that may be described as a "twilight sleep," whereby the patient may be aroused if necessary through stimulation or by administering a chemical agent to reverse the effects of sedation. Commonly, a combination of a sedative benzodiazepine such as midazolam (Versed) and an opioid narcotic such as fentanyl is used. Although midazolam relaxes the patient and eases him or her to sleep, fentanyl provides pain control as well as cough suppression. These drugs are chosen for their quick on-and-off action. Benzodiazepines are good amnestic agents also, so even when the patient is uncomfortable during the procedure, he or she often does not remember it afterward. Some bronchoscopists also give codeine to further suppress the cough and atropine to decrease the secretions about 30 minutes before the procedure. As soon as the patient relaxes and appears to be asleep, and all preparation is done, the bronchoscopy can begin.

## PROCEDURE

For spontaneously breathing patients, the bronchoscope is passed through the nares. This allows for more stable scope position and less likelihood of the patient biting and damaging the optical fibers. In some patients, the nasopharynx is too small for the bronchoscope, or previous trauma or surgery does not allow the scope to be passed. In this case, an oral airway or "bite block" is inserted into the mouth and the bronchoscope advanced through it. Special types of "bite blocks" are used for orally intubated patients to prevent the patient from biting through the airways and the bronchoscope.

Once the bronchoscope passes through the pharynx (nasopharynx, oropharynx, or artificial airway, as the case may be), the epiglottis and then the vocal cords come into view. A small amount of lidocaine is injected to numb the cords and allow easy passage of the bronchoscope through them. Sometimes, especially in patients with suspected cancer, the bronchoscopist will ask the patient to say "eeeee" to see the vocal cords adduct (close). Patients with cancer infiltrating the recurrent laryngeal nerve may be unable to fully adduct their vocal cords.

Once the cords have been anesthetized, the patient is asked to take deep breaths. This will allow a full abduction (opening) of the vocal cords and passage of the bronchoscopy through them. It is common for the cough reflex to close the vocal cords and not allow the advancement of the scope.

Once in the trachea, the scope is advanced firmly to avoid being bounced back by the strong cough. Nearly all spontaneously breathing patients will start coughing at this point, requiring large, sometimes repeated doses of local or IV anesthetic.

Once the main stem bronchi are identified and examined, the plan of action is devised. If the disease is unilateral, the normal side is examined first to avoid cross-contamination (e.g., infection, tumor material). In general, the extent and the order of the procedures performed will vary depending on the nature and etiology of the disease being evaluated during bronchoscopy.

## SPECIMEN COLLECTION AND PROCESSING

Some pathologists prefer cytology specimens fixed on slides. There should be four sets of frosted slides placed back to back and labeled legibly with the patient's name, medical record number, physician number (if applicable), and date. Two slide bottles with 90% alcohol and one biopsy specimen bottle containing 10% formalin should be available. Other pathologists prefer cytology specimens preserved in Saccomanno solution.

An 80-mL mucus specimen trap is placed in-line between the suction source and the bronchoscope. Standard biopsy forceps, a brush holder loaded with a disposable wire brush, and an aspiration needle accompanied by a 10-mL syringe filled with 5 mL 0.9% NaCl should be available, depending on the specimens the bronchoscopist needs to collect.

To obtain a lung brushing, the bronchoscopist gently brushes the abnormal-appearing area and then withdraws the brush from the scope. The assistant rubs the brush lightly on the frosted side of a slide, making a smear about the size of a dime. This slide is then placed in the slide bottle containing 90% alcohol (or the brush is agitated in the Saccomanno solution). This procedure should take no longer than 10 seconds.

Lung biopsy specimens are placed into a labeled specimen bottle filled with formalin. Usually, four to six samples are obtained. Formalin is an airway irritant, so if any amount of it ends up on the forceps, it is usually removed by rinsing the forceps in saline. It is often necessary for the assistant to tease the small piece of tissue out of the biopsy cusps with a needle. Some bronchoscopists prefer to "evaluate" the quality of biopsy specimens by visually inspecting the specimens in formalin and observing whether they float. Although commonly practiced, the clinical value and accuracy of such evaluation are hard to ascertain.

Obtaining a needle aspiration sample requires the bronchoscopist to place two or three drops of specimen on the frosted side of a slide (or into Saccomanno solution). The assistant then places a second slide, frosted side down, on top of the original slide containing the specimen and slowly slides it across this slide. Both slides should be placed into a slide bottle containing 90% alcohol. This procedure is repeated with each new specimen collected.

BAL is performed with repeated instillations of 20 to 30 mL of preservative-free 0.9% NaCl. The instillations are followed by suctioning into an 80-mL mucus specimen trap. It is usually sent for smears and cultures (e.g., routine, acid-fast bacilli, fungal) when infection is suspected, cell count and differential when interstitial lung disease is suspected, or cytology when malignancy is suspected. The sample is usually split into different cups (all need to be appropriately labeled) to be sent to the different parts of the laboratory. Contamination should be avoided, especially for the sample sent to the microbiology laboratory.

### SIMPLY STATED

After patient safety, collection of samples and their careful management is the most important job of the RT or other clinician assisting with the procedure.

## POSTPROCEDURE CONSIDERATIONS

On completion of the bronchoscopy, the patient is monitored closely while recovering. Vital signs, including blood pressure, heart rate, respiratory rate, and $SpO_2$, are monitored and recorded by the RT or RN every 5 to 15 minutes. The bronchoscopist must be notified of significant changes in any of these parameters. It is essential to recognize signs of increased discomfort, bleeding, or respiratory distress. The IV site should be examined periodically for signs of infiltration or blockage until its discontinuation.

Once the patient is alert and oriented, usually within an hour of the procedure's completion, the patient is given a small sip of water to see whether the gag reflex and sensation in the throat have returned to normal. If these parameters are normal, the IV is removed, and a final set of vital signs is obtained. The following criteria should be met before discharge:

- The patient is alert and oriented.
- Gag reflex is present.
- Sensation in the throat has returned to normal.
- Vital signs are stable.
- No significant bleeding is present.

At this time, the bronchoscopist can explain the findings to the patient and patient's family and tell the patient that he or she might cough up small amounts of blood or develop mild fever for up to 24 hours after the procedure. Larger amounts of blood, sudden shortness of breath, pain, or high-grade fever should prompt a call to seek medical attention. Arrangements are made for a return visit in 5 to 7 days to review the findings from the patient's specimens and to make recommendations.

The patient can then be liberated from all monitors and assisted in dressing. A wheelchair should be available to transport the patient out to his or her attendant. It is imperative to remind the patient not to drive for several hours. The patient and attendant are also informed that if any unusual bleeding, shortness of breath, fever, or pain occurs, they are to seek medical attention immediately.

All specimens must be handled appropriately for transport to the laboratory. Biopsies, brushings, needle aspirations, and lung washings should be labeled with the patient's name, medical record number, ordering physician name, date, and site of origin. Necessary pathology or laboratory slips should also contain similar data, including what tests should be performed.

Finally, any additional documentation should be completed, signed by the bronchoscopist, and filed in the patient's medical record. The bronchoscopist must also make his or her own notes of the entire procedure, including indications, medications given, specimens collected, tests requested on the specimens, any intraoperative complications, and postoperative impression.

## OUTPATIENT VERSUS INPATIENT BRONCHOSCOPY

With the increasing demand for more cost-effective ways to render care, the outpatient clinic has been shown to be a safe and inexpensive site for routine flexible bronchoscopy.

The outpatient bronchoscopy room should be equipped with adequate suction capability; electrocardiographic, arterial oxygen saturation ($SpO_2$), and blood pressure monitoring; an oxygen source; a bag-valve-mask system; and a code/crash cart with defibrillator and appropriate drugs, in the event that cardiopulmonary resuscitation is needed. Specifically, naloxone and flumazenil (direct antagonists to opiates and benzodiazepines, respectively) should be immediately available.

A complete history and physical examination are performed to assess the patient and the appropriateness of the bronchoscopy. Box 17.3 lists contraindications to performing the bronchoscopy in the outpatient setting.

In many hospitalized patients, especially the ones in the ICU, bronchoscopy may be performed via an artificial airway such as an endotracheal (ET) or a tracheostomy tube. Although many of the steps described earlier apply to both spontaneously breathing outpatients and those in the hospital with artificial airways on mechanical ventilation, there are several modifications to remember. In intubated patients, the procedure is often done at the bedside because they are

### BOX 17.3   Contraindications for Outpatient Flexible Bronchoscopy

- Recent myocardial infarction
- Lack of patient cooperation
- Unstable severe asthma
- Severe hypoxemia and/or severe hypercapnia
- Bleeding disorders
- Potentially lethal cardiac arrhythmias
- Lung abscess
- Renal failure
- Immunosuppression
- Obstruction of the superior vena cava

often too unstable to travel to the endoscopy suite. A special adaptor is placed between the ET tube and the ventilator circuit to allow passage of the bronchoscope without interrupting ventilation, and a bite block is placed in the patient's mouth to prevent biting down on the bronchoscope. Special consideration must be given to the size of the ET tube in relation to the size of the bronchoscope. Most standard bronchoscopes can easily pass through the size 8.0 ET tube. A smaller bronchoscope will need to be used in a patient with smaller ET tubes. Using an inappropriately large bronchoscope may be dangerous not only for the obvious reason of being wedged inside the tube but also by obstructing a large percentage of the airway lumen and making mechanical ventilation difficult. Once the right-sized bronchoscope is chosen for a given ET tube, it can be advanced through the artificial airway and into the trachea without much difficulty. In addition, many patients (especially those in the ICU) may already be adequately sedated for the purposes of the bronchoscopy.

### SIMPLY STATED

There are specific contraindications to performing flexible bronchoscopy in the outpatient setting as opposed to the hospital. Because there is less support in an outpatient clinic if complications occur, these guidelines must be applied carefully to patient selection to ensure patient safety.

## ROLE OF THE RESPIRATORY THERAPIST

As suggested previously, it is common for the RT to be involved in assisting the physician with many aspects of the preparation, performance, and postprocedure considerations associated with bronchoscopy. These may include reviewing the medical record for proper documentation, preparing the equipment, assisting with the procedure, and monitoring the patient's clinical status before, during, and after the procedure (Fig. 17.7). Table 17.2 summarizes the common functions of the RT before, during, and after the bronchoscopy.

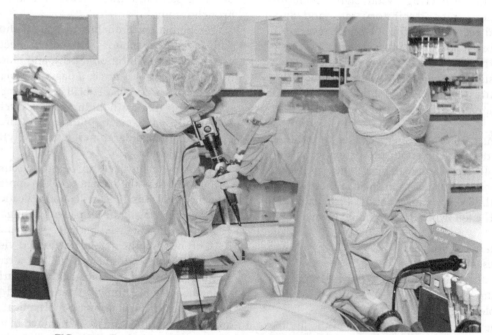

**FIG. 17.7** Typical outpatient setup for performing flexible bronchoscopy.

| TABLE 17.2    Respiratory Therapist's Role When Assisting with Bronchoscopy | |
|---|---|
| **Therapist's Function** | **Purpose** |
| **Before the Procedure** | |
| Help identify potential need for a bronchoscopy | Determine which patients may benefit from the procedure |
| Review chart to confirm the following: physician order, signed consent form, no contraindications | Confirm physician's order, that the patient has consented to it and that it is not contraindicated, and any special considerations |
| Prepare/ensure proper function of equipment, including bronchoscope, light source, monitor, video recorder, medications, specimen traps | Minimize unnecessary delay and likelihood of patient harm from procedure |
| Prepare patient, providing patient education and premedication | Minimize untoward delays and ensure patient's well-being |
| Ensure time-out to confirm correct patient and procedure | Minimize patient harm and medical errors |

**TABLE 17.2   Respiratory Therapist's Role When Assisting with Bronchoscopy—cont'd**

| Therapist's Function | Purpose |
|---|---|
| **During the Procedure** | |
| Ensure proper functioning of all equipment (bronchoscope, light source, TV monitor) needed during procedure | Minimize unnecessary delay from equipment failure |
| Assist physician in obtaining specimens; help with medication preparation | Minimize unnecessary delay and likelihood of patient harm from procedure |
| Monitor patient vital signs and overall clinical status; respond to adverse reactions | Minimize patient harm from adverse reactions |
| **After the Procedure** | |
| Monitor patient's vital signs and clinical status | Ensure the patient has tolerated procedure and detect adverse reactions |
| Ensure specimens are properly labeled and sent to laboratory | Help obtain accurate diagnosis and treatment |
| Clean, disinfect/sterilize equipment, and ensure it is properly stored | Minimize nosocomial infection risk and potential damage to equipment |
| Record results in chart and other pertinent records | Maintain medical and legal record of procedure and patient response |

## KEY POINTS

- Rigid bronchoscopes allow good access to large airways and allow ventilation during the procedure. However, rigid bronchoscopy requires general anesthesia for patient comfort.
- Today, flexible fiberoptic bronchoscopes allow better access to small airways and are comfortable enough that only light to moderate sedation is needed. The patient can breathe spontaneously during the procedure.
- The standard flexible bronchoscope has an external diameter of 5.3 mm and a total length of 605 mm.
- The flexible fiberoptic bronchoscope has greatly expanded the practice of pulmonary medicine, allowing inspection of the airways, removal of many different foreign bodies, and biopsy of airway and peripheral lung tissue.
- The most common indication for flexible bronchoscopy is to diagnose the cause of an abnormality seen on a chest radiograph. These abnormalities include infiltrates of any size or location, atelectasis, masses or lesions.
- The flexible fiberoptic bronchoscope can be used to reach to the periphery of the lung and remove a small piece of lung biopsy for submission to the pathologist. In certain clinical scenarios, this is helpful in the diagnosis of interstitial lung disease.
- If a large foreign body has been inhaled into the airway, a large-bore rigid bronchoscope inserted during general anesthesia is most useful to remove the object.
- Sometimes the aspirated object is small and passes beyond the reach of a rigid scope. In these cases, the flexible fiberoptic bronchoscope is used.
- Few complications are associated with fiberoptic bronchoscopy. When they do occur, they are most often associated with medications used in the procedure, not the procedure itself.
- Bleeding, pneumothorax, and respiratory failure are the potential major complications associated with bronchoscopy, especially when tissue biopsy is performed.
- RTs commonly provide technical support for bronchoscopy procedures.
- RT activities include setting up the bronchoscopy suite, providing medications for the physician, operating biopsy forceps, collecting specimens and preparing them for presentation to the pathologist, cleaning the bronchoscope and biopsy equipment, and preparing the suite for the next procedure.

## ASSESSMENT QUESTIONS

1. In most patients, the standard adult bronchoscope can visualize to a maximum of what depth in the airways?
   a. Third-level bronchi
   b. Fourth-level bronchi
   c. Fifth-level bronchi
   d. Sixth-level bronchi
2. Double-sided brushes are used during bronchoscopy to:
   a. Clean the fiberoptics
   b. Obtain microbiologic samples
   c. Assist in cleaning the smaller airways of mucous plugs
   d. Assist in diagnosing malignancies
3. The purpose of using lasers during bronchoscopy is to:
   a. Obliterate obstructing tumors
   b. Stop excessive bleeding
   c. Open mucous-plugged airways
   d. Improve visualization of smaller airways
4. The most common indication for the use of a bronchoscope is:
   a. To retrieve inhaled foreign objects
   b. To obtain microbiologic samples
   c. To help diagnose abnormalities seen on chest radiograph
   d. To treat hemoptysis

5. The rigid bronchoscope most likely is used for:
   a. Pneumonia
   b. Massive hemoptysis
   c. Tumors
   d. Interstitial lung disease
6. The most common complication associated with bronchoscopy is:
   a. Side effects of the medications used in the procedure
   b. Pneumothorax
   c. Secondary infection
   d. Excessive bleeding
7. Use of excessive suctioning during bronchoscopy is discouraged because:
   a. It removes mucus that has a protective role
   b. It may cause atelectasis and hypoxia
   c. It requires additional sedation
   d. It may lead to arrhythmias

8. In addition to lidocaine and normal saline, the most commonly used medication to be delivered into the airways during bronchoscopy is:
   a. Acetylcysteine (Mucomyst)
   b. Epinephrine
   c. Sterile water
   d. Midazolam (Versed)
9. The most common sign of lidocaine overdose during bronchoscopy is:
   a. Tachycardia
   b. Bradycardia
   c. Seizures
   d. Apnea
10. It is safe to discharge a postbronchoscopy patient with the following finding:
    a. Poor gag reflex
    b. Sputum with small flecks of blood
    c. Respiratory distress
    d. Confusion and disorientation

# BIBLIOGRAPHY

Bolliger CT, Mathur PN, Beamis JF, et al. ERS/ATS statement on interventional pulmonology. *Eur Respir J*. 2002;19:356.

Du Rand IA, Blaikley J, Booton R, et al. British Thoracic Society guideline for diagnostic flexible bronchoscopy in adults. *Thorax*. 2013;68(suppl 1):i1.

Kacmarek RM, Stoller JK, Heuer AJ. *Egan's fundamentals of respiratory care*. 11th ed. St. Louis: Mosby-Elsevier; 2017.

Meyer KC, Raghu G, Baughman RP, et al. An official American Thoracic Society clinical practice guideline: the clinical utility of bronchoalveolar lavage cellular analysis in interstitial lung disease. *Respir Crit Care Med*. 2012;185:1004.

Özdilek A, Beyoglu CA, Esquinas AM. Fibreoptic bronchoscopy in patients with acute respiratory distress syndrome. *Anesthesia*. 2016;71:729.

Silvestri GA, Feller-Kopman D, Chen A, et al. Latest advances in advanced diagnostic and therapeutic pulmonary procedures. *Chest*. 2012;142:1636.

Various Authors: Best of ATS video lectures. Series on bronchoscopy. Available at https://www.thoracic.org/professionals/clinical-resources/video-lecture-series/procedures/.

# 18

# Nutrition Assessment

*Jane E. Ziegler and Janet Reid-Hector*

## LEARNING OBJECTIVES

*After reading this chapter, you will be able to:*

1. Recognize how nutrition and respiration and pulmonary status are interrelated.
2. Recognize the functional importance of oxygen in nutrition.
3. Identify the nutritional significance of measuring oxygen uptake.
4. Identify the value of determining the resting energy expenditure.
5. Recognize how starvation affects the following:
   a. Body weight
   b. Muscle mass (diaphragm and other respiratory musculature)
   c. Forced vital capacity, forced expiratory volume in 1 second, and diffusing capacity of the lung for carbon dioxide
   d. Surfactant production
6. Recognize how some respiratory treatment modalities may inhibit the nutritional status of patients.
7. Identify the byproducts of anaerobic (without oxygen) metabolism.
8. Identify oxygen's importance in terms of adenosine triphosphate production.
9. Recognize how fat, carbohydrate, and protein metabolism affect the respiratory quotient.
10. Recognize the daily nutritional requirements for carbohydrate, protein, and fat.
11. Identify the protein requirements for normal and severely catabolic patients.
12. Recognize the significance of measuring nitrogen balance.
13. Recognize the problems associated with a low-protein diet.
14. Recognize the advantages and disadvantages of a high-carbohydrate diet in regard to the pulmonary system.
15. Identify the importance of vitamins and minerals in respiratory function.
16. Recognize the methods available for meeting nutritional requirements and their advantages and disadvantages.
17. Recognize the methods for assessing nutritional status.
18. Identify the role of the respiratory therapist in nutritional assessment in relation to inspection, auscultation, and laboratory and pulmonary function findings.

## OUTLINE

## KEY TERMS

adenosine triphosphate (ATP)
anabolism
anemia
basal energy expenditure (BEE)
basal metabolic rate (BMR)
body mass index (BMI)
cachectic
catabolism
creatine phosphate
creatinine
creatinine-height index (CHI)
diet-induced thermogenesis

direct calorimetry
gluconeogenesis
glycolysis
ideal body weight
indirect calorimetry
kilocalories
lactic acid
metabolic cart
metabolism
nitric oxide
nitrogen balance
oncotic pressure

oxygen uptake
parenteral
parenteral nutrition (PN)
phytochemicals
protein-energy malnutrition
  (PEM)
respiratory quotient (RQ)
resting energy expenditure (REE)
serum albumin
serum transferrin
skinfold measurement

The pulmonary system has a synergistic relationship with nutrition throughout life, beginning with the fetus and extending through adulthood. Although nutritional status and pulmonary function are interdependent, a healthy pulmonary system supports the body through its ability to obtain oxygen needed for cellular demands of the metabolism of the three macronutrients: carbohydrates, proteins, and lipids. Provision of adequate nutrition to maintain optimal nutritional status assists in ensuring growth, as well as development and maintenance of the pulmonary system, including its supporting structures. The skeletal and respiratory muscles, as well as the nervous system and immune system, are supported and maintained through optimal nutrition. A person's nutritional status and ability to metabolize carbohydrates, proteins, and fats is directly related to a healthy pulmonary system.

Pulmonary dysfunction or changes in pulmonary status can occur throughout life, beginning with the premature infant with bronchopulmonary dysplasia, to the child with asthma or the adolescent with an eating disorder, to adulthood and the elderly. Pulmonary disorders with significant nutrition concerns include asthma, cystic fibrosis, bronchopulmonary dysplasia, chronic obstructive pulmonary disease (COPD), and emphysema, as well as acute respiratory distress syndrome. The nutritional needs and nutritional status of patients with pulmonary disease have emerged as major factors influencing acute and long-term patient outcomes. The major function of the pulmonary system is gas exchange, with the lungs providing oxygen for cellular metabolic demands and allowing for removal of carbon dioxide from these metabolic processes. Lungs also assist in the regulation of acid-base balance, synthesize surfactant and arachidonic acid, and convert angiotensin I to angiotensin II.

Breathing provides the oxygen necessary for metabolism of nutrients to meet the energy needs of individuals. Nutrition affects the efficiency of the metabolic processes and influences the amount of oxygen needed and the amount of carbon dioxide exhaled. Nutrition influences the immune defense mechanisms, thereby affecting the patient's susceptibility to infection and ability to deal with physiologic stress. Understanding the role of and need for nutrition in maintaining normal respiratory function and in treating pulmonary disease is important for today's respiratory therapist (RT).

## MALNUTRITION AND THE PULMONARY SYSTEM

Malnutrition adversely affects the structure, elasticity, and function of the lungs, as well as the mass, strength, and endurance of muscles involved in the respiration process. Malnutrition-altered lung function includes decreased strength, power, and endurance of respiratory muscles and increased respiratory muscle fatigue. In addition, skeletal muscle relaxation slows, and muscle mass is diminished due to specific reduction in muscle fiber size and type. During starvation or malnutrition, respiratory muscles and skeletal muscles are subject to catabolism, providing energy to the body at the expense of muscle mass. The resultant reduction in the mass of the diaphragm, diminished inspiratory and expiratory muscle strength, and decreased vital capacity and endurance result in impaired pulmonary function. Inadequate nutrition or an increase in energy needs due to disease process can result in malnutrition, leading to alterations in pulmonary muscle function.

Within days, protein deficits in the diet result in a decline in respiratory muscle function. Low levels of proteins in the blood (hypoalbuminemia) contribute to pulmonary edema as colloid osmotic pressure is decreased, allowing a fluid shift into the interstitial space. Extravascular lung water, the amount of water contained in the lungs outside the pulmonary vasculature, increases, resulting in a decrease in functional residual capacity and pulmonary reserve. Low serum albumin levels can result in an increase in extracellular fluid volume and a reduction in the intracellular space. Surfactant provides the low surface tension at the air-liquid interface, preventing the atelectasis, alveolar collapse, alveolar flooding, and severe hypoxia that result in respiratory distress. Even short periods of starvation result in a decreased synthesis and secretion of surfactant. A reduction of surfactant, which is synthesized from proteins and phospholipids, contributes to the collapse of alveoli, resulting in an increased effort of breathing. Also, airway mucus is composed of glycoproteins, water, and electrolytes. Malnutrition results in depletion of liver and muscle glycogen and energy-rich compounds used to provide cellular energy, resulting in metabolic and muscular endurance dysfunction. This reduction in respiratory muscle function often coexists with increased energy requirements, resulting in a deterioration of gas exchange and an increased work of breathing, which can lead to pulmonary failure.

Micronutrients consist of vitamins and minerals. Micronutrient imbalances and deficiencies can affect pulmonary function in several ways. Iron deficiency can result in low hemoglobin levels, thus reducing the oxygen-carrying capacity of the blood. Low levels of other micronutrients, such as potassium, phosphorus, calcium, and magnesium, affect cellular processes. Collagen, composing the supporting connective tissue of the lungs, requires vitamin C for synthesis. Low levels of phosphorus result in neuromuscular dysfunction and can exacerbate pulmonary failure. A reduction in 2,3-diphosphoglycerate (2,3-DPG) in the red blood cells due to reduced phosphorus levels decreases oxygen delivery to tissues and decreases the contractibility of respiratory muscles. Muscle strength is reduced in the presence of magnesium deficiency. Deficiencies in vitamin A, pyridoxine, and zinc may impair immune status and increase risk for pulmonary infections. Antioxidant nutrients, including vitamins A, C, and E and flavonoids, have been reviewed for their relationship to the pathogenesis or exacerbations in patients with COPD. Reduced serum or tissue levels of antioxidant vitamins were found in people with COPD; however, other studies did not show significant effects. Malnutrition has been found to be an independent predictor of higher morbidity and mortality in respiratory disease.

## EFFECT OF PULMONARY DISEASE ON NUTRITIONAL STATUS

Diseases of the pulmonary system can increase energy requirements. In addition, complications and treatment of pulmonary disease affect the ability to ingest and digest adequate food and affect the circulation, cellular use, storage, and excretion of most nutrients. The increased work of breathing, chronic infection, and medical treatments used to treat pulmonary diseases, such as chest physical therapy and some medications, increase energy requirements. Medications such as bronchodilators, steroids, and antibiotics used to treat disease may have other nutritional implications and need to be considered in the nutritional evaluation and intervention. Patients with pulmonary disease usually present with a reduced nutritional intake attributed to fluid restrictions, gastrointestinal discomfort, vomiting, anorexia, shortness of breath, and decreased oxygen saturation when eating. A reduced ability to prepare foods because of fatigue and shortness of breath, impaired feeding skills, altered metabolism, and financial limitations all result in additional difficulties

in achieving adequate nutritional intake. Also, some diseases, such as cystic fibrosis, affect not only the lungs but also the pancreas, resulting in inadequate production of certain enzymes necessary in the digestion of proteins, carbohydrates, and particularly fats. This puts patients with cystic fibrosis at risk for malnutrition, unless certain dietary supplements and pancreatic enzymes are taken to compensate.

## INTERDEPENDENCE OF RESPIRATION AND NUTRITION

Respiration and nutrition are interdependent (Fig. 18.1). Air and food share common pathways during ingestion and then separate only briefly during "digestion," with air going to the lungs for distribution and food to the stomach and intestinal tract for digestion and absorption. Oxygen and nutrients then combine in the blood and are distributed to the tissues of the body. The use of food for energy at the cellular level requires oxygen to support a controlled combustion process that produces energy

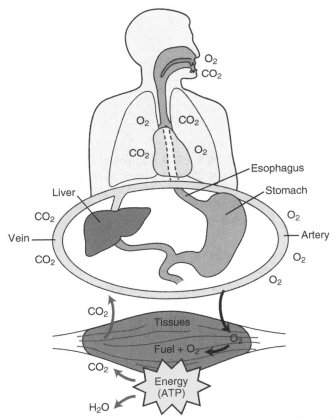

FIG. 18.1 Nutrition and breathing are interrelated. Air and food share common pathways of entry during ingestion and then separate only briefly during "digestion," with air going to the lungs for distribution and food to the stomach and intestinal tract for digestion and absorption. Oxygen and nutrients then combine in the blood and are distributed to the tissues of the body. The use of food for energy at the cellular level requires oxygen to support a controlled combustion process that produces energy molecules of adenosine triphosphate (ATP), which is used in all of the body processes for energy, carbon dioxide, and water.

**FIG. 18.2** Functions of adenosine triphosphate (ATP) are as follows: muscle contraction and relaxation, active transport of substances across membranes, substrate for cyclic adenosine monophosphate, energy for synthesis of various chemical compounds, and energy storage.

**FIG. 18.3** Block diagram illustrating components of the respiratory system. The neurologic component drives and controls respiration at the lungs by the respiratory muscles. It also affects the cardiovascular system by altering heart function and circulatory resistance. All components are necessary to achieve respiration. Nutritional quality and quantity directly affect the functioning of each system.

molecules of adenosine triphosphate (ATP), which are used in all of the body processes for energy (Fig. 18.2).

Body heat is a result of a combustion process called metabolism. Metabolism requires fuel in the form of food. For combustion to occur, oxygen must be present, provided through the process of breathing. Unless oxygen is delivered to the cells, the food eaten cannot be used. Nutrition and respiration are truly interdependent because breathing and oxygenation are considered part of the process of providing nutrition to the body's tissues.

Titrating the proper amount of oxygen and eliminating carbon dioxide (the metabolic "smoke" of the combustion process) is the job of the respiratory system, coupled closely with the cardiovascular system. The respiratory system must be sensitive to the metabolic needs of the entire body. This process requires the integration of several organ systems. The respiratory system consists of neurologic components, cardiovascular components, respiratory muscles, and lungs (Fig. 18.3).

The metabolic rates of the tissues dictate the amount of oxygen needing to be picked up in the lungs. Oxygen uptake ($\dot{V}O_2$) is a respiratory factor that can be measured in the laboratory

or at the bedside using specialized equipment. Nutritionally speaking, it is this measure that indicates the patient's energy requirement. If $\dot{V}O_2$ is measured while a person is in a resting, nonstressed state, the basal metabolic rate (BMR) or basal energy expenditure (BEE) can be calculated. The BEE is the measure obtained when a person is at absolute rest with no physical movement, which is not clinically possible in the hospitalized patient. The term resting energy expenditure (REE) is used when a person is at rest upon waking. REE is the measurement used in hospitalized patients and is about 10% higher than BEE because measurements are done when the patient is awake and at rest but not at basal conditions. A variety of predictive equations have been developed for use in estimating REE. For the purposes of predicting energy needs through predictive equations in nonobese critically ill patients when indirect calorimetry is not available, four equations were considered precise and unbiased in this population. In nonobese critically ill patients younger than 60 years and in those older than 60 years, respectively, the equations and their accuracy are as follows: Penn State equation (69%, 77%), Brandi equation (61%, 61%), Mifflin–St. Jeor equation × 1.25 (54%, 54%), and Faisy equation (65%, 37%). For obese critically ill patients the Penn State equation predicted resting metabolic rate (RMR) with 70% accuracy in obese patients. For a subset of obese critically ill patients ≥60 years old, the modified Penn State equation predicted RMR with 74% accuracy. All other predictive equations have lower accuracy rates among this population.

Because calculating the REE produces only an estimate, it is preferable to measure the actual metabolic rate by indirect calorimetry in order to know the patient's true energy needs. This eliminates some of the guesswork, especially when treating critically ill or metabolically challenged patients, and helps to prevent overfeeding or underfeeding.

Adequate nutrition support depends on the ability to determine a patient's energy needs. There are several ways to determine energy needs, including direct and indirect calorimetry and whole body potassium measurement. Total daily energy expenditure is usually divided into three components:

1. REE, which includes metabolic rate at rest while the patient is awake
2. Diet-induced thermogenesis
3. Energy cost of physical activity

Energy production generates heat, and heat is measured in calories. Direct calorimetry directly measures the heat given off by the body in a carefully designed room. This measurement is not practical in clinical settings and cannot be used with compromised patient populations. Indirect calorimetry is the method most commonly used in clinical environments. Indirect calorimetry is the calculation of energy expenditure using measured respiratory parameters of oxygen consumption ($\dot{V}O_2$) and carbon dioxide production ($\dot{V}CO_2$). $\dot{V}O_2$ and $\dot{V}CO_2$ require precise measurements of inspired and expired gas concentrations and volume. $\dot{V}O_2$ and $\dot{V}CO_2$ are converted to energy expenditure through the application of the abbreviated Weir equation:

$$\text{Energy expenditure (kcal)} = [(\dot{V}O_2 \text{ L/min})(3.941) + (\dot{V}CO_2 \text{ L/min})(1.11)]1440$$

where $\dot{V}O_2$ and $\dot{V}CO_2$ are expressed in liters per minute, and 1440 is the number of minutes in a day.

Because oxygen is not stored in the body, the measurement of oxygen uptake ($\dot{V}O_2$) correlates directly with energy (ATP) creation and use. Metabolism (REE) can then be measured by oxygen consumption and is directly related to the energy (calories) used. Indirect calorimetry may be clinically beneficial in the identification of patients who will not be able to sustain spontaneous ventilation because of excessive pulmonary work. The work of breathing is attributable to about 2% to 3% of the REE in the normal adult; however, in the pulmonary-compromised patient, as much as 25% of the REE can be attributed to the work of breathing. The respiratory quotient (RQ) ($\dot{V}CO_2/\dot{V}O_2$) is also obtained from indirect calorimetry, which is used in the interpretation of net substrate use and as an indicator of test validity. The normal RQ range in humans is 0.67 to 1.2. Because energy measurements by indirect calorimetry are respiratory measurements, the RT is one of the members of the patient care team who commonly performs these measures in clinical settings. The RT who is trained to perform indirect calorimetry measurements is an important contributor to the assessment of the nutritional needs of patients.

Indirect calorimetry measurements are usually performed using a metabolic cart, although different types of calorimeters exist. A metabolic cart is a computer-controlled unit composed of oxygen and carbon dioxide gas analyzers and flow transducers. The cart automatically measures patients' airflow and expiratory volumes, applies correction factors, and prints out and graphs the results. Different types of gas collection devices, such as a face mask, mouthpiece with nose clip, or canopy, can be used as long as rigorous control is used and no air leaks occur.

Having an understanding of this procedure will help the RT better understand what is automatically calculated by a metabolic cart. The following is a summary of the traditional energy measurement procedure:

1. Collect expired gas in a bag or Tissot spirometer for several minutes.
2. Analyze for carbon dioxide and oxygen (or oxygen and nitrogen).
3. Measure the volume of the gas collected in the bag.
4. Calculate:
   a. If oxygen and carbon dioxide are measured:

$$\dot{V}O_{2(STPD)} = \frac{\dot{V}_{E(ATPS)} \times (P_B - H_2O) \times 21.55}{\text{Collection time} \times (273 + \text{temp in } °C)}$$
$$\times \left[ \frac{1 - F_eO_2 - F_eCO_2 \left(\frac{PH_2O}{P_B}\right)}{1 - \frac{FIO_2}{FIO_2}} \right] - F_eO_2$$

$$\text{Note:} \frac{(273°K \times 60 \text{ sec})}{760 \text{ mm Hg}} = 21.55$$

If gas is analyzed with desiccant (a drying agent) in line, then

$$PH_2O/P_B = 0$$

where $\dot{V}O_{2(STPD)}$ = oxygen uptake, standard conditions
$\dot{V}_{E(ATPS)}$ = minute volume; ambient temperature and pressure, saturated
$P_B$ = barometric pressure
$F_eO_2$ = fraction of expired oxygen
$F_eCO_2$ = fraction of expired carbon dioxide
$PH_2O$ = water vapor pressure
$FIO_2$ = fraction of inspired oxygen
   b. $\dot{V}CO_2 = \dot{V}_E \times (F_eCO_2 - 0.0003)$

where $\dot{V}CO_2$ = carbon dioxide production
   c. $RQ = \dot{V}CO_2/\dot{V}O_2$

where RQ = respiratory quotient
   d. If only oxygen and nitrogen are measured,

$$\dot{V}O_2 = \dot{V}_E \times (F_eN_2/F_IN_2) \times F_IO_2 - \dot{V}_E \times F_eO_2$$

where $F_eN_2$ = fraction of expired nitrogen
$F_IN_2$ = fraction of inspired nitrogen

For patients confined to a hospital bed, portable equipment is used. For patients who are not intubated and whose condition does not allow them to cooperate with the procedure using a nose clip and mouthpiece, a special hood or canopy apparatus becomes necessary. The RT's interactions with the nutritional support team for metabolic measurements is most helpful because respiratory therapy departments are usually equipped and therapists are trained for such measurements.

In nutrition, energy is quantified in terms of kilocalories (kcal); 1 kcal is the amount of energy it takes to raise the temperature of 1 kg of water 1°C. (Although kilocalories have been used most frequently in clinical nutrition, the kilojoule [kJ] is often used in research because kJ is the international unit for energy. To convert kcal to kJ, multiply kcal by 4.184.) For approximately every 5 kcal burned, 1 L of oxygen is used by the tissues. Therefore if a patient's $\dot{V}O_2$ is measured as 300 mL of oxygen per minute, 300 mL of oxygen × 60 minutes × 24 hours equals 432 L of oxygen required per day and 5 kcal × 432 L of oxygen/day equals 2160 kcal/day that should be given to the patient. If less than this amount of energy is given, the patient must use body energy stores (glycogen, adipose tissue, and lean muscle mass), which are often already depleted in chronically ill patients. The abbreviated Weir equation is used for more precise conversion of $\dot{V}O_2$ to kilocalories, as follows:

$$kcal/min = \left(3.94 \times \dot{V}O_2 \; L/min\right) + \left(1.11 \times \dot{V}O_2 \; L/min\right)$$
$$Energy \; expenditure = kcal/min \times 1440 \; min \; (per \; day)$$

## Nutritional Depletion and Respiration

A patient who is not ingesting food enterally (through the gastrointestinal tract) probably will be placed on intravenous (IV) therapy. An IV solution of 5% dextrose running at 3 L/day will provide the patient with only 600 kcal/day (0.05 × 3000 mL × 3.41 kcal/g of glucose). (Note: glucose, when given in hydrated form [IV $D_5$/W and so on], yields 3.41 kcal/g; otherwise the yield is about 4 kcal/g of carbohydrate.) This is far from what is needed to meet a person's energy needs and does not include requirements for protein, essential fatty acids, vitamins, and minerals.

Blood glucose levels are maintained from liver glycogen (carbohydrate) stores between meals and during fasting. The liver's glycogen stores come from the carbohydrates (starches and sugars) that are eaten in the diet and converted to glucose and stored as glycogen. However, liver glycogen will be depleted within 12 to 16 hours unless sufficient carbohydrate is provided again. When the liver glycogen is depleted, the body obtains sugar (glucose) by converting protein (amino acids) to sugar (glucose). This process is called gluconeogenesis (gluco, meaning "glucose sugar"; neo, meaning "new"; and genesis, meaning "to create"). The protein used for gluconeogenesis is obtained from functional proteins (muscles, serum proteins and enzyme systems) because protein is never stored like fat in the body. Protein in the body is always a part of structural or functional tissue, organ, enzyme, or other biochemical action molecule or is in an "amino acid pool" in circulation while waiting to be incorporated into body systems. Therefore in patients who have a consistently inadequate nutritional intake, protein, instead of serving a functional role, must be used for more and more of the body's

energy needs. This leads to a loss of functional tissue. Skeletal muscle tissues, including the diaphragm and other respiratory muscles, lose muscle mass, with a resultant decrease in endurance and strength. In malnourished states, respiratory muscle strength can diminish, producing a decrease in forced vital capacity (FVC) and forced expiratory volume in 1 second ($FEV_1$) because the muscles of respiration, as well as other skeletal muscles, are being catabolized for energy. In malnutrition, a decrease in carbon monoxide diffusing capacity ($D_{LCO}$) also occurs, which reflects a diminished gas exchange capacity of the lungs. The decline in $FEV_1$ also correlates with a decreased creatinine-height index (CHI), indicative of loss of muscle mass. Because immune antibodies are composed of proteins, persistent inadequate calorie and protein intake will also compromise the immune system, thereby limiting the body's ability to fight pneumonia or other infections.

If the calorie intake is less than needed, there will be a decrease in weight, as is commonly seen in patients with COPD. Patients with emphysema are more commonly underweight, appearing thin and often cachectic (nutritionally depleted) compared with those with chronic bronchitis, who may be of normal weight and often are overweight. Emphysema produces a catabolic state that usually results in weight loss and mild hypoxemia. Nutritional depletion is evidenced by low body weight or body mass index (BMI) and a reduced triceps skinfold thickness measurement. Lean body mass may be decreased, although weight may be stable. BMI alone may not be indicative of a patient's nutritional status, and body composition measurement is preferred in this population to detect alterations in body compartments. Body composition can help differentiate lean body mass from adipose tissue and overhydration from dehydration because changes in hydration status can hide actual body wasting. In patients who retain fluids, it is important to carefully assess physical findings, anthropometric measurements, and biochemical measurements in light of fluid status.

Measures of REE are consistently higher in malnourished emphysematous patients; however, studies report that the total daily energy needs of individuals with COPD are highly variable. An increased REE leads to nutritional depletion and eventually malnutrition. Malnutrition can exacerbate symptoms of COPD by decreasing respiratory muscle strength and exercise tolerance and can compromise immune function, leading to increased respiratory infections. Energy expenditure is usually elevated related to pulmonary complications, including the degree of airway obstruction and resultant increased work of breathing. Respiratory inflammation, carbon dioxide retention, gas diffusing capacity, and other mediators, including hormones and cytokines, affect energy expenditure. In addition, insufficient absorption of some nutrients may lead to muscle wasting and malnutrition. Adequate protein intake is needed to maintain or restore lung and muscle strength in these patients. COPD presenting with chronic hypoxia and oxidative stress could be responsible for the catabolic state seen in these patients. Systemic inflammation, anorexia, and muscle dysfunction may all relate to the hypoxia. Correction of the hypoxia by oxygen supplementation seems to allow weight gain and in the short term improve exercise tolerance. This improvement is usually not sustained because the underlying metabolic increase is not reversed, and the patient's appetite is not improved.

---

**SIMPLY STATED**

Chronic nutritional depletion eventually weakens the muscles of breathing and can contribute to the onset of respiratory failure, especially in patients with chronic lung disease.

---

If an increased amount of food is consumed, weight can begin to normalize, but emphysematous patients are not comfortable eating larger quantities of foods. In one study, it was necessary to increase intake above 140% of the BMR before improvement of the nutritional status of COPD patients was achieved. In patients with COPD who have a low BMI (under 20 kg/m$^2$), unintentional weight loss, or reduced oral intake or who are at nutritional risk, provision of medical food supplements is suggested. Medical food supplementation for 7 to 12 days results in increased energy intake in this population.

If not continuously encouraged to do so, patients typically return to eating their normal amount, which is insufficient to maintain a normal weight. In addition, patients with malnutrition experience higher morbidity and mortality rates. With loss of body protein, there is a subsequent loss not only of muscle and various enzyme systems but also of immunoglobulins (IgA, IgG, and IgM). Thus susceptibility to respiratory infections is increased because of decreased immunocompetence.

### Therapeutic Interactions of Respiration and Nutrition

Nutritional repletion in respiratory patients is often compromised by some of the necessary therapeutic actions. Bronchodilators may produce nausea; oxygen by nasal cannula disturbs the sense of smell and therefore taste because olfaction plays a dominant role in the taste of foods. Medications the patients are taking may also interact with nutrients and render them less available for absorption or even inhibit specific metabolic enzymes. An intubated patient complicates the process of eating, requiring specialized feeding approaches. Furthermore, eating large meals expands the stomach, thereby limiting the movement of the diaphragm, the main muscle of respiration. Because of this, frequent small meals may be necessary, requiring greater effort in food preparation. These factors, along with shortness of breath, fatigue, increased work of breathing, and a greater prevalence of peptic ulcers, increase the risk for malnutrition. Being knowledgeable about these factors can help the patient to improve both nutritional status and respiratory function.

The respiratory response to the body's need for oxygen and carbon dioxide elimination is usually regulated by the carbon dioxide produced ($\dot{V}CO_2$). At the oxygen sensor level, increased hydrogen ion ($H^+$) concentration in addition to carbon dioxide drives ventilation; this occurs when the amount of oxygen present is insufficient with respect to metabolic need, resulting in lactic acidosis. Oxygen levels, when low enough, become an important stimulus for breathing. A malnourished state can decrease hypoxic drive, compromising a patient even further.

Oxygen uptake and carbon dioxide excretion are as much a part of nutrition as are eating and the elimination of food byproducts through the gastrointestinal tract and kidneys. Usually, respiration is not thought of in this way because of the abundance of air and the minimal effort involved in its continuous "ingestion" (breathing). However, patients with respiratory disease often find themselves needing higher levels of the "nutrient" oxygen or assistance in getting rid of the metabolic waste, carbon dioxide. Under these conditions, breathing becomes a more conscious and deliberate effort. In critical care patients, both feeding and breathing often require continuous assistance. Just as patients require intubation when the ventilatory status is compromised sufficiently, they may also require enteral feeding tubes or parenteral (into a vein) nutrition feeding. Matching a patient's energy and nutritional needs with ventilatory needs can become a challenge. Meeting this challenge is necessary to achieve better survival for the patient.

## RESPIRATORY SYSTEM AND NUTRITIONAL NEEDS

For optimal ventilatory function, proper nutrition is needed for all components of the respiratory system (see Fig. 18.3).

### Neurologic Component

The neurologic component drives and controls ventilation. The higher the $\dot{V}CO_2$ level, the greater the blood carbon dioxide concentration and therefore the greater the stimulus to the chemoreceptors. $\dot{V}CO_2$ is increased in the body by metabolism, buffering of fixed acids, or both. This in turn increases the electrical activity in the respiratory centers of the central nervous system (CNS), resulting in increased minute ventilation. The nervous system's fundamental requirement is for glucose. The energy derived from glucose is used to maintain an electrical charge across the nerve cell membrane, allowing for depolarization (action potential) and subsequent repolarization. The neurotransmitters at the synaptic ends are amino acids or derivatives of them, and their presence is necessary for the relay of information from one neuron to another and from nerve to muscle. Apparently, the sensitivity of the respiratory centers (either peripheral or central chemoreceptors) is affected by the amount and quality of protein ingested. The respiratory response to carbon dioxide or low levels of oxygen is improved with higher protein intake.

### Respiratory Muscle Component

The respiratory muscles make up the pump that drives the lungs. They receive the final stimulus from the CNS and produce the appropriate breathing rate and tidal volume as dictated by the CNS and local feedback pathways. The muscles require energy for contraction and relaxation. This energy is derived from blood glucose, free fatty acids from fat stores, muscle glycogen, and, at times, branched-chain amino acids.

The muscle glycogen stores are the most readily available source of energy for the muscles; however, the amount of glycogen stored depends on the level of carbohydrate in the diet as well as the exercise history of the muscle. A muscle that has been exercised has a greater ability to store glycogen (muscle carbohydrate) after a meal than when one eats without having exercised first. In any case, for the body to store muscle glycogen, there must be an adequate amount of carbohydrate in the diet. The diaphragm, being the main muscle of respiration, needs adequate glycogen stores to be able to meet the metabolic demand of breathing.

## Cardiovascular Component

The heart and the circulatory system are vital for pumping the blood through the lungs and throughout the body, carrying both nutrients and oxygen to all the tissues. The requirements of the cardiovascular system for food energy for the heart muscle are similar to those of the respiratory muscles.

### Protein

Protein is needed to maintain and build up the heart muscle and other structural components of tissue. Protein is also a part of buffering actions, clotting factors in the blood, and transport of lipids and iron. Oncotic pressure (a form of osmotic pressure that tends to pull water into the blood vessels from the tissue) in the blood is maintained primarily through albumin, the major blood protein produced by the liver. Arginine, one of the amino acids that make up proteins in the body, is the main contributor of nitrogen for the crucial vasodilating molecule nitric oxide (NO). NO plays the key role in relaxing the smooth muscles around the artery walls, resulting in vasodilation and thereby regulating blood flow throughout the body. NO is also involved in some end processes of the immune system. Arginine is found in highest concentrations in plant-based proteins.

### Carbohydrate

Carbohydrate is the major fuel for heart muscle. Carbohydrate metabolism is also the source of 2,3-DPG that facilitates oxygen release in the tissue. 2,3-DPG, synthesized by the red blood cells, is an important regulator for the affinity of hemoglobin for oxygen. Phosphorus is also a crucial nutrient in the synthesis of this compound. Blood sugar levels come primarily from dietary carbohydrate and release of stored liver glycogen between meals. Regulation of blood sugar (glucose) is key to normal metabolic function.

### Fat

Fat is an important component of all cell membranes and is a part of packaging of molecules that are produced by cells. Fat is also a source of fuel for heart muscle, especially when blood glucose levels or muscle glycogen runs low. Essential fatty acids are the backbone of prostaglandins and help regulate blood lipid levels, blood glucose levels, and blood pressure. The fat in nuts also appears to have antiarrhythmic properties and contains omega-3 fatty acids as found in flaxseed and fish oils. A diet that meets the adequate intake (AI) for omega-3 fatty acids should be consumed; however, there is not adequate evidence to support intakes of omega-3 fatty acids above the AI.

### Vitamins and Minerals

Vitamins and minerals are needed to maintain the metabolic pathways, integrity of cell membranes, and antioxidant activity of cells. They are major players in all body enzyme and metabolic systems. Iron is a major mineral that is a structural part of the heme of hemoglobin and is where oxygen attaches and is carried by the blood. Phosphate stores are commonly depleted in patients with COPD, and medications used in the treatment of COPD, such as corticosteroids, diuretics, and bronchodilators, are associated with phosphate depletion and may contribute to these low stores. Serum phosphate levels should be closely monitored. A diet that meets the recommended dietary allowances (RDA) for vitamin A, vitamin C, and vitamin E is recommended. Reduced serum or tissue levels of vitamin A, vitamin C, and vitamin E have been reported in individuals with COPD; however, evidence does not support intake above the RDA.

### Fluids

Water is the major constituent of the blood and body cells. Sufficient water intake is necessary for proper circulation, clearing of waste from the body, and maintenance of blood pressure. What is eaten or drunk has a vital effect on the cardiovascular system.

## Gas Exchange Component (Lungs)

The lungs, which introduce air from the atmosphere into the circulatory system, require a delicate balance of various systems to achieve efficient gas exchange. Alveolar ventilation must be matched with alveolar circulation to allow the efficient transfer of gases between blood and air. To prevent alveolar collapse, surfactant is needed to lessen the surface-active forces that promote collapse of the lung. Malnutrition leads to decreased surfactant synthesis, as well as emphysematous changes in the lung. Humidity and mucociliary performance in the lung require adequate hydration. Smooth muscle function, macrophage activity, and secretion of immunoglobulins (e.g., IgA) into mucus all depend on good nutrition. Obesity changes the physiology of several organ systems. Decreased compliance of the lungs is caused by accumulation of fat tissue around the chest wall, ribs, diaphragm, and abdomen, resulting in impaired lung expansion. Compliance of the pulmonary system declines with increasing BMI. Results of decreased compliance include shallow and rapid breathing and an increased work of breathing. Functional residual capacity declines with increasing BMI, resulting in small airway closure, right-to-left shunting, and arterial hypoxemia. High levels of adipose tissues result in increased metabolic activity of the fat cell and in increased oxygen consumption and $CO_2$ production. Gas exchange is severely impaired postoperatively and when in a supine position. Obstructive sleep apnea leads to hypoxemia and hypercapnia.

## METABOLISM

Because basic requirements for both oxygen and nutrients are determined by the cellular metabolic rate, an understanding of metabolism is essential for both respiratory and nutritional assessment.

Metabolism is the body's way of transferring energy from food to the body's energy currency molecules: ATP. The metabolic process can be divided into two pathways: those that break down molecules as energy is released (catabolism) and those that build up new molecules (anabolism) to be used in a structural or a functional role. The catabolic pathways produce ATP, which is used for energy to drive the anabolic pathways for growth and maintenance of the organism or simply for the organism's movement in the environment. Therefore energy is the fundamental need of the body. If sufficient food is eaten, the body can maintain its equilibrium and satisfy the demands placed on it by changes in the environment. However, if too little food is ingested, the body must rely on energy previously stored. If the stored energy—fat and carbohydrate (glycogen)—is not sufficient, the body will break down protein to produce ATP. As mentioned previously, this condition is undesirable because the protein comes from functioning tissue and therefore lessens the functional capability of the organism.

If too much food energy is taken in, the body must use some of its energy to convert the excess carbohydrate or protein so that it can store the excess in the form of fat. As the level of body fat increases, the metabolic cost of moving and breathing increases along with the risk for various diseases. Again, the functional capability of the organism is decreased.

A basic understanding of the metabolic pathways is essential when planning nutritional and ventilatory support. Fig. 18.4 illustrates schematically the major energy-producing pathways used by almost every cell of the body. The reader is encouraged to refer to biochemistry or physiology texts for a more complete discussion of metabolism.

The metabolic process can be viewed as having four major phases (see Fig. 18.4). The first is the digestive phase, in which the food substrates are broken down to the basic components: fat (fatty acids and glycerol), carbohydrates (sugars), and protein (amino acids). The food components are then absorbed from the gastrointestinal tract into the blood and then to the liver, from which they eventually travel to every cell in the body.

The second phase involves the catabolism of the food components within the cell down to a common molecule, acetyl coenzyme A (acetyl-CoA). A small amount of the food energy is used directly to produce a few ATP molecules or transferred to molecular energy shuttles (energy intermediates) in this phase, but acetyl-CoA still contains the bulk of the food energy. It is also possible for the metabolic pathways in this phase to go in the opposite direction, from acetyl-CoA to form the basic food components again. However, molecules move in this anabolic direction only when the cell has plenty of energy currency (ATP) available. Also note that anaerobic metabolism (energy—ATP—being formed without the presence of oxygen) can occur only in this second phase of metabolism, in the pathway labeled glycolysis. In anaerobic metabolism, pyruvate produces lactate (lactic acid) rather than acetyl CoA. The greater the energy production without sufficient oxygen, the more lactic acid produced. This can result in lactic acidosis. If this occurs, the acid must be buffered with bicarbonate ($HCO_3^-$), and carbon dioxide is produced in the process. This requires increased minute ventilation to eliminate the carbon dioxide generated.

Whereas the phases just described have different pathways for each of the food components, the third phase uses the same tricarboxylic acid (TCA) pathway (also called the *Krebs* or *citric acid cycle*), regardless of the origin of the acetyl CoA. The rest of the food energy is removed in the TCA phase, again transferring the energy to molecular energy shuttles. It is here that most of the energy-depleted carbon "skeletons" are discarded as carbon dioxide. For the TCA cycle to be active, the energy shuttles, nicotinamide adenine dinucleotide (NAD) and flavoprotein adenine dinucleotide (FAD), must be able to unload their energy-rich hydrogen and electrons into the respiratory transport chain (oxidative phosphorylation). This requires the presence of oxygen. Without it, the TCA cycle grinds to a halt.

The fourth phase occurs in the cell's mitochondria and is the final destination of the molecular energy shuttles, in which they "dump" their energy-rich loads of hydrogen and electrons into the oxidative phosphorylation system where ATP molecules are mass produced. This is also the final destination of the oxygen that was inhaled. Here, the energy is extracted from the hydrogen and electrons; in the energy-depleted form, the hydrogen and electrons combine with oxygen to form water.

It is in the metabolic pathways just outlined where the body's oxygen is used and carbon dioxide is produced. The oxygen used can be measured and is expressed as the oxygen uptake per minute ($\dot{V}O_2$). The measured carbon dioxide produced per minute is expressed as the $\dot{V}CO_2$. The ratio of $\dot{V}CO_2$ to $\dot{V}O_2$ is the RQ. The RQ is an indirect measure of substrate utilization. Pure fat oxidation has an RQ of 0.71 (more oxygen used than carbon dioxide produced), protein oxidation has a value of 0.82, and carbohydrate oxidation has a value of 1.0 (an even ratio, where one carbon dioxide molecule is produced for each molecule of oxygen used). A mixture of the three different types of foods used for energy at the same time results in an RQ of about 0.85. (This is the R value used most often in the alveolar air equation.) In indirect calorimetry, the RQ should be used as a measure of test validity; measures in the range of 0.6 to 1.2 are within the normal physiologic range.

## NUTRITIONAL REQUIREMENTS

The basic nutritional requirements include carbohydrate, protein, fat, vitamins, minerals, and water. In light of the present discussion, it would not be wrong to include oxygen as a nutrient because food is of no value unless oxygen

**FIG. 18.4** Four major phases of metabolism are schematically illustrated. Phase I: digestion and nutrient absorption of fat, carbohydrate, and protein. Phase II: breakdown of fatty acids, glucose, and amino acids to acetyl CoA, which either can go on to synthesize (directly or indirectly) fat, carbohydrate, or amino acids, as need be, or can have more energy extracted from it in phases III and IV. Phase III: tricarboxylic acid cycle, where most of the body's carbon dioxide is produced and where most of the molecular energy shuttles (nicotinamide adenine dinucleotide [NAD] and flavoprotein adenosine dinucleotide [FAD]) receive their energy supply in the form of hydrogen atoms. Shuttles transport energy to the respiratory chain. Phase IV: inner mitochondrial membrane where oxidative phosphorylation (production of adenosine triphosphate [ATP] in the presence of oxygen) occurs. Oxygen is the final acceptor of the now energy-depleted electrons and hydrogen ions. *2,3-DPG,* 2,3-Diphosphoglycerate; *FADH,* flavoprotein adenine dinucleotide dehydrogenase; *NADH,* nicotine adenine dinucleotide dehydrogenase.

is present, although traditionally it is not included in discussions of nutritional requirements. Carbohydrate, protein, and fat provide the energy the body needs, as well as the basic chemical skeletons on which structural and functional body systems are built. Vitamins, being part of coenzymes, work

along with enzymes in various metabolic pathways and allow specific reactions to occur. Minerals often are elements of specific molecules such as hemoglobin, cytochromes, and thyroxin and may function as cofactors in enzyme systems. Water is the medium in which the various chemical reactions take place within cells. It is also responsible for the fluidity of the blood, which allows blood to circulate. It is not surprising that 50% to 70% of the body's weight is made up of water.

The optimal amount of each of the nutritional components has not been determined precisely, especially for those required in trace amounts. There is agreement that a minimum nutrient level should be high enough so that deficiency symptoms cannot be detected and low enough to prevent toxicity. Within this range, there is much discussion as to what is the right amount because nutritional requirements vary from person to person. Greater or lesser amounts of specific nutrients may be needed because of genetically induced enzyme defects, various disease states, varying amounts of energy expenditure, and various drug-nutrient interactions. Because of the complexity of nurturing the body, a careful nutritional assessment by a nutritional support team, composed of at least a physician and dietitian, is essential. A clinical pharmacologist, for nutrition given parenterally and to evaluate drug interactions with enteral and parenteral feedings, and an RT, for assessing $\dot{V}CO_2$ and $\dot{V}O_2$, are important additions to the team.

## Energy

Energy requirements of people with COPD are variable owing to differences in REE and levels of physical activity. COPD, whether stable or in exacerbation, results in an increase in inflammation and thus an increase in REE. Other influences on energy needs include the efficiency of breathing, thermic effect of food and medications, and others that are beyond the scope of this text. To meet these energy needs and the overall nutritional requirements of the body, a proper balance of macronutrients (carbohydrates, protein, and fat) and micronutrients (vitamins and minerals) is required.

The macronutrient food component that should compose the largest amount of the dietary intake is carbohydrate. Carbohydrates are sometimes broadly classified as complex or simple. The complex carbohydrates are starches (sugar molecules linked together in long branching chains) readily found in a variety of foods; the best sources are grains, vegetables, and fruits. Foods high in complex carbohydrates usually contain the vitamins required in the metabolic pathways for catabolism. In addition, these foods provide water, fiber, protein, and chemical components that are associated with a decrease in chronic disease processes. Simple carbohydrates are free sugars; in natural foods, the largest amounts of simple carbohydrates are found in fruits. However, the majority of sugar consumed comes from processed, refined foods and sugar-sweetened beverages. Ingestion of simple carbohydrates (not including fruits) should be at a minimum because their nutritional value is quite low, but their metabolic demand is quite high (i.e., they travel down the glucose metabolic pathway or go to fat synthesis but do not "pay any taxes" in the form of vitamins or minerals for the maintenance of the metabolic machinery). They can provide a quick form of energy, but when ingested alone, they can stimulate an exaggerated insulin response because of their rapid absorption from the intestinal tract. Complex carbohydrates tend not to trigger this response because they have to be broken down to free sugars, which takes time, before they are absorbed. Various complex carbohydrate foods differ from one another in their effects on blood sugar levels.

Carbohydrate has often been contrasted with fat. Because the $\dot{V}CO_2$ with fat metabolism is lower than that with carbohydrate, it has been suggested by some that minimizing the dietary intake of carbohydrate is to the advantage of the patient with respiratory disease. A patient's response to carbohydrate should be evaluated so that adverse effects can be avoided. It appears, however, that when high levels of carbohydrate are given enterally to patients with COPD who retain carbon dioxide, elevated arterial carbon dioxide tension ($PaCO_2$) levels do not always occur. In fact, there are even some advantages. A load of ingested carbohydrate can elevate the arterial blood oxygen level ($PaO_2$) by a modest amount of 7 to 9 mm Hg. This is of definite benefit to patients with low oxygen saturations. When the oxygen saturation is low, small increases in $PaO_2$ can produce significant increases in oxygen content. In addition, a high-carbohydrate diet can significantly increase endurance and allow a given amount of work to be performed with less oxygen than with low-carbohydrate diets. The low $\dot{V}CO_2$ advantages of a high-fat diet may be offset in some patients by the increased oxygen requirement for a given work rate. The major problem that has arisen with carbohydrate intake in patients with respiratory disorders occurs when glucose has been given in excess. The increased $\dot{V}CO_2$ (a result of both the high RQ of glucose metabolism and its conversion to fat) has induced respiratory difficulty in patients being weaned from mechanical ventilators. This has been observed primarily when glucose has been administered by the parenteral (IV) route.

### SIMPLY STATED

Excessive glucose intake leads to an increase in carbon dioxide production, and the respiratory system must work harder to rid the body of this extra carbon dioxide.

Clearly, the problem with glucose lies not in its use but in its "abuse" or overuse. It is recommended that with the use of parenteral nutrition in critically ill patients, fat should be infused along with the glucose. The infused fat not only helps provide energy but also inhibits the fat synthesis pathway, thereby preventing excessive carbon dioxide production.

Despite the advantages of carbohydrates, diets must be individualized for each patient. Identification of the causes of reduced or inadequate intake is required to develop a nutrition plan that will be effective. Patients with more severe COPD often do better with a higher fat content in the diet and less carbohydrate because there is less carbon dioxide production. But this does not lessen the importance of carbohydrates. Various carbohydrate and dietary fat percentages should be tried until the best combination is found for each patient. This point is stressed because there is a tendency to simply put patients with COPD on a high-fat diet without determining how much carbohydrate they can handle before their condition becomes compromised. Generally, carbohydrates should make up about 55% to 60% of the caloric intake of enterally fed patients. If a patient is having difficulty weaning from mechanical ventilation, a higher fat diet (55% fat) may be useful during the weaning process, in particular those with high $Pco_2$ and $CO_2$ levels. Follow-up assessment of patients by a registered dietitian familiar with COPD allows proper dietary adjustments.

## Protein

Protein should make up 12% to 15% of the caloric intake. The RDA of protein for a healthy person has been set at 0.8 g/kg of body weight each day. Thus a 70-kg person should obtain about 56 g of protein each day. Typically, a person who ingests an adequate number of calories each day, from a variety of foods, will get sufficient protein. In general, protein intake should be sufficient to establish positive nitrogen balance in patients who are nutritionally compromised. A nitrogen balance of +2 g/24 hours is desirable for repletion.

Protein is determined by calculating grams of protein per kilogram of body weight (actual or ideal, whichever is lower):
- 0.8 g/kg for the normal healthy adult
- 1.2 to 1.5 g/kg for the initial provision of protein in the pulmonary compromised patient; if protein depletion is present, assessing nitrogen balance and reassessing protein needs is critical
- 2.0 to 2.5 g/kg for severe catabolic conditions

### Nitrogen

Nitrogen values are often referred to in discussion of protein requirements because nitrogen is only found in the amino acids that make up proteins. Thus measuring nitrogen, which is a simple laboratory measure, is the easiest way to measure protein intake or excretion. Amino acids make up all the proteins. Amino acids contain an acid group, COOH, and an amino group, $NH_2$. The amino group is the nitrogen-containing portion of the amino acid. Specific laboratory methods are used to measure nitrogen in the blood (blood urea nitrogen [BUN]) or in the urine (urinary urea nitrogen [UUN]). Because every 100 g of proteins contains approximately 6.25 g of nitrogen, grams of nitrogen can readily be converted to grams of protein by multiplying by 6.25. Conversely, to find how much nitrogen there is in a given amount of protein, in grams, divide by 6.25 (or the appropriate factor for the specific protein).

### Protein Quality and Adequacy

When considering adequacy of protein intake, both quantity and quality of the protein must be considered. The quality of a protein is determined by the amount of each essential amino acid it contains. Essential amino acids cannot be synthesized by the body in sufficient quantities to meet body needs or cannot be synthesized at all. Of the 20 amino acids, 9 are considered essential for the healthy adult: histidine, isoleucine, leucine, lysine, methionine, phenylalanine, threonine, tryptophan, and valine. By definition, the greater the number of essential amino acids contained in a protein, the higher its quality. The ratio of various key amino acids is emerging as an important factor in nutritional health. Soy protein is considered a high-quality protein, along with milk or egg protein; however, soy protein has an additional benefit of lower insulin stimulation and a lowering of cholesterol. With milk or egg protein, there is an opposite effect. Plant-based proteins lower many of the risk factors for many chronic diseases. Most of the plant proteins have lower essential amino acid profiles than do animal proteins, but when combined with other complementary plant protein, complete essential amino acid profiles can be obtained.

### Effects and Consequences of Extreme Intakes of Protein

As with anything else, the extremes of protein intake, either too little or too much, can have detrimental effects. Too little protein compromises the immune system, contributes to edema and ascites, produces generalized wasting of muscle tissue, and retards growth and proper development in children. Too much protein, although not as harmful, increases the requirements for some other nutrients, notably calcium and water. In addition, there may be an increase in the work of breathing, as noted previously, and increased stress on the liver and kidneys (of concern mostly in patients with liver or renal insufficiency).

### Acid-Base Balance

The final consideration involves the body's acid-base balance. Protein is the major source of fixed acids that are ingested (fixed acids must be cleared by the kidney; volatile acids, like carbon dioxide, can be cleared by the lungs). Patients with COPD who are in a state of respiratory acidosis may experience more difficulty if an increased fixed acid load (large quantity of protein) is ingested. Protein from plant-based sources is more alkaline in nature. In fact, fruits and vegetables leave an alkaline residue in the body after metabolism, and they help buffer the acids from the proteins. Without sufficient fruits and vegetables, more calcium must be pulled from the bones, forming calcium carbonate, which is then used to buffer the fixed acids from the proteins. So, in patients who have respiratory acidosis and are in need of more protein intake, the acid-base balance is better regulated by adding more plant-based foods in the diet.

### Nitrogen Balance

To establish the optimal amount of protein, a patient needs the measurement of protein intake (nitrogen intake) and nitrogen excretion. A patient whose intake of nitrogen equals excretion of nitrogen is said to be in nitrogen balance. If more nitrogen is excreted than ingested, negative nitrogen balance exists. Conversely, positive nitrogen balance exists when the nitrogen intake is greater than the nitrogen excretion. Patients who are severely ill or who are simply not getting enough calories are often in negative nitrogen balance. This is undesirable because it indicates that body protein is being used for energy. Patients who are nutritionally depleted need to be in positive nitrogen balance to build up body tissues. In the well-nourished patient, the clinical goal is to maintain nitrogen balance.

## Fat

Dietary fat plays a number of important roles in the body. The fat-soluble vitamins, A, D, E, and K, are carried in fats and oils. These vitamins are involved in immunity, antioxidant activity, blood clotting, and bone and arterial health. Fat is energy dense and contains twice as many calories per gram weight as carbohydrate or protein. Because of this, fat is the best storage form of energy, and this is why the body stores excess calories in the form of fat or triglycerides in the adipose tissue. Fat is also the most efficient way to provide more calories to hospitalized patients when they are fluid restricted or cannot tolerate large volumes of food. Fat provides a feeling of fullness (satiety), improves palatability of food, and is digested more slowly than proteins and starches. There are two essential fats, linolenic (omega-3) and linoleic (omega-6), that the body must obtain from the diet. These fats are needed for modulation of inflammatory processes, nerve function, and other essential chemical activities.

### Key Functions of Fat

Within the body, fat is involved in many different functions. Notably, fat is a component of all cell membranes, provides energy storage and organ protection, and is the major component of surfactant (dipalmitoyl lecithin). However, these tasks do not require much fat to be eaten. The typical American diet is composed of more than 30% of calories from fat. This is more than necessary. With excess dietary fat comes increased risk for heart disease, breast cancer, colon cancer, and lung cancer in women. Increased fat also decreases oxygenation of the tissues, impairs pulmonary gas diffusion ($D_{L}CO$), and hinders capillary circulation by promoting the clumping of red blood cells. However, these outcomes do not always occur because the effects seen depend on the amount of fat that is circulating, the rate of clearance of fat, and possibly the type of fat. As the fat content of the diet increases, there is a measurable decrease in $\dot{V}CO_2$. For many patients with COPD, this results in less dyspnea and improved function.

### Types of Dietary Fats and Health Implications

The main concern of nutritionists is to determine the optimal percentage of calories that should come from carbohydrate and protein. With that established, the remaining number of calories required can come from fat.

With the quantity of fat determined, one must be concerned with the quality of fat. Fat can be either saturated (no double bonds present in the fatty acid chain) or unsaturated (some of the fatty acid carbons contain double bonds). The two types of unsaturated fats are polyunsaturated (more than two double bonds in the fatty acid chain) and monounsaturated (only one double bond present). Most diets are too high in saturated fat, and a higher intake of monounsaturated fat is recommended. Monounsaturated fat, found in olives, nuts, and avocados, has numerous health benefits. This type of fat lowers total and low-density lipoprotein (LDL) cholesterol with no adverse effect on the high-density lipoprotein (HDL) cholesterol, thereby lowering the risk for heart disease. Monounsaturated fat also helps regulate both blood sugar and blood pressure. Olive oil and canola oil are the recommended choices. Despite all the information available about the advantages and disadvantages of given foods and optimal combinations of carbohydrate, fat, and protein, dietary patterns established early in life are difficult to change in later years. Patients should be encouraged to eat foods that provide good nutrition and do not aggravate a compromised respiratory condition. However, some patients will not adapt to a change in diet, and in these cases, any nutrition is better than no nutrition.

## Vitamins, Minerals, Phytochemicals, and Other Nutrients

Vitamins can be classified into two main categories: water soluble and fat soluble. Water-soluble vitamins are those of the B group and vitamin C. The fat-soluble vitamins are A, D, E, and K. Vitamins are cofactors in the enzyme systems needed for various metabolic pathways and body processes. The minerals can be divided into either macronutrient elements or micronutrient (trace) elements. Minerals are used in all of the body chemical reactions and are part of numerous enzyme systems serving as cofactors. It is just as important to supplement with minerals as it is with vitamins when there appears to be a deficient food intake.

For most people who eat a variety of foods each day, ingesting the recommended amounts of vitamins and minerals is not difficult. But when physiologic functioning has been altered by a disease process, an increased need for specific nutrients may arise. Vitamin and mineral supplementation will also be more necessary when there is a decreased consumption of food because of, for example, loss of appetite. The less food eaten, the more difficulty there will be in obtaining all the different nutrients. Furthermore, various medications can interact with the absorption, function, or excretion of some nutrients, thereby altering the required amount. Studies show that in older people, supplementation with a basic vitamin and mineral results in fewer infections and more days of wellness each year. However, not all studies confirm these findings. The differing results might be due to different levels or combinations of supplementations. There appears to be a consistent finding that higher antioxidant levels in the blood correlate with improved lung function, but this may be more likely from the diet rather than the supplements. Subjects with higher plasma β-carotene are shown to have higher FVC levels, and vitamin D is linked to improved lung function. Higher intakes of vitamin C or β-carotene are protective for $FEV_1$ and FVC. These observations are important for COPD patients because there is a decrease in plasma antioxidants in people who smoke; this is associated not only with decreased lung function but also with greater mortality. It has also been found that a deficiency of vitamins C and E is associated with more wheezing symptoms. Higher levels of dietary intakes of antioxidants appear to be associated with higher skeletal muscular strength in elderly persons. This relationship would apply to the respiratory muscles, which are skeletal muscles.

A few nutrients deserve special mention because of their importance in patients with lung disease. Iron's role in oxygen transport and use in hemoglobin and myoglobin and within the respiratory transport chain makes it necessary to maintain iron at normal levels. It has also been found that anemia is associated with decreases in muscular strength. Vitamin A promotes optimal functioning of mucous membranes and helps promote resistance to respiratory tract infections. Vitamin A depletion induced by cigarette smoking has been associated with development of emphysema in rats. Carotene, a vitamin A precursor, and vitamin C have been found to be associated with a decreased risk for certain types of lung cancers. A number of studies show that the benefits from these nutrients are better realized from eating the fruits and vegetables that contain them than from simply supplementing the isolated vitamin. Vitamins E and C and selenium, which are antioxidants, appear to help lessen the effects of oxygen toxicity and ozone on lung tissue. Vitamin D in the form of $D_3$ (also known as cholecalciferol) has come to the forefront in recent years because of numerous benefits: improved lung function, immunity and resistance against some cancers and viruses, bone density, calcium uptake, muscle strength, and relief of aches and pains. Vitamin D is the "sunshine" vitamin, and proper exposure to the sun can help a person achieve sufficient levels; however, in many areas, sufficient exposure to the sun is not readily available, and oral supplementation should be used to optimize the amount of vitamin D received. Monitoring blood levels of vitamin D is recommended so that proper dosing adjustments can be made as needed.

Any chronically ill patient may have altered eating habits that are insufficient to meet nutrient requirements. The severity of nutritional depletion appears to be related to the severity of COPD despite an adequate caloric intake. This may result in a need for supplementation of some or all of the vitamins and minerals.

Phytochemicals are plant components that make up plant colors and other active components of plants. Intake of plant phytochemicals, as would be obtained from eating whole plant foods, lowers risk for chronic diseases, including asthma. Flavonoids and other phytochemicals, which are only found in plant foods, especially fruits, vegetables, and berries, have potent antioxidant tissue-protective effects that are vital to health and disease prevention. Diets need to ensure generous amounts of these types of foods.

COPD patients, as with other patients with chronic diseases, are often found to have an underlying inflammatory component. Skeletal muscle loss in COPD appears to be linked with systemic inflammation. It is also known that the underlying problem with asthma is airway inflammation, which leads to bronchoconstriction. Dietary omega-3 polyunsaturated fatty acids, which are found in flaxseeds and fish oils, have important antiinflammatory effects in the body and may benefit patients with lung disease.

## Fluids and Electrolytes
### Fluid Concerns

Adequate fluid intake is extremely important for patients with respiratory disorders. Proper function of the lung's mucociliary clearance mechanism requires good hydration. Although the body is composed of about 60% water by weight, it is constantly losing water through urine, feces, sweat, breathing, and, in patients with respiratory problems, expectoration. This requires continual fluid replacement.

Patients with respiratory problems often develop heart failure (right or left, or eventually both), which complicates the fluid replacement process. The need for fluids must be carefully balanced with the need to restrict fluids because of the fluid retention resulting from the heart problem. In a patient who has a heart problem, both fluid and sodium intake must be monitored. Sodium levels determine how much water the body will retain; therefore dietary sodium often must be limited.

### Water

Water is the best fluid to provide hydration. However, fruit or vegetable juices add some variety, as well as some nutrition and more calories for those who need additional caloric intake. Low-sodium juices can be obtained. Drinks containing caffeine promote bronchodilation to some extent because caffeine is in the same family as theophylline; both are xanthines. If a patient is using theophylline-type bronchodilators and is also a heavy user of drinks containing caffeine, there is a greater chance of side effects. Because the ingestion of alcohol has been correlated with decreased FVC and $FEV_1$, bronchoconstriction, impairment of lung defenses, and increased likelihood of sleep apnea, its use is contraindicated. Good nutrition for the respiratory system involves not only getting enough of that which is essential but also avoiding that which is harmful.

### Intravenous Fluids

Patients receiving IV fluids must have the input and output amounts monitored continually so that neither too much nor too little is given. Fluid overload often results in pulmonary congestion or edema, further complicating a poorly functioning lung.

In addition to serum sodium levels, potassium, phosphorus, and chloride values should be checked. All of these electrolytes play an important role in acid-base balance and nerve function. Potassium also plays an important role in heart, muscle, and nerve function, as well as in stimulation of aldosterone secretion (along with angiotensin II) from the adrenal cortex.

One must not forget that fluid and sodium intake can occur with medication and normal saline nebulization. Nebulized fluid retention is most critical when dealing with small children and infants, especially when an ultrasonic nebulizer is used.

## Phosphorus

Respiratory insufficiency may occur in some patients with severe hypophosphatemia, particularly when the underlying cause is malnutrition. It has also been shown to increase mortality by fourfold. Serum phosphate ranges from 2.5 to 4.5 mg/dL (0.81 to 1.45 mmol/L) in adults. Hypophosphatemia is defined as mild (2 to 2.5 mg/dL, or 0.65 to 0.81 mmol/L), moderate (1 to 2 mg/dL, or 0.32 to 0.65 mmol/L), or severe (<1 mg/dL, or 0.32 mmol/L). Phosphate depletion causes reduction of ATP and increased affinity for oxygen to hemoglobin, resulting in decreased oxygen delivered to tissues. Inadequate dietary intake of phosphate is a rare cause of hypophosphatemia because of wide availability in foods. Dietary sources of phosphate include fruits, vegetables, meats, and dairy products. Vitamin D enhances the absorption of both phosphate and calcium. Certain conditions such as anorexia nervosa or chronic alcoholism may also lead to hypophosphatemia, as well as losses via increased renal excretion. Certain medications and disease states precipitate hypophosphatemia. Patients with acute respiratory distress due to asthma or COPD exacerbations requiring intense, sustained nebulized (such as albuterol) treatments activates the β-adrenergic receptor, which can move phosphate into the cells, thus lowering serum phosphate levels. Most important, patients requiring mechanical ventilation for asthma or COPD may develop respiratory alkalosis, which is a common cause of hypophosphatemia and contributes to failure to wean patients from mechanical ventilation.

---

### SIMPLY STATED

Excessive intake of sodium can lead to fluid retention, especially in the patient with heart failure. The association between hypophosphatemia and failure to wean from mechanical ventilation in patients on ventilator support requires monitoring of serum phosphate levels and treatment to prevent severe hypophosphatemia.

---

# METHODS OF MEETING NUTRITIONAL REQUIREMENTS

Nutritional requirements are not always achieved easily. Registered dietitian nutritionists often work against patient factors such as loss of appetite, dyspnea that is increased with eating, inability to eat normal amounts of solid food, fluid restrictions, inability to take food by mouth, and a comatose state. Careful evaluation of a patient's nutritional needs, food preferences, educational and economic status, cooking facilities, and self-help level is necessary. All factors influence a patient's ability to reach the nutritional goals set.

The routes of nutritional administration can be either enteral or parenteral. The preferred route is enteral. If a patient is intubated and cannot take food by mouth, enteral tube feeding is instituted. The last resort, when all other attempts at feeding are unsuccessful or not recommended, is parenteral nutrition (PN). PN is the feeding of patients by direct infusion of nutrients into either a peripheral or a central vein. There is a reluctance to feed patients by PN because it is not as efficient as the enteral route, it is expensive, and there are increased risks for complications such as infection. However, because nutrition is so important, it is used. Nutritionally depleted or catabolic patients should never go without nutritional support for more than a day.

## Condition-Specific Nutritional Considerations

There are some respiratory disorders that require special nutritional considerations. Some of the more common such disorders and considerations are as follows.

### Chronic Obstructive Pulmonary Disease

Patients with emphysema are often underweight and need to gain weight, whereas those with chronic bronchitis are likely to be overweight and need to lose weight. Patients with COPD may find it uncomfortable to eat a large meal because a flattened diaphragm along with a full stomach makes it even more difficult to function. To avoid this problem, frequent small meals may be helpful. The goal for a patient with emphysema is a positive nitrogen balance and an increase in caloric intake because respiratory muscle function improves with an increase in weight (muscle mass). The goal for an overweight patient with bronchitis is maintenance of nitrogen balance with decreased caloric intake because respiratory muscle function improves with a loss of weight due to fat.

### Patients Receiving Mechanical Ventilation

In addition to the previously noted association between hypophosphatemia and failure to wean, patients being assisted by continuous mechanical ventilation provide an additional nutritional challenge. Positive-pressure breathing can affect splanchnic (internal organs of the abdomen) circulation and can cause increased resistance to portal blood flow to the liver, increased resistance to bile flow down the bile duct, and decreased blood flow to the kidneys. These effects are increased as the pressure is increased and are most pronounced with the use of continuous positive airway pressure (CPAP) or positive end-expiratory pressure (PEEP). However, these effects may reach significance only for a minority of patients. Yet any alteration in blood flow in the gastrointestinal tract, liver, or kidneys can have an effect on the nutritional status of the patient, thus making it more difficult to meet his or her nutritional requirements.

### Cystic Fibrosis

In addition and as previously indicated, a disease such as cystic fibrosis (CF) affects not only the lungs but also other organ systems, including the pancreas. As a result, patients with CF tend to have a deficiency of certain digestive enzymes produced in the pancreas and needed for digesting fats. To address this and enable the body to better digest and absorb fats, such patients generally need to take digestive enzyme supplements.

## Guidelines for Nutritional Management of Cystic Fibrosis

Although a diet high in fat is often recommended, it has disadvantages for patients with CF. The omega-6 fatty acid arachidonic acid found in these foods may adversely affect CF patients by precipitating oxidative stress and induce a proinflammatory effect in lung tissue through an increase in leukotriene B4. Omega-3 fats offer clinical benefit in patients with CF. Reduction of sputum volume, improved lung function, decrease in leukotriene B4, and decrease in use of antibiotics have been observed in eicosapentaenoic acid/docosahexaenoic acid (EPA/DHA)-supplemented patients. Increasing the intake of plant sources of omega-3 fats (alpha-linolenic acid) and monounsaturated fats (e.g., flax, canola, soy) is an alternative approach to improving fatty acid nutrition in CF patients.

## Nutrition Guidelines

- Energy intake of 120% to 150% of the RDA for normal growth and adequate protein intake/kg/body weight
- Oral pancreatic enzymes to facilitate digestion of fats and proteins and absorption of vitamins
- Supplements of vitamins A, D, E, and K to replace the fat-soluble vitamins
- High-calorie shakes/supplements to provide adequate nutrients
- A high-salt diet or salt supplements before exercising
- Nocturnal enteral nasogastric/gastrostomy feedings to provide additional calories
- Adequate calcium and vitamin D to aid in the management of osteoporosis associated with CF

---

### SIMPLY STATED

Patients with cystic fibrosis tend to have a deficiency of enzymes produced in the pancreas and need for the digestion of fats. As a result, most patients with cystic fibrosis need to take digestive enzyme supplements to minimize the likelihood of a certain type of malnutrition.

---

## NUTRITIONAL ASSESSMENT

The RT is not responsible for the nutritional assessment of the patient but should be familiar with the process and may actually participate in it. Because the RT and the nurse usually spend the most time with a patient, their observations are valuable. A complete nutritional assessment is performed by the registered dietitian nutritionist and may include some factors assessed by other members of the health care team. The components of nutritional assessment consist of medical and diet histories, including medications with nutritional considerations, anthropometric measurements (weight, body composition, skinfold, and waist and limb circumferences),

biochemical evaluations, energy and macronutrient and micronutrient evaluations, and immunologic evaluations. The areas to be assessed in determining the patient's nutritional profile are summarized in Box 18.1.

## Data Gathering and Interpretation
### History

Conditions that should be discovered in the medical history are as follows:

- Multiple surgical or nonsurgical trauma
- Fever
- Infection (acute and chronic)
- Burns

---

### BOX 18.1   Areas Requiring Assessment to Determine a Patient's Nutritional Profile

**Physiologic**
- Types of diseases present
- Severity of illness
- Metabolic stress of disease
- Medications being used (both prescription and over the counter)
- Botanical and/or herbal therapies
- Genetic deficiencies
- Activity level
- Resting energy expenditure (REE)
- Food allergies and intolerances
- Current nutritional status
  - Anthropometric
  - Biochemical
  - Immunologic

**Psychosocial**
- Mental state (mood, alertness)
- Culture
- Food preparation skills
- Appetite
- Learned eating behaviors/habits (food preferences)
- Motivation
- Habits: alcohol, smoking
- Education
- Income
- Support system

**Environmental**
- Mechanical hindrances to eating (continuous mechanical ventilation and tracheostomy)
- Food availability
- Temperature
- Humidity

**Suggested Measurements**
- Skinfold thickness
- Skinfold + arm circumference = arm, muscle circumference, muscle and fat area
- Body mass index (BMI)
- Percent body fat
- Percent lean body mass—body protein reserves (an indicator of protein energy nutrition)
- Body fat stores (an indicator of energy reserves)
- Result of long-term nutritional status

---

- Long bone fractures
- Hyperthyroidism
- Prolonged corticosteroid therapy

These conditions increase a patient's metabolic rate or caloric and other nutrient requirements. Such metabolic challenges pose a serious threat to the homeostatic maintenance of a marginally nourished patient with COPD. A patient with one of these conditions should be evaluated further with an REE using indirect calorimetry.

During the patient interview, the following information is collected:

- Smoking or other tobacco habits
- Occupation and usual daily activity
- Use of supplemental oxygen
- Usual energy and nutrient intake through 24-hour recall, usual daily intake or food frequency pattern
- Special diet restrictions at home
- Food aversions, intolerances, and allergies
- Medications (prescription and over the counter); nutritional, botanical, and herbal supplements
- Mechanical feeding problems (e.g., biting, chewing or swallowing, mouth sores)
- Changes in appetite
- Changes in food intake or food patterns
- Gastrointestinal problems (e.g., anorexia, nausea, vomiting, or heartburn)
- Elimination pattern and consistency of stool
- Maximal weight attained and how long ago it was attained
- Usual weight, recent weight changes
- Alcohol intake

This information is usually obtained from the patient or family members during the initial evaluation.

## Physical Examination

The physical examination often yields clues to the patient's nutritional status; however, many signs of nutritional deficiency can be missed by the inexperienced RT or other member of the patient care team.

- Look at the health of the patient's hair, and check for sparseness, dyspigmentation, or easy pluckability.
- Assess the skin for areas of drying, flaking, cracking, or pigment change.
- Swollen parotid glands, changes in saliva production, or an enlarged liver may indicate concern for nutritional status.
- Weight loss, temporal wasting or general muscle wasting, edema, mental apathy, and confusion all can lead the clinician to suspect malnutrition. Although signs of malnutrition, they are rather nonspecific and therefore only suggestive of malnutrition. When these signs are present in a patient, more sensitive and objective methods of assessment should be used to confirm or rule out compromised nutritional status.

The following is a summary of some basic anthropometric measurements and their nutritional assessment value.

### Anthropometric Measurements of Physical Assessment

The assessment most commonly used and easiest to perform during the physical examination involves weighing and measuring stature and body circumference. Measurements of weight, height, and arm and waist circumference require little effort or time yet give important information. Because height and weight can vary with the time of day and the amount of clothing, the measurements should be performed in the same way each time and the pertinent information recorded so that serial measurements are meaningful. Bed scales can be used for weighing ventilator-dependent patients. The weight of any ventilator tubing or other devices and dressings should be subtracted from the total weight. A weight loss of 5% of the usual body weight or an unintentional weight loss of 10 lb or more indicates increased nutritional risk. Although body weight has limited value in detecting malnutrition, low body weights correlate with poor medical outcomes. The patient care team should evaluate for edema and ascites when assessing weight status, which can result in misinterpretation of actual weight status. If a fluctuation or change in weight of several pounds is observed during a 24-hour period, it is most likely caused by water retention or loss.

*Body mass index.* The body mass index (BMI) is the primary method for assessment of the appropriateness of weight for a given height. The BMI is determined by weight (kg)/height (m²). Fig. 18.5 is a table for finding the BMI without having to calculate it.

- A BMI in the range of 20 to 25 is considered optimal.
- A BMI from 25 to 30 is considered overweight.
- A BMI from 30 to 35 is stage 1 obesity.
- A BMI from 35 to 40 is stage 2 obesity.
- A BMI from 40 to 45 is stage 3 obesity, also known as morbid obesity.

As the BMI exceeds 27, the risk for weight-related problems begins to increase. BMIs that are below 19 are associated with malnutrition problems and increased pneumonia infections. BMI is shown to be significantly associated with $FEV_1$ and $FEV_1$ divided by vital capacity. In patients with COPD, the best survival outcomes are associated with those who have higher BMIs and in whom low BMI is an independent risk factor for dying. Prevalence of malnutrition may be as high as 30% in people with COPD (BMI <20 kg/m²), and the risk for COPD-related death doubles with weight loss. Body composition differs from healthy controls even in those with BMI greater than 20 kg/m². Fat-free mass and bone density are lower in people with COPD. A quick estimate of ideal body weight can be determined from the following (Hamwi equation): allow 106 lb for the first 5 feet of height and 6 lb for each additional inch (men). For women, start with 100 lb for the first 5 feet, and add 5 lb for each additional inch. This does not account for variations in frame size but is useful for rapid estimation as to appropriateness of a patient's weight. The ideal body weight can also be used for estimating a patient's anatomic dead space (1 mL/lb ideal body weight) or for determining a starting tidal volume for a ventilator-dependent patient (5 to 7 mL/lb ideal body weight). The term ideal body weight simply refers to the weight the patient probably should weigh.

Body weight is often divided into two types: fat weight and lean body weight (lean body weight = total weight − fat

Height in Inches

| ↓ | 56 | 57 | 58 | 59 | 60 | 61 | 62 | 63 | 64 | 65 | 66 | 67 | 68 | 69 | 70 | 71 | 72 | 73 | 74 | 75 | 76 |
|---|----|----|----|----|----|----|----|----|----|----|----|----|----|----|----|----|----|----|----|----|----|
| 100 | 22 | 22 | 21 | 20 | 20 | 19 | 18 | 18 | 17 | 17 | 16 | 16 | 15 | 15 | 14 | 14 | 14 | 13 | 13 | 13 | 12 |
| 105 | 24 | 23 | 22 | 21 | 21 | 20 | 19 | 19 | 18 | 18 | 17 | 16 | 16 | 16 | 15 | 15 | 14 | 14 | 14 | 13 | 13 |
| 110 | 25 | 24 | 23 | 22 | 22 | 21 | 20 | 20 | 19 | 18 | 18 | 17 | 17 | 16 | 16 | 15 | 15 | 15 | 14 | 14 | 13 |
| 115 | 26 | 25 | 24 | 23 | 23 | 22 | 21 | 20 | 20 | 19 | 19 | 18 | 18 | 17 | 17 | 16 | 16 | 15 | 15 | 14 | 14 |
| 120 | 27 | 26 | 25 | 24 | 23 | 23 | 22 | 21 | 21 | 20 | 19 | 19 | 18 | 18 | 17 | 17 | 16 | 16 | 15 | 15 | 15 |
| 125 | 28 | 27 | 26 | 25 | 24 | 24 | 23 | 22 | 22 | 21 | 20 | 20 | 19 | 18 | 18 | 17 | 17 | 17 | 16 | 16 | 15 |
| 130 | 29 | 28 | 27 | 26 | 25 | 25 | 24 | 23 | 22 | 22 | 21 | 20 | 20 | 19 | 19 | 18 | 18 | 17 | 17 | 16 | 16 |
| 135 | 30 | 29 | 28 | 27 | 26 | 26 | 25 | 24 | 23 | 23 | 22 | 21 | 21 | 20 | 19 | 19 | 18 | 18 | 17 | 17 | 16 |
| 140 | 31 | 30 | 29 | 28 | 27 | 27 | 26 | 25 | 24 | 23 | 23 | 22 | 21 | 21 | 20 | 20 | 19 | 19 | 18 | 18 | 17 |
| 145 | 33 | 31 | 30 | 29 | 28 | 27 | 27 | 26 | 25 | 24 | 23 | 23 | 22 | 21 | 21 | 20 | 20 | 19 | 19 | 18 | 18 |
| 150 | 34 | 33 | 31 | 30 | 29 | 28 | 27 | 27 | 26 | 25 | 24 | 24 | 23 | 22 | 22 | 21 | 20 | 20 | 19 | 19 | 18 |
| 155 | 35 | 34 | 32 | 31 | 30 | 29 | 28 | 28 | 27 | 26 | 25 | 24 | 24 | 23 | 22 | 22 | 21 | 20 | 20 | 19 | 19 |
| 160 | 36 | 35 | 34 | 32 | 31 | 30 | 29 | 28 | 28 | 27 | 26 | 25 | 24 | 24 | 23 | 22 | 22 | 21 | 21 | 20 | 20 |
| 165 | 37 | 36 | 35 | 33 | 32 | 31 | 30 | 29 | 28 | 28 | 27 | 26 | 25 | 24 | 24 | 23 | 22 | 22 | 21 | 21 | 20 |
| 170 | 38 | 37 | 36 | 34 | 33 | 32 | 31 | 30 | 29 | 28 | 27 | 27 | 26 | 25 | 24 | 24 | 23 | 22 | 22 | 21 | 21 |
| 175 | 39 | 38 | 37 | 35 | 34 | 33 | 32 | 31 | 30 | 29 | 28 | 27 | 27 | 26 | 25 | 24 | 24 | 23 | 23 | 22 | 21 |
| 180 | 40 | 39 | 38 | 36 | 35 | 34 | 33 | 32 | 31 | 30 | 29 | 28 | 27 | 27 | 26 | 25 | 24 | 24 | 23 | 23 | 22 |
| 185 | 42 | 40 | 39 | 37 | 36 | 35 | 34 | 33 | 32 | 31 | 30 | 29 | 28 | 27 | 27 | 26 | 25 | 24 | 24 | 23 | 23 |
| 190 | 43 | 41 | 40 | 38 | 37 | 36 | 35 | 34 | 33 | 32 | 31 | 30 | 29 | 28 | 27 | 27 | 26 | 25 | 24 | 24 | 23 |
| 195 | 44 | 42 | 41 | 39 | 38 | 37 | 36 | 35 | 34 | 33 | 32 | 31 | 30 | 29 | 28 | 27 | 27 | 26 | 25 | 24 | 24 |
| 200 | 45 | 43 | 42 | 40 | 39 | 38 | 37 | 36 | 34 | 33 | 32 | 31 | 30 | 30 | 29 | 28 | 27 | 26 | 26 | 25 | 24 |
| 205 | 46 | 44 | 43 | 41 | 40 | 39 | 38 | 36 | 35 | 34 | 33 | 32 | 31 | 30 | 29 | 29 | 28 | 27 | 26 | 26 | 25 |
| 210 | 47 | 46 | 44 | 43 | 41 | 40 | 38 | 37 | 36 | 35 | 34 | 33 | 32 | 31 | 30 | 29 | 29 | 28 | 27 | 26 | 26 |
| 215 | 48 | 47 | 45 | 44 | 42 | 41 | 39 | 38 | 37 | 36 | 35 | 34 | 33 | 32 | 31 | 30 | 29 | 28 | 28 | 27 | 26 |
| 220 | 49 | 48 | 46 | 45 | 43 | 42 | 40 | 39 | 38 | 37 | 36 | 35 | 34 | 33 | 32 | 31 | 30 | 29 | 28 | 28 | 27 |
| 225 | 51 | 49 | 47 | 46 | 44 | 43 | 41 | 40 | 39 | 38 | 36 | 35 | 34 | 33 | 32 | 31 | 31 | 30 | 29 | 28 | 27 |
| 230 | 52 | 50 | 48 | 47 | 45 | 44 | 42 | 41 | 40 | 38 | 37 | 36 | 35 | 34 | 33 | 32 | 31 | 30 | 30 | 29 | 28 |
| 235 | 53 | 51 | 49 | 48 | 46 | 44 | 43 | 42 | 40 | 39 | 38 | 37 | 36 | 35 | 34 | 33 | 32 | 31 | 30 | 29 | 29 |
| 240 | 54 | 52 | 50 | 49 | 47 | 45 | 44 | 43 | 41 | 40 | 39 | 38 | 37 | 36 | 35 | 34 | 33 | 32 | 31 | 30 | 29 |
| 245 | 55 | 53 | 51 | 50 | 48 | 46 | 45 | 43 | 42 | 41 | 40 | 38 | 37 | 36 | 35 | 34 | 33 | 32 | 32 | 31 | 30 |
| 250 | 56 | 54 | 52 | 51 | 49 | 47 | 46 | 44 | 43 | 42 | 40 | 39 | 38 | 37 | 36 | 35 | 34 | 33 | 32 | 31 | 30 |
| 255 | 57 | 55 | 53 | 52 | 50 | 48 | 47 | 45 | 44 | 43 | 41 | 40 | 39 | 38 | 37 | 36 | 35 | 34 | 33 | 32 | 31 |
| 260 | 58 | 56 | 54 | 53 | 51 | 49 | 48 | 46 | 45 | 43 | 42 | 41 | 40 | 38 | 37 | 36 | 35 | 34 | 33 | 33 | 32 |
| 265 | 60 | 57 | 56 | 54 | 52 | 50 | 49 | 47 | 46 | 44 | 43 | 42 | 40 | 39 | 38 | 37 | 36 | 35 | 34 | 33 | 32 |
| 270 | 61 | 59 | 57 | 55 | 53 | 51 | 49 | 48 | 46 | 45 | 44 | 42 | 41 | 40 | 39 | 38 | 37 | 36 | 35 | 34 | 33 |
| 275 | 62 | 60 | 58 | 56 | 54 | 52 | 50 | 49 | 47 | 46 | 44 | 43 | 42 | 41 | 40 | 38 | 37 | 36 | 35 | 34 | 34 |
| 280 | 63 | 61 | 59 | 57 | 55 | 53 | 51 | 50 | 48 | 47 | 45 | 44 | 43 | 41 | 40 | 39 | 38 | 37 | 36 | 35 | 34 |

*Weight in Pounds*

FIG. 18.5 The body mass index (BMI) is determined by aligning a patient's weight with his or her height. The BMI is found where the row of weight intersects the column of height. See text for more explanation. (From http://www.niddk.nih.gov.)

weight). The problem is never simply a weight problem. A patient weighs too much only when the percentage of total body weight made up of fat exceeds about 23% for males and 28% for females. A method for estimating the percent of body fat is the skinfold measurement.

*Triceps skinfold thickness.* Measurement of skinfold thickness with the use of calipers is a fairly simple procedure (proper technique is important) that yields data on the fat and protein reserves in the body. The triceps skinfold is the most common place of measurement; however, several other sites can be used, usually in addition to the triceps area. Skinfold thickness, coupled with measurements of the upper arm circumference, arm muscle circumference, and arm muscle area, provides accepted estimates of protein-energy malnutrition (PEM). The arm fat area may also be calculated and improves the body fat weight estimate when used along with triceps skinfold measurements. These measurements are all compared with standard normal values to assess the degree of malnutrition. As with other tests, the exact value obtained with any one measurement may not be as important

## TABLE 18.1 Current Laboratory Biochemical Tests and Guidelines for Interpretation

| Measurement of Index | Deficient | Normal | Sensitivity |
|---|---|---|---|
| Creatinine-height index (CHI) (%) | 40 | 60 | Poor |
| Serum albumin level (g/dL) | 2.5 | 3.5-5.0 | Limited because of long half-life (20 days) and because a negative acute phase protein will respond negatively to any physiologic stress |
| Serum transferrin level (mg/dL) | 100 | 200-400 | Poor; unpredictable response to refeeding |
| Total iron-binding capacity (TIBC) (mg/dL) | <250 | 250-350 | Poor; increased in pregnancy, iron deficiency, oral contraceptive use; iron may bind to proteins other than serum transferrin |
| Nitrogen balance | Negative balance | Equilibrium | Good, although nitrogen excretion often underestimated; must be carefully measured to be helpful |
| Thyroxin-binding prealbumin (TBPA) (mg/dL) | <10 | 10-20 | Limited; half-life short (2 days) but is a negative acute phase protein |
| Retinol-binding protein (RBP) (μg/dL) | <3 | 3-6 | Limited; half-life short (12 h) but is a negative acute phase protein |
| Total lymphocyte count (cells/mm$^3$) | <1200 | 2000-3500 | Limited; decreased in injury, chemotherapy, radiotherapy, surgery; increased in infection |
| Differential count for lymphocytes (%) | | 20-45 | Limited |
| Skin antigen testing | Negative | Positive | Good |

as the trend seen with serial measurements. It is important to establish baseline data for a patient when first admitted. Then the first signs of malnutrition can be detected and appropriate treatment implemented before serious deficiency symptoms occur.

*Other methods to assess body composition.* Other, more accurate methods for assessment of body fat include underwater weighing, body volume displacement, and electrical bioimpedance measurements. Only the last has a role in the hospital setting because underwater weighing requires the patient to be healthy and to be able to hold the breath under water for a period of time, and body volume displacement requires the patient to be confined in a small chamber. Electrical bioimpedance readings can be obtained at the bedside.

### Laboratory Biochemical Tests

Laboratory biochemical tests have been used in the past to assess nutritional status, specifically protein nutriture. It was once thought that serum proteins reflected protein status; however, we now know that they are not directly linked to nutritional status and should not be relied upon as indicators of nutritional status or recovery. Table 18.1 summarizes their relative sensitivities to body nutritional change and suggests guidelines for interpretation. There are four commonly identified serum transport proteins: albumin, transferrin, prealbumin, and retinol-binding proteins. Historically they have been used to assess protein status among individuals, but it is now understood that these serum proteins are not reflective of protein status and should not be used as a marker of nutritional adequacy. They can identify the presence of inflammation, which causes about a 25% decrease in the synthesis of serum proteins.

Creatine phosphate is used in muscle as an energy reserve molecule. When there is an increased demand for ATP, creatine donates a phosphate to adenosine diphosphate (ADP), making ATP. The more muscle mass there is in the body, the more creatine there will be. Creatine is metabolized to creatinine, the form in which it is largely excreted. The clearance of creatinine from the blood by the kidneys is a good indicator of renal function. Measurement of 24-hour urinary excretion of creatinine correlates with the patient's lean body weight (muscle mass): the greater the muscle mass, the higher the urinary excretion of creatinine. When expressed in terms of height, a measure generally unaffected by malnutrition, urinary excretion of creatinine can be used as a general measure of malnutrition. The CHI is a predictor of muscle mass but may not correlate well with arm muscle circumference, probably because of the many factors that govern the excretion of creatinine.

Nitrogen balance measurements, using 24-hour urine specimens, are valuable for assessment of protein intake and are useful in acute care settings. However, an underestimation of nitrogen excretion can occur in patients with burns, diarrhea, vomiting, or other nitrogen-losing conditions. During critical illness the urea nitrogen urine concentration increases radically, which reflects protein catabolism seen in the inflammatory process; therefore even if the patient is in positive nitrogen balance, he or she may still be catabolic. A commonly used clinical estimation is as follows:

$$\text{Nitrogen balance} = \text{grams of nitrogen intake} - (24\text{-hr grams of UUN} + 4\text{ g})$$

Malnutrition can lead to a decline in immunocompetence. Total lymphocyte count (lymphocytes make the immunoglobulins) or their function can be measured. An easy test of their function (which requires them to have adequate protein to make their antibodies) is to challenge them with skin antigen testing. Antigens used are those to which a patient is most likely to have been previously exposed. With these, a quick antigen-antibody reaction should be seen at the skin-testing site, much like a positive tuberculin skin test reaction. However, if the patient is protein deficient, the skin test reaction will be greatly diminished or absent. However, because of the inflammatory response seen in many critically ill patients there measures are rarely used in clinical practice. It should be noted that an iron deficiency can also diminish the response.

As can be seen, no one test constitutes a perfect assessment of a patient's nutritional status. But with the appropriate use of selected anthropometric and biochemical measurements, along with astute observations by respiratory care practitioners, an adequate nutritional profile can be developed. Other sources should be consulted for further discussion of nutritional assessment.

---

### SIMPLY STATED

No single measurement can determine the patient's nutritional status. A combination of the history, physical examination, and laboratory tests is often needed to determine the patient's nutritional needs.

---

## ROLE OF THE RESPIRATORY THERAPIST IN NUTRITIONAL ASSESSMENT

Alert members of the patient care team not involved in direct nutritional assessment, including RTs, can contribute significantly to achieving good nutrition for patients with respiratory disorders. Signs or symptoms of potential nutritional problems should be sought during routine patient care.

In examining a patient with respiratory problems, the first step is to observe. Although malnutrition can never be

diagnosed by simple inspection (except in extreme cases), much information can be learned by simply looking. During this time, various differential diagnoses can be formulated, which subsequent findings will confirm or disprove.

### Inspection Findings

One should note the effects of body mass on breathing efficiency. Cachectic (nutritionally depleted) patients have readily outlined bony structures with depression of the intercostal spaces. Accessory muscles of respiration are often visible in these patients. Because severe muscle wasting can decrease lung function in those without lung disease, malnourished patients with COPD have compounded breathing difficulties. Patients who are obese have difficulty breathing in direct proportion to their excess fat weight. Obesity imposes a restrictive condition on top of whatever lung condition already exists. Fig. 18.6 illustrates the effects of excess fat weight on the mechanics of breathing. Note the increased energy that must be expended during inspiration. Pregnancy can produce similar interference with the mechanics of breathing.

During inspection of the patient, the amount of effort that can be generated during coughing should be observed. Muscle weakness accompanies poor nutrition. Also, the viscosity of the sputum should be noted. This, along with jugular venous pressure (JVP) estimation, can give clues to fluid balance. Of course, in patients with right ventricular heart failure the JVP will be elevated by factors other than simple fluid overload. In addition, a distended abdomen, as with ascites

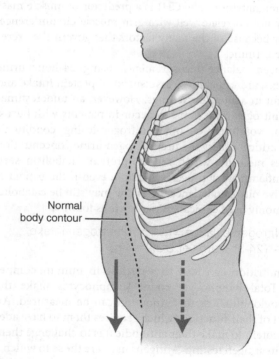

Normal body contour —

A

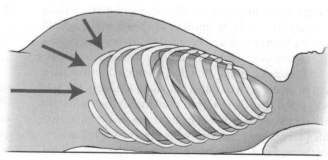

B

**FIG. 18.6** Effects of obesity on mechanics of breathing. **A,** In normal-weight persons, the weight of viscera is borne by the pelvic area, and the net weight force is in the direction of the *dotted arrow.* However, in obese people, the net force of the weight *(solid arrow)* is not supported by the pelvic area, and weight pulls directly down on the ribs. This favors the expiratory phase, making inspiration more difficult. **B,** In the supine position, the weight of viscera pushes up on the diaphragm, again making inspiration difficult.

(fluid retention), may cause fluid balance and breathing problems. Edema of the extremities should also be noted; when present, it may require alterations in the patient's fluid and sodium intake.

## Auscultation Findings

Coarse or fine crackles in the lung bases on auscultation can indicate either fluid overload or a loss of blood protein (oncotic pressure). Wheezing may be associated with some food intolerances or foods that contain yellow food coloring. As previously mentioned, alcohol can produce wheezing in some people. Aspirated food can also produce wheezing. The fine, late inspiratory crackles of atelectasis may result from decreased surfactant production resulting from malnutrition. Hearing the $S_3$ heart sound of congestive heart failure could suggest that fluid may be accumulating in the lungs. An $S_4$ heart sound can be associated with severe anemia.

## Laboratory Findings

Decreases in pulmonary function measures, such as FVC or $FEV_1$, may indicate malnutrition. In morbidly obese patients, decreased FVC can also occur with excess adipose tissue weight because of adipose tissue's restrictive effects. Decreases in peak expiratory pressure (PEP) and peak inspiratory pressure (PIP) are also associated with poor nutrition. Altered lung compliance, as measured in the laboratory, or effective compliance, as measured when taking ventilator parameters, can result from fluid and serum albumin changes acutely or from chronic malnutrition.

Arterial blood gas (ABG) values can be altered with nutrition, as mentioned previously. Increased $Paco_2$ levels can result from excess parenteral infusion of glucose or simply from insufficient muscle energy to achieve adequate ventilation. The chemoreceptor set point can also be altered by changes in protein (amino acid) intake, thereby altering

sensitivity to $Paco_2$ levels. Oxygenation parameters (oxygen saturation, oxygen content, hemoglobin) are all affected by nutritional status. Anemias can result from deficiencies in iron, folic acid, or vitamin $B_{12}$. Some patients may not be able to tolerate high intakes of fat or lipid infusions because of the resulting lowered $Pao_2$.

Changes in pH can indicate changes in dietary intake of potassium, sodium, or foods that leave an alkaline or acidic residue. Low $Pao_2$ levels, with subsequent lactate production, can lower pH as well. As alluded to earlier, any change in the $Paco_2$ set point can alter acid-base balance.

The RT can become directly involved in the nutritional assessment of patients by measuring $\dot{V}o_2$ in determining energy needs. In addition, the eating environment and conditions that may affect the eating process should be assessed. An effort should be made to have clean equipment in the patient's room, to empty suction bottles, and to remove or hide sputum cups during mealtimes. A prerequisite to good nutrition is a good appetite, and a good appetite is hard to invoke unless the surroundings are pleasant. The RT can further assist by helping patients receive adequate oxygen therapy during and after meals and by scheduling breathing treatments to not interfere with mealtimes. Patients who are using oxygen masks should have an order for oxygen via cannula while eating. Attending to the oxygenation of the patient is of great nutritional importance. A decrease in oxygen saturation while eating can occur in patients with severe COPD. A patient who is short of breath may not eat, and if the patient does eat, food metabolism may be compromised.

A respiratory problem is rarely caused by poor nutrition alone; however, the RT will often see nutritional deficiencies complicating an existing lung problem. Being alert to the effect of nutrition on respiratory function may help stabilize the condition of a patient with lung disease that was previously deteriorating because of nutritional neglect.

## KEY POINTS

- The use of food for energy at the cellular level requires oxygen to support a controlled combustion process that produces energy molecules of ATP, which are used in all of the body processes for energy.
- The metabolic rates of the tissues dictate the amount of oxygen needing to be picked up in the lungs. Oxygen uptake ($\dot{V}o_2$) is a respiratory factor that can be measured in the laboratory or at the bedside.
- If $\dot{V}o_2$ is measured while a person is in a resting state, on awakening, the REE or RMR can be calculated.
- If the calorie intake is less than needed, there will be a decrease in weight, as is commonly seen in patients with COPD.
- Nutritional repletion in respiratory patients is often hindered by some of the necessary therapeutic actions. Bronchodilators may produce nausea; oxygen by nasal cannula disturbs the sense of smell and therefore taste because 70% of the taste of food is contributed by the sense of smell.
- The diaphragm, as the main muscle of respiration, needs adequate glycogen stores to be able to meet the metabolic

- demand of breathing, especially when the work of breathing is elevated.
- Protein is needed for maintaining the heart muscle, buffering acids, helping to make clotting factors in the blood, and transporting lipids and iron in the blood.
- Oncotic pressure (a form of osmotic pressure that tends to pull water into the blood vessels from the tissue) in the blood is maintained primarily by albumin, the major blood protein produced by the liver.
- Water is the major constituent of the blood and body cells. Sufficient water intake is necessary for proper circulation, clearing of waste from the body, and maintenance of blood pressure.
- The metabolic process can be divided into two pathways: those that break down molecules as energy is released (catabolism) and those that build up new molecules (anabolism) to be used in a structural or a functional role.
- The basic nutritional requirements include carbohydrate, protein, fat, vitamins, minerals, and water. Carbohydrate, protein, and fat provide the energy the body needs, as well

as the basic chemical skeletons on which structural and functional body systems are built.

- Patients with more severe COPD often do better with a higher fat content in the diet and less carbohydrate because there is less carbon dioxide production.
- Patients with cystic fibrosis tend to lack certain enzymes produced in the pancreas and needed for the digestion and absorption of fats. As a result, such patients generally need to take dietary supplements to compensate.
- Adequate fluid intake is extremely important for patients with respiratory disorders. Proper function of the lungs' mucociliary clearance mechanism requires good hydration.
- The routes of nutritional administration can be either enteral or parenteral. The preferred route is enteral. If a patient is intubated and cannot take food by mouth, tube feeding is instituted through a nasogastric tube.
- When all other attempts at feeding are unsuccessful, the last resort is TPN. TPN is the feeding of patients by direct infusion of nutrients into either a peripheral or a central vein.

- The BMI is the primary method for assessment of the appropriateness of weight for a given height. The BMI is determined by weight (kg) divided by height ($m^2$).
- Cachectic (nutritionally depleted) patients have readily outlined bony structures with depression of the intercostal spaces. Accessory muscles of respiration are often visible in these patients.
- Patients who are obese have difficulty breathing in direct proportion to their excess fat weight. Obesity imposes a restrictive condition on top of whatever lung condition already exists.
- The association between hypophosphatemia and failure to wean from mechanical ventilation in patients on ventilator support requires monitoring of serum phosphate levels and treatment to prevent severe hypophosphatemia.

## CASE STUDY

The patient, FM, is a 58-year-old white female who presents to the emergency department (ED). She is retired from a cashier's position at a large chain store. She lives with her husband who is 59 years old and has a history of myocardial infarction (MI). Her chief complaints are extreme fatigue and difficulty completing activities of daily living (ADLs). Her past medical history reveals the following:

- Diagnosed with emphysema 4 years ago, before she had frequent episodes of bronchitis and upper respiratory infections
- Medications include ipratropium bromide and albuterol sulfate
- Smoker: 1 pack/day for more than 44 years; quit 1½ years ago
- Family history: significant for lung cancer in father and uncle
  A physical examination shows the following:
- General appearance: female in no acute distress
- Vitals: temperature, 98.6°C; heart rate 90 beats/min; respiratory rate, 23 breaths/min; blood pressure, 134/85 mm Hg
- Heart: regular rate and rhythm; mild jugular distention
- Neurologic: alert and oriented; cranial nerves intact
- Skin: warm and dry
- Extremities: mild pitting edema, 1+; no clubbing or cyanosis
- Chest/lungs: breath sounds decreased; on percussion, hyperresonant; wheezing with prolonged expiration; rhonchi; use of accessory muscles at rest
- Abdomen: normal examination
- Weight: 120 lb = 54.5 kg
- Height: 5 ft, 3 in
- Usual body weight: 140 to 150 lb (3 years ago)
- Ideal body weight: 115 lb
- BMI: healthy range
- Significant weight loss since diagnosis of COPD
- Edentulous with poorly fitting dentures
  Patient was admitted to the hospital with an admitting diagnosis of acute exacerbation of COPD, increasing dyspnea, hypercapnia, rule out pneumonia
  The plan includes the following:
- $O_2$ at 1 L/min via nasal cannula; $O_2$ saturation 90% to 92%
- IV fluids started at $D_5$ half-normal saline with 20 mEq KCl at 75 mL/h
- Medications: methylprednisolone (Solu-Medrol)

- Antibiotic: cephalosporin (Ancef)
- Bronchodilator: ipratropium bromide and albuterol sulfate
- ABGs q6h, chest radiograph, sputum cultures, and Gram stain
  The diagnosis is acute exacerbation of COPD with bacterial pneumonia, progressive COPD.

### Laboratory Values
#### Chemistry Laboratory

| Values | FM Values | Normal Range |
|---|---|---|
| Albumin (g/dL) | 3.3 ↓ | 3.5-5.0 |
| Prealbumin (mg/dL) | 15 ↓ | 16-40 |
| Transferrin (mg/dL) | 215 | 200-400 |
| Sodium (mEq/L) | 138 | 135-145 |
| Potassium (mEq/L) | 3.8 | 3.5-5.0 |
| Chloride (mEq/L) | 102 | 96-106 |
| $PO_4$ (mg/dL) | 3.3 | 3.0-4.5 |
| Magnesium (mEq/L) | 1.9 | 1.3-2.1 |
| Total $CO_2$ (mEq/L) | 31 ↑ | 23-29 |
| Glucose (mg/dL) | 90 | |
| Total bilirubin (mg/dL) | 0.5 | 0.3-1.9 |
| BUN (mg/dL) | 10 | 10-20 |
| Uric acid (mg/dL) | 4.0 | 3.5 and 7.2 |
| Calcium (mg/dL) | 9.3 | 8.5-10.2 |

#### Hematology Laboratory

| Values | FM Values | Normal Range |
|---|---|---|
| WBC × $10^3$ ($mm^3$) | 14 | 4.5-10 |
| RBC × $10^6$ ($mm^3$) | 4.5 | 4.2-5.4 |
| Hgb (g/dL) | 11.6 | 12.3-15.3 |
| Hct (%) | 34.9 | 36.1-44.3 |

| ABG Values | Admission Values | Day 3 | Normal Range |
|---|---|---|---|
| pH | 7.28 | 7.5 | 7.38-7.42 |
| $Paco_2$ (mm Hg) | 51 | 41 | 38-42 |
| $Pao_2$ (mmHg) | 74 | 91 | 75-100 |
| $SO_2$ (%) | 92 | 95 | 94-100 |
| $HCO_3^-$ (mEq/L) | 23 | 28 | 22-28 |

## CASE STUDY—cont'd

Her usual nutritional intake includes the following:
Breakfast: tea with sugar, ½ cup oatmeal
Lunch: ½ cup cottage cheese, small amount of canned fruit
Dinner: soup and crackers, eggs, and toast
Drinking juices or caffeinated colas throughout the day
Complains of poor appetite, taste changes, and weight loss, fatigue when cooking meals
Her nutritional diagnosis is inadequate oral/food intake and involuntary weight loss.

### Interventions
Educate the patient regarding use of bronchodilators and caffeine intake.
Provide suggestions to ease preparation of foods/meals.

Increase intake of food throughout day, including small, frequent meals.
Increase nutrient density of meals and snacks without increasing volume.
Rest before and after meals.
Improve $O_2$ status before and after meals.
Schedule treatments at least 1 hour before meals; improve physical conditioning.

## ASSESSMENT QUESTIONS

1. What gas is required for the optimal production of ATP?
   a. Carbon dioxide
   b. Oxygen
   c. Nitrous oxide
   d. Argon
2. Which of the following is an indicator of the energy requirements of the patient?
   a. $Pao_2/Pao_2$ ratio
   b. Minute ventilation
   c. $\dot{V}o_2$ per minute
   d. Vital capacity
3. Which of the following is true about the REE?
   a. It requires a $\dot{V}o_2$ measurement to calculate
   b. It gives an exact estimate of the patient's nutritional needs
   c. It cannot be measured in mechanically ventilated patients
   d. It should be measured daily
4. Measuring the patient's energy expenditure using oxygen consumption is referred to as which of the following?
   a. Direct calorimetry
   b. Indirect calorimetry
   c. Simple calorimetry
   d. Complex calorimetry
5. Which of the following is a pulmonary effect of malnutrition?
   a. Increased $D_{LCO}$
   b. Increased $FEV_1$
   c. Increased risk for pneumonia
   d. Catabolism of fats to meet glucose needs
6. Which of the following in excess quantities contributes to the most $CO_2$ production?
   a. Protein
   b. Carbohydrates
   c. Fat
   d. Calories

7. What element must be stored in sufficient quantities to meet the metabolic demands of the diaphragm?
   a. Arginine
   b. Glycogen
   c. 2,3-DPG
   d. Fat
8. Which of the following is true about anaerobic metabolism?
   a. It can cause a metabolic acidosis
   b. It results in reduced lactate production
   c. It results in reduced production of carbon dioxide
   d. It requires oxygen to take place
9. What is the RQ value of a patient on a pure carbohydrate diet?
   a. 0.60
   b. 0.70
   c. 0.85
   d. 1.00
10. In feeding the patient with pulmonary disease, how many grams of protein per kilogram of body weight are initially required?
    a. 1.5 to 2.0
    b. 1.2 to 1.5
    c. 0.8 to 1.0
    d. 0.6 to 0.8
11. Which of the following may be more difficult to achieve with a high-carbohydrate feeding?
    a. Oxygenation
    b. Cellular gas exchange
    c. Oxygen transport
    d. Weaning from mechanical ventilation
12. Nitrogen balance is useful in determining:
    a. The possible need for increased protein
    b. The adequacy of fat intake
    c. The need for vitamin supplementation
    d. Fluid and electrolyte balance

13. Which of the following is associated with a low-protein diet?
    a. Increased work of breathing
    b. Increased fixed acid load
    c. Immune compromise
    d. Increased stress on the kidneys

14. Which of the following is not associated with a high-fat diet?
    a. Increased risk for heart disease
    b. Decreased tissue oxygenation
    c. Decreased DLCO
    d. Increased carbon dioxide production

15. What mineral plays a very important role in oxygen transport?
    a. Calcium
    b. Iron
    c. Zinc
    d. Magnesium

16. What route of nutritional feeding is considered as the first choice in feeding patients?
    a. Enteral
    b. Parenteral
    c. Intravenous
    d. Subcutaneous

17. Which of the following is not associated with an increased metabolism?
    a. Severe burns
    b. Severe infection
    c. Trauma
    d. Hypothyroidism

18. Which of the following might indicate poor nutritional status?
    a. BMI at normal weight
    b. Nitrogen balance
    c. Positive response to skin antigen testing
    d. Negative nitrogen balance

19. What factor may contribute to decreased colloid osmotic pressure and pulmonary edema?
    a. Hypoalbuminemia
    b. High-fat diet
    c. High magnesium levels
    d. Essential fatty acid deficiency

20. How does the cachectic patient appear physically?
    a. Central obesity only
    b. Very thin and malnourished
    c. Edematous around the face
    d. Very short of breath

## BIBLIOGRAPHY

Academy of Nutrition and Dietetics: Evidence analysis library, chronic obstructive pulmonary disease. Available at https://www.andeal.org/topic.cfm?menu=5301. Retrieved July 9, 2016.

Academy of Nutrition and Dietetics: Evidence analysis library, critical illness. Available at http://preview.andeal.org/topic.cfm?menu=5302&pcat=4106&cat=4524. Retrieved July 9, 2016.

Albertine KH. Anatomy of the lungs. In: *Murray and Nadel's textbook of respiratory medicine*. 6th ed. Philadelphia, PA: Elsevier Saunders; 2015:37–60.

Alsumrain MH, Jawad SA, Imran NB, et al. Association of hypophosphatemia with failure-to-wean from mechanical ventilation. *Ann Clin Lab Sci*. 2010;40(2):144–148.

Benjamin I, Griggs RC, Wing EJ, et al. *Andreoli and Carpenter's Cecil essentials of medicine*. 9th ed. Philadelphia, PA: Saunders; 2015.

Benott RN, Bistrian B. Metabolic and nutritional aspects of weaning from mechanical ventilation. *Crit Care Med*. 1989;17:181.

Budweiser S, Meyer K, Jorres RA, et al. Nutritional depletion and its relationship to respiratory impairment in patients with chronic respiratory failure due to COPD or restrictive thoracic disease. *Eur J Clin Nutr*. 2008;62:436.

Chen R, Tunstall-Pedoe H, Bolton-Smith C, et al. Association of dietary antioxidants and waist circumference with pulmonary function and airway obstruction. *Am J Epidemiol*. 2001;153:157.

Cohen RI, Marzouk K, Berkoski P, et al. Body composition and resting energy expenditure in clinically stable, non-weight losing patients with emphysema or chronic bronchitis in acute respiratory failure. *Chest*. 2003;124:1365.

Doley J, Mallampalli A, Sandberg M. Nutritional management for the patient requiring prolonged mechanical ventilation. *Nutr Clin Pract*. 2011;26:232.

Federspiel C, Itenov T, Thormar K, et al. The effect of low phosphate levels on respiratory failure and mortality in critically ill patients. *Am J Respir Crit Care Med*. 2016;193:A3648.

Fiaccadori E, Coffrini E, Fraccia C, et al. Hypophosphatemia and phosphorus depletion in respiratory and peripheral muscles of patients with respiratory failure due to COPD. *Chest*. 1994;105:1392.

Fletcher AE, Breeze E, Shetly PS. Antioxidant vitamins and mortality in older persons: findings from the nutrition add-on study to the Medical Research Council Trial of Assessment and Management of Older People in the Community. *Am J Clin Nutr*. 2003;78:999.

Girardet JPH, Viola S. Nutrition and severe chronic respiratory diseases: pathophysiologic mechanisms. *Pediatr Pulmonol Suppl*. 2001;23:20.

Haugen HA, Chan LN, Li F. Indirect calorimetry: a practical guide for clinicians. *Nutr Clin Pract*. 2007;22:377.

Jozwiak M, Teboul JL, Monnet X. Extravascular lung water in critical care: recent advances and clinical applications. *Ann Intensive Care*. 2015;5(1):38. http://dx.doi.org/10.1186/s13613-015-0081-9.

Khan SH, Karhik AM. Medical nutrition therapy for pulmonary diseases. In: *Krause's food and the nutrition care process*. 14th ed. St. Louis: Saunders; 2017.

Koehler F, Doehner W, Hoernig S, et al. Anorexia in congestive obstructive pulmonary disease: association to cachexia and hormonal derangement. *Int J Cardiol*. 2007;119:83.

Lev S, Cohen J, Singer P. Indirect calorimetry measurements in the critically ill patient: facts and controversies—the heat is on. *Crit Care Clin*. 2010;26:e1.

Lewandowski K, Lewandowski M. Intensive care in the obese. *Best Pract Res Clin Anaesthesiol*. 2011;25:95.

Mason PJ, Dobbs LG. Alveolar epithelium and pulmonary surfactant. In: *Murray and Nadel's textbook of respiratory medicine*. 6th ed. Philadelphia, PA: Elsevier Saunders; 2015: 37–60.

McClave SA, Snider HL. Use of indirect calorimetry in clinical nutrition. *Nutr Clin Pract*. 1992;7:207.

Murciano D, Rigud D, Pingleton S, et al. Diaphragmatic function in severely malnourished patients with anorexia nervosa: effects of renutrition. *Am J Respir Crit Care Med*. 1994;150:1569.

Orozco-Levi M. Structure and function of the respiratory muscles in patients with COPD: impairment or adaptation? *Eur Respir J*. 2003;22(suppl 46):415.

Raguso CA, Luthy C. Nutritional status in chronic obstructive pulmonary disease: role of hypoxia. *Nutrition*. 2011;27:138.

Schwartz DD. Pulmonary and failure. In: *Contemporary nutrition support practice*. 2nd ed. Philadelphia, PA: Saunders; 2003.

Stacy KM. Pulmonary alterations. In: Urden LD, Stacy KM, Lough ME, eds. *Priority in critical care nursing*. 7th ed. St. Louis: Mosby; 2015.

Stallings VA, Stark LJ, Robinson KA, et al. Ad Hoc Working Group: evidence-based practice recommendations for nutrition-related management of children and adults with cystic fibrosis and pancreatic insufficiency: results of a systematic review. *J Am Diet Assoc*. 2008;108(5):832–839.

Swartz DB. Malnutrition in congestive obstructive pulmonary disease. *Respir Care Clin North Am*. 2006;12:S21.

Vitale J. *Impact of nutrition on immune function: nutrition in disease series*. Columbus, OH: Ross Laboratories; 1979.

Weir JBV. New methods for calculating metabolic rate with special reference to protein metabolism. *J Physiol*. 1949;109(1).

Wooley JA, Sax HC. Indirect calorimetry: applications to practice. *Nutr Clin Pract*. 2003;18:434.

Yen EH, Quinton H, Borowitz D. Better nutritional status in early childhood is associated with improved clinical outcomes and survival in patients with cystic fibrosis. *J Pediatr*. 2013;162(3):530–535.

Zhao Y, Li Z, Shi Y, et al. Effect of hypophosphatemia on the withdrawal of mechanical ventilation in patients with acute exacerbations of chronic obstructive pulmonary disease. *Biomed Rep*. 2016;4(4):413–416.

# 19

# Sleep and Breathing Assessment

*Pooja Raju and Zaza Cohen*

## LEARNING OBJECTIVES

*After reading this chapter, you will be able to:*

1. Discuss the importance of sleep disorders in the United States.
2. Describe the normal stages of sleep with associated physiologic changes in the cardiopulmonary system.
3. Describe the role of the respiratory therapist in the assessment of patients for potential sleep disordered breathing. Explain the correlation among sleep apnea, snoring, and excessive daytime sleepiness.
4. List the criteria used with the Epworth Sleepiness Scale and the Berlin Questionnaire surveys in assessing the presence of a sleep disorder.
5. Describe the expected findings in the assessment of patients with sleep disordered breathing. List the clinical

and assessment criteria for obstructive and central sleep apnea.
6. Describe the role of a polysomnogram in providing a differential diagnosis for sleep disordered breathing.
7. Describe the typical physiologic parameters monitored on a polysomnogram montage.
8. List the criteria used to classify sleep apnea as mild, moderate, or severe.
9. Discuss the treatment options and their mechanisms of action in patients with obstructive sleep apnea.
10. Identify the symptoms and assessment characteristics for children with sleep apnea.

## OUTLINE

## KEY TERMS

apnea-hypopnea index (AHI)
arousal
Berlin Questionnaire
central sleep apnea (CSA)
delta-wave sleep
EEG arousal
electroencephalogram
Epworth Sleepiness Scale (ESS)
excessive daytime sleepiness/
  somnolence (EDS)
hypopnea

Mallampati score
micrognathia
mixed sleep apnea (MSA)
montage
non–rapid eye movement
obstructive sleep apnea (OSA)
polysomnogram
rapid eye movement
respiratory effort–related arousal
  (RERA)
retrognathia

sleep apnea
sleep architecture
sleep disordered breathing
slow-wave sleep
snoring
STOP-BANG analysis
sudden infant death syndrome
  (SIDS)

According to the National Sleep Foundation, approximately 40 million Americans suffer from some type of sleep disorder. The National Heart, Lung, and Blood Institute estimates that of those with sleep disorders, nearly 18 million have some form of sleep disordered breathing (SDB), such as sleep apnea. Many experts suggest that the prevalence of sleep disorders is often underestimated and underreported. With a staggering number of Americans afflicted with sleep-related illnesses, respiratory therapists (RTs) must be prepared to identify sleep disorder symptoms in their patients. Critical thinking skills that relate a patient's known cardiopulmonary history to the presenting complaints and symptoms are key to identifying sleep-related complications or comorbidities.

RTs, sleep technologists, and sleep technicians are important members of the patient care team responsible for conducting a sleep assessment study, or polysomnogram (PSG), and related functions in sleep disorder centers throughout the country. Clinicians working in these centers provide the diagnostic and therapeutic expertise needed to provide primary care physicians, board-certified sleep specialists, and other physicians with the information necessary to correctly diagnose and treat sleep disorders.

There are several pathways to entering the sleep profession. Although on-the-job trainees can function without licenses or credentialing in some states, an increasing number of states are requiring credentialing, licensure, or both. At least part of the reason for this is that the Centers for Medicare and Medicaid Services requires that only specifically credentialed professionals perform sleep studies for Medicare beneficiaries. An individual can be credentialed to perform sleep studies by several boards. The Board of Registered Polysomnographic Technologists grants the credential of Registered Polysomnographic Technologist. The American Board of Sleep Medicine (ABSM) offers credentialing as a Registered Sleep Technologist.

In addition, licensed and credentialed RTs can perform sleep studies, noninvasive positive-pressure titration, and related functions in all 50 states. Many RTs are employed in sleep disorder centers, and their specific background in ventilation, pulmonary anatomy and physiology, pharmacology, and cardiopulmonary diseases makes them valuable assets to the sleep community.

It is recommended that an average adult should spend approximately 8 hours a day sleeping to ensure physical and mental restoration. However, sleep may be a frustrating experience for many individuals with sleep disorders. With sleep occupying one-third of our life, the quality and quantity of sleep have long-range health and quality-of-life implications. Worse yet, sleep disorders can actually exacerbate or compromise preexisting disease conditions, such as diabetes and hypertension, and present life-threatening scenarios. This chapter provides the reader with information on normal sleep staging, the physiologic changes seen during normal sleep, the assessment of SDB, and a brief discussion of selected sleep disorders.

## NORMAL STAGES OF SLEEP

Although dictionary definitions of sleep may suggest a "suspension of consciousness and muscular activity" or a "reduction of one's awareness of the environment," in reality, sleep is an active process with continuous stimulation of specific regions of the brain throughout the night.

Historically, sleep has been classified in various ways; however, current nomenclature recognizes only two primary states of sleep for adults and children: non–rapid eye movement (NREM) and rapid eye movement (REM). There are special states for newborns and infants up to 6 months of age because their brain wave patterns do not yet conform to standard adult classification. They include definitions such as wake, NREM, REM, and transitional sleep. In adults, during a normal 8-hour sleeping period, NREM and REM stages cycle back and forth every 60 to 90 minutes for a total of four or five cycles.

### Non–Rapid Eye Movement Sleep

Sleep normally begins with NREM and progresses to REM sleep. While in NREM, electroencephalogram (EEG) tracings demonstrate diminishing brain activity, suggesting a resting or restorative state. NREM stages are broken into N1, N2, and N3, the "N" standing for non-REM. Each stage is differentiated by the amplitude, or wave height, and the frequency, or speed, of the EEG tracings (Fig. 19.1). With each progressive stage of NREM, the state of sleep is deeper.

As sleep progresses, children and adults normally begin with stage N1. During stage N1, slow rolling eye movements and low-amplitude and mixed-frequency EEG waves are noted. Only 5% to 10% of the sleep period is normally spent in N1. Subsequently, sleep usually progresses to stage N2. Stage N2 is characteristic of EEG tracings showing *K complexes* and *sleep spindles* (see Fig. 19.1). In adults, about 40% to 50% of the total sleep period is spent in stage N2.

Stage N3 is considered the deepest stage of sleep and is about 25% of the sleep period. The EEG demonstrates slow-wave sleep or delta-wave sleep, which is characterized by high-amplitude waves. While in N3, sensitivity to external stimuli is diminished, and it is difficult to awaken a person out of this stage of sleep. Essential growth hormones are also released during this stage during childhood and adolescence, especially during the first half of the night.

With age, the percentage of time spent in stages N1 and N2 progressively increases, whereas stage N3 sleep decreases dramatically, dropping by as much as 50% after puberty. Because stages N1 and N2 are lighter stages of sleep, a higher incidence of insomnia is understandably reported with age.

### SIMPLY STATED

NREM occupies about 75% of the sleep period normally and includes restorative sleep known as slow-wave sleep.

Awake-low voltage-random, fast

$50\ \mu v$

$1\ sec$

Drowsy: 8-13 CPS, alpha waves

Stage N1: 4-7 CPS, theta waves

Theta waves

Stage N2: 12-14 CPS, sleep spindles and K complexes

Sleep spindle

K complex —

Stage N3: 0.5-2 CPS, delta waves, amplitude >75 $\mu$V

REM Sleep-low voltage-random, fast with sawtooth waves

Sawtooth waves  Sawtooth waves

**FIG. 19.1** Human sleep stages. *CPS,* Cycles per second; *REM,* rapid eye movement. (Adapted from Hauri P: *The sleep disorders: current concepts,* ed 2, Kalamazoo, MI, 1982, Upjohn. Used with permission from Pfizer Inc.)

## Rapid Eye Movement Sleep

REM is named for the presence of the rapid fluttering or rolling of the eyes and is characterized by the loss of muscle tone. The brain is very active, and dreaming almost always occurs during this stage. Throughout the night, REM episodes increase in duration and normally account for about 25% of the total sleep period. EEG tracings demonstrate low-amplitude mixed-frequency waves, similar to those seen in N1 sleep (see Fig. 19.1), except that patients in REM have rapid eye movements and a substantial decrease in muscle tone. Chin tone is lowest during REM, and electromyography (EMG) monitoring of muscles of the chin (representative of skeletal muscle tone) demonstrates measurements that are similar to a paralyzed state. This partial paralysis decreases the minute ventilation in healthy adults and children, producing associated episodes of relative hypoxemia

and hypercapnia. Additional cardiovascular changes during REM sleep include great variability of blood pressure and heart rate.

Understandably, the physiologic effects of REM may be more profound in patients with preexisting pulmonary or cardiac disease. Normal physiologic changes associated with REM may precipitate increased complications associated with altered ventilation, blood pressure, and heart rate for these particular patients.

### SIMPLY STATED

REM occupies 25% of the sleep period and is characterized by a high level of brain activity, dreaming, and partial paralysis of skeletal muscles.

**FIG. 19.2** Histogram showing normal sleep architecture for each stage of the sleep period for a young, healthy adult, beginning with the patient's awake state (WAKE). Note the cycling of stages throughout the sleep.

A histogram is a graph representing the pattern of sleep architecture and is part of each sleep study (Fig. 19.2). Although the approximate percentage of sleep time spent in the three phases of NREM and REM previously described are representative of normal sleep architecture, each person has a distinct pattern particular to his or her own sleep cycle. This pattern can also vary on a day-to-day basis based on the person's overall tiredness, physical exertion during waking hours, and overall lifestyle.

In summary, during normal sleep, we begin at stage N1, progress to stage N2, and then reach stage N3 as sleep deepens. During NREM, the brain is in a state of rest, while the body can still move and respond to stimuli. Once REM sleep is initiated, the brain becomes more active, and the body experiences partial skeletal muscle paralysis, with variability in ventilation, blood pressure, and heart rate.

## PHYSIOLOGY DURING SLEEP

Respiration is controlled metabolically and behaviorally during wakefulness. During sleep, only metabolic control is present. Therefore there is a decrease in hypoxic and hypercapneic ventilatory responses. As a result, the $Pao_2$ decreases by 2 to 12 mm Hg, oxygen saturation drops by about 2%, and $Paco_2$ rises by 2 to 8 mm Hg. During NREM sleep there is a decrease in heart rate, cardiac output, and blood pressure. During REM there are fluctuations in heart rate, blood pressure, and respiratory drive. The heart rate variability is increased, and cardiac arrhythmias are commonly seen. During sleep there is reduced esophageal motility; however, gastric acid secretion tends to peak between 10 PM and 2 AM. There is reduced urine volume during sleep due to increased water reabsorption. Release of growth hormone is mainly during N3 sleep stage, and sleep deprivation suppresses this hormone. Cortisol levels are lowest during sleep.

## SLEEP DISORDERS

Sleep disorders can occur at any age. Various sleep-related illnesses affect quality and/or quantity of sleep and lead to signs and symptoms of physical and mental disorders, in addition to sleep deprivation and somnolence. Sleep disorders can be broadly classified into sleep-related breathing disorders, insomnia, hypersomnolence disorders, circadian rhythm disorders, parasomnias, and sleep-related movement disorders. Sleep-related breathing disorders include obstructive sleep apnea (OSA), which is the cessation of airflow for more than 10 seconds due to complete anatomic upper airway closure, and hypopnea, which is generally characterized by a substantial but not total decrease in airflow due to relaxation of upper airway tissue. These and other sleep-related breathing disorders are reviewed in detail later in this chapter; the rest of the sleep disorders are briefly discussed here.

Disorders of insomnia relate to persistent difficulty with sleep initiation, duration, consolidation, or quality of sleep despite adequate opportunity and circumstances for sleep. Hypersomnolence disorders relate to patients who have symptoms of excessive sleepiness and include narcolepsy.

Circadian rhythm disorders result when there is disruption of the normal 24-hour sleep-wake cycle and include jet lag and shift work disorder. Parasomnias are undesirable physical events or experiences that occur during sleep such as REM behavior disorder, night terrors, sleep walking, and others. Sleep-related movement disorders include disorders that involve movements that disturb sleep such as restless legs syndrome and periodic limb movement disorder.

Treatment of these various sleep disorders depends on the underlying etiology, and these treatments can often overlap. The approach to treatment is usually multimodal, ranging from behavioral modifications to utilization of medical equipment and use of medications.

## EVALUATION OF SLEEP DISORDERS

When assessing a patient who presents for evaluation of a sleep disorder, a thorough history and physical examination are invaluable to the health care personnel. Diagnoses can often be narrowed down by this simple evaluation. Additional tests may also be required and are discussed later in the chapter.

Everyone has experienced the difficulty of staying awake after a night of interrupted or shortened sleep. For individuals with sleep disorders, poor and inadequate sleep is likely to be a daily experience that leads to a key symptom of sleep-related disorders—excessive daytime sleepiness/somnolence (EDS). Daytime somnolence often interferes with the patient's ability to function during the day and ultimately increases the possibility of workplace or school accidents and has a negative impact on overall productivity and quality of life. Additional symptoms that patients may experience are snoring, daytime fatigue, early morning headaches, difficulty with memory, and unrefreshing sleep. However, many patients have these findings for many years before seeking medical assistance and often do not mention their symptoms, considering them a part of "normal" life. Certain tools have been developed that can provide additional valuable information and insight. They include the Epworth Sleepiness Scale (ESS), the Berlin Questionnaire, and the STOP-BANG Assessment. The usefulness of the ESS and the Berlin

Questionnaire is critical to the assessment of a possible sleep disorder. Inclusion of one or both surveys during the patient assessment will provide the RT with information crucial to identifying patient symptoms.

## Epworth Sleepiness Scale

The ESS is a simple, eight-item questionnaire that measures daytime sleepiness and is essential for initial screening of sleep disorders in adults. The ESS was developed by Dr. Murray Johns of the Epworth Hospital in Melbourne, Australia, in 1991. The survey presents eight situations, and the patient is asked to rate the chances of dozing in each situation, with the value of 0 representing no chance of dozing; 1, a slight chance of dozing; 2, a moderate chance of dozing; and 3, a high chance of dozing (Fig. 19.3). The sleepiness score is totaled, and if the ESS total is

---

**Epworth Sleepiness Scale**

Name: _____ Today's date: _____

Your age (Yrs): _____ Your sex (Male=M, Female=F): _____

How likely are you to doze off or fall asleep in the following situations, in contrast to feeling just tired?

This refers to your usual way of life in recent times.

Even if you haven't done some of these things recently try to work out how they would have affected you.

Use the following scale to choose the most appropriate number for each situation:

> 0 = would never doze
> 1 = slight chance of dozing
> 2 = moderate chance of dozing
> 3 = high chance of dozing

*It is important that you answer each question as best you can.*

| **Situation** | **Chance of Dozing (0-3)** |
|---|---|
| Sitting and reading _____ | ___ |
| Watching TV _____ | ___ |
| Sitting, inactive in a public place (e.g., a theatre or a meeting) _____ | ___ |
| As a passenger in a car for an hour without a break _____ | ___ |
| Lying down to rest in the afternoon when circumstances permit ____ | ___ |
| Sitting and talking to someone _____ | ___ |
| Sitting quietly after a lunch without alcohol _____ | ___ |
| In a car, while stopped for a few minutes in the traffic_____ | ___ |

**THANK YOU FOR YOUR COOPERATION**

© M.W. Johns 1990-97

---

**FIG. 19.3** Epworth Sleepiness Scale (ESS) developed by Dr. M. W. Johns. An ESS score of 9 or greater suggests the need to see a sleep specialist because excessive daytime sleepiness is present. (Courtesy M. W. Johns, 1990-1997. For information and permission to use, please contact: Mapi Research Trust, Lyon, France. – Internet: https://eprovide.mapi-trust.org. Johns MW. A new method for measuring daytime sleepiness: the Epworth Sleepiness Scale. *Sleep* 1991;14(6):540–545.)

1 to 6, sleep is appropriate and no EDS is noted. If the ESS total is 7 or 8, the score is considered average. An ESS score of 9 or greater indicates that the individual should consult a sleep specialist because there is evidence of EDS. The ESS questionnaire has been shown to have a high degree of reliability and internal consistency as an evaluation instrument.

## Berlin Questionnaire

The Berlin Questionnaire is an outcome of the 1996 Conference on Sleep in Primary Care held in Berlin, Germany. More than 120 pulmonary and primary care physicians developed the questionnaire from the literature to identify behaviors consistent with the presence of SDB. The focus of the instrument is deliberately limited to risk factors associated with sleep apnea in adults. The 10-item survey is divided into three categories, with category 1 addressing snoring, category 2 identifying EDS, and category 3 assessing current blood pressure and body mass index (BMI) (Fig. 19.4). To be classified as at high risk for sleep apnea, an individual must qualify for at least two categories. The Berlin Questionnaire has a high degree of sensitivity and specificity for predicting sleep apnea in individuals.

## STOP-BANG Assessment

Created in 2008 by a group of anesthesiologists, the STOP-BANG assessment is rapidly becoming the standard for

**Berlin** *Questionnaire*

© 1997 IONSLEEP

SLEEP EVALUATION IN PRIMARY CARE

**Category 1**

1. Complete the following:
   Height _____ Age _____
   Weight _____ Male/female ___

2. Do you snore?
   ☐ Yes
   ☐ No
   ☐ Don't know

*If you snore:*

3. Your snoring is?
   ☐ Slightly louder than breathing
   ☐ As loud as talking
   ☐ Louder than talking
   ☐ Very loud. Can be heard in adjacent rooms.

4. How often do you snore?
   ☐ Nearly every day
   ☐ 3-4 times a week
   ☐ 1-2 times a week
   ☐ 1-2 times a month
   ☐ Never or nearly never

5. Has your snoring ever bothered other people?
   ☐ Yes
   ☐ No

6. Has anyone noticed that you quit breathing during your sleep?
   ☐ Nearly every day
   ☐ 3-4 times a week
   ☐ 1-2 times a week
   ☐ 1-2 times a month
   ☐ Never or nearly never

**Category 2**

7. How often do you feel tired or fatigued after your sleep?
   ☐ Nearly every day
   ☐ 3-4 times a week
   ☐ 1-2 times a week
   ☐ 1-2 times a month
   ☐ Never or nearly never

8. During your waketime, do you feel tired, fatigued, or not up to par?
   ☐ Nearly every day
   ☐ 3-4 times a week
   ☐ 1-2 times a week
   ☐ 1-2 times a month
   ☐ Never or nearly never

9. Have you ever nodded off or fallen asleep while driving a vehicle?
   ☐ Yes
   ☐ No

   If yes, how often does it occur?
   ☐ Nearly every day
   ☐ 3-4 times a week
   ☐ 1-2 times a week
   ☐ 1-2 times a month
   ☐ Never or nearly never

**Category 3**

10. Do you have high blood pressure?
    ☐ Yes
    ☐ No
    ☐ Don't know

    BMI =

**Scoring questions:** Any answer within box outline is a positive response.

**Scoring categories:**
Category 1 is positive with 2 or more positive responses to questions 2-6 ☐
Category 2 is positive with 2 or more positive responses to questions 7-9 ☐
Category 3 is positive with 1 positive response and/or a BMI >30 ☐

**Final result:** 2 or more positive categories indicates a high likelihood of sleep disordered breathing.

**FIG. 19.4** The Berlin Questionnaire predicts risk factors associated with sleep apnea. (The Berlin Questionnaire is the outcome of the Conference on Sleep in Primary Care held in Berlin, Germany, April, 1996.)

quickly and effectively identifying a person's likelihood of having obstructive sleep apnea. The questions revolve around different factors—some symptomatic, some physical features. These symptoms and features include snoring, high blood pressure, observed pauses in breathing, daytime sleepiness, BMI, age, neck size, and gender. These factors are measured by asking eight questions. The likelihood of SDB is based on the respondent's answering more than or less than three questions positively. The major factors considered in a STOP-BANG assessment are summarized in Box 19.1.

> ### SIMPLY STATED
> The ESS assesses daytime sleepiness, and the Berlin Questionnaire and the STOP-BANG assessment tool identify sleep apnea risk factors.

## PHYSICAL EXAMINATION

On physical examination, patients with SDB most commonly present with obesity and increased neck circumference. When interviewing the patient, symptoms of EDS may be present, and if left undisturbed the patient may begin to quickly doze during an assessment. In some cases, the loss of sleep can produce lethargy or inability to concentrate on tasks and questions. Many patients will have oral airway crowding due to anatomic reasons such as tonsillar hypertrophy, retrognathia, or micrognathia. During the physical examination, the patient's throat should be visualized and the Mallampati score documented.

> ### SIMPLY STATED
> Although the physical examination may appear normal for the SDB patient, the role of the RT is pivotal during routine patient assessment through questioning the patient's sleeping habits.

The Mallampati score was first described by Dr. S. R. Mallampati to categorize the amount of open space in the oropharynx when certain anatomic structures are visualized by looking in the mouth. Scoring of the Mallampati from direct visualization is as follows: class 1—full visibility of tonsils, uvula, and soft palate; class 2—visibility of hard and soft palate, upper portion of tonsils, and uvula; class 3—soft and hard palate and base of the uvula are visible; and class 4—only hard palate is visible (Fig. 19.5). A Mallampati score of class 1 would be considered normal. Although it was initially developed and still widely used as a tool to evaluate a difficult airway before intubation, a high Mallampati score has been correlated with a high risk for OSA, especially in the presence of nasal obstruction.

---

### BOX 19.1    STOP-BANG Questionnaire

1. **Snoring**
   Do you snore loudly (louder than talking or loud enough to be heard through closed doors)?
   Yes   No
2. **Tired**
   Do you often feel tired, fatigued, or sleepy during daytime?
   Yes   No
3. **Observed apnea**
   Has anyone observed you stop breathing during your sleep?
   Yes   No
4. **Blood pressure**
   Do you have or are you being treated for high blood pressure?
   Yes   No
5. **BMI**
   Is your body mass index more than 35 kg/m²?
   Yes   No
6. **Age**
   Are you older than 50 years?
   Yes   No
7. **Neck circumference**
   Is the circumference of your neck greater than 40 inches?
   Yes   No
8. **Gender**
   Are you a male?
   Yes   No

Answering yes to three or more of these questions indicates a high likelihood for having sleep disordered breathing.

From Chung F, Yegneswaran B, Liao P, et al: STOP questionnaire: a tool to screen patients for obstructive sleep apnea, *Anesthesiology* 108:812-821, 2008.

Class 1          Class 2

Class 3          Class 4

**FIG. 19.5** Mallampati scores.

In addition, signs and symptoms of common systemic illnesses, such as cardiovascular and endocrine disorders, should be elicited. Systemic arterial blood pressure is elevated in more than 50% of patients with OSA, and the resting blood pressure should be assessed. Sleep evaluation has become a routine assessment in patients with difficult to control hypertension. Finally, signs of left- and right-sided heart failure should be assessed.

### Additional Testing

More often than not, symptoms of sleep disorders overlap, and therefore these diagnoses are then confirmed with appropriate testing modalities such as polysomnography, home sleep study, positive airway pressure (PAP) titration studies, mean sleep latency test, maintenance of wakefulness test, and actigraphy. This chapter discusses the PSG in detail.

### The Polysomnogram

Guidelines for conducting and evaluating sleep studies are established by the American Academy of Sleep Medicine (AASM) and specifically pertain to Medicare patients but also provide insight regarding best practices for all patients. The term *polysomnogram* is best understood by dissecting the word for its root meaning: *poly* means "many," *somno* means

"sleep," and *gram* means "writing." Combined together, these terms mean "many sleep writings," which is an accurate description of how the test looks on the computer screen. The arrangement or configuration of the various physiologic tracings on the PSG page or screen is called a montage. A typical montage has a minimum of 17 channels of information or tracings, similar to an electrocardiogram (ECG) tracing (Fig. 19.6). In fact, the ECG channel is always monitored during a PSG study, along with at least three channels recording the EEG tracings to identify NREM or REM sleep stages, two channels documenting right and left eye movement, one channel monitoring chin movement, two channels recording right and left leg movement, and seven more channels recording snoring, airflow, thoracic-abdominal movement, $SpO_2$, heart rate, and body position (Fig. 19.7).

An EEG is the documented record of brain wave activity collected from electrodes placed on the head and face, using a measuring system referred to as the *international 10-20 system,* or simply "10-20," so-named because it uses percentages of 10 and 20 in relation to physical landmarks on the human head. The EEG waveforms, when used for sleep purposes, are to identify the levels or stages of sleep during a sleep study or to evaluate for any underlying seizure-like activity that is the root of the sleep disorder.

**FIG. 19.6** A typical montage of physiologic data recorded during a polysomnogram study.

When indicated, a PSG study should be ordered directly by the physician or through a referral to a board-certified sleep specialist. When the patient arrives at the sleep center, the RT or sleep technologist obtains a brief history and performs a brief physical examination, reviews clinical documentation, and then attaches electrodes with electrolyte gel in specific locations on the patient's body to gather the physiologic data during the sleep study. As the patient sleeps, the PSG records physiologic changes during the sleep period. At the conclusion of the sleep study the next morning, the patient is awakened and instructed to check with his or her prescribing physician for the final PSG report. The RT, sleep technologist, or other qualified clinician then analyzes the EEG tracings and scores the sleep study by staging the NREM and REM periods. All abnormal breathing events, movement events, arousals, and desaturations are also scored, and calculations are made relative to each event. Software allows for apneas and hypopneas to be counted during each hour of the sleep study and specific calculations made. The primary index defining the presence of apneas and hypopneas is the apnea-hypopnea index (AHI), or the number of hypopneas and apneas per hour of sleep time. Other criteria and symptoms must also be considered by the sleep specialist to completely evaluate or score a patient's sleep study. The scored sleep study is then forwarded to a physician trained in interpreting sleep studies, such as a board-certified sleep physician. Sleep physicians may have a background in neurology, pulmonary medicine, internal medicine, otolaryngology, cardiology, or other related areas. Once the PSG study is interpreted, the results are returned to the prescribing physician, and the patient is informed of the results. If the PSG study demonstrates the need for treatment, such as PAP, the sleep laboratory or physician will either order an in-laboratory titration study or contact a durable medical equipment (DME) company for autotitrating PAP therapy. The DME employs RTs, who will fit the patient with the proper continuous PAP (CPAP) or bilevel PAP interface (nasal mask or pillows), instruct the patient how to use the PAP equipment, and provide education on the patient's specific SDB. Patient follow-up is provided by the DME and sleep physician for PAP or treatment compliance issues.

> **SIMPLY STATED**
>
> A sleep study continuously records physiologic data from at least 17 sources (channels) on the patient's head and body. The arrangement of these data on a single page is called a *montage*.

Some patients will undergo a so-called split-night study. During this type of PSG, a patient with severe sleep apnea is identified, and a presumptive diagnosis is made by the sleep technician in the first half of the study. Given the severity of the underlying disease and potential serious complications, the second half of the study is spent on adjusting the mask size and PAP setting for appropriate treatment. RTs and sleep technologists conducting PSG studies must strictly adhere to specific criteria to properly complete the study and titrate PAP to the appropriate treatment pressure to correct patient apneas and hypopneas. Patients with a pulmonary or cardiac disease history in addition to sleep apnea will present a more complicated patient scenario and require additional assessment for treatment options.

> **SIMPLY STATED**
>
> The AHI is the primary diagnostic calculation used to confirm the presence of sleep apnea and to classify its severity. All patients with abnormal AHI scores should be further assessed and if necessary, offered appropriate treatment.

**FIG. 19.7** Patient with sleep disordered breathing ready for a sleep study with electrodes attached to detect chest and abdominal movement, electrocardiogram (ECG) leads on the chest, electroencephalogram (EEG) leads on the head and face, electrodes above and below the eyes and on the chin and cheek, and leads going down to the right and left legs.

# SLEEP DISORDERED BREATHING

SDB development may be related to anatomic or chemical predisposing factors or both combined. The RT will frequently encounter cardiopulmonary patients with sleep disorder issues, whether diagnosed or undiagnosed. Like patients with COPD, sleep disorder patients have symptoms that may not always be blatantly present. The role of the clinician assessing the patient with SDB is to evaluate for overt and occult findings associated with the disease. In addition to sleep-related signs and symptoms, this assessment may include respiratory, cardiovascular, endocrine, and psychiatric evaluation.

## Obstructive Sleep Apnea

By far the most common form of SDB in adults is OSA. Risk factors associated with OSA include a BMI of 25 or higher, alcohol consumption before bedtime, smoking, nasal congestion at night, and large tonsils (Box 19.2).

As REM sleep is approached and partial paralysis of skeletal muscles occurs throughout the body, the decrease in muscle tone and relaxation of muscles throughout the oropharyngeal region result in a progressive narrowing in the airway lumen. Snoring is the noise produced during inspiration during sleep as a result of soft tissue vibrations in the palate and pillar regions of the narrowed oropharynx. Patients may not be aware that they have sleep apnea but may comment that they often awaken from sleep with a gasp, snort, or loud snore. Not all patients who snore have OSA, but snoring can be a halmark sign of OSA and therefore must be closely evaluated. Because patients are not aware of their snoring problem, apneas, or arousals, a sleep partner or family member may be more likely to provide this portion of the medical history. Regardless of the patient's knowledge, the obstructive events (apneas, hypopneas, and associated arousals) are often repeated throughout the night, leading to unrefreshing sleep, as well as repeating cycles of stress hormone release, causing a variety of physical, mental, and behavioral abnormalities, as described throughout this chapter.

---

### SIMPLY STATED

OSA occurs when an obstruction of airflow in the upper airway causes air movement into the lungs to cease while thoracic-abdominal efforts to breathe continue.

---

### BOX 19.2   Risk Factors for Obstructive Sleep Apnea

- Excessive body weight (BMI ≥25)
- Alcohol consumption before bedtime
- Smoking
- Nasal congestion at night
- Increased neck size (≥17 inches in males and ≥16 inches in females)
- Large tonsils
- Males >40 years of age

*BMI,* Body mass index.

## Signs, Symptoms, and Additional Health Consequences

During apnea, the patient with OSA will continue to make ventilatory efforts despite airway obstruction. PSG tracings reflect no airflow and active thorax contractions working in opposition to abdominal movement with a declining $SpO_2$ (Fig. 19.8). In addition, the drop in $SpO_2$ results in an EEG arousal, and the patient often gasps and sits up in bed to open the airway.

Symptoms and signs of OSA in adults may include EDS, loud snoring, apnea periods (as reported by sleep partners), chronic morning tiredness regardless of the length of sleep, morning headaches, recent weight gain, limited attention, memory loss, changes in judgment or personality, lethargy or sluggishness, hyperactive behavior, the need to take naps, depression, slowed responses, decreased libido, frequent falling asleep while driving, high blood pressure, automatic behavior (performing actions by rote), and swelling of the feet or legs. Symptoms associated with apnea and hypopnea are generally most profound when the sleeping patient is supine and can be worsened if the patient is suffering from sleep deprivation, has consumed alcohol before going to bed, or has used sedatives.

Aside from EDS and other sleep-related signs and symptoms, the additional health consequences of untreated OSA are significant. Beyond daytime somnolence, disruption of normal sleep cycles can result in impaired mental function and psychosocial problems. It is suspected that disruption of sleep-wake cycles and frequent periods of hypoxia may increase the release of stress hormones, resulting in abnormalities in cardiovascular and endocrine systems. Common consequences include coronary artery disease, myocardial

**FIG. 19.8** Polysomnogram representation of obstructive sleep apnea with absence of airflow for 10 seconds and paradoxic movement of the rib cage and abdomen in response to an obstructed airway. The electroencephalogram arousal signals the patient gasping for breath to reestablish the airway and resume ventilation. (From Kacmarek RM, Stoller JK, Heuer AJ: *Egan's fundamentals of respiratory care,* ed 11, St. Louis, 2016, Mosby.)

## BOX 19.3　Obstructive Sleep Apnea Quick Facts

### Signs and Symptoms of Untreated OSA
- Habitual, loud snoring
- Breathing pauses while asleep
- Falls asleep while driving
- Struggles to stay awake when inactive, such as when watching television or reading
- Difficulty paying attention or concentrating at work, school, or home
- Performance problems at work or school
- Often told, "you look sleepy"
- Difficulty remembering information
- Slowed responses
- Difficulty controlling emotions
- Need to take naps almost every day
- Morning tiredness and feeling a lack of rest even after sleeping
- Morning headaches
- Depression

### Consequences of Untreated OSA
- Daytime sleepiness impairing ability to operate machinery or a vehicle
- Decreased physical performance
- Decreased academic performance due to attention issues
- Diabetes
- Psychosocial problems
- Erectile dysfunction and decreased libido
- Decreased ability to concentrate
- Reduced quality of life
- High blood pressure
- Coronary artery disease
- Myocardial infarction
- Cor pulmonale
- Heart failure
- Stroke

infarction, heart failure, stroke, insulin resistance, and erectile dysfunction. Furthermore, decreases in alveolar ventilation during repeated apneic periods can contribute to pulmonary vasoconstriction and polycythemia, which can lead to cor pulmonale. Box 19.3 summarizes the signs, symptoms, and other health consequences of untreated OSA. RTs and other clinicians should be aware of these conditions associated with OSA because with proper diagnosis and treatment, they can be effectively treated in most cases.

## SIMPLY STATED

Clinicians evaluating patients with suspected or diagnosed OSA should be aware of the conditions associated with OSA and frequently screen for them.

Classifying SDB severity involves many factors, but sleep specialists generally agree that the degree of AHI corresponds to the severity of sleep apnea. An AHI of less than 5 means the sleep study documented fewer than five

hypopneas and apneas per hour, which is within normal range. According to the AASM, an AHI of 5 to 15 is termed *mild sleep apnea* and does not necessarily warrant treatment unless the patient is symptomatic or has comorbidities. An AHI of 15 to 30 describes moderate sleep apnea, and an AHI greater than 30 denotes severe sleep apnea in the adult population, both of which typically need to be treated. Patient compliance is important to improve quality of life.

### Children and Infants with Obstructive Sleep Apnea

As with adults, the primary symptom of OSA in children is snoring. The presentation of OSA in children and infants is quite different from that in adults. Certainly, anatomic features of the airway lumen are the primary issue, but OSA can be found in children of any body size. Symptoms are also quite different from those in adults, and the clinical features addressed in the ESS and Berlin Questionnaire are not applicable to children. Children with OSA may present as sleepy or hyperactive, which may confuse parents and teachers. Another important clinical symptom is secondary enuresis (bedwetting). Unlike primary enuresis, patients with this condition develop bedwetting after achieving bladder control. Additionally, OSA may cause children to exhibit social withdrawal, poor academic performance, and aggressive behavior.

For infants and children, an AHI greater than 1 is considered abnormal.

## SIMPLY STATED

Children with OSA present with different symptoms than expected with adults and may include hyperactivity, aggressive behavior, social awkwardness, poor attention span, poor academic performance, or characteristics of attention-deficit/hyperactivity disorder (ADHD).

### Obstructive Sleep Apnea Treatment Options

A full diagnostic PSG study is required to accurately diagnose OSA and its severity. Once diagnosed, multiple treatment modalities are available to the patient. These therapies include PAP and non-PAP therapies. In certain cases, both maybe used. The type of therapy that is used will depend on severity of SDB, patient tolerance and comfort, and patient compliance. Regardless of the treatment modality used the goal in the treatment of all SDB is to minimize arousals and sleep disruptions, helping to normalize sleep architecture. This is usually achieved by keeping the airway open during sleep by administration of increased airway pressure (PAP therapies) or by altering the upper airway anatomy to relieve the airway obstruction (non-PAP therapies).

Clinicians can titrate PAP devices to relieve SDB and return the patient to more normalized sleep architecture. This can be done in the laboratory, and the patient is monitored for respiratory events on each pressure tested. The pressure is titrated to achieve AHI of less than 5. PAP therapies include continuous positive airway pressure (CPAP), which delivers a single continuous pressure; bilevel positive airway pressure (BiPAP), which delivers a separate inspiratory and expiratory pressure; auto-PAP (APAP), which will automatically adjust pressure, without a clinician's input, based on the internal analysis of the respiratory events; and adaptive servoventilation (ASV), which can provide a fully assisted breath in patients with central sleep apnea (discussed later in this chapter).

Non-PAP therapies include behavioral modification, oral appliances, and surgical options. Behavioral modifications include weight loss, proper sleep habits, and avoidance of respiratory depressants such as narcotics and alcohol. However, these modifications are typically not enough to improve the AHI unless the patient has mild OSA. Oral appliances include mandibular reposition and tongue retaining devices. Sleep studies must be repeated with the oral appliance in place to evaluate the efficacy of the device. PAP therapy tends to give the most benefit in terms of long-term health outcomes, but oral appliances are a reasonable first-line therapy in patients with mild to moderate OSA. Conventional surgical options are uvulopalatopharyngoplasty (UPPP) and maxillofacial surgery in patients with facial anatomy that is amenable to surgery.

One of the newest treatment modalities is hypoglossal nerve stimulation. Here, the upper airway dilator muscles are stimulated during sleep with a pacemaker-like system. A pulse generator is placed in an infraclavicular pocket, and a remote control allows the patient to turn it on at bedtime. This therapy appears to be gaining momentum, and studies are currently ongoing. The ultimate therapy for OSA is tracheostomy, but this is seldom required given other treatment options. It is typically reserved for patients with life-threatening arrhythmias during periods of sleep apnea.

## Upper Airway Resistance Syndrome

As previously defined, hypopnea (Fig. 19.9) is characterized by decreased airflow associated with a partial upper airway closure, until an EEG arousal causes airflow to be established. However, incomplete airway obstruction that cannot be classified as apnea or hypopnea may be classified as respiratory effort–related arousal (RERA) (Fig. 19.10). This tends to be caused by minor airway resistance but not to the degree of an obstructive event such as apnea or hypopnea. During RERAs, the thorax and abdomen move in a diminished, asynchronous manner, although the SpO2 remains stable. RERAs usually result in an EEG arousal, and the patient's sleep stage is disrupted. The clinical importance of RERAs is debatable, and many sleep laboratories choose not to report them during PSG evaluation.

## Central Sleep Apnea

Central sleep apnea (CSA) is sleep apnea in which there is a lack of thoracic-abdominal effort in addition to complete airflow obstruction for at least 10 seconds (Fig. 19.11). The basis for the apnea is not obstruction of the airway; rather, it is the physiologic lack of the drive to breathe. CSA is typically observed during transitional sleep stages, such as N1 or REM sleep. The cause of CSA can be quite varied and complex. The neurologic control of breathing, located in

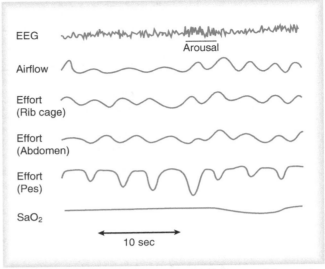

FIG. 19.9 Hypopnea with decreased airflow and increasing respiratory efforts until an electroencephalogram arousal occurs to awaken the patient as the airway is reestablished. (From Kacmarek RM, Stoller JK, Heuer AJ: *Egan's fundamentals of respiratory care,* ed 11, St. Louis, 2016, Mosby.)

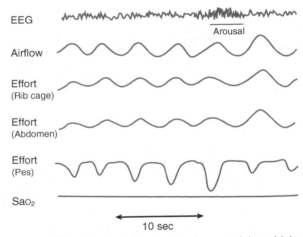

FIG. 19.10 Respiratory effort–related arousal in which airflow, chest, and abdominal movements appear normal, but respiratory efforts increase until an electroencephalogram arousal reestablishes the airway. (From Kacmarek RM, Stoller JK, Heuer AJ: *Egan's fundamentals of respiratory care,* ed 11, St. Louis, 2016, Mosby.)

the brainstem, may be impaired because of stroke, brainstem lesion, encephalitis, neurodegeneration, radiation treatments to the cervical spine region, or congestive heart failure (CHF).

The drive for ventilation, called the *hypercapnic drive,* is normally controlled by the amount of $CO_2$ dissolved in the blood. The secondary, or backup, ventilation drive mechanism, termed the *hypoxic drive,* is based on the amount of oxygen in the blood. During sleep, both the hypoxic and hypercapnic ventilatory drive mechanisms are suppressed. It is thought that, during sleep, the control of ventilation is

**FIG. 19.11** Central sleep apnea in which there is cessation of airflow for at least 10 seconds in the absence of thoracic and abdominal movement until an electroencephalogram arousal resynchronizes respiratory effort. (From Kacmarek RM, Stoller JK, Heuer AJ: *Egan's fundamentals of respiratory care,* ed 11, St. Louis, 2016, Mosby.)

closely associated with metabolic pathways, making body chemistry primarily responsible for ventilation.

> **SIMPLY STATED**
>
> CSA results from a lack of physiologic stimulation to breathe causing cessation of airflow and is characterized by the absence of thoracic-abdominal efforts.

### Signs and Symptoms of Central Sleep Apnea

The signs of CSA are not as apparent as those of OSA. Individuals with CSA are most often not obese and do not have a large neck circumference. Snoring is not usually present; however, EDS may be reported as a result of the lack of restorative sleep from frequent awakenings during apnea periods. CSA usually has an underlying cause such as use of narcotics, underlying cardiac or neurologic disorders, periodic breathing, or emergent central apnea.

Cheyne-Stokes respirations are periodic breathing in which respiratory efforts gradually increase in depth and frequency, followed by a decrease in depth and frequency, punctuated by an apneic period. The pattern of increasing and decreasing depth and rate is also known as the *waxing and waning* or *crescendo-decrescendo pattern.* The proper way to describe the Cheyne-Stokes event during an assessment is to record the time of the waxing and waning phase and the apneic episode. It is not uncommon for the apnea periods or waxing and waning phases to vary, with each cycle lasting at least 40 seconds. In some patients with OSA, as PAP is being titrated to relieve the obstructive apneas, an underlying CSA episode emerges (hence the term *emergent* CSA). Once the patient's OSA component is treated with PAP, the CSA component can be addressed by providing a backup rate controller on the PAP device.

### Mixed Sleep Apnea

As the name implies, mixed sleep apnea (MSA) is the combination of OSA and CSA in the same patient. Typically, the diagnostic sleep study presents with a CSA component initially, followed by an OSA phase (Fig. 19.12). Without the PSG diagnostic and titration study, MSA is virtually impossible to confirm. Once the MSA patient's OSA component is treated with PAP, the CSA component can be addressed by providing a backup rate controller on the PAP device.

Comparison of the PSG tracing of airflow through the nose or mouth with respiratory effort tracings is the primary way to differentiate among OSA, CSA, and MSA. During OSA, the obstructed airway results in the cessation of airflow while respiratory efforts continue. During CSA, neither airflow nor respiratory efforts are present. With MSA, the tracings reflect the typical CSA lack of airflow or respiratory effort followed by respiratory effort and no airflow, as seen with OSA.

### Children with Central Sleep Apnea

Although CSA is much less common in children, it more often found found in infants born before 37 weeks of gestation or can be found in infants of at least 37 weeks of gestation secondary to developmental conditions or medical conditions. Multiple disorders may precipitate CSA in children and infants, including neuromuscular, neurologic, metabolic, gastrointestinal, or hematologic abnormalities or an infection with an accompanying fever. As with adults, hypercapnic drive centers in the brainstem may be insensitive or too immature to trigger corrective breathing commands to respiratory muscles, resulting in periods of apnea.

Sudden infant death syndrome (SIDS) is thought by some experts to be associated with CSA, but no clinical evidence that the two are linked has been presented to date. SIDS is defined as "the sudden death of an infant under

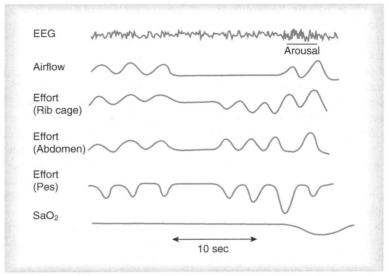

**FIG. 19.12** Mixed sleep apnea in which an initial central sleep apnea episode gives way to an obstructive sleep apnea episode until an electroencephalogram arousal reestablishes the airway and resynchronizes respiratory efforts. (From Kacmarek RM, Stoller JK, Heuer AJ: *Egan's fundamentals of respiratory care*, ed 11, St. Louis, 2016, Mosby.)

1 year of age, which remains unexplained after a thorough case investigation, including performance of a complete autopsy, examination of the death scene, and review of the clinical history." Although the etiology is unknown, the majority of reported SIDS cases occur in the first 6 months of age, with a peak incidence between 2 and 4 months of age. SIDS has been shown to have a familial relationship to OSA, positional sleeping, and families with a history of apparent life-threatening events rather than CSA. SIDS research during the past decade has linked it to significant risk factors such as prone sleeping position, bed sharing, maternal substance abuse, and cigarette smoking. Despite a decrease in SIDS incidence by 38% in the United States, it remains the leading cause of death in children younger than 1 year.

## Hypoventilation Syndromes

There are multiple hypoventilation syndromes of which the most notable is obesity hypoventilation syndrome. This may be seen in patients with BMIs >30 who have elevated $Paco_2$ during wakefulness of greater than 45 mm Hg. The majority of these patients have comorbid OSA. The underlying cause is not completely understood. It is thought that the hypoventilation syndromes are due to blunted hypercapneic ventilator response in the brain, allowing this hypercapnia to persist during the day. Extreme obesity and difficulty moving the chest wall due to decreased chest wall compliance may also play a role. To make the diagnosis, daytime hypercapnia must be present. Treatment typically includes BiPAP or other modes of backup ventilation, in addition to weight loss.

## KEY POINTS

- Approximately 1 in 6, or more than 40 million, Americans suffer from some type of sleep disorder, with an estimated 18 million having some form of sleep apnea.
- RTs are valuable assets to the sleep community because they are a major segment of the workforce conducting sleep studies in sleep disorder centers throughout the country, and they have a unique background in ventilation, pulmonary anatomy and physiology, pharmacology, and cardiopulmonary diseases.
- Clinical assessment skills and awareness of the impact of unidentified and untreated sleep disorders are more critical than ever. During the patient interview and assessment process, a few simple questions regarding the quality and quantity of the patient's sleep may redirect the physical assessment.
- The two major states of sleep, NREM and REM, cycle back and forth every 60 to 90 minutes for a total of four

- or five cycles during a normal 8-hour sleeping period. Usually, sleep begins at stage N1, progresses to stage N2, and is followed by stage N3 as sleep deepens. In NREM, the brain is in a state of rest while the body can move and respond.
- In REM sleep, the brain becomes more active, and the body experiences partial skeletal muscle paralysis with changes in ventilation, blood pressure, and heart rate.
- EDS is difficulty staying awake during the day. Patients with sleep apnea will be very conscious of the effects of daytime somnolence on their lifestyle.
- The ESS is an eight-item questionnaire that measures daytime sleepiness for the initial screening of sleep disorders. The Berlin Questionnaire focuses on the risk factors associated with sleep apnea and is a good measure for predicting sleep apnea.

- The STOP-BANG assessment is rapidly becoming the standard for a quick way to effectively identify a person's likelihood of having obstructive sleep apnea.
- Although a physical assessment may not initially reveal SDB, additional investigation may demonstrate that associated signs and symptoms may be present. They may include lethargy, poor concentration, obesity, large or short neck, retrognathia or micrognathia, morning headache, loss of memory or concentration, recent weight gain, erectile dysfunction, nocturnal enuresis, pedal edema, or general tiredness regardless of how many hours of reported sleep.
- A typical polysomnographic montage has a minimum of 17 channels of physiologic data, including ECG, EEG, right and left eye movement, chin movement, right and left leg movement, snoring, airflow, thoracic movement, abdominal movement, $SpO_2$, heart rate, and body position.
- During an obstructive apneic event, the obstructed airway results in the cessation of airflow while respiratory efforts continue. With central apnea, neither airflow nor respiratory efforts are present. Mixed apnea tracings reflect the typical central apnea lack of airflow or respiratory effort, followed by respiratory effort and no airflow as seen with obstructive apnea.
- Based on the PSG study, a calculated AHI of less than 5 is considered within normal range. Mild sleep apnea is defined by an AHI of 5 to 15, moderate sleep apnea describes an AHI between 15 and 30, and an AHI greater than 30 denotes severe sleep apnea in adults.
- Snoring is the noise produced during inspiration during sleep as a result of soft tissue vibrations in the palate and pillar regions of the oropharynx and may eventually lead to the development of significant sleep apnea.
- The primary symptom of OSA in children is snoring, but children with OSA may present as hyperactive or sleepy; exhibit social withdrawal, poor academic performance, or aggressive behavior; or be misdiagnosed as having ADHD.
- Beyond daytime somnolence, disruption of normal sleep cycles that comes with OSA can result in impaired mental function, psychosocial problems, diabetes, hypertension, heart failure, stroke, and other conditions.

## CASE STUDY

A 23-year-old man who plays football for a local university as a defensive lineman has difficulty staying awake in class and in football meetings, where he quickly falls asleep. Complaining of severe fatigue, he visits his attending physician. A teammate accompanying him states that when the team is on road trips, none of the other team members can sleep in the same room with him because of his very loud snoring with pauses in breathing and gasping. He has a present medical history of hypertension and a past history of a nasal fracture, which was corrected with nasal surgery. His physician ordered a diagnostic sleep study to determine the potential presence of SDB.

### Physical Assessment

The patient is 76 inches tall and weighs 350 lb for a BMI of 42.6 kg/m². He is a nonsmoker who consumes one caffeinated beverage daily and three to four alcoholic beverages weekly. He gets regular exercise 4 days per week. His vital signs at rest are blood pressure: 145/88 mm Hg; respiratory rate: 26 breaths/min; and heart rate: 112 beats/min.

On inspection, the patient has a short, 19-inch neck. His enlarged tonsils and the narrowed hypopharynx result in a Mallampati score of class 3, and he appears to be primarily a mouth breather. Chest assessment reveals a large, muscular thorax with normal, bilateral chest wall movement noted. There is no digital clubbing or cyanosis present. Palpation reveals bilateral chest wall movement with normal intercostal spacing for thorax size. Tactile fremitus is somewhat diminished because of the large BMI. Percussion is all within normal limits for thorax size. Auscultation reveals somewhat diminished but normal breath sounds. No abnormal heart sounds were noted.

The ESS and Berlin Questionnaire were administered, with an ESS score of 22 and three positive categories for the Berlin survey. When asked to comment on his sleeping habits, he stated that he is always tired regardless of how much time he spends in bed trying to get rest. The patient also stated that he usually awakes about 2:00 or 3:00 AM and has a difficult time going back to sleep. He stated he has difficulty driving during the day or night without "dozing at the wheel."

### Polysomnogram

A complete PSG with a digital sleep system was used, along with the international 10-20 system of electrode placement for recording EEG, EMG, electrooculogram (EOG), ECG, respiratory effort, oximetry, body position, airflow, snoring sound, pulse rate, and limb movement channels. Sleep study results revealed the following:

| | |
|---|---|
| Total REM sleep | 16% (normal 15%-20%) |
| Stage N1 | 6.1% (normal 5%-10%) |
| Stage N2 | 63% (normal 40%-50%) |
| Stage N3 | 14.9% (normal 25%) |

### Interpretation and Impression

The patient meets diagnostic criteria for OSA, upper airway resistance, periodic limb movement syndrome, and primary snoring. Severe OSA is present with an AHI of more than 40. The arousal index of 76.1 per hour substantiates the patient's complaint of EDS. Sleep distribution and sleep architecture are abnormal and consistent with frequent arousals. Delta sleep during stage N3 is limited, with prolonged N2 sleep.

### Recommendations

- PAP titration PSG study ordered
- Clinical follow-up
- Dietary consultation not appropriate at this time because of sports involvement

## CASE STUDY

A 44-year-old woman who complains of chronic fatigue and morning headaches made an appointment with her physician. Her husband states that she snores very loudly during the night with frequent pauses in her breathing that frighten him. He has tried to awaken her to take a deep breath, but sometimes it takes several attempts to wake her up. He is not resting well himself because of her sleeping habits. Her present medical history includes hypertension, hypothyroidism, and CHF. After the patient interview and assessment, her physician ordered a split-night PSG study that will include a diagnostic sleep study and a PAP titration trial, if indicated.

### Physical Assessment

The patient is 61 inches tall and weighs 235 pounds for a BMI of 63.5 kg/m². She is a nonsmoking mother of two teenagers who consumes six to seven caffeinated beverages daily and one to two alcoholic beverages weekly. She does not regularly exercise. Her resting vital signs are blood pressure: 162/90 mm Hg; respiratory rate: 24 breaths/min; and heart rate: 122 beats/min.

On inspection, she has a short, thick neck that is 17.5 inches in circumference. She has large tonsils, a large tongue, and a long uvula with a Mallampati score of class 4. Her neck and throat area seem enlarged for her body size. Chest assessment reveals normal, bilateral movement with no digital clubbing or cyanosis. All other findings are within normal limits. Her feet and legs appear to be edematous. Palpation reveals bilateral chest wall movement and diminished tactile fremitus. Her feet and legs show 2+ pitting edema. Percussion is all within normal limits, and auscultation reveals diminished, normal breath sounds. A pronounced $P_2$ heart sound is noted over the precordium.

The ESS score for the patient was 18, and she had three positive categories for the Berlin survey, indicating EDS and significant sleep apnea factors, respectively. She also states she was diagnosed with hypothyroidism several years ago but has not been taking her medication. She reports a weight gain of 60 lb in the past 3 years.

### Polysomnogram

A standard PSG study with a digital sleep system was performed with the international 10-20 system of electrode placement for recording EEG, EMG, EOG, ECG, respiratory effort, oximetry, body position, airflow, snoring sound, pulse rate, and limb movement channels. After 4 hours, the sleep study results revealed the following:

| | |
|---|---|
| Total REM sleep | 2% (normal 15%-20%) |
| Stage N1 | 4% (normal 5%-10%) |
| Stage N2 | 76% (normal 40%-50%) |
| Stage N3 | 18% (normal 25%) |

### Pretreatment Interpretation and Impression

The patient meets diagnostic criteria for OSA, hypoxemia, upper airway resistance, absence of REM sleep, periodic limb movement syndrome, and primary snoring. Severe OSA is present with an AHI of more than 40. The arousal index of 83.4 per hour substantiates the patient's complaint of EDS. Sleep distribution and sleep architecture are abnormal, consistent with frequent arousals. Delta sleep during N3 is limited with prolonged N2 sleep, and REM sleep is essentially absent.

### PAP Titration Study

After the 4-hour PSG study, the technician fitted the patient with an appropriate nasal CPAP mask, and after lights out, the patient was returned to sleep. At 12:35 AM, CPAP was initiated at 5 cm $H_2O$ and increased incrementally to BiPAP of 19/16 cm $H_2O$. At this level of PAP support, only one hypopnea was recorded, and the AHI was reduced to 2.4. The lowest $Spo_2$ recorded at this setting was 92%, and the mean $Spo_2$ was 94%. The therapeutic pressure to reverse sleep apnea was a BiPAP setting of 19/17 cm $H_2O$.

### Recommendations

- BiPAP for home use with a preset pressure of 19/17 cm $H_2O$
- Clinical follow-up
- Dietary consultation with nutritionist
- Consult with endocrinologist for thyroid condition
- Consult with cardiologist for CHF
- Recommend exercise program

## ASSESSMENT QUESTIONS

1. Which of the following will assist the RT in predicting daytime sleepiness?
   a. ESS
   b. Berlin Questionnaire
   c. Inspection of the chest
   d. ECG

2. All of the following are symptoms of OSA in adults *except:*
   a. Morning headaches
   b. Memory loss
   c. Hyperactive behavior
   d. Depression

3. In which stage of sleep is "restorative sleep" thought to occur?
   a. N1
   b. N2
   c. N3
   d. REM

4. To meet the definition criteria for sleep apnea, how many seconds of airflow cessation during sleep must be documented?
   a. 4 seconds
   b. 6 seconds
   c. 8 seconds
   d. 10 seconds

5. Which of the following is *not* a physiologic parameter routinely monitored during the PSG study?
   a. Spo$_2$
   b. ECG
   c. EEG
   d. Arm EMG

6. If on assessment the Mallampati score is class 4, the patient would be at high risk for which type of SDB?
   a. CSA
   b. OSA
   c. MSA
   d. SIDS

7. A reduction in airflow greater than 30% for 10 seconds during sleep defines which of the following?
   a. Apnea
   b. RERA
   c. Arousal
   d. Hypopnea

8. Which of the following diagnostically defines the presence of moderate sleep apnea?
   a. AHI of 3
   b. AHI of 12
   c. AHI of 28
   d. AHI of 44

9. Which of the following is *not* true regarding SIDS?
   a. Involves infants younger than 1 year
   b. Peaks at 8 months of age
   c. Familial relationship to OSA
   d. Incidence has decreased by 35% in the United States

10. Which of the following is the most common complaint in patients with SDB?
   a. Snoring
   b. EDS
   c. Obesity
   d. Hypertension

## BIBLIOGRAPHY

Berry RB, Budhiraja R, Gottlieb DJ. Rules for scoring respiratory events in sleep: update of the 2007 AASM Manual for the Scoring of Sleep and Associated Events. *J Clin Sleep Med.* 2012;8:597.

Cooksey JA, Balachandran JS. Portable monitoring for the diagnosis of OSA. *Chest.* 2016;149:1074.

Kacmarek RM, Stoller JK, Heuer AJ. *Egan's fundamentals of respiratory care.* 11th ed. St. Louis: Mosby; 2016.

Mokhlesi B, Tulaimat A. recent advances in obesity hypoventilation syndrome. *Chest.* 2007;132:1322.

Nagappa M, Liao P, Wong J, et al. Validation of the STOP-BANG questionnaire as a screening tool for obstructive sleep apnea among different populations: a systematic review and meta-analysis. *PLoS ONE.* 2015;10. e0143697.

Opperer M, Cozowicz C, Bugada D, et al. Does obstructive sleep apnea influence perioperative outcome? *Anesth Analg.* 2016;122:1321.

Simon S, Collop N. Latest advances in sleep medicine: obstructive sleep apnea. *Chest.* 2012;142:1645.

Spriggs WH: *Principles of polysomnography.* Salt Lake City, 2003, Sleep Ed.

Various authors for American Thoracic Society Sleep Education for Pulmonary Fellows and Practitioners. Available at http://www.thoracic.org/professionals/clinical-resources/sleep/sleep-modules/.

# 20

# Assessment of the Home Care Patient

*Albert Heuer and Dave Gourley*

## LEARNING OBJECTIVES

*After reading this chapter, you will be able to:*

1. Describe the evolution and advantages of respiratory home care.
2. Identify the types of patients who receive home respiratory care.
3. Describe the role of the respiratory therapist in home care.
4. List major tools and resources used in respiratory home care assessment.
5. Identify the key elements involved in assessing the respiratory home care patient.
6. Identify the components of the initial evaluation of the patient and home environment.
7. Describe respiratory equipment commonly used to assess and treat patients at home.
8. Explain the purpose and the procedures for developing a plan of care.
9. Describe strategies for educating patients in the home care setting.
10. Explain the importance of follow-up care.

## OUTLINE

## KEY TERMS

eHealth (electronic health)
home medical equipment (HME)
Hospital Readmissions Reduction Program (HRRP)

mHealth (mobile health)
oxygen concentration indicators (OCIs)
portable oxygen concentrator (POC)

respiratory home care
telemedicine
telemonitoring
The Joint Commission

---

Legislation that established Medicare in the 1960s also introduced a reimbursement structure for health care services provided in the home and at other alternate settings. As a result of this and other factors, including our aging population, the number of patients receiving care at home increased to over 12 million in 2010. Many patients needing home care suffer from respiratory conditions such as chronic obstructive pulmonary disease (COPD), which is ranked as the third most common cause of death in the United States. Patients with acute exacerbations of disease, such as COPD, asthma, or cystic fibrosis, are initially treated in a hospital or a similar facility. However, a common goal of the care plan for such patients is to successfully treat their acute illness and discharge them to an alternate site, often to the home setting. Home care is not only cost-effective but also enhances patients' quality of life, can have a positive influence on their psychosocial well-being, and minimizes their exposure to nosocomial infections and in-hospital hazards.

The American Association for Respiratory Care (AARC) defines respiratory home care as the "prescribed respiratory services provided in a patient's personal residence." It should be noted that the term *home care* is not limited to care provided in a patient's house, condo, or apartment and may also include other forms of personal residences such as group homes and assisted living facilities. In addition, many of the concepts in this chapter can be applied to other alternative settings such as skilled nursing facilities. The AARC also states in regard to home care that "prescribed respiratory care services include, but are not limited to, patient assessment and monitoring, diagnostic and therapeutic modalities and services, disease management and patient and caregiver education." On the surface, these services may appear to be similar to those provided in traditional acute care facilities. However, the way in which such services are performed and the resources immediately available require adjustments when applied by the respiratory therapist (RT) in a home care environment. In fact, there are career opportunities for RTs in home care, primarily with home medical equipment (HME) companies. However, success as a home care RT not only depends on clinical competency in patient assessment and treatment but also requires strong skills related to patient education, communication, time management, ability to work independently, and resources. These and other qualifications of the RT working in home care are discussed in more detail later in this chapter.

## IMPORTANCE OF RESPIRATORY HOME CARE

As a result of skyrocketing medical costs, pressure from third-party payers, such as Medicare, Medicaid, and health insurance companies, and the desire to enhance the patient's quality of life, strong emphasis is now placed on reducing the length of a patient's stay in an acute care facility. Some suggest that the plan to discharge patients from a hospital or similar setting to their home should begin when they are first admitted and stabilized. This significant increase in the number and complexity of home care patients has affected respiratory home care. In essence, there are now more respiratory patients being cared for at home, and they tend to be sicker and need a greater variety of medical interventions. A greater number of patients are receiving relatively common modalities, such as home oxygen therapy, while others require procedures that were once only performed in an acute care facility. In addition, tracheostomy tube changes, aerosolized antibiotic treatments, and ventilator weaning are now being done in the patient's home. The availability of such services and the personnel to perform them not only enable physicians to discharge their patients earlier, and perhaps not admit them at all. This presents RTs in home care with some interesting challenges.

In addition to offering the advantage of decreased medical costs, home care tends to enhance a patient's quality of

life by enabling a patient to participate in his or her own care, spend more time with loved ones and friends, and potentially avoid the need to be placed in a long-term care or similar facility. When coupled with the fact that respiratory diseases account for the fourth and fifth largest reimbursement category under Medicare, it is expected that home care will continue to provide RTs with opportunities for the future. However, to successfully pursue such opportunities, RTs need to excel in many areas, including those relating to assessing the patient and the environment of care as discussed in the next sections.

More recently, the Hospital Readmissions Reduction Program (HRRP) of the federal government now penalizes hospitals for excessively high, short-term readmission rates for selected diagnoses, including COPD and pneumonia. To comply with these programs, hospitals and affiliated providers, including home care companies, have established protocols that include patient follow-up and education aimed at care plan compliance. Patient assessment in the home can act as an early warning system to help identify a smaller problem such as a change in clinical status or the need for patient education, thus preventing a larger problem and a hospital readmission. As a result, respiratory home care companies and the RTs working in this environment are well situated to play an important role in such protocols and help reduce short-term readmissions.

## THE HOME CARE PATIENT

The notion of a typical home care patient does not exist because all are unique in some way. However, there are certain diseases and therapeutic modalities that are much more likely to be found in alternate settings, including the home. Thus assessments and care plans done for home care patients should address clinical findings most commonly associated with such conditions.

From the standpoint of such diseases, the home care RT most often sees patients with some form of a chronic lung condition. Emphysema, asthma, and chronic bronchitis are health problems the RT is likely to encounter daily. Sleep disordered breathing, infant apnea, neuromuscular diseases, and other debilitating illnesses are also frequently seen. Box 20.1 lists some of the most common respiratory disorders seen in home care.

---

**SIMPLY STATED**

The home care RT sees a great variety of patients at home; they tend to be medically complex and often require several treatment modalities.

---

Oxygen is the most common respiratory therapy modality seen in home care. A patient with an acute exacerbation of his or her COPD may need short-term home care services designed to instruct and evaluate the patient on the use of home oxygen equipment, compressor nebulizer therapy, or a new medication schedule.

## BOX 20.1 Disorders Commonly Encountered in Respiratory Home Care

- COPD
- Acute and chronic bronchitis and bronchiolitis
- Stable and unstable asthma
- Acute and resolving pneumonia
- Restrictive lung disease
- Sleep disordered breathing
- Acute upper respiratory infections
- Airway clearance problems
- Neuromuscular and other ventilator insufficiency disorders
- Infant apnea, apnea of prematurity

Assessments should be performed to determine need, response to therapy, and compliance and to identify emergent problems that could lead to a rebound hospitalization.

Goals might relate to assisting the patient in becoming independent with his or her care: to self-administer nebulizer treatments as prescribed, to use and maintain the oxygen equipment as instructed, to know when to call the oxygen provider, and to know how to respond to emergency situations. Once these goals are accomplished, the patient would generally be discharged from services.

Conversely, a patient needing mechanical ventilation for life support requires home care services for as long as he or she remains at home. The technical nature of home ventilators and ancillary equipment necessitates that evaluation and maintenance be done often to ensure that they function properly. Home ventilator users also require periodic physical assessment to determine adherence with treatment, response to therapy, and to identify emergent problems.

In the middle of the spectrum are patients who require limited home care services for days, weeks, or months for the treatment of infections, management of a tracheostomy, newly prescribed oxygen therapy, or stabilization of a program of noninvasive ventilation. Home care services are terminated once the need no longer exists; however, the patient whose condition has changed or who has had a change in caregivers, environment, or equipment may need to have those services restarted.

## HOME CARE ASSESSMENT TOOLS AND RESOURCES

The home care RT uses many of the methods of assessment available in the acute care setting. Several of the techniques of physical examination described earlier in this book are used in home care (see Chapters 4 and 5). Likewise, the equipment used in assessing the home care patient is also similar to that employed in the bedside evaluation of many hospitalized patients. However, the home care RT needs to become especially proficient in the use of basic equipment (e.g., stethoscope) and techniques because of the limited availability of high-tech assessment resources such as radiographic images (x-rays) or computed tomography scans, bronchoscopy, serial arterial blood gases, and complete pulmonary function tests

(PFTs). The absence of such advanced resources in home care means that each available resource needs to be used correctly and all the results properly considered by the RT.

Some of the most important assessment resources available to RTs are their own senses, including what they see, hear, feel, and smell. Changes in the patient's overall appearance, skin color, breath sounds, and chest expansion are strong clues that the care plan needs adjustment.

## SIMPLY STATED

The limited availability of high-tech assessment tools, such as radiographic images (x-rays), in home care means that each assessment tool and technique available needs to be used correctly and all results properly considered by the RT.

The devices most commonly used to assess home care patients are a stethoscope, sphygmomanometer, and pulse oximeter. Peak flowmeters and respirometers may also be useful in assessing basic pulmonary function on select patients such as patients with asthma and neuromuscular disease, as well as ventilator-assisted patients. End-tidal carbon dioxide ($ETCO_2$) monitors and portable diagnostic sleep-recording devices are used for select patients. Beyond patient assessment, other devices, such as oxygen analyzers, flowmeters, and calibrated pressure gauges, are used to monitor the function of home respiratory equipment, including oxygen concentrators and home ventilators.

It is important to understand the limitations of these portable assessment instruments used in the home and other alternate sites. Most important, each parameter assessed must be taken as part of the whole, and the RT must understand that an abnormal reading may not be abnormal for a particular patient, given the patient's baseline values. For example, a chronically ill patient's baseline vital sign measurements may be slightly above the normal ranges such as a COPD patient whose heart rate and respiratory rate are typically 110 beats/min and 22 breaths/min, respectively. This is why it is essential to perform an initial assessment on each patient and establish baseline parameters.

The tools themselves have limitations. Blood pressure measurements usually are done using an aneroid sphygmomanometer and cuff. Blood pressure measurements can be inaccurate if performed improperly. Using a cuff that is too narrow or applying the cuff too tightly results in erroneous readings. Some automated blood pressure monitoring devices are prone to error. The RT should also take care not to press on the brachial artery too forcefully with the head of the stethoscope because this could result in erroneously high diastolic pressure readings. Some patients use self-administered blood pressure units to monitor their blood pressure. Used correctly, these units are generally accurate. However, it is fairly easy to use them incorrectly, which can give the patients inaccurate results. The RT should review the patient's technique and review the manufacturer's instructions to ensure that the equipment is being used properly. It is also useful to periodically compare an automated unit's readings with those using the RT's blood pressure cuff. It is important for the patient to take his or her blood pressure readings at the same time each day, using the same arm, after a short rest period, and sitting in the same position each time.

Peak flowmeters are commonly used for generally stable patients at home. In fact, daily peak flow measurements are often included in asthma management programs, particularly for children. Reductions in peak flow readings may be a good indicator of changes in airway reactivity and patency associated with asthma. Proper technique is essential to obtain accurate readings, and the patient should be instructed to use the peak flowmeter on waking in the morning before using a bronchodilator. Each patient should have his or her own peak flowmeter; however, there is variability among models and brands that may lead to inconsistent results.

Pulse oximetry is also used in home care as an indicator of the adequacy of hemoglobin oxygen saturation ($SpO_2$). It is generally considered medically unnecessary for most home care patients to have ongoing or continuous pulse oximetry monitoring, and most insurance companies will not pay for oximeters for home use. Consequently, the home care RT or nurse may simply bring a pulse oximetry unit to monitor $SpO_2$ during periodic visits. However, a few home care patients on more sophisticated modalities, including mechanical ventilation, may have a pulse oximeter at home. In such instances, the patient or caregiver will need to be instructed on how to obtain an accurate reading and how to avoid inaccurate readings. For example, if the patient's hands are cold, the oximetry readings could be erroneously low or unobtainable. If the patient smokes, the readings could be erroneously high. Excessive movement, high levels of ambient light, or a low battery in the oximeter can also result in inaccurate readings. The user must understand these issues and be instructed to interpret the oximetry readings as part of a whole assessment; recommended changes should not be based on oximetry readings alone.

Oxygen analyzers are commonly used in home respiratory care, but like oximeters, they are not necessary for continuous monitoring in most cases. Oxygen analyzers are used most often to evaluate the function of oxygen equipment during servicing or troubleshooting. They must be calibrated according to the manufacturer's recommendations, and the RT must use care when carrying an oxygen analyzer in his or her car to avoid damaging it.

Other equipment used in respiratory home care includes $ETCO_2$ monitors, which can be particularly useful in patients with COPD and neuromuscular disorders. In rare instances, arterial blood sampling and analysis is performed in the home by mobile blood gas laboratories or by using point-of-service analyzers. Sputum and venous blood samples can be collected, and even electrocardiograms are occasionally obtained in the home. Once again, all of the devices used in assessing the home care respiratory patient have limitations and should be used with these issues in mind. On the other hand, the ability to properly use these tools may eliminate the need to transport the patient to a health care facility for

a diagnostic procedure. More important, the ability to collect an array of clinical information often helps form a "clinical picture" and may warrant that the RT recommend a change to the patient's care plan that may avoid hospitalization of the patient.

## ROLE AND QUALIFICATIONS OF THE HOME CARE RESPIRATORY THERAPIST

The role of the home care RT depends in part on whether the HME company provides only HME services or if it also handles clinical respiratory services under The Joint Commission accreditation guidelines. The Joint Commission is a private organization recognized by the federal government that surveys and evaluates a large number of HME companies in the United States for accreditation. If a home care company is accredited to provide only HME services, the RT's role is mainly educating and ensuring safe use of home respiratory equipment such as oxygen concentrators (discussed later in this chapter). However, if the HME company also provides clinical respiratory services, the RT's function typically includes performing clinical patient assessment and testing and administering treatment to patients at home.

The primary role of the home care RT is to help set up respiratory equipment and train the patient and caregiver on the equipment's safe and effective use and maintenance. The RT also monitors the patient's overall clinical status and changes in his or her condition, as well as the patient's response to home therapy. Several skills and qualifications are needed to fulfill this role. Foremost, a home care RT must have outstanding clinical abilities to properly train and assess the home care patient, as well as being well versed in all respiratory therapy modalities. In applying their clinical skills, RTs must be extremely resourceful and versatile and possess good critical thinking skills because home care RTs generally perform most of their daily work functions without the presence of other clinicians. Being "on the road," the home care RT mainly has access to the medical equipment and devices that he or she brought or that have been previously delivered to the patient's home. It is not uncommon for the job to require creative adjustments or adaptions within the realm of appropriate clinical care. Despite operating by himself or herself, the home care RT must also be a team player, understanding that the home care RT represents just one of several health disciplines responsible for devising and executing the patient care plan. Other members of the health care team often include home health nurses; speech, physical, and occupational therapists; social workers; dietitians; home health aides; lay caregivers; and, most important, the patient. Cooperation and collaboration among team members is vital to optimizing outcomes; the home care RT must also excel in communication and interpersonal skills. Communication skills coupled with an organized approach, attention to detail, and sensitivity to cultural and age-specific considerations are helpful in teaching a patient to use, maintain, and troubleshoot a complex piece of medical equipment. These same skills will also help the RT uncover changes in clinical status and promptly recommend appropriate modifications in the plan of care. In extreme situations, such as a patient whose condition has worsened since the last home care visit, the RT may need to use several skills simultaneously, within the context of the patient's limitations. The RT should quickly recognize the seriousness of the situation and promptly activate emergency medical services (calling 911), administer cardiopulmonary resuscitation if appropriate, and later notify other team members, including the physician.

Finally, it is helpful for the home care RT to have basic skills relating to insurance reimbursement. The acute care RT has little need to know the cost of the therapy or a medical device or reimbursement limits and procedures. However, the home care RT should have a general understanding of the rules and guidelines for reimbursement and keep abreast of the periodic changes to reimbursement. The RT who knows the major relevant provisions of Medicare and private health insurance can help provide efficient quality care to home care patients that maximizes the use of limited resources.

---

### SIMPLY STATED

The home care RT must be thoroughly familiar with respiratory care procedures, as well as possess some familiarity with many nursing care procedures, nonrespiratory equipment, and reimbursement policies.

---

## ASSESSMENT AND THE HOME VISIT

Assessment is one of the most important aspects of respiratory home care because it can affect all aspects of the patient's care. The home care RT needs to be proficient in assessing both the patient and the environment of care. A thorough evaluation includes assessing the type of equipment required, instruction needs of the patient and caregivers, whether other medical services are necessary, the type of monitoring and follow-up needed, and the safety and adequacy of the home environment. This section covers proper clinical assessment of the home care patient and describes the major considerations in evaluating the home care environment.

In general, the RT makes an initial home visit because the patient has a respiratory problem that can be treated at home with the appropriate respiratory equipment. After the physician writes the order for home therapy, a referral is typically made to the HME provider, who contacts the insurance company or Medicare to verify that the patient meets the qualifications for the specific equipment and to receive approval. Medicare has implemented a system called "competitive bidding" for some home medical equipment, including oxygen, nebulizers, and continuous positive airway pressure (CPAP). Medicare will only reimburse for these services if provided through an approved competitive bid vendor. In the case of home oxygen, the patient's home oxygen levels will need to be assessed to ensure that they meet criteria to qualify for insurance or Medicare reimbursement. It is important to

---

### BOX 20.2  Key Elements of the Initial Evaluation

| Patient | Environment |
|---|---|
| Past and current medical history | Cleanliness, safety hazards |
| Symptom profile | Smoke detector, fire extinguisher |
| Medication review | Adequate electricity |
| Physical examination | Heating, cooling |
| Evaluation of functional limitations | Space for equipment, supplies |
| Psychosocial evaluation | Adequate cleaning facilities |
| Nutritional status | Telephone |
| Caregiver evaluation | Emergency access |
| Advance directives | Equipment needs |

---

note that in such instances, the assessment of blood oxygen levels should not be performed by the RT working for the HME provider to avoid any possible conflict of interest. Once approval is received by the HME company, arrangements are made to deliver the equipment and the RT is notified to schedule an initial visit. It should be noted that health insurance reimbursement in most cases is only permitted for the rental or purchase of respiratory equipment and that generally no payments are made to the HME company for the RT's hourly wage.

### Initial Visit and Assessment

The purpose of the initial visit is to assess the patient and home environment, as well as to set up the prescribed respiratory equipment if not already done and instruct the patient and caregivers on how to use it. In some instances, the equipment has already been set up before the RT's arrival. Most HME providers use specially trained service technicians to deliver, set up, and train the patient in the use of certain types of respiratory equipment such as home oxygen equipment. The RT then sees the patient, usually within 24 to 48 hours.

Once the equipment has been set up and the patient and caregiver have been properly instructed, the RT will then generally perform a comprehensive evaluation of the patient. The results of this assessment affect all other aspects of the patient's home care program. It also establishes a baseline against which the patient is compared during subsequent visits. Box 20.2 highlights the elements of the comprehensive initial evaluation.

### Medical History

If possible, the RT begins reviewing the portions of the medical record received by the HME provider before the initial visit to become familiar with the patient's medical history and current medical condition. This previsit review can also help the RT anticipate if there will be additional equipment or services needed. To build on this foundation, the RT interviews the patient and caregivers and then examines the patient during the initial visit. The patient interview is conducted to help disclose relevant existing conditions and establish the patient's current medical status and symptom profile. Smoking status, pulmonary risk factors, and previous medical history (including preexisting conditions, surgeries, and hospitalizations) should be determined. Any treatments or therapies the patient is undergoing should also be identified. The RT should also ask the patient whether his or her immunization record for influenza and pneumococcal vaccines is current and to identify any drug allergies. A medical history of the patient's family should also be obtained and recorded because certain respiratory conditions (such as cystic fibrosis) are believed to have a genetic link.

## Physical Examination

Once the medical history has been obtained, the RT should assess the patient's cardiopulmonary status and examine other clinical findings. Initially, the patient's age, height, weight, and general appearance are recorded followed by an assessment of vital signs, including blood pressure, pulse rate, respiratory rate and quality, and pulse oximetry, as previously noted. It is important to note that pulse oximetry should generally be done only with a physician's order. Often, this is handled by ensuring that the physician's standing orders that allow the RTs to perform oximetry on their patients are in place. Auscultation, palpation of the chest, and observation for cyanosis, clubbing, and peripheral edema are also done. Abnormal findings or those that suggest a change in clinical status should be documented and reported to the physician, if appropriate. Many of these examination techniques are similar to those used in an acute care setting and described throughout this text.

Some aspects of the physical examination may need to be altered to protect the patient's privacy. The home care therapist may be the only person in the room with the patient when the examination is being performed. Therefore it may be considered improper for the RT to ask the patient to disrobe for auscultation of the lungs, especially when an RT examines a patient of the opposite gender. In such cases, auscultation must be performed over the patient's shirt or nightclothes, keeping in mind that extraneous sounds may occur when the patient's clothing rubs against the chest piece of the stethoscope. Obtaining the patient's permission to perform the physical examination is essential to making the encounter comfortable for both the patient and the RT.

Part of the physical examination often includes some form of diagnostic testing. Basic PFTs, such as peak flow, tidal volume, negative inspiratory force, and forced vital capacity, may be appropriate for patients with asthma or certain neuromuscular disorders. It is also becoming more common for an $ETCO_2$ breath sampling to be ordered for a patient with suspected ventilatory insufficiency. A change in sputum production may prompt a physician's order for sputum sample collection and analysis.

HME providers that are accredited by The Joint Commission for clinical respiratory services can allow the RT to perform a patient's initial physical assessment without a physician's order; however, the RT can only perform ongoing physical assessments of the patient under written orders by the patient's physician.

## Physical and Functional Limitations

Evaluation of physical and functional limitations is performed to identify any physical or functional problems that could reduce the patient's ability to care for himself or herself. In addition, such problems predispose the patient to falling and sustaining related injuries. Consequently, specific precautions should be followed to minimize the risk of falls and other household accidents.

To help reveal such limitations, the RT should become aware of preexisting conditions noted in the medical record, as well as examine the patient to uncover physical deficits in eyesight, hearing, speech, strength, endurance, and mobility. The RT must also evaluate a patient's cognitive abilities. Any physical or cognitive problems could affect the patient's ability to perform self-care and limit his or her ability to safely manage any medical equipment that has been prescribed. If the patient has other caregivers assisting with his or her care, consideration must be given to any functional or physical limitations those caregivers may have.

Several functional areas must be considered. The patient's ability to independently perform basic activities of daily living should be assessed. Such activities include personal care, cooking, and independent or assisted mobility within the home. For example, the patient with COPD may appear unkempt because he or she cannot bathe and dress without severe shortness of breath. The patient may not use his or her portable oxygen tank because he or she does not have the hand strength to turn on the oxygen regulator. Perhaps he or she cannot walk from the living room to the bathroom without stopping or does not have enough strength to get up out of a chair. The same patient may have difficulty seeing the calibration markings on an oxygen tank or medication eyedropper. The RT may even have had difficulty scheduling the initial visit because the patient could not hear the telephone ringing. The presence of any of these limitations should be noted in the initial assessment, and the RT can follow up to ensure that they have been properly addressed.

It is also important to assess cognitive function. A patient with short-term memory problems may have difficulty remembering the RT's instructions on how to fill the portable oxygen tank. A patient who is depressed may not listen to instructions or may refuse the oxygen altogether. Cognitive impairment caused by stroke or even some types of medications can interfere with the patient's ability to use HME safely or without caregiver assistance. It is also important to note that moderate to severe hypoxemia or hypercarbia may cause acute cognitive impairment and may signify that the patient's condition has worsened or that the equipment has either malfunctioned or is not being used properly. Any of these circumstances would require immediate action by the

RT and a prompt modification to the care plan. Finally, caregivers in the home will need a basic evaluation to ensure that they have the cognitive abilities to help manage the patient's care and equipment.

## Medication Review

The RT and other clinicians, such as home health nurses, should review the patient's current medication regimen. This review identifies all prescriptions, over-the-counter, and herbal remedies the patient is taking. Special attention should be given to medications that have similar names, such as salmeterol and Solu-Medrol. The RT evaluates the patient's level of understanding about how he or she should be taking each medication and assesses the patient's compliance with the treatment plan. It may be helpful to ask the patient how he or she keeps track of medications and suggest the use of a medication scheduling pill holder for simplification, if needed. The RT should also ask to see the patient's technique for using metered-dose inhalers, dry powder inhalers, and medication nebulizers. If the RT determines that the patient is not using his or her medications as prescribed, the RT should inform the patient's physician and document this point. The RT can also recommend that the patient consult with a pharmacist for advice and clarification. Issues regarding medications should be communicated to other members of the patient care team, such as a home health nurse, and addressed in the patient's care plan.

## Psychosocial Evaluation

It is relatively common for patients with chronic lung disease to also have psychosocial issues such as anxiety and depression. As a result of this and because such issues can affect other aspects of the patient's health, a review of the home care patient's psychosocial status should be included in the initial home patient assessment. This assessment includes the patients' self-image, outlook on his or her present and future situation, home status and support systems, and work history. Home care patients can be anxious, embarrassed, angry, or depressed over their state of health and may feel that they are a burden to their families. They may have difficulty coping with being dependent on others for help with basic activities of daily living, particularly when this dependence involves role reversal. For example, a male patient who has always had control and authority may have difficulty coping with losing that control and having to be assisted by his wife or being told what to do by health care workers. This patient may deny his condition or try to exert control by not complying with treatment regimens or refusing treatment altogether, to the detriment of his health.

Patients forced to retire due to declining health may be depressed at the loss of their role as breadwinner. They may become so concerned about finances that they refuse their medications or equipment because they feel they cannot afford them. They feel that they have become a physical and financial burden on their families. Depression can lead to hostility toward caregivers, refusal of care and treatment, and verbal expression of suicide thoughts. Anxiety can lead

### BOX 20.3   Signs and Symptoms of Psychosocial Problems in the Home

- Seemingly unwarranted fear
- Signs of excessive shame or embarrassment
- Evidence of depression
- Evasive answers
- Socially isolated behavior
- Physical signs of abuse
- Evidence of verbal abuse

to medication abuse, increased shortness of breath, insomnia, and other health problems.

Caregivers in the home can also suffer from depression, anxiety, and burnout. The spouse of a patient with COPD may have to quit work to care for the patient and may be concerned with financial problems while also having to worry about the patient's health. The asthmatic child's mother may overuse emergency services because of her fear of a life-threatening asthma attack.

It is important that the RT look for signs of caregiver depression, anxiety, and burnout such as abuse and neglect. Box 20.3 lists some behavioral clues the RT should look for during this evaluation.

The RT should notify the patient's physician of any psychosocial problems, and ultimately the involvement of a mental health clinician, such as a social worker, may be indicated. The social worker can assist the patient and family with financial issues, caregiver burnout, and adjustment problems. The social worker can also assist the patient and family with decisions about advance directives if these have not been made.

### QUESTIONS TO ASK

**Physical and Functional Limitations in Patients and Caregivers**

Ask yourself the following questions when assessing the limitations of patients and caregivers:

- Is the patient able to walk with or without a walker, cane, or other ambulatory aid?
- Does the patient experience shortness of breath at rest, while in any positions, or during exertion? Is the patient able to climb a flight of stairs if the home has stairs?
- Does the patient have any weakness, arthritis, pain, swelling, or reduced range of motion in his or her feet, ankles, or legs?
- Does the patient have arthritis in his or her hands? Is the patient able to make a fist? Does the patient need assistance when performing an activity with his or her hands? Do the patient's hands shake? Does the patient have the strength to lift a portable oxygen cylinder or nebulizer?
- Does the patient have any hearing, speech, or vision problems? Can the patient read medication containers accurately? Is the patient able to read gauges, flowmeters, or other indicators on the HME? Can the patient read the written instructions provided with his or her medications and equipment? Can the patient hear the alarms made by the equipment? Can the patient hear the telephone, doorbell, or normal speaking voices?

*Continued*

**QUESTIONS TO ASK—cont'd**

- Can the patient shower or bathe without assistance? Is the patient exhausted or short of breath after bathing or going to the toilet? Does the patient using oxygen need a higher flow rate during these activities?
- Is the patient able to make his or her own bed? Does the patient do his or her own house cleaning and laundry?
- Is the patient able to prepare meals? Does the patient need assistance with food shopping? How many meals does the patient eat per day? What does the patient typically eat during each meal?
- Does the patient have difficulty remembering how to use any of the medical equipment, such as oxygen, CPAP, other? Does the patient remember which HME company has provided his or her equipment and how the company can be contacted? Can the patient remember when his or her last bronchodilator treatment was? Can the patient remember what medications are prescribed, as well as their dose and frequency?
- Do the patient's breathing problems limit his or her lifestyle or that of the patient's family in any way? Is the patient homebound?

## Nutritional Review

The patient's nutritional status is also evaluated in the initial visit, and the RT should inquire about any dietary restrictions (e.g., sodium, sugar, fat, or calories). The RT should determine how many meals the patient eats per day mainly because it is common for patients with pulmonary disease to eat poorly or decline food rather than suffer the dyspnea associated with its preparation and consumption. Such a patient would benefit from instruction in energy conservation techniques to help him or her prepare food and eat it. An important question to ask during the nutritional assessment is whether the patient wears his or her oxygen cannula during cooking and eating. It is common to discover that patients remove their oxygen cannula while cooking because they are afraid of the danger of using oxygen around sources of heat. Many patients also remove their oxygen cannula during meals, often for cosmetic reasons. Identifying these issues would prompt problem solving by the RT and patient. For example, a visit by a home health dietitian could be suggested or the patient could be encouraged to use a local meal preparation and delivery service (e.g., meals on wheels). A review of oxygen safety while cooking would also be appropriate. Chore workers or personal attendants can be hired to assist the patient with meal preparation. The dietitian may ultimately recommend that the patient be started on parenteral or enteral nutrition. The RT can also reinforce any dietary recommendations that have already been made for the patient.

## Cultural, Ethnic, and Religious Considerations

Cultural, ethnic, and religious beliefs can also affect the patient's home care program. Language barriers can make it difficult for the patient and the RT to communicate. The RT may need to locate an interpreter or use an outside service to translate; however, there may be a family member available who can also assist in this role. Additionally, many equipment user manuals and other written instructional materials are now written in several languages to help overcome this problem.

Some cultures encourage extended families to live together in a single dwelling. This can be advantageous because it increases the number of potential caregivers and reduces the feeling of isolation suffered by some patients. It can be less of an advantage when care must be divided among a limited number of family members, particularly if this involves small children. Some customers dictate that shoes be removed before entering the home. Other patients may have religious beliefs and customs that require an alteration in the home care program (e.g., a patient may decline visits on days of worship or may decline treatment on religious grounds). A patient may request religious counsel as part of his or her health care team or request that prayers be said for him or her. In all cases, the RT should try to identify and respect the patient's spiritual, cultural, and ethnic customs and preferences.

## Environmental Assessment

An environmental assessment is done to determine whether problems exist in the physical environment that would affect patient care. The home is inspected to identify health, fire, and safety hazards. The home's walkways should be free of anything that could cause the patient to stumble and fall (e.g., throw rugs should be removed if the patient has gait problems or uses an ambulatory aid, such as a walker). Halls and doorways should be wide enough for the patient to pass through, particularly when he or she uses a walker. Emergency exit routes must be identified, and a plan for the quick removal of the patient should be developed and posted for all caregivers and emergency personnel.

Many older homes have electrical outlets that are not grounded properly. Patients often use multiple-plug adapters that are overloaded or in ill repair. Depending on the amount of medical equipment the patient needs, the home may not supply enough amperage on a circuit to power the equipment and the other appliances the patient wants to use. In extreme cases, some patients do not have electricity at all or "borrow" it from neighbors via extension cords. Inspection by a professional electrician may be needed to determine whether modifications are necessary to support the patient's equipment needs. In extreme cases, it may not be possible to safely place equipment in the home.

The home should be inspected for functioning smoke detectors and fire extinguishers. There should be plenty of room for all equipment and supplies the patient will need; this is critical when oxygen is going to be used. Oxygen equipment must be placed at least 6 feet away from any heat sources and should not be placed on or near heater vents or in closets. Equipment powered by compressors, such as oxygen concentrators, nebulizers, and ventilators, must have enough free space around it to allow for adequate air intake and cooling. Other furniture may need to be removed to make space for hospital beds and other large equipment.

The home should have a working telephone. Touch-tone telephones with oversized numbers are available for patients with poor vision, and telephones with amplifiers or lights are helpful to patients with hearing deficits. Cordless and cellular telephones are ideal for patients who become short of breath trying to get to a ringing phone. Cordless and cellular phones are also handy to keep at the patient's bedside; this enables the caregiver to stay at the patient's side instead of having to leave the room to make a call, particularly in an emergency. However, cordless phones and other electronic devices should not be placed on or too close to equipment, such as ventilators or apnea monitors, because of the potential for electromagnetic interference, which can affect the functioning of such equipment.

Patients with pulmonary impairment may not tolerate wide fluctuations in ambient temperature, so the home should be evaluated for its heating and cooling systems. Wood-burning stoves and fireplaces can aggravate lung problems, particularly asthma, as do stoves or heaters that are not vented. When inspecting the home of an asthmatic patient, the RT must be particularly careful to identify possible triggers such as old carpeting, pets, mold, and wood fires.

### SIMPLY STATED

The home care RT must ensure that the home environment is safe and suitable for the type of equipment in use.

## Home Care Equipment

The nature of the patient's illness generally dictates the respiratory and other medical equipment needs of the home care patient. Respiratory equipment commonly used at home is listed in Box 20.4. However, the practitioner's assessment of the patient and the home environment may reveal that equipment-related modifications or additions should be pursued. For example, the RT's assessment may show that the functional ability of a patient with an oxygen concentrator may have improved and as a result, a portable oxygen concentrator (POC) or home fill system may be a good option because it facilitates ambulation. Careful observation of where and how the equipment will be used is essential.

The patient using a home ventilator will need battery-powered equipment as a backup in the event of a power outage. A patient who lives in a small mobile home may not have enough room for a hospital bed, and if that patient suffers from orthopnea, arthritis, or another need for frequent changes in body position, it will be necessary to find other ways to elevate the head during sleep or to facilitate positioning.

If the functional assessment reveals that the patient has difficulty with personal care, such as bathing or using the toilet, adaptive equipment can make these activities less taxing and, more important, less hazardous. Bath seats, shower chairs, handheld shower attachments, and grab bars can make bathing and washing safer and much easier. In such instances, the RT can recommend that a physical therapist do

### BOX 20.4　Respiratory Equipment Necessitating a Home Care Respiratory Therapy Visit

- Oxygen therapy equipment
- Invasive and noninvasive ventilators
- Compressor nebulizers
- Bland aerosol therapy
- Continuous positive airway pressure (CPAP) and bilevel pressure devices
- Suction machines for oral, endotracheal, and intermittent gastric suction
- Mechanical airway clearance devices (percussors, flutter valves, or exsufflation devices)
- Apnea monitors
- Portable sleep-recording devices
- Oximeters
- End-tidal $CO_2$ monitors
- Airway adjuncts (tracheostomy tubes, laryngectomy tubes, or transtracheal oxygen catheters)

a home evaluation to ensure that the patient's environment permits him or her to function as independently and safely as possible.

### Equipment Maintenance

An essential aspect of home care is ensuring proper maintenance of home respiratory equipment. As a result, the RT not only needs to assess the patient and set up the equipment but also should instruct the patient and caregiver and evaluate their ability to use and maintain the equipment (see next section). To accomplish this, equipment maintenance and basic troubleshooting should be thoroughly covered on the initial visit and reinforced during subsequent visits.

With regard to medical equipment maintenance, it is important to note that each manufacturer has specific guidelines for periodic preventive maintenance and servicing. Home ventilators must also be exchanged periodically for more extensive maintenance, usually after specified hours of operation or a specific time period. Oxygen equipment also needs monitoring and maintenance. Output concentration and flow rates of oxygen concentrators must be checked and external and internal filters replaced. An electrical safety check should be performed on all electrically powered equipment at least every 12 months.

Some types of home oxygen equipment include monitoring devices to assist with equipment maintenance. Oxygen concentrators are commonly equipped with oxygen concentration indicators (OCIs) that alert the user if the concentration output drops below a certain level. OCIs are helpful in ensuring that the patient is always receiving an adequate concentration of oxygen (e.g., an oxygen concentrator without an OCI may still put out the prescribed flow of 2 L/min, but the concentration of that flow may be 80%, 75%, or even lower). In this instance, the patient has no way to know that the inspired oxygen level is too low except that he or she may not feel as good. As a result, patients and caregivers should be instructed on the significance of OCIs.

## Patient Education and Training

Assessment is one of the most important skills that an RT can have, although the ability to teach runs a close second. Part of the initial and subsequent home visits should be spent training the patient and caregivers on basic assessment techniques and how to use and maintain the prescribed medical equipment, as well as performing the related respiratory care procedures. Indeed, RTs have been shown to be uniquely effective in teaching patients. The RT must be able to convey technical information in a simple and meaningful way and to verify that what was taught was also understood. Each patient learns differently, and the RT must determine how each particular person learns best. Some patients learn best by visualization or by reading. Others learn best by listening, and some learn best by doing. The RT probably will use a combination of these methods during training. In any event, it is generally useful to give the patient printed material that covers the key points in an easily understandable manner. Some patients and caregivers may benefit from audiovisual or web-based educational resources. It may also be helpful to select a "teachable moment," which is a moment relatively free from outside stimuli and other distractions. Box 20.5 outlines some useful teaching strategies.

In general, the caregivers and even the patients can be taught to obtain and record basic vital signs, such as heart and respiratory rate and regularity, blood pressure, and temperature. They should also be instructed on basic emergency procedures, including those to follow in a natural catastrophe or an apparent medical emergency. In addition, patients and caregivers should be taught to use, maintain, and perform basic troubleshooting on respiratory equipment in place at the home. If the patient has a functional limitation that prevents him or her from doing the procedure or using the equipment, he or she may still be involved in the training.

Whether the training or education involves assessment, equipment use, or emergency procedures, it is important that the RT evaluate how much the patient and caregiver have understood and provide additional training as necessary. Generally, competency to perform such procedures can be shown through a return demonstration given by the caregiver or patient and recorded by the RT. To get to that point, however, it may be necessary for the RT to visit the patient's home two or three times to continue the training sessions, particularly when there are several concepts to be covered relating to assessment and multiple pieces of equipment. It is common for patients and families to be overwhelmed during the RT's initial visit and for them not to remember all the instructions the RT may give them. It is important for the RT to factor this into the plan of care and use follow-up visits to provide additional training and monitor the patient's condition and the caregiver's ongoing performance.

**BOX 20.5    Helpful Strategies to Use during Patient Education and Training**

- Select a "teachable moment" to ensure the learner's attention
- Present only the necessary information
- Use simple or lay terms
- Demonstrate the procedure exactly as it should be performed
- Have the learner practice several times
- Ask for a return demonstration from the patient or caregiver
- Try to limit each training session to 30 to 60 minutes
- Encourage the learner to ask questions
- Use video, audio, and web-based material
- Leave printed instructions
- Leave a 24-hour telephone number

## Plan of Care

One of the primary objectives of the initial assessment and evaluation is for the RT to gather information that will help develop an individualized plan of care for the patient. The plan of care is developed from the issues and problems identified during the initial evaluation. From there, goals and desired outcomes are identified along with activities that will help achieve them. Goals should be specific, measurable, attainable, realistic, and within a specified time frame. As time passes and the patient has been home for some time, the plan of care is generally modified to reflect changes in the patient's condition, needs, or environment of care. Likewise, the physician's orders should reflect the initial goals, and the RT should recommend any appropriate changes over time.

For example, during the initial evaluation, the RT may notice that the patient is having difficulty reading the flowmeter on the oxygen concentrator or that the patient is too weak to carry a portable oxygen cylinder. In other cases, the patient may admit to the RT that he or she is embarrassed to wear an oxygen cannula in public, so he or she refuses to use the portable oxygen system outside the house. In these instances, the plan of care should list these issues or problems and include goals and corrective actions. Table 20.1 shows a sample plan of care for a patient with home oxygen based on the physician's order for treatment.

## Follow-up Care

The plan of care or service should also include the RT's plan for follow-up care. Based on the issues identified during the initial evaluation and the desired outcomes, the patient may or may not need ongoing physical assessment and evaluation. This is usually a function of how ill or unstable the patient is or what type of equipment the patient is using. For example,

**TABLE 20.1 Sample Plan of Care**

| Problem | Goal | Action |
|---|---|---|
| Hypoxia by $O_2$ saturation | Patient will maintain $O_2$ saturation above 90% | Monitor $O_2$ saturation by pulse oximetry monthly and as needed |
| Patient cannot see flowmeter on concentrator | Patient will use $O_2$ at 1 L/min at rest and 2 L/min with activity | Instruct patient's family in how to change flow rate on concentrator as prescribed |
| Patient cannot carry portable $O_2$ cylinder | Patient will use portable $O_2$ as prescribed when away from home | Supply patient with smallest aluminum $O_2$ cylinder with conserving device, or portable oxygen concentrator |
| Patient refuses to wear cannula in public | Patient will wear $O_2$ as prescribed | Review health problems associated with hypoxia, provide patient with clear nasal cannula, encourage patient to carry portable cylinder in backpack or other carrying bag |

**TABLE 20.2 Interpretation of Signs and Symptoms in the Home Care Patient**

| Finding | Possible Causes | Action |
|---|---|---|
| Dyspnea, cyanosis | Malfunction of equipment, poor compliance with treatment, change in physical status | Check $O_2$ equipment, assess patient, review energy conservation techniques and pursed-lip breathing, contact physician |
| Wheezing | Bronchospasm, congestive heart failure, pulmonary infection | Examine patient, verify compliance with medication regimen, review medication nebulizer procedures, contact physician |
| Increased sputum or change in sputum color | Lung or airway infection | Assess patient, check temperature, check compliance with therapy and cleaning of equipment, contact physician |
| Pedal edema | Heart failure, fluid overload | Assess patient, verify function of $O_2$ equipment, check compliance with $O_2$ therapy, verify compliance with medication regimen |
| Poor appetite | Depression, dyspnea, fever | Assess patient, examine medication schedule, review energy conservation techniques, contact physician |

the RT probably would not perform ongoing assessments on a patient using a compressor nebulizer or, if follow-up was indicated, it would be for a short duration. The RT may have found during the initial evaluation that the patient seemed to have difficulty remembering how to schedule his or her treatments, and a follow-up visit would be made. Once it is established that the patient is taking treatments as prescribed, he or she no longer needs regular follow-up.

It is ideal to reassess the patient completely during each follow-up visit, particularly when the home visits are done less frequently. The RT often will identify something that has changed from the initial evaluation, and emergent problems are found this way. It may be during a periodic visit to evaluate the oxygen equipment that the RT notices a change in the patient's shortness of breath or an increase in pedal edema. The RT may have found that the patient is using portable cylinders faster than expected or that the patient is not using as much oxygen as he or she should as evidenced by the hour meter on the concentrator. The essence of the follow-up visit is that the RT generally will find something that has changed about the patient, equipment, or environment; thus the plan of care is continually evolving based on the goals that are met and new issues that arise. Table 20.2 reviews physical changes that may be found during a follow-up visit and the recommended actions for the RT.

### Discharging the Patient

Most home care patients are not followed by the RT indefinitely. The ultimate goal of respiratory home care is to provide the patient with the tools to manage his or her own care. These tools include the knowledge base, equipment, procedures, and self-monitoring capability.

The plan of care is established to work through the problems and issues found during the RT's home visits. As problems are identified, goals are set to achieve desired outcomes and correct the problems. For most patients, the goals are achieved and the patient becomes capable of self-monitoring. At this point, the patient is discharged from respiratory care services.

If the patient continues to use medical equipment, such as oxygen, ventilators, and apnea monitors, he or she will at least continue to need service visits to monitor the function of that equipment. Those services may or may not be performed by the RT. Some HME providers use specially trained service technicians to make these service calls, and others use RTs to service life support equipment and service technicians to monitor oxygen and nebulizer equipment. These service technicians are trained to identify and report back any problems that might require patient contact by the RT.

## TELEMEDICINE, TELEMONITORING, AND EHEALTH

A growing trend in health care and in home care is telemedicine, now commonly referred to as eHealth (electronic health). Telemedicine refers to the use of electronic and telecommunication technologies to support health care at a geographically different location from the patient, increasing access to specialty and patient care. Telemedicine can allow for the evaluation, diagnosis, treatment, monitoring, triage, consultation, and follow-up of patients without travel. According to the Centers for Medicare and Medicaid Services (CMS), telemedicine seeks to improve a patient's health by permitting two-way, real-time interactive communication between the patient and the physician or practitioner at a distant site. This electronic communication means the use of interactive computerized telecommunications equipment that generally includes audio and video equipment. Telemedicine is viewed as a cost-effective alternative or supplement to the more traditional in-person way of providing medical care, including home care patient follow-up.

A form of telemedicine is telemonitoring, which involves the use of telecommunications and information technology to provide access to health assessment, diagnosis, intervention, consultation, supervision, and information across distance. A related concept is mHealth (mobile health), which specifically refers to the use of mobile applications (apps) for such monitoring and for access to health resources or data.

Though best practices in this area are still emerging, telemedicine and telemonitoring are gaining ground in respiratory care and home care. In some cases, it has facilitated the timely diagnosis and treatment of patients with limited access to health care facilities. In particular, patients with limited mobility such as ventilator-dependent individuals, as well as those with severe COPD or neuromuscular disease, have benefited from telemedicine. Computer interfaces for telemonitoring facilitate patient assessment through the two-way

transmission of key clinical data such as vital signs, pulmonary function measures and patient-ventilator data, and even the patient's physical appearance captured by computer webcams. Similar monitoring can also facilitate the early detection of, and intervention for, any deterioration in the patient's condition. Such inventions have been shown to be helpful in reducing doctor's visits and hospital admissions, a benefit both to the patient and to the economics of health care.

In addition, telemedicine has proven useful in facilitating the patient's participation in computer-based disease management programs, including COPD and asthma. In particular, selected telemedicine applications have been created that bundle patient education, disease management, interactive communication, and other features. In particular, telemedicine has helped facilitate the participation of COPD patients in remote access pulmonary rehabilitation programs within which they otherwise would not have been able to participate. Furthermore, their participation in such computer-aided rehabilitation programs has permitted these patients to achieve similar benefits associated with traditional rehabilitation programs such as demonstrable enhancement in their tolerance for activities of daily living.

Like many aspects of eHealth, telemedicine seems to be in its infancy. As health care resource limitations and cost-containment pressures continue, and eHealth applications improve, it appears inevitable that the use of this and related technologies will expand and become commonplace in respiratory care and home care.

## KEY POINTS

- Several factors, including technologic advancements, our aging population, and increasing demands on our health care resources, have resulted in a greater number of patients who receive respiratory therapy at home.
- For RTs, home care is a viable career path and an alternative to working in an acute care facility.
- In addition to outstanding clinical abilities, the successful home care RT needs to possess an array of other competencies, including critical thinking skills and resourcefulness, as well as time management and communication skills.
- Respiratory conditions that are commonly encountered in home care include COPD, sleep disorders, and neuromuscular diseases.
- Treatment modalities that are often used in home care include long-term oxygen, continuous positive airway pressure (CPAP), and mechanical ventilation.
- The initial assessment of a home care patient should include an evaluation of the medical history, a physical examination, review of medications, and an assessment of psychosocial and nutritional status, as well as cultural, ethnic, and religious needs.

- An environment of care evaluation done by the RT should focus on identifying and addressing potential hazards, ensuring the adequacy of space and electrical service, and devising a plan for responding to emergencies such as power outages and fires.
- Patient and caregiver training/education initiatives done by the RT should focus on basic patient assessment, as well as proper usage, cleaning, and maintenance of all respiratory equipment.
- The RT should ensure that an appropriate plan of care be developed that includes attainable goals and activities focused on achieving those goals and should recognize active participation by the patient and/or the caregiver(s).
- To optimize care and help ensure the best possible quality of life for the patient, the plan of care should be periodically reviewed and revised based on changes uncovered through patient follow-up.
- Telemonitoring enables the RT to monitor the patient and equipment remotely and to review patterns over a period of time, thus increasing clinical efficiency.

## ASSESSMENT QUESTIONS

1. All of the following factors have contributed to the rise in respiratory home care *except:*
   a. Legislation facilitating reimbursement
   b. Desire to enhance quality of life for chronically ill patients
   c. Home care is easier for the RT than acute care
   d. Cost-effectiveness

2. Which of the following conditions is/are commonly seen in the home care setting?
   a. COPD
   b. Sleep disorders
   c. Neuromuscular patients with ventilator insufficiency
   d. All of the above

3. All of the following respiratory modalities are commonly found in home care *except:*
   a. Long-term oxygen therapy
   b. Continuous positive airway pressure (CPAP)
   c. Bronchodilator therapy
   d. High-frequency jet ventilation

4. All of the following are important attributes of the home care RT *except:*
   a. Outstanding clinical assessment skills
   b. Extensive knowledge of home care respiratory equipment
   c. In-depth understanding of the history and evolution of home care
   d. Excellent communication and interpersonal abilities

5. Which of the following procedures generally would *not* be assessed during a respiratory home care visit?
   a. Vital signs
   b. Mixed venous blood gas analysis
   c. Physical inspection of the patient
   d. Breath sounds

6. When should an RT working for an HME provider assess pulse oximetry specifically to determine if the patient qualifies for home oxygen reimbursement under Medicare?
   a. Never
   b. If they first sign a disclaimer
   c. Only if the HME company gets to set up oxygen on that patient
   d. If the patient had a lung transplant

7. Which of the following is/are potential signs and symptoms of psychosocial problems in the home?
   a. Evasive answers
   b. Physical signs of abuse
   c. Unwarranted fear
   d. All of the above

8. Which of the following is true about the RT's evaluation in an initial home care visit?
   a. It never includes clinical evaluation of the patient
   b. It is performed by a physician
   c. It involves educating the patient and caregiver on equipment and ongoing care
   d. Both a and c

9. Which of the following is true about the patient's plan of care?
   a. It identifies issues and establishes goals for the patient
   b. It includes activities consistent with attaining such goals
   c. It should be reviewed and updated to reflect changing patient needs
   d. All of the above

10. Which of the following would *not* be part of the environmental assessment?
    a. Assessment of vital signs
    b. Determining adequacy of electrical service to accommodate electrically powered equipment
    c. Identifying potential safety hazards and recommending potential remedies
    d. Evaluating space requirements for ambulation and equipment

11. Which of the following is part of follow-up care?
    a. Helping the patient become actively involved in his or her care as much as possible
    b. Reviewing and modifying the treatment plan
    c. Assessing the patient's compliance with the therapy
    d. All of the above

12. Appropriate ways to help ensure that patients or caregivers are competent to perform a procedure are which of the following?
    a. Instruct them thoroughly
    b. Let them practice and ask questions
    c. Have them do a good return demonstration
    d. All of the above

# BIBLIOGRAPHY

Ball J, Dains J, Flynn JA, et al. *Mosby's guide to physical examination*. 8th ed. St. Louis: Mosby-Elsevier; 2015.

Coughlin S, Liang WE, Parthasarathy S. Retrospective assessment of home ventilation to reduce rehospitalization in COPD. *J Clin Sleep Med*. 2015;11(6):663–670.

DesJardins T, Burton GG. *Clinical manifestations and assessment of respiratory disease*. 7th ed. St. Louis: Mosby-Elsevier; 2016.

Jarvis C. *Physical examination and health assessment*. 7th ed. St. Louis: Mosby-Elsevier; 2016.

Kacmarek RM, Stoller JK, Heuer AJ. *Egan's fundamentals of respiratory care*. 11th ed. St. Louis: Mosby-Elsevier; 2017.

Mohktar MS, Redmond SJ, Antoniades NC, et al. Predicting the risk of exacerbation in patients with chronic obstructive pulmonary disease using home telehealth measurement data. *Artif Intell Med*. 2015;63(1):51–59.

Shah T, Churpek MM, Coca Perraillon M, et al. Understanding why patients with COPD get readmitted: a large national study to delineate the Medicare population for the readmissions penalty expansion. *Chest*. 2015;147(5):1219–1226.

Vitacca M, Fumagalli LP, Borghi G, et al. Home-based telemanagement in advanced COPD: who uses it most? Real-life study in Lombardy. *COPD*. 2016;13(4):491–498.

# 21

# Documentation

*Samone Norsworthy and David Gourley*

## LEARNING OBJECTIVES

*After reading this chapter, you will be able to:*

1. Recognize the general reasons why documentation is important.
2. Identify the expectations for documentation in the patient's medical record required by The Joint Commission standards.
3. Explain the legal definition of negligence.
4. Identify the three major types of medical record documentation for respiratory therapists.
5. Describe the use of the subjective, objective, assessment, and plan method for documentation in the patient's medical record.
6. Explain the assessment, plan, implementation, and evaluation method and the problem, intervention, and plan method for documentation of patient assessment data.
7. Review the use of the situation, background, assessment, and recommendation format in patient assessment.
8. Explain the federal electronic medical record mandate.
9. Identify the advantages and disadvantages of the electronic health record.

## OUTLINE

## KEY TERMS

Centers for Medicare and Medicaid Services (CMS)
confidentiality
critical thinking
electronic health record (EHR)
electronic medical record (EMR)

negligence
objective
privacy
situation, background, assessment, and recommendation charting (SBAR)

subjective
subjective, objective, assessment, and plan charting (SOAP)
The Joint Commission (TJC)

## THE JOINT COMMISSION

This chapter describes the reasons that so much time and energy are spent documenting patient care. The time spent documenting may appear counterproductive because it takes time away from providing direct patient care. However, documentation of the care provided and the patient's response is an essential element of the entire process of health care. This chapter reviews the medicolegal aspects of patient care documentation, with emphasis on The Joint Commission (TJC) requirements. The recent requirements for an electronic medical record are also reviewed.

There is no one method of documentation that is preferred or required. Several different charting methods are presented here. The reader will appreciate how good documentation is essential from a legal perspective and, more important, how it provides better communication among members of the health care team and ultimately improves patient care.

## GENERAL PURPOSES OF DOCUMENTATION

Once the respiratory therapist (RT) has completed the bedside patient assessment, consulted other members of the health care team, taken notes, reviewed the information in the medical record, and discussed the information with the patient's physician, it is time to record the assessment and plan into the medical record. The process of collecting the data involves the mental process called critical thinking. The critical thinking process requires many skills, including interpretation, analysis, evaluation, inference, explanation, and self-regulation. The difficult part of assessment is over, and now all the RT has to do is describe the findings and thoughts in a concise and professional manner. Because the medical record is a legal document, the RT needs to understand some fundamental principles before making an entry into the patient's medical record.

The reasons for creating a record of the patient's interactions with any health care organization (HCO) include the following:

- To serve as a legal record of the care and service provided. The medical record is more than just a collection of data; it is a legal document.
- To collect evidence in support of the patient's problems and needs. When the clinical facts about the patient's condition are collected, the correct diagnosis can be confirmed, and the patient's clinical progress can be better monitored.
- To provide communication among members of the health care team. The clinical notes, reports, flow sheets, vital signs, and test results enable the physician and other members of the team to document that the patient has received high-quality care according to each profession's standards of care or hospital policies. Each discipline has unique perspectives to bring to the discussion of a patient's care plan.
- To support appropriate reimbursement. The hospital is a business that must collect revenues. As a result, the medical record is also a financial document. The medical record must clearly show the nature of the patient's needs in the form of the diagnosis. Hospital coders use the medical record to review information and assign appropriate codes to produce a bill. Medicare and other payers reimburse the hospital based on the patient's diagnosis.
- To support the operation of the HCO and its allocation of internal resources and to provide documentation of compliance with TJC and regulatory standards of care. This type of documentation provides data for legally mandated reports to state and federal governmental agencies. These reviews of the medical records and related financial records, as well as the subsequent reports from these reviews, are used to show the hospital's administration that the business is functioning effectively and in compliance with accreditation and regulatory bodies.
- To serve as an educational tool. Every health care professional must learn how to use the medical record correctly. At first the medical record can be intimidating, but with time it becomes more familiar. The initial problem is often just finding the information you need. The medical record provides documentation of the clinical manifestations, course of the disease process, and the patient's responses to interventions. For this reason, even the experienced health care worker can learn from a good medical record. By reviewing a patient's record, you can learn what has and has not been effective for this particular patient. Furthermore, by reviewing large numbers of patient medical records, the RT and other members of the patient care team can learn how to more accurately describe each patient's condition and determine how to better treat patients with specific diseases. Most human research is based on or related to medical records. Extracting data from medical records is a complex process that requires skill, diligence, and attention to detail.

As noted, the patient's medical record is subject to review by different professionals for multiple reasons. By far the most common and compelling reason to scrutinize a patient's record, or the HCO's handling of medical records in general, is to monitor and improve the quality of medical care.

> ### SIMPLY STATED
>
> A retrospective review of patient charts can provide RTs and other health care professionals with the opportunity to see how patients with a certain problem were diagnosed, what treatment was given, and how the patients responded to that treatment.

## THE JOINT COMMISSION AND LEGAL ASPECTS OF THE MEDICAL RECORD

The Joint Commission (TJC), formerly known as the *Joint Commission on Accreditation of Healthcare Organizations (JCAHO)*, is the largest accreditation organization in the United States. It is an independent, nonprofit organization that accredits more than 19,000 health care providers and programs in all care settings. Its mission is "to continuously improve health care for the public, in collaboration with other stakeholders, by evaluating health care organizations and inspiring them to excel in providing safe and effective care of the highest quality and value." TJC's vision statement is "All people always experience the safest, highest quality, best-value health care across all settings," and its position statement is "Helping Health Care Organizations Help Patients."

TJC performs on-site surveys of HCOs to assess the quality of patient care and improve patient safety. If any HCO fails to comply with TJC standards, it will require action plans, follow-up, and evidence of compliance. If an HCO does not meet the requirements of TJC, the organization may be denied accreditation. TJC is authorized by the Centers for Medicare and Medicaid Services (CMS) to monitor hospitals for compliance with the federal conditions of participation; thus hospitals not accredited by TJC risk losing reimbursement through Medicare and Medicaid. In addition, many state health departments use TJC survey as their on-site inspection, so there could be regulatory ramifications as well.

TJC surveyors review patient records for documentation of safe and high-quality patient care. The Information Management and Record of Care, Treatment, and Services sections of The Joint Commission Comprehensive Accreditation Manual for Hospitals (CAMH) outlines how the organization "manages internal and external information, including the medical record, and includes the components of a complete medical record." The individual elements required in the medical record are provided and organized in common groups. The chapter also includes the medical record structure and details for management of the medical record. How each organization accomplishes these tasks is left up to that facility. TJC's on-site survey team evaluates an HCO's compliance with these requirements and reviews patients' medical records to assess the level of compliance. The survey team members may also provide consultation, including samples of how other organizations have complied with the standards. TJC survey team's objective is to assist the HCO to comply with the standards, not to be punitive toward individuals or the organization.

The following are TJC standards from their CAMH regarding the required medical record elements. Periodically, there are revisions to these standards, but the basic principles of information management and documentation have remained unchanged.

- IM.02.01.01 The organization protects the privacy of health information.
- IM.02.01.03 The organization maintains the security and integrity of health information.

These standards are directed toward guarding the patient's rights to privacy (the individual's right to limit the disclosure of personal information) and confidentiality (the safekeeping of data and information so as to restrict access to individuals who have need, reason, and permission for such access). These standards are consistent with both state and federal laws and regulations. Violations of these standards, or of related laws and regulations, can result in legal action with fines for the institution or civil or criminal prosecution of the offenders (depending on the details of the incident). This legal action could result in personal fines, loss of job, loss of professional license, and possibly even jail time. The federal law, known as the Health Insurance Portability and Accountability Act of 1996 (HIPAA), details the legal expectations and professional standards regarding the transmission (verbal, written, or electronic) of Protected Health Information (PHI).

In summary, these professional standards state that what you learn about a patient is on a "need to know" basis and you are not to share that information outside of that professional context. Generally, the RT needs to refer almost all questions coming from relatives and friends to the other professional team members such as the nurse, social worker, and physician. These issues become complex at times, particularly when dealing with a culturally diverse environment.

- IM.02.02.01 The organization effectively manages the collection of health information.

This standard describes the use of standardized terminology, definitions, abbreviations, and symbols, including abbreviations that are prohibited.

- RC.01.01.01 The organization maintains complete and accurate patient records for each individual patient. This standard describes the general components of the medical record.
- RC.01.02.01 Entries in the medical record are authenticated.

This standard describes who can make entries into the medical records and how the entries are authenticated.

- RC.01.03.01 Documentation in the patient record is entered in a timely manner.
- RC.02.01.01 The patient record contains information that reflects the patient's care, treatment, and services.

This standard defines in detail demographic and clinical information that must be contained in the patient record. It also includes a listing of additional documents that are required, when applicable.

- RC.02.03.07 Qualified staff receive and record verbal orders.

Communication problems during the receipt of verbal and telephone orders have resulted in serious medical errors. This alarming problem has resulted in TJC including the expectation that all verbal orders are to be read back to the person giving the order as part of the National Patient Safety Goals. This is meant to verify that the complete and correct order is being recorded and implemented. The person who gave the order, within a specified time frame, must authenticate all verbal orders. Because of these inherent problems regarding verbal orders, there is a general movement in the health care industry to discourage the use of verbal orders.

Guidelines regarding the authority to accept verbal orders are outlined in the respiratory care practice acts in most states. The general rule is that RTs can accept orders only for those treatments and services that they directly provide. This excludes drugs that RTs do not directly administer. RTs can, however, take orders for routine laboratory tests, chest radiographs, and standardized multidisciplinary protocols that are related to respiratory care practice.

All orders (written and verbal) must be dated and timed and must identify the names of the individuals who gave and received the order. Under certain circumstances, two persons should be present to take a verbal order or be on the phone line, and then one of these persons needs to repeat the order back to the physician before recording and carrying out the order. Both persons who heard the verbal directive should cosign the order in the medical record. The medical record must also indicate who implemented the order and what time the order was carried out.

- PC.01.02.01 The organization assesses and reassesses its patients.
- PC.01.02.03 The organization assesses and reassesses the patient and his or her condition according to defined time frames.
- PC.01.03.01 The organization plans the patient's care.
- PC.02.02.01 The organization coordinates the patient's care, treatment, or services based on the patient's needs.

RTs should integrate the information from various assessments of the patient, such as those of the physician, nurse, and other allied health professionals, to identify and assign priorities to the patient's care needs. Then the RT should base care decisions on the identified patient needs and care priorities. Attention should be paid to treating symptoms, such as dyspnea, and using accepted professional standards of practice, such as the American Association for Respiratory Care (AARC) Clinical Practice Guidelines.

TJC also requires that there be reassessments at regular intervals in the course of care to determine a patient's response. Furthermore, any significant change in a patient's condition should result in a reassessment, and the results or observations should be communicated to the other health care team members as appropriate.

These professional expectations are scrutinized carefully when the patient or family believes that the patient did not receive high-quality care or, more specifically, when it is believed that there has been some form of negligence.

Negligence is defined as an instance of failure to use the reasonable standard of care ("ordinary prudence") that results in injury or damages to another. Negligence has been committed when someone (who becomes the defendant) has failed to live up to a required duty of care owed to another person (the plaintiff). Generally, the legal definition of negligence requires the presence of the following four conditions:

- The defendant owed a duty of care to the plaintiff.
- The defendant breached that duty.

- The plaintiff suffered a legally recognizable injury.
- The defendant's breach of duty of care caused the plaintiff's injury.

As an RT, you have a duty of care to your patients. The scope of your duty to a patient is outlined by your professional standards (e.g., the AARC Clinical Practice Guidelines, your state's respiratory care practice act and regulations, and TJC standards). Your scope of practice is further defined or limited by your job description in your place of employment. Functioning within your job description, the limits of your state's practice act, and the professional expectations keeps you professionally safe.

Concerns regarding ethical situations or clinical conflicts among disciplines should not be entered into the patient's medical record. These issues need to be referred to the institution's quality assessment or risk management department. Every HCO is required by TJC to have a performance improvement process that ensures that patient safety and quality of care issues can be brought up in a manner that is not punitive and that every employee is instructed on how to report or access this process.

- The absence of information or the lack of documented recognition of specific problems could constitute malpractice. Essentially, if a treatment, assessment finding, or clinical problem was not charted, it is generally considered not to have been done or detected.

If it was not charted, it was not done. For example, if it was not recognized that a patient on a ventilator had severe chronic obstructive pulmonary disease (COPD) and was at very high risk for auto–positive end-expiratory pressure (auto-PEEP) and the patient suffered injury or death possibly as a result, the potential exists for legal liability. However, if the following occurred:

- Clinical notes show that auto-PEEP was being monitored with every ventilator parameter
- There was documentation of communication among the patient care team members, including the RT, physician, and nurse, about the auto-PEEP problem
- Bronchodilator therapy was started and ventilator changes were made (both in an attempt to decrease auto-PEEP)

then the presumption would be that appropriate care was taken and the patient's injury or death was not caused by neglect or malpractice in this regard.

The medical record must accurately reflect the course and results of the patient care provided. Therefore the accurate recording of the date, time, and place of events is essential. Late entries into the medical record are sometimes necessary but not a recommended practice. The standard calls for all information to be entered into the medical record in a timely manner. The definition and interpretation of *timely* are not always clear. In one case (*Joseph Brant Memorial Hospital v. Koziol* [1978]), a nurse did not chart her observations for 7 hours for a postoperative patient who then died during her shift. The delay in charting was interpreted by the court as the nurse not having made the observations. Vital signs and parameters should be charted immediately. Late entries of clinical notes or observations should be clearly marked as late entries and show the time entered and the time or period covered in the note.

---

### SIMPLY STATED

Important information about patient assessment must be entered into the medical record in a timely fashion. If a therapeutic or diagnostic intervention is not charted, it is generally assumed not to have been done.

---

## TYPES OF MEDICAL RECORDS

The different kinds of entries into the medical record depend on the purpose of that entry. The major types that are most familiar to the RT are treatment records, flowcharts or parameter sheets, and test results.

Treatment records are concerned with a single event at a specific time. The treatment record shows when, how, and with what drugs or equipment a treatment was given. The patient's response to the therapeutic intervention must also be included in the treatment record. The record can contain patient-subjective information on the response to the treatment, but most of the treatment record is objective information. This type of documentation should include the following:

- Date and time of test or treatment
- Type of test or treatment
- Drugs and their dosages, if used
- Result, or response to treatment, including adverse reactions
- Goals, objectives, or end-point criteria for the treatment

This type of documentation is ideal for aerosolized medications, secretion clearance therapy, and tracheostomy care.

Flowcharts or parameter sheets have similar requirements for dates, times, changes in equipment settings, and, most important, the patient's responses to the therapeutic intervention. Flowcharting and parameter charting have become increasingly important in the sophisticated environment of the intensive care unit (ICU). This type of documentation is designed to show that the clinician assessed and responded to data or trends identified. In addition, it shows that the RT responded to opportunities to reduce invasive procedures and medications or adverse events. Busy clinicians often overlook the importance of recording accurate ventilator and monitor alarm settings. If a patient were to die from a massive tension pneumothorax after a period of high peak pressures with an inappropriately set high peak pressure alarm, a strong case could be made for malpractice. However, accurate and timely documentation will verify that the RT appropriately assessed the patient-ventilator interface. This type of documentation is best suited for ventilator parameter monitoring, serial vital signs, or oximetry readings.

Tests are mostly objective observations of clinical laboratory results (e.g., arterial blood gas [ABG] levels or electrolytes) or physiologic responses to clinical challenges (e.g., fluid challenges or optimal PEEP studies). Because tests are seen as integral to the clinical course of the patient's care, the date and time of the test and its subsequent reporting to the physician are very important.

Treatment records, parameter sheets, and test result forms are standard practice in most hospitals and typically do not pose a problem for most members of the patient care team. However, some RTs find documentation of patient assessments to be a challenge. Assessment notes, medical histories, and clinical notes are extremely important in conveying information and documenting that appropriate care has been given. These types of documentation demonstrate the efforts to collect all of the information about the patient and determine his or her medical needs.

### Electronic Health Records

Historically, the medical record was a binder or similar device stored in the nurses' station, containing all the required and appropriate paper documents. However, over the past several years a transformation has taken place whereby medical records formerly maintained primarily in paper form are now almost exclusively computerized and are maintained as part of the patient's electronic health record (EHR). A closely related but different term is the electronic medical record (EMR), which represents the computerized record that is produced every time the patient (or consumer) uses health services. The EHR is the sum of all EMRs produced by a patient during the different encounters with various health care entities throughout a lifetime. Unlike the EHR, which is owned by the patient, the EMR (the "chart") is owned by the hospital or health care delivery organization. The terms *EHR* and *EMR* are so closely related that for simplicity, we will use the term *EHR* to describe both concepts for the rest of this chapter.

It should be noted that some health care organizations and facilities are still operating with a "hybrid," or combination of electronic and paper records. However, this has been rapidly changing to the full EHR model for most such organizations. This shift has been motivated by the many obvious advantages to the EHR. In addition, the federal government also introduced financial incentives to implementation of a full EHR. Under the Health Information Technology for Economic and Clinical Health (HITECH) Act, enacted as part of the American Recovery and Reinvestment Act of 2009 (ARRA), Medicare and Medicaid payments will require "meaningful use" of an EHR, accredited by a proper certification authority. As of 2015 the widespread use of EHRs throughout patient care facilities was required to avoid losing a portion of Medicare reimbursement.

The advantages of the EHR include the following:

- Legibility
- Increased storage capacity for longer periods of time

- Accessibility from remote devices and sites
- Real-time clinical data input and accessibility
- Built-in "alert" systems for critical tests and values
- Customized views for various users
- Increased management monitoring capabilities
- Increased accuracy
- A potential data repository for process improvement and research

As a result of these advantages, EHRs decrease the time it takes for clinicians to properly diagnose patients. Diagnosis becomes more accurate as a result of the accessibility to information in real time. When EHRs are used with decision support clinical applications, treatment plans and disease management are more effective.

Although the advantages of EHRs are significant, implementation and use of EHRs is not without challenges. TJC outlined some of these concerns in Sentinel Event # 42 titled "Safely Implementing Health Information and Converging Technologies." The disadvantages of the EHR include the following:

- High start-up and maintenance costs
- Significant learning curve for staff
- Confidentiality and security
- Lack of standardization among systems

## ORGANIZING PATIENT INFORMATION

There is no single best way to document medical information, especially patient assessment. The challenge that RTs face clinically is to organize patient information and assessment in a logical, professional presentation.

One of the most frequently used methods of documenting patient assessments is the subjective, objective, assessment, and plan charting (SOAP) method. We will start with the SOAP format to demonstrate how to document a patient assessment because this format is an excellent teaching tool.

### Step 1: Data Collection

As one astute physician has pointed out, "Data collection has been likened to picking flowers rather than mowing a lawn" (author unknown). For novices, a great deal of time and effort goes into collecting and organizing data without knowing its relevance. Novices do this because they do not know which information is valuable and which is not. As members of the patient care team become more experienced, they spend less time and effort in the collection of data because they know which data are clinically meaningful. The collection and organization of relevant data to make correct decisions are complex. The goal of data collection is to come to an accurate conclusion about the patient's condition, problems, and needs. To do so, it is necessary to start with proper bedside examination techniques. Poor examination methods lead to invalid data and inaccurate conclusions.

The first two steps of this system call for subjective and objective data collection (the S and O of SOAP). Subjective information is what the patient can tell you about how he

or she feels. According to experts, obtaining a good medical history from the patient can give you a reasonable chance of correctly identifying a patient's problem before doing a single test. It is also evidence of the patient's level of consciousness. If the patient is comatose, that is all the subjective information you can gather; any additional information must be objective. Other people's observations can be included in this section because they may be able to answer some of the following questions. Remember, when another person's report about a subjective issue is used, it is always hearsay. Hearsay information can be entered into the SOAP only if the RT documents who was the source of the information.

The major questions to answer in the subjective section include the following:

- What is the patient's level of consciousness?
- What is the patient's chief complaint?
- How does the patient feel at the time of the assessment?
- Can the patient contribute any information that affects his or her diagnosis or treatment plan?

### SIMPLY STATED

Subjective data are limited to what the patient tells you about his or her medical problems. Such documentation often is best put in terms of what the patient actually says during the interview.

The O in SOAP stands for objective. This is everything the RT or other member of the patient care team can measure and learn from tests and procedures. This part of the data collection can include the following:

- Vital signs (see Chapter 4)
- Physical examination of the head and neck, abdomen, and extremities for physical evidence of respiratory abnormality
- Physical examination of the thorax (heart and lungs) by inspection, palpation, percussion, and auscultation (see Chapter 5)
- Review of clinical laboratory studies (see Chapter 7)
- Review of ABG levels (see Chapter 8)
- Review of pulmonary function tests (see Chapter 9)
- Review of radiologic procedures, such as chest radiographs, computed tomography, and magnetic resonance imaging (see Chapter 10)
- Review of electrocardiograms (ECGs) (see Chapter 11)
- Review of ICU vascular pressure and cardiac outputs (see Chapters 15 and 16)
- Review of respiratory mechanics monitoring (see Chapter 14)

### Step 2: Assessment

The RT's assessment of the patient's data involves critical thinking. This includes applying clinical and scientific reasoning processes and forming a hypothesis about the nature and cause of the patient's problems. This hypothesis is used to form a "problems/needs list," which helps focus on the patient's problems and needs. Case Study 21.1 is used to illustrate how to develop a problems/needs list (Box 21.1).

## BOX 21.1 Assessment and Development of a Problems/Needs List

How do you organize and report the information in Case Study 21.1 so that you can quickly identify the patient's problems and needs? All of this information can be used as the subjective and objective information of the SOAP. You can start with almost any sign or symptom you want; just make sure you use all the information you have. As you review each piece of information, ask yourself the following questions:

- Are the data normal or abnormal? (As a corollary, are the data normal in an abnormal setting?) As an example, a $Paco_2$ of 40 mm Hg is textbook normal, but if it is associated with a minute ventilation of 15 L, the patient probably has a severe dead space disease process. In this case, a $Paco_2$ of 32 mm Hg is not normal for a patient with dyspnea and a low $Pao_2$.
- If the findings are abnormal, are they mildly, moderately, or severely out of the norm? In this case, the acid-base and carbon dioxide levels are mildly out of line with normal ABG values, but the $Pao_2$ of 53 mm Hg is moderately reduced.
- Is this an acute or chronic problem for the patient? Does the patient have an acute episode superimposed on a chronic problem? For example, in this case the hypoxemia may be a worsening of a chronic problem. More data are needed for further evaluation.
- Are any of these signs and symptoms related to each other? In this case, the patient is complaining of pain in his right elbow, but this sign probably is not related to his primary cardiopulmonary disease process. However, his fine inspiratory crackles and the leg pain have a high probability of being related to his cardiopulmonary disease process.
- Do the data indicate that there is something you can do about the patient's condition? Obviously, you can do something about the oxygenation problem, but you may not be able to administer the needed intravenous drugs because your scope of practice limits what you can and cannot give the patient.

Problems can also fit into the following additional categories:

- Current versus potential problems. Potential problems include events or outcomes that RTs want to prevent, such as volutrauma, tracheoesophageal fistulas, and reduced cardiac outputs from excessive mechanical ventilation.
- Respiratory versus nonrespiratory problems. The nonrespiratory problems that RTs are interested in include cerebral blood flow, infections, ascites, and causes of metabolic acidosis. RTs need to know enough about these and similar topics to identify how nonrespiratory problems result in cardiopulmonary signs and symptoms.

Another important factor is to not confuse the cause or diagnosis with the patient's problem. For example, the cause is smoking, the diagnosis is heart and lung disease, and the patient's problem is chronic hypoxemia.

Ultimately, it is up to the physician to make an official diagnosis. However, the RT and other members of the patient care team may assist in making an accurate diagnosis by objectively identifying patient problems and describing their signs and symptoms. There may be a subtle difference at times, but it is a necessary distinction for medicolegal reasons. If RTs perform in a competent manner within their areas of expertise and scope of practice, they will generally be on safe medicolegal ground.

RTs can define the problems they identify using the following five major types:

- *Airway management:* from the nose and mouth down to the terminal respiratory bronchiole. This includes any problem that can be treated with artificial airways, pulmonary hygiene, cough assisting, suctioning, postural drainage, and, in some circumstances, PEEP.
- *Ventilation:* the act of ventilating the patient's lungs. Acute and chronic hypoventilation problems fall into this area and can be treated with invasive or noninvasive positive-pressure ventilation.
- *Oxygenation:* the process of delivering oxygen ($O_2$) down to the cellular level. This includes cardiac output as a component of delivered oxygenation. These conditions would typically be treated with $O_2$ therapy.
- *The work of breathing (WOB):* the mechanics of both spontaneous and artificial ventilation of the lungs. Most respiratory treatments have a direct or indirect positive effect on WOB; for instance, $O_2$ therapy reduces the amount of cardiopulmonary work the patient must perform to maintain a certain amount of ventilation or partial pressure of arterial $O_2$ ($Pao_2$). RTs can measure the WOB for a mechanically ventilated patient in joules per breath or joules per minute, but measuring the $O_2$ cost of breathing is generally too difficult to perform clinically.
- *Signs of acute cardiopulmonary problems that do not have a respiratory cause:* a good example is diabetic ketoacidosis with Kussmaul breathing in which the pulmonary manifestation is relieved with the administration of insulin.

From this perspective, it is clear that RTs provide a highly specialized focus on a fairly narrow scope of practice. Furthermore, this short problem list is clearly integrated into the full range of therapeutic interventions, from life support and emergency issues to daily supportive therapies such as simple $O_2$ therapy.

Documenting the problem in the medical record helps to prioritize patient needs and improve communication among the different disciplines. This method of linking the data with problem identification is a crucial learning step and cannot be stressed enough. If the RT documents the relationships between the data and the identified problem, other members of the health care team can follow your logic (Box 21.2).

## SIMPLY STATED

The assessment part of the SOAP record is not used by RTs to diagnose the patient's problem but rather to formulate a list of the patient's cardiopulmonary problems and needs in order of severity.

---

**BOX 21.2 Problem List for the Patient in Case Study 21.2**

1. Hypoxemia: $Pao_2$, 56 mm Hg; $Sao_2$, 89%; cyanosis of the lips
2. SOB, pursed-lip breathing, and tachypnea
3. Fine crackles in both bases
4. Unresponsiveness to bronchodilators: peak flow 50% before and after treatment
5. Edema of the lower extremities
6. Tachycardia with irregular beats

---

## Step 3: The Plan

Now that the patient's problems have been listed, each patient problem should indicate an intervention and therapeutic objective. For example, in Case Study 21.1, the hypoxemia should be treated with $O_2$. The amount of $O_2$ and the therapeutic objective must be discussed with the physician. The physician's order becomes the plan (e.g., "$O_2$ at 2 L/min via nasal cannula continuously; titrate to keep $Spo_2$ at 92% or greater").

Consulting with the physician regarding orders is very important. The RT who repeatedly demonstrates effective data collection, problem identification, and appropriate therapeutic suggestions and communicates effectively with the physician will build a professional relationship based on trust. This trust between the physician and the therapist contributes to the reputation of the respiratory care department and our profession.

The following information is evident in Case Study 21.1 from the data gathered:

- The patient is acutely ill and requires interventions that may necessitate admission to the hospital for further evaluation.
- This may not be primarily a respiratory problem, and further information is needed to identify the underlying cause of the patient's symptoms.

A good medical plan must include a goal to measure against. Factors to consider when establishing or evaluating an objective include the following:

- *The purpose of the treatment.* By stating a goal for the treatment or therapy, the RT is meeting the expectations of the ordering physician and the needs of the patient. Every RT should know how to judge the effectiveness of the therapies he or she is administering and be able to guide both physicians and nurses in understanding the rationale for these goals.
- *Responsiveness of the patient.* If the therapy is administered correctly, the patient should respond in a predictable fashion. Assuming that the treatment was done correctly, if the patient does not meet the therapeutic goal, there are the following two basic possibilities:
  - The patient problem was not identified correctly, and the patient has a different problem.
  - The patient's condition is worse than originally thought. A good example would be status asthmaticus, which is asthma that does not respond to conventional treatment.

---

**BOX 21.3 The Plan (Physician Orders) for the Patient in Case Study 21.1**

1. $O_2$ via nasal cannula at 2 L/min continuously; titrate to keep $Spo_2$ 92% or greater; ABG to follow
2. Morning ABG, also PRN if condition worsens; $Spo_2$ q4h
3. CBC, CPK, electrolytes
4. Chest radiograph
5. ECG
6. Four puffs Atrovent qid
7. Four puffs Proventil, q4h PRN for SOB
8. Lasix 40 mg PO bid
9. Monitor I&O of fluids

*ABG,* Arterial blood gas; *CBC,* complete blood count; *CPK,* creatine phosphokinase; *ECG,* electrocardiogram; *I&O,* intake and output; *PO,* by mouth; *PRN,* as needed; *SOB,* shortness of breath.

---

Objectives are critical for knowing when to make decisions or perform further interventions. When ordered to give a $\beta_2$-adrenergic bronchodilator to improve the shortness of breath (SOB), it might be wise to evaluate the patient's responsiveness by comparing the current peak expiratory flow (PEF) against the prior PEF. Objectives can be used as end-point criteria for the termination of the therapy. For example, if a patient reaches a $Pao_2$ of 110 mm Hg on 1 L/min nasal cannula, it is probably time to discontinue the $O_2$.

A number of barriers to correctly setting up patient plans are as follows:

- Inadequate data collection to make correct decisions (most common)
- Failure to recognize patient problems
- False assumptions about relationships between the data and the identified problem
- Confusing the disease with the problem, or confusing the cause with the problem; this barrier leads to ineffective intervention

The physician has continued the assessment by including additional tests (information collection) to assess cardiac signs and symptoms (e.g., ECG, chest radiograph, creatine phosphokinase [CPK], and heart sounds) and to confirm or eliminate additional diagnoses (Box 21.3). The physician has recognized that there is a high probability that there is a cardiac problem. The RT cannot state that there is a cardiac problem because that is a diagnosis and out of the RT's scope of practice. An RT, however, can correctly relate the signs of a cardiac problem (e.g., tachycardia, irregular heartbeat, and edema of the lower extremities) and the signs of cellulitis.

## Step 4: Implementation of the Plan

The next step is to actually give the treatment or perform the test. During the administration of bedside treatment, the RT still has to use critical thinking skills to perform the procedure or test correctly. Furthermore, the RT needs to keep in mind the technical aspects of equipment operation necessary for safe and effective care.

As the RT does the treatment or test, he or she continues to collect data through assessment to move on to the next step of evaluating the effectiveness of the plan.

## Step 5: Evaluation of the Results of the Plan and Implementation

An important question to ask is whether the problem has been correctly identified. To answer this, it is necessary to go through another couple of questions, as follows:

- Was there any evidence of adverse effects?
- Was the response expected, given your knowledge of the patient and the technology used?

By actively seeking answers to these and similar questions and then acting on the observed results, the RT is returning to the data collection, assessment, plan, and implementation steps outlined earlier. This cycling through the steps of the scientific process is essential for good patient care.

### SIMPLY STATED

RTs and other members of the patient care team who blindly follow physician orders are doing a disservice to their patients. The competent RT is constantly evaluating the effects of therapy and documenting the results in the patient's medical record. It may be necessary to contact the physician if serious adverse effects occur or if the patient requires a change in therapy.

## CHARTING METHODS

Most charting systems in use today are based on some variation of the problem-oriented medical record. All of the following charting systems require a clear outline of the patient's problems and corresponding physician orders or professional care plans to address those problems. Patient assessments can be written either on profession-specific forms or in the multidisciplinary progress notes, depending on the hospital standards. Four popular formats for writing progress notes are described in this section. The HCO will determine which of the following methods is acceptable.

### SIMPLY STATED

The RT typically documents the results of tests and treatment on treatment records, flowcharts, and test records. Failure to do so may call into question whether the tests or treatments were actually done.

### Subjective, Objective, Assessment, and Plan Charting

As noted earlier, SOAP charting is one of the most frequently used documentation methods, in part because it is believed to be the best presentation of the patient's conditions and clearly shows how the physician or other member of the patient care team arrives at his or her professional conclusions.

### Assessment, Plan, Implementation, and Evaluation Charting

A primary goal of the assessment, plan, implementation, and evaluation (APIE) method is to condense the data-collection statements and emphasize evaluation of the effectiveness of the interventions.

### Problem, Intervention, and Plan Charting

At the other extreme from the detailed presentation of SOAP charting is the minimalist approach: problem, implementation, and plan (PIP) charting. PIP charting is based on the assumption that the data collection has already been done in the medical record and that the subjective and objective information gathering of SOAP charting is redundant. Some people dislike this method because they like to see the evidence and logic leading to the assessment and resulting order. However, the PIP method works well for the experienced clinician who is pressed for time, wants to meet charting requirements, and needs to be brief. Under the "Problem" section, the patient's problem is stated simply, often with reference to the evidence that brought the author to this conclusion. Next is the "Intervention" section, which describes what is being done for the patient. This is often identical with the physician orders or standards of care for the services being provided. The "Plan" section shows how the intervention will be assessed or carried out, depending on the intervention.

### Situation, Background, Assessment, and Recommendation Charting

The situation, background, assessment, and recommendation charting (SBAR) is one of the newer methodologies for communication in health care. The SBAR format was originally modeled in aviation and military handoff. Poor communication is identified as one of the root causes in the majority of sentinel events reported to TJC; thus the SBAR method was well received in the health care community. The use of a standardized communication and documentation technique for all health care team members will ensure patient safety and quality outcomes. The SBAR format is meant to promote a structured situational briefing, regardless of different communication styles. The parts of the acronym SBAR stand for the following:

- *Situation:* What is happening now? (chief complaint or acute change)
- *Background:* What factors led to this event? (admitting diagnosis, history, vital signs, laboratory results, or other pertinent clinical findings)
- *Assessment:* What do you see? What do you think is going on?
- *Recommendation:* What action do you propose? What do you think should be done?

The SBAR method has proved highly successful in critical situations and has been promoted with the implementation of *medical emergency teams,* also known as *rapid response teams.* It is most successful for summary information with less than five key points. It is not as effective for broad communication or for in-depth coverage of many related topics.

See the Case Studies for illustrations of each of these different charting styles.

## KEY POINTS

- The role of the RT in the documentation of the patient assessment is well defined. The RT must be able to not only assess the patient's condition accurately but also document the findings in the patient's medical record using a prescribed format that meets HCO, TJC, and legal requirements.
- The documentation of patient assessments serves a variety of purposes that are important to the business of the HCO.
- The absence of information or the lack of documented recognition of specific problems could constitute malpractice.
- If a treatment, assessment finding, or clinical problem was not charted, it is generally considered not to have been done or detected.

- A variety of documentation formats are available, each of which has its own advantages. Regardless of the method chosen, each recording in the patient chart must be accurate, concise, and available to other clinicians for review.
- Subjective information is what the patients can tell you about how they feel, whereas objective information is what you can measure, such as laboratory test results or vital signs.
- High-quality documentation after each patient encounter promotes improved communication within the HCO and promotes improved patient outcomes.

### CASE STUDY 21.1

You are called to the emergency department to see a patient who is complaining of SOB. An order has been written for bronchodilator treatment. On arrival, you find a 65-year-old moderately obese man sitting upright on the examination table in a single-patient examination room. You observe that his respiratory rate is about 20 breaths/min, with pursed-lip breathing and slight cyanosis around the lips, and he is unable to say more than a few words per breath. He is complaining of right elbow pain. His heart rate is 126 beat/min and irregular. On auscultation, you hear fine crackles in both lung bases. He reports a nonproductive cough for the past 2 days, with increasing SOB, an inability to lie flat, and increasing leg pain. You notice that he is unable to tie his shoes because his feet are swollen and that his legs are very red, shiny, and painful to the touch. His current PEF is 50% of predicted. A room air ABG was done before your arrival: pH, 7.47; $Paco_2$, 32 mm Hg; $Pao_2$, 53 mm Hg; $HCO_3^-$, 23 mEq; BE, 0; $Sao_2$, 89%. No chest radiograph has been ordered yet.

You give the ordered bronchodilator treatment with $O_2$, but the patient reports no subjective relief. No changes in vital signs are noted. His color does improve a little during the treatment ($O_2$ at 6 L/min via small-volume nebulizer), and his breath sounds are unchanged. His cough is nonproductive, and there is no measurable change in the peak flow after treatment.

**SOAP Format Example**
Date: 2/27/12
Time: 0950
S: Pt. c/o SOB and right elbow pain
O: Patient is a moderately obese male, orthopneic, pursed-lip breathing with cyanosis around lips. Can only speak a few words per breath. Fine crackles at bases, nonproductive cough × 2 days. Heart rate 126 beats/min and irregular. Bilateral pedal edema noted and painful to touch. $Pao_2$ 53 on room air.
A:
   1. Hypoxemic with $Pao_2$ 53 on room air. Slight hyperventilation
   2. Crackles auscultated with nonproductive cough
   3. Pedal edema with pain to touch
   4. Reduced peak flow, unchanged with bronchodilator

P:
   1. Chest radiograph to be performed ASAP
   2. Start on 2 L/min nasal cannula: done
   3. Repeat ABG on $O_2$
   4. ECG stat
   5. Repeat bronchodilator

**APIE Format Example**
Date: 2/27/12
Time: 0950
A:
   1. Signs and symptoms of respiratory distress and hypoxemia
   2. Probable bronchospasm, unrelieved by bronchodilator
   3. Tachycardia at 126, irregular
   4. Pedal edema, painful to touch
P:
   1. Chest radiograph ASAP
   2. $O_2$ at 2 L/min nasal cannula
   3. Repeat ABG
   4. ECG
I:
   1. Consultation with physician
   2. $O_2$ at 2 L/min nasal cannula started
   3. ECG performed
E: At 1030: Patient continues SOB, color improved. $Pao_2$ increased to 68 mm Hg on $O_2$

**PIP Format Example**
Date: 2/27/12
Time: 0950
P:
   1. Signs and symptoms of respiratory distress and hypoxemia
   2. Fine crackles, probably bronchospasm
   3. Tachycardia at 126, irregular
I:
   1. $O_2$ at 2 L/min nasal cannula: $Pao_2$ increased to 68 mm Hg on $O_2$
   2. Chest radiograph ASAP
   3. ECG stat
P:
   1. Continue $O_2$ therapy and monitor patient's ABG
   2. Consult with physician for ongoing bronchodilator therapy

## CASE STUDY 21.1—cont'd

**SBAR Format Example**

Date: 2/27/12

Time: 0950

S: Patient is dyspneic and orthopneic, with nonproductive cough, severe pedal edema, painful to touch

B: Patient is an obese male. Nonproductive cough × 2 days

A: Patient is orthopneic at 20 breaths/min. Heart rate 126/min and irregular. $Pao_2$ 53 on room air. Fine crackles bilaterally with nonproductive cough. Pedal edema severe and painful to touch. Peak flow 50% predicted, unchanged postbronchodilator

R: $O_2$ at 2 L/min via nasal cannula

Stat ECG

Repeat ABG

Continue bronchodilator therapy

## CASE STUDY 21.2

The charge nurse calls you to the medical floor on the night shift because a patient has awakened with SOB. You find a 65-year-old man sitting upright in his bed, leaning forward on the nightstand. He is pursed-lipped and using accessory muscles to breathe, with a prolonged expiratory phase, at a rate of 16 to 18 breaths/min. In the dim light of his semiprivate room, it is hard to see his color, but his skin is warm and moist over his upper torso, and his chest has an increased anteroposterior diameter. His $Spo_2$ is 86% on room air. On auscultation, you hear fine crackles in the right base and expiratory low-pitched wheezing in the upper lung fields bilaterally. Breath sounds in the left lung base are diminished. He has expectorated at least 10 mL of thick greenish-yellow sputum; no blood is seen. By palpation, his pulse is rapid and occasionally irregular. He was admitted 6 hours earlier for a knee fracture incurred during a fall that afternoon. When interviewed, he relates that he has COPD but has not been receiving any treatment for it for the past 6 months. When he was taking medication, it was only one metered-dose inhaler, 4 puffs in the early morning and afternoon, but he does not remember the name of the medication. The physician has been called, and you are awaiting a return phone call. You and the nurse agree to do the following:

1. Start $O_2$ therapy at 2 L/min via nasal cannula
2. Repeat $Spo_2$ after $O_2$ therapy
3. Get an ECG stat
4. Call the physician again and call the nursing and respiratory supervisors

Immediately after completing these interventions and telling your supervisor what you have done, you sit down to chart your assessment and what has transpired.

**SOAP Format Example**

Date: 2/27/12

Time: 0130

S: "I can't breathe," "I'm not on any inhalers at this time," "I have COPD."

O: Patient has SOB, skin is warm and moist. Using accessory muscles, pursed-lip breathing, and long expiratory phase. Expectorated 10 mL of thick yellow and greenish sputum. Fine crackles in right base, left base diminished, low-pitched wheezing throughout. $Spo_2$ on room air 86%.

A:
1. Signs and symptoms of respiratory distress and hypoxemia
2. Retained secretions, possible bronchospasm

P:
1. Call physician and appropriate supervisors: done
2. Start on 2 L/min nasal cannula: done
3. Repeat $Spo_2$: done at 0155: 89%
4. ECG: done at 0145

5. Request orders for above, stat ABG, bronchodilator therapy, and sputum culture and sensitivity

**APIE Format Example**

Date: 2/27/12

Time: 0130

A:
1. Signs and symptoms of respiratory distress and hypoxemia
2. Retained secretions, possible bronchospasm

P:
1. Call physician and hospital supervisors
2. Start on 2 L/min nasal cannula
3. Repeat $Spo_2$
4. ECG
5. Request orders for above, stat ABG, bronchodilator therapy, and sputum C&S

I:
1. Calls made
2. Started on 2 L/min nasal cannula
3. ECG done

E: At 0210: Patient's SOB decreased but not totally reversed; $Spo_2$ 89% on $O_2$

**PIP Format Example**

Date: 2/27/12

Time: 0130

P:
1. Signs and symptoms of respiratory distress and hypoxemia
2. Retained secretions, possible bronchospasm

I:
1. Call physician and hospital supervisors: done
2. Start on 2 L/min nasal cannula: done and $Spo_2$ 89% at 0155
3. ECG: done at 0145

P:
1. Continue $O_2$ therapy and monitor patient's level of SOB and $Spo_2$
2. Request orders for above, stat ABG, and bronchodilator therapy

**SBAR Format Example**

Date: 2/27/12

Time: 0130

S: Patient has increased SOB

B: Patient has a history of COPD. He was admitted today after a fall that resulted in a fractured knee.

A: Patient is orthopneic: 18 breaths/min. Skin is warm and moist. $Spo_2$ is 86% on room air. Breath sounds diminished. He is expectorating green-yellow sputum.

R: $O_2$ at 2 L/min via nasal cannula. Stat ECG. Repeat pulse oximetry.

## CASE STUDY 21.3

You are just starting your morning shift in the adult ICU, and you have been assigned a 22-year-old woman with a history of acute asthma. The shift report to you is that she has been on q1h bronchodilator therapy with 2.5 mg albuterol in 3 mL normal saline for 18 hours; concurrently she has been receiving 50% via air-entrainment mask, with a "PRN ABG for SOB" order and with a continuous pulse oximeter and ECG. She has been alert and cooperative, and her SOB had diminished through the night shift. Her admission ABG levels on 50% $Fio_2$ were pH, 7.46; $Paco_2$, 30; $Pao_2$, 70; $HCO_3^-$, 22; BE, 1; $Sao_2$, 94%; Hb, 12.0; COHb, 0.7%.

When you arrive in the ICU, you note a slightly sleepy but easily aroused cooperative young adult. Her $Spo_2$ is reading 94% on 50% $O_2$, heart rate is 126 beats/min, and respiratory rate is 20 breaths/min without accessory muscle use. Auscultation reveals that she has bilateral inspiratory and expiratory wheezing. Her chest radiograph report states that there is hyperinflation noted bilaterally, with patchy infiltrates and atelectasis in the right lung base. Her radial pulses are strong and unaffected by her respiratory pattern. Her stat morning electrolyte levels are all within normal limits; her complete blood count (CBC) shows eosinophilia but otherwise is within normal limits. You start her treatment at 0700 and finish at 0715; vital signs and breath sounds are unchanged throughout the treatment. You finish your charting and go to your next patient.

At 0745, the nurse calls you and asks you to come see the same asthmatic patient. You immediately recognize that her ECG rate and respiratory rate have increased in the past 30 minutes, and her accessory muscle use has increased. She is becoming restless, pulling her air-entrainment mask off and complaining of increasing SOB. You cannot hear any breath sounds over her right lower lobe. With the nurse helping hold the patient's arm steady, you draw an arterial sample. Her $Spo_2$ is now 89% on the air-entrainment mask when she keeps it on. Before you go to analyze the ABG levels, you put her on a nonrebreather mask per physician orders. Her ABG levels are pH, 7.26; $Paco_2$, 52 mm Hg; $Pao_2$, 50 mm Hg; $HCO_3^-$, 22; BE, 5; $Sao_2$, 87%; Hb, 12.0. On your return, the patient's physician is at the bedside, and she tells you the patient is going to be intubated and placed on a ventilator. The anesthesiologist is called to intubate as you leave to get the ventilator. The patient is successfully intubated and placed on the ventilator per physician initial orders. Before you start an in-line bronchodilator treatment, you note and report that her auto-PEEP is 12 cm $H_2O$ at a respiratory rate of 14 breaths/min with an inspiratory/expiratory (I/E) ratio of 1:2.5. After the in-line treatment, the breath sounds, peak pressures, and auto-PEEP are all unchanged, but the $Spo_2$ has improved to 95%.

According to hospital policy, you now have to write an assessment in the medical record.

### SOAP Format Example

Date: 2/27/12

Time: 0850

S: "I can't breathe!" "Help me!"

O: Increasing SOB, despite q1h bronchodilator treatments; increasing $Paco_2$ to 52 mm Hg with falling pH, $Pao_2$ decreasing to 50 mm Hg concurrently, right lung sounds much more diminished than at start of shift. Patient was intubated and placed on a ventilator. Initial settings: respiratory rate of 14

breaths/min with an I/E ratio of 1:3.5; $V_T$, 700 mL; $Fio_2$, 70%; $Spo_2$, 95%. Auto-PEEP is 12 cm $H_2O$ initially on ventilator.

A:

1. Acute hypercapnia, respiratory acidosis
2. Hypoxemia despite $O_2$ therapy
3. Increased work of breathing with profound SOB
4. Greatly diminished breath sounds in RLL area

P:

1. Intubate and place on ventilator: done
2. Increase $Fio_2$: done
3. Repeat ABG: pending
4. Continue bronchodilator therapy in-line, q1h: started
5. Monitor sedation needs and effectiveness
6. Monitor auto-PEEP
7. Check tube placement on chest radiograph
8. Adjust the ventilator settings, post-ABG, to new settings per physician orders

### APIE Format Example

Date: 2/27/12

Time: 0850

A:

1. Acute hypercapnia and respiratory acidosis
2. Hypoxemia despite $O_2$ therapy
3. Increased work of breathing with profound SOB
4. Greatly diminished breath sounds in right lower lobe area

P:

1. Intubate and place on ventilator
2. Increase $Fio_2$
3. Repeat ABGs
4. Continue bronchodilator therapy in-line q1h
5. Monitor sedation needs and effectiveness
6. Monitor auto-PEEP
7. Check tube placement on chest radiograph
8. Adjust the ventilator settings, post-ABG, to new settings per physician orders

### APIE Format Example

A:

1. Acute hypercapnia and respiratory acidosis
2. Hypoxemia despite $O_2$ therapy
3. Increased work of breathing with profound SOB
4. Greatly diminished breath sounds in right lower lobe area

P:

1. Intubate and place on ventilator
2. Increase $Fio_2$
3. Repeat ABGs
4. Continue bronchodilator therapy in-line q1h
5. Monitor sedation needs and effectiveness
6. Monitor auto-PEEP
7. Check tube placement on chest radiograph
8. Adjust the ventilator settings, post-ABG, to new settings per physician orders

I:

1. Intubated and placed on ventilator with the following settings: respiratory rate of 14 breaths/min, with an I/E ratio of 1:2.5; $V_T$ at 700 mL; $Fio_2$, 70%
2. Increased $Fio_2$: done
3. Continue bronchodilator therapy in-line q1h: done
4. Monitor auto-PEEP

## CASE STUDY 21.3—cont'd

E:
1. Patient is resting on ventilator, sedated
2. ABG: pending
3. $SpO_2$ is 95% currently
4. Breath sounds unchanged

**PIP Format Example**
Date: 2/27/12
Time: 0850
P:
1. Acute hypercapnia and respiratory acidosis
2. Hypoxemia despite $O_2$ therapy
3. Increased work of breathing with profound SOB
4. Greatly diminished breath sounds in right lower lobe area

I:
1. Intubated and placed on ventilator
2. Increased $FiO_2$
3. Repeat ABG: pending
4. Continue bronchodilator therapy in-line q1h: done

P:
1. Monitor sedation needs and effectiveness
2. Monitor auto-PEEP

3. Check tube placement on chest radiograph
4. Adjust the ventilator settings, post-ABG, to new settings per physician orders

**SBAR Format Example**
Date: 2/27/12
Time: 0130
S: Increased shortness of breath and accessory muscle usage. Patient is restless.
B: History of asthma. Has been receiving bronchodilators q1h and is on 50% air-entrainment mask.
A: $PaO_2$ has decreased to 50 mm Hg on 50% air-entrainment mask. $PaCO_2$ increased to 52 mm Hg, and pH is 7.26. Respiratory rate and heart rate are increased. Absent breath sounds over RLL.
R: Intubate patient
   Continue bronchodilators
   Repeat ABG
   Monitor auto-PEEP
   Check tube placement on chest radiograph

## ASSESSMENT QUESTIONS

1. The patient's medical record is all of the following *except:*
   a. A financial document
   b. A legal document
   c. An educational tool
   d. A contract

2. Which of the following organizations specifies what is required to be documented in a patient's medical record?
   a. FDA
   b. CMS
   c. Financial intermediary
   d. The patient's family

3. What is the primary goal of The Joint Commission?
   a. Monitor financial reimbursement of hospitals
   b. Review HCOs to improve the quality of health care
   c. Provide health care workers with a safe work environment
   d. Monitor the ethical practice of medicine at HCOs

4. Which of the following statements is most appropriate for the RT to document in the assessment section of the SOAP documentation?
   a. Onset of asthma
   b. Viral pneumonia
   c. Hypoxemia on room air
   d. Diabetic ketoacidosis

5. Which of the following is *not* true regarding the legal definition of negligence?
   a. The defendant owed a duty of care to the plaintiff
   b. The defendant breached that duty
   c. The plaintiff suffered a legally recognizable injury
   d. The defendant's breach of duty of care did not cause the plaintiff's injury

6. Which of the following is *not* a type of medical record entry that the RT needs to perform in his or her daily routine?
   a. Treatment record
   b. History and physical examination
   c. Flowchart
   d. Test results

7. Which of the following outlines your medicolegal duties to the patient?
   a. TJC standards
   b. Your state's respiratory care practice act
   c. Your job description and employer's policies and procedures
   d. All of the above

8. All of the following are examples of "objective" data *except:*
   a. Laboratory results
   b. Observation of the patient's sleep apnea
   c. The patient's report of the amount of sputum he or she produces daily
   d. The physician's interpretation of the patient's ECG

9. What does the letter "I" stand for in the APIE method of documentation?
   a. Implementation
   b. Impact
   c. Inconsistencies
   d. None of the above

10. Which method of documentation is probably best for a clinician pressed for time?
   a. SOAP
   b. APIE
   c. PIP
   d. SBAR

# BIBLIOGRAPHY

Cohen MF. Impact of the HITECH financial incentives on EHR adoption in small, physician-owned practices. *Int J Med Inform.* 2016;94:143–154.

Davis KA, Smith LB. Ethical considerations about EHR-mediated results disclosure and pathology information presented via patient portals. *AMA J Ethics.* 2016;18(8):826–832.

Davis RL. Using SBAR as a reconference reporting tool for nursing students. *Nurse Educ.* 2016;41(2):74.

Ford RM. Therapist-driven protocols: new incentives for change. *Respir Care.* 2015;60(5):757–759.

Kacmarek RM, Stoller JK, Heuer AJ. *Egan's fundamentals of respiratory care.* 11th ed. St. Louis: Mosby-Elsevier; 2017.

Pearce PF, Ferguson LA, George GS, et al. The essential SOAP note in an EHR age. *Nurse Pract.* 2016;41(2):29–36.

Sebelius K. Major progress in doctors, hospital use of health information technology. Available at http://www.hhs.gov/news/press/2012pres/02/20120217a.html. Retrieved March 9, 2012.

Sittig DF, Singh H. Legal, ethical, and financial dilemmas in electronic health record adoption and use. *Pediatrics.* 2011;127(4):e1042–e1047.

Sullivan D. *Guide to clinical documentation.* 2nd ed. Philadelphia: FA Davis; 2011.

The Joint Commission. *Comprehensive accreditation manual for hospitals.* Oakbrook Terrace, IL: TJC ; 2015.

# GLOSSARY

**6MWD**   6-minute walk distance, the distance a patient can walk in the 6-minute walk test; used to help determine the degree of dyspnea and quality of life (Ch 9)

## A

**abdominal paradox**   paradoxic movement of the abdomen during breathing, associated with diaphragm fatigue (Ch 5)

**abortion**   termination of pregnancy, either spontaneous (natural interruption from abnormalities of the fetus, placenta, uterus, or mother) or therapeutic (induced interruption) (Ch 12)

**acceptability**   as pertaining to pulmonary function tests, meeting prespecified criteria that ensure the validity of the results, such as the forced vital capacity maneuver being free of artifacts (Ch 9)

**accessory muscles**   muscles of the neck, back, and abdomen that may assist the diaphragm and the internal and external intercostal muscles in respiration, especially in some breathing disorders or during exercise (Ch 5)

**acidemia**   as pertaining to arterial blood, an abnormally high hydrogen ion concentration, indicated by a pH less than 7.35 (Ch 8)

**acidosis**   a respiratory or metabolic process causing acidemia or an abnormally decreased pH (Ch 8)

**acrocyanosis**   a bluish discoloration of the extremities usually caused by inadequate circulation; also known as peripheral cyanosis (Chs 5, 12)

**action plan**   a written plan that involves patients in the goal-setting and self-care activities needed to help manage their disease process (Ch 1)

**action potential**   a brief reversal in the electrical potential difference across a nerve cell or muscle fiber membrane that occurs in response to a stimulus (Ch 10)

**adenosine triphosphate (ATP)**   the body's energy currency molecules (Ch 18)

**adventitious**   refers to adventitious lung sounds, abnormal lung sounds superimposed on the basic underlying normal sounds (Ch 5)

**afferent**   pertaining to nerves, those transporting impulses to the central nervous system (Ch 6)

**afterload**   the resistance to blood flow out of a ventricle during systole (Ch 16)

**ageism**   discrimination against older people (Ch 13)

**air bronchogram**   abnormal radiographic finding that occurs when the air-filled bronchi are surrounded by consolidated alveoli (Ch 10)

**airway hyperresponsiveness (AHR)**   state of airways that causes them to constrict abnormally in response to stress or insults (e.g., exercise, inhaled materials such as dust or allergens) (Ch 9)

**airway resistance**   opposition to the movement of air in the respiratory tract; defined as pressure difference across the airway divided by the flow (the reciprocal of airway conductance) (Chs 9, 14)

**alkalemia**   as pertaining to arterial blood, an abnormally low hydrogen ion concentration, indicated by a pH greater than 7.45 (Ch 8)

**alkalosis**   a respiratory or metabolic process causing alkalemia or an abnormally elevated pH (Ch 8)

**alveolar dead space**   alveoli that are ventilated but not perfused (Ch 14)

**anabolism**   the constructive phase of metabolism in which more complex structures are made out of simple ones (Ch 18)

**analyte**   a sample of blood or body fluids that undergoes chemical analysis (Ch 7)

**analytic error**   error occurring during the analysis or measurement phase of a laboratory test (Ch 8)

**anasarca**   widespread tissue edema (Ch 12)

**anatomic dead space**   the volume of air in the trachea and other airways not in intimate contact with pulmonary capillaries (Ch 14)

**anemia**   an abnormal decrease in the circulating red blood cells and/or hemoglobin (Chs 7, 8, 18)

**anergy**   impaired reaction to antigens administered by skin test (Ch 7)

**anaerobic threshold**   the point during incremental exercise at which blood lactate and $CO_2$ levels increase due to anaerobic metabolism occurring in the muscles (Ch 9)

**angina**   chest pain associated with inadequate coronary blood flow (Ch 3)

**angle of Louis**   slightly oblique angle where the manubrium articulates with the body of the sternum (Ch 5)

**anion gap**   the difference between the measured cations and anions in serum, used to help differentiate among causes of metabolic acidosis (Ch 8)

**anisocoria**   one pupil is larger than the other (Ch 6)

**anterior fontanel**   the largest of the spaces between the bony plates of the skull in newborn infants, which close over the first few years of life (Ch 12)

**anteroposterior (AP) view**   a chest radiograph in which the x-ray beam is directed from the front of the thorax, with the film or sensor placed at the back (Ch 10)

**Apgar score**   a 10-point score used to evaluate the well-being of infants at birth and after delivery (Ch 12)

**apical lordotic view**   a radiographic technique in which the patient is positioned at a 45-degree angle to better visualize the right middle lobe or the lung apices (Ch 10)

**apnea**   the cessation of breathing; during sleep, the pause in breathing must be at least 10 seconds for apnea to be present (Ch 12)

**apnea-hypopnea index (AHI)**   the total number of apneas and/or episodes of reduced airflow occurring per hour of sleep (Ch 19)

**arousal**   an abrupt change in sleep stage from a deeper level to a lighter one, typically accompanied by an increase in EMG activity (Ch 19)

**arterial-to-alveolar tension ratio ($Pao_2/PAo_2$)**   the ratio of arterial oxygen partial pressure to the alveolar oxygen partial pressure; normally >0.90 (Ch 14)

**arterial-to-mixed venous oxygen content difference ($C[a-\dot{v}]o_2$)**   the difference between the oxygen content of the arterial blood and the oxygen content of the mixed venous sample; normally 3.5 to 5.0 mL/100 mL of blood (Ch 14)

**ascites**   the accumulation of serous fluid in the abdominal cavity (Chs 5, 12)

**ataxia**   loss of muscle coordination (Ch 6)

**ataxic breathing**   an irregular and unpredictable breathing pattern that indicates that all brain function above the medulla is absent (Ch 6)

**atelectasis**   collapse of normally expanded lung tissue (Ch 10)

**atrial kick**   the added filling of the ventricles during diastole caused by atrial contraction (Ch 11)

**attenuation**   the decrease in the frequency range of sounds as they travel through lung tissue to the chest wall (Ch 5)

**auscultation**   the act of listening to bodily sounds, for example, heart or lung sounds (Ch 5)

**automaticity**   the ability of cardiac tissue to stimulate depolarization spontaneously (Ch 11)

**auto–positive end-expiratory pressure (auto-PEEP)**   positive pressure remaining in the alveoli after exhalation not associated with its therapeutic application; most often due to high expiratory airway resistance combined with inadequate expiratory times (Ch 14)

## B

**Babinski sign**   dorsiflexion of the great toe with fanning of remaining toes during testing of the plantar reflex; a sign of neurologic disease (Ch 6)

**back-extrapolated volume**   a measure used to judge the validity of a forced expiratory volume (FEV) vs. time curve; equals the volume at time 0, which is defined as the point at which the tangent to the steepest portion of the FEV curve crosses the X-axis (Ch 9)

**barotrauma**   physical injury sustained as a result of exposure to ambient pressures above normal, most commonly secondary to positive-pressure ventilation (e.g., pneumothorax, pneumomediastinum) (Ch 14)

**barrel chest**   the abnormal increase in anteroposterior chest diameter (Ch 5)

**basal energy expenditure (BEE)**   the measure obtained when a person is at absolute rest with no physical movement (Ch 18)

**basal metabolic rate (BMR)**   rate of oxygen consumption at rest (Ch 18)

**base excess (BE)**   measures changes in total blood buffer base above or below normal (Chs 8, 12, 21)

**basophilia**   an abnormal elevation of the blood basophil count (Ch 7)

**Berlin Questionnaire**   a screening questionnaire used to identify the risk for sleep disordered breathing (Ch 19)

**biologic control**   as pertaining to pulmonary function testing, a healthy subject for whom quality control data are available (Ch 9)

**Biot breathing**   breathing characterized by irregular periods of apnea alternating with periods in which four or five breaths of identical depth are taken (Ch 5)

**blasts**   early cells that produce the formed elements in the blood (Ch 7)

**body mass index (BMI)**   one's weight in kg divided by the square of one's height in cm; the primary method for assessment of the appropriateness of weight for a given height (Ch 18)

**bradycardia**   a decrease in the heart rate below normal range (<60 beats/min in adults) (Chs 4, 12)

**bradypnea**   an abnormal decrease in the rate of breathing (Chs 4, 12)

**brain death**   irreversible cessation of all functions of the brain, including the brainstem (Ch 6)

**breathing reserve**   proportion of the maximum voluntary ventilation (MVV) that is unused after reaching maximum minute ventilation at peak exercise; typically exceeds 30% (Ch 9)

**bronchial breath sounds**   harsh breath sounds with an expiratory component equal to the inspiratory component (Ch 5)

**bronchoalveolar lavage**   the instillation of sterile fluid and its recollection from a portion of the lung via fiberoptic bronchoscopy, with the fluid analyzed by cytologic or microbiologic methods (Ch 17)

**bronchophony**   an increase in intensity and clarity of vocal resonance (Ch 5)

**bronchoprovocation testing**   a specialized pulmonary function test that uses substances such as methacholine or histamine to "provoke" the airways into contracting; a measure of airway hyperreactivity (Ch 9)

**bronchopulmonary dysplasia (BPD)**   chronic lung disease of newborns, usually premature (Ch 12)

**bronchoscope**   highly specialized medical device that allows for examination of the patient's airways using a long tube with a fiberoptic light bundle and an open channel running its entire length; used for irrigating distal airways, suctioning, and obtaining specimens using brushes and biopsy forceps (Ch 17)

**bronchoscopy**   the procedure in which the patient's airways are examined with a bronchoscope (Chs 10, 17)

**bruit**   a cardiovascular term associated with the sound of blood passing through a site of obstruction (Ch 12)

**bulging**   the opposite movement of the skin between the ribs during exhalation (Ch 5)

## C

**cachectic**   a state of poor health resulting from malnutrition (Ch 18)

**calibration**   exposing a measurement device to two or more known levels of measurement to confirm proper zeroing, gain, and linearity (Chs 8, 9)

**capnography**   monitoring the concentration of exhaled carbon dioxide using a graph (Ch 14)

**capnometry**   the general process of monitoring exhaled carbon dioxide (Ch 14)

**carbon dioxide production ($\dot{V}CO_2$)**   the amount of carbon dioxide produced by metabolism per minute (Ch 14)

**cardiac index (CI)**   the cardiac output indexed to a patient's body surface area (Ch 16)

**cardiac output**   the amount of blood pumped out of the left ventricle in 1 minute (Ch 16)

**cardiac work**   a measurement of the energy the heart uses to eject blood against the aortic or pulmonary pressures (resistance) (Ch 16)

**cardiac work index**   the work per minute per square meter of body surface area for each ventricle (Ch 16)

**catabolism**   the destructive phase of metabolism that breaks complex structures into simple ones (Ch 18)

**Centers for Medicare and Medicaid Services (CMS)**   a federal agency within the U.S. Department of Health and Human Services that administers Medicare, Medicaid, the State Children's Health Insurance Program (SCHIP), and health insurance portability standards (Chs 20, 21)

**central cyanosis**   a bluish discoloration of the trunk or oral mucosa usually due to low arterial $O_2$ content and high proportions of deoxygenated hemoglobin (Ch 5)

**central nervous system (CNS)**   that part of the nervous system consisting of the brain and spinal cord (Ch 6)

**central sleep apnea (CSA)**   pauses in breathing resulting from a temporary loss in the drive to breathe (Ch 19)

**central venous pressure (CVP)**   the pressure measured in the right atrium (Chs 15, 16)

**cerebral perfusion pressure (CPP)**   the pressure difference across the cerebral circulation; equals mean arterial pressure minus intracranial pressure (Ch 6)

**chest radiograph**   an x-ray image of the chest; a posteroanterior view and a lateral, or side, view are routinely obtained (Ch 10)

**chest ultrasound**   a noninvasive procedure using transmission and reflection/detection of high-frequency sound waves to assess the organs and structures within the chest, such as the lungs, mediastinum, and pleural space (Ch 10)

**Cheyne-Stokes respiration**   an abnormal breathing pattern that consists of phases of hyperpnea that regularly alternate with episodes of apnea; often caused by an intracranial lesion (Ch 6)

**cholestasis**   the cessation or blockage of bile flow from the liver to the duodenum (Ch 12)

**chronologic age**   the age of an infant in days, weeks, months, or years from birth (Ch 12)

**closed-loop communication**   repeating an oral order back to ensure its accuracy (Ch 1)

**clubbing**   painless enlargement of the terminal phalanges of the fingers and toes (Ch 5)

**coarctation of the aorta**   abnormal narrowing of the internal diameter of the aorta; usually around the ductus arteriosus (Ch 12)

**compliance**   a measure of relative stiffness of the lung that is defined as volume change per unit change in pressure (Chs 9, 14)

**computed tomography (CT)**   a highly advanced means of imaging in which x-ray shadows are enhanced by using a computer (Ch 10)

**confidentiality**   the ethical and legal obligation to maintain the privacy of protected health information except as allowed by the patient or as needed by other authorized persons (Ch 21)

**content of consciousness**   the sum of cognitive and affective mental functions, including awareness of one's existence, as well as memory and thinking processes (Ch 6)

**contractility**   as pertaining to the heart, the force with which myocardial fibers shorten during systole (Ch 16)

**corneal reflex**   used to test the afferent cranial nerve V and the efferent cranial nerve VII, performed by lightly touching the cornea with a cotton swab; normal response is that the patient should blink both eyes (Ch 6)

**cough**   a forceful expiratory maneuver designed to clear the larger airways; a common complaint of patients with lung disease (Ch 3)

**crackles**   discontinuous adventitious lung sounds (Ch 5)

**cranial sutures**   the open space between any two of the flat bones of the skull in the newborn and young infant (Ch 12)

**creatine phosphate**   an energy reserve molecule in muscle (Ch 18)

**creatinine**   a waste product of metabolism (Ch 18)

**creatinine-height index (CHI)**   a predictor of muscle mass (Ch 18)

**crepitus**   a grating or popping sound or sensation; when felt under the skin, indicates trapped air (subcutaneous emphysema), often a sign of pneumothorax (Ch 13)

**critical congenital heart disease (CCHD)**   a category of heart defects present at birth that cause serious, life-threatening symptoms and typically require immediate intervention; includes hypoplastic left heart syndrome, tetralogy of Fallot, and transposition of the great arteries (Ch 12)

**critical thinking** the process of analyzing and/or evaluating empirically gathered information as a guide to action (Ch 21)

**croup** a disorder most often affecting small children that causes inflammation of the upper airway and trachea resulting from viral infection (Ch 12)

**crying vital capacity (CVC)** gas volume moved while an infant is crying; this is the closest measurement of vital capacity possible in infants (Ch 12)

**culturally competent communication** the application of general communication skills, self-awareness, situational awareness, and adaptability to identify and respond appropriately to the cultural cues affecting the clinical encounter (Ch 1)

**Cushing triad** an increasing systolic blood pressure with a widening pulse pressure, bradycardia, and bradypnea (Ch 6)

**cyanosis** a bluish cast to the skin that clinically may be difficult to detect, especially in a poorly lighted room and in patients with dark-pigmented skin (Ch 5)

**cytology** the study of cells of the body (Ch 7)

## D

**daytime somnolence** an increased desire to sleep and associated lack of energy during the day as reported by a patient; a symptom of sleep disordered breathing (Ch 3)

**dead space–to–tidal volume ratio ($V_D/V_T$)** the ratio of the dead space volume to the total amount of gas inhaled (Ch 14)

**dead space ventilation** ventilation that does not participate in gas exchange; includes both the volume of the conducting airways (anatomic dead space) and ventilated alveoli that are not perfused by the pulmonary circulation (physiologic dead space) (Ch 8)

**decerebrate posture** posture in which the upper extremity is in pronation and extension and the lower extremity is in extension (Ch 6)

**decorticate posture** a recognizable posture, caused by an upper motor neuron lesion, in which the patient's thumb is tucked under flexed fingers in a fisted position, with pronation of forearm and flexion at the elbow and the lower extremity in extension with foot inversion (Ch 6)

**deep sulcus sign** hyperlucency of the lateral costophrenic angle seen on chest x-ray of some patients in the supine position; suggests the presence of a pneumothorax (Ch 10)

**deep tendon reflexes** a physical examination test to evaluate spinal nerves; includes the triceps, biceps, brachioradialis, patellar, and Achilles tendon (Ch 6)

**delirium** an abnormal mental state characterized by confusion, incoherent speech, and hallucinations (Ch 6)

**depolarization** an electrical change in an excitable cell in which the inside becomes positive; associated with contraction of cardiac muscle cells (Ch 11)

**diaphoresis** excessive sweating (Chs 3, 5)

**diastolic blood pressure** the pressure in the arteries during relaxation of the ventricles (Ch 4)

**dicrotic notch** a secondary rise in the descending part of the arterial pulse pressure waveform that corresponds to closure of the aortic valve (Ch 15)

**diet-induced thermogenesis** the conversion of dietary calories in excess of those required to meet immediate metabolic needs into heat rather than being stored as fat (Ch 18)

**diffusing capacity** the ability of the lung to exchange oxygen between the alveoli and the pulmonary capillary blood; usually measured using low concentrations of carbon monoxide gas and expressed in mL/min/mm Hg (Ch 9)

**diplopia** blurred or double vision (Ch 5)

**direct calorimetry** measurement of metabolism by quantifying the total heat given off by the body when in an enclosed chamber (Ch 18)

**doll's eyes reflex** a neurologic test in which the physician turns the patient's head briskly from side to side; the eyes should turn to the left while the head is turned to the right, and vice versa; if this reflex is absent, there will be no eye movement when the patient's head is moved side to side (Ch 6)

**do not attempt to resuscitate (DNAR)/do not resuscitate (DNR) order** a physician's order based on a patient's legally authorized advance directive specifying that resuscitation should not be attempted in the event of a cardiorespiratory arrest (Ch 2)

**dynamic compliance** represents the total impedance to gas flow into the lungs (Ch 14)

**dynamic hyperinflation** a problem seen with severe airway obstruction in which mechanical breaths are stacked on one another (Ch 14)

**dyshemoglobin** any abnormal form of hemoglobin, such as carboxyhemoglobin or methemoglobin (Ch 8)

**dyspnea** shortness of breath as perceived by the patient (Ch 3)

**dysrhythmia** any deviation of the heart's normal sinus rhythm (Ch 11)

## E

**early inspiratory crackles** abnormal high-pitched, discontinuous lung sounds heard early in inspiration and associated with obstructive airway diseases such as COPD and asthma (Ch 5)

**ectopic impulse** a heartbeat originating outside the SA node (Ch 11)

**edema** excessive fluid in tissue (Ch 3)

**EEG arousal** an abrupt shift in EEG frequency during sleep, usually lasting 3 seconds or more and commonly associated with the end of sleep-related obstructive events (Ch 19)

**efferent** as pertaining to nerves, those transporting impulses from the CNS to effector sites, such as muscle tissue (Ch 6)

**eHealth** telemonitoring of health care to help monitor patients and equipment remotely (Ch 20)

**ejection fraction (EF)** the portion of the end-diastolic volume ejected during systole; normally about 60% to 70% (Ch 16)

**electroencephalogram (EEG)** the tracing of brain waves made by an electroencephalograph (Chs 3, 5)

**electromagnetic navigation bronchoscopy** an electromagnetic computerized procedure that tracks the position of a sensor incorporated into a flexible catheter advanced through a bronchoscope, used to reach and increase the biopsy yield from lesions in the smaller airways and mediastinum (Ch 17)

**electronic medical record (EMR)** an electronically accessible and cumulative record of patient health information generated by the various encounters occurring across the spectrum of care delivery; also known as the *electronic health record (EHR)* (Chs 2, 21)

**encephalopathy** a general term referring to any disorder or disease of the brain (Ch 6)

**end-diastolic pressure (EDP)** the pressure in a heart chamber at the end of diastole (Ch 16)

**end-diastolic volume (EDV)** the volume of blood in a heart chamber just before systole (Ch 16)

**endoscopy** a medical procedure in which a physician looks into the body of the patient using a scope (Ch 17)

**end-tidal Pco₂ (Petco₂)** the partial pressure of $CO_2$ during the end-expiratory plateau phase of the capnogram (Ch 14)

**eosinophilia** an abnormal increase in the presence of eosinophils (Ch 7)

**epiglottitis** infection of the upper airway resulting from bacteria; most often seen in children (Ch 12)

**Epworth Sleepiness Scale** a short patient questionnaire used in diagnosing sleep disorders that assesses the magnitude of daytime somnolence (Ch 19)

**escape beat** a heartbeat that originates outside the sinus node after a period of SA node inactivity (Ch 11)

**estimated date of confinement (EDC)** estimated date of a term delivery of a pregnant woman (Ch 12)

**excessive daytime sleepiness/somnolence (EDS)** an abnormal increased desire to sleep during the day as reported by a patient; a symptom of sleep disordered breathing (Ch 19)

**expiratory reserve volume (ERV)** the amount of gas that can be forcefully exhaled after a passive tidal exhalation (Ch 9)

**expiratory view** in chest radiography, an image taken during or after exhalation; the resulting reduction in lung volume can make small pneumothoraces more evident (Ch 10)

**extremely low birth weight (ELBW)** refers to newborns weighing less than 1000 g (Ch 12)

**exudate** when used to describe a pleural effusion, fluid with a high (>3 g/L) protein content (Ch 10)

## F

**F$_E$NO** the fraction of expired nitric oxide in the exhaled breath, measured in parts per billion (ppb) (Ch 9)

**fetal hemoglobin (HbF)** hemoglobin present in the fetus in utero; has a higher affinity for oxygen than does adult hemoglobin; allows the fetus to survive and grow in the relatively low-oxygen environment of the uterus (Ch 12)

**fetid** foul smelling (Ch 3)

**fever** an increase in body temperature above normal (Chs 3, 4)

**fiberoptic bronchoscope** a long, thin, flexible tube consisting of a light-transmitting fiberoptic bundle and a channel used for examining a patient's airways; the channel allows the clinician to irrigate distal airways, suction fluids, and pass brushes or biopsy forceps to obtain tissue samples (Ch 17)

**Fick principle** a method for measuring cardiac output using oxygen consumption and the oxygen content difference between arterial and venous blood (Ch 14)

**first-degree block** a dysrhythmia in which the PR interval is prolonged, exceeding 200 ms; there are no missed beats, and the rhythm typically is regular (Ch 11)

**flail chest** the paradoxic motion seen as a sinking inward of the affected region with each spontaneous inspiratory effort and an outward movement with subsequent exhalation (Ch 5)

**flow-volume loop** a graphic plot of a patient's flow (Y-axis) vs. volume (X-axis) during a forced inspiratory and expiratory maneuver (Ch 9)

**fluoroscopy** the use of x-rays projected through the body onto a fluorescent screen to observe internal structures and their activity (such as swallowing) in real time (Ch 10)

**focus** the site within the heart from which an ectopic impulse originates (Ch 11)

**forced vital capacity (FVC)** the maximum amount of air the patient exhales after a full, deep inspiration (Ch 9)

**fractional saturation** the amount of hemoglobin that is saturated compared with the total amount of hemoglobin present (Ch 14)

**fremitus** internal vibrations sensed at the body surface with the flat of the hand (Ch 13)

**frothy** descriptive term referring to a fluid with air bubbles (Ch 3)

**functional lung volume** lung volume in open communication with the airways (Ch 9)

**functional residual capacity (FRC)** the resting lung volume defined mechanically as the volume at which the expanding tendency of the chest wall is exactly counterbalanced by the contractile tendency of the lung; equals the sum of the residual and the expiratory reserve volumes (Chs 9, 14)

**functional saturation** the amount of hemoglobin that is saturated compared with the amount of hemoglobin that is capable of being saturated (Ch 14)

## G

**gag reflex** a test performed by gently inserting a tongue depressor into the back of the throat; directly assesses the function of cranial nerve IX and more generally a patient's level of consciousness and upper airway protective reflexes (Ch 6)

**gait** the manner of walking (Ch 6)

**gallop rhythm** an abnormal condition in which a third or fourth heart sound is present (Ch 5)

**gastroesophageal reflux disease (GERD)** abnormal movement of stomach contents into the esophagus or mouth; acid from the stomach may be aspirated into the lung and cause asthma-like symptoms (Ch 3)

**gestational age** the age of a fetus; estimated as the time in weeks from the last menses and typically measured using ultrasonic dimensions of the crown-to-rump length (up to 12 weeks of gestation) or the diameter of fetal head (after 12 weeks of gestation) (Ch 12)

**Glasgow Coma Scale (GCS)** a clinical assessment scale used to quantify the degree of neurologic impairment (Ch 6)

**gluconeogenesis** converting protein (amino acids) to sugar (Ch 18)

**glycolysis** process of converting glucose into pyruvic acid (Ch 18)

**glycosuria** excessive sugar in the urine (Ch 7)

**granulocytes** a category of cells known for their prominent granules, including neutrophils, eosinophils, and basophils (Ch 7)

**gravida** number of prior pregnancies experienced by a woman (Ch 12)

**grunting** the sound heard when an infant exhales against a partially closed glottis; represents an effort to increase airway pressures and overcome the decrease in lung volumes associated with some neonatal respiratory disorders (Ch 12)

## H

**harsh breath sounds** breath sounds with increased intensity (Ch 5)

**heart block** a category of dysrhythmias caused by defective transmission of the heart's electrical impulses through its conducting system (Ch 11)

**heave** a forceful, systolic thrust occurring during systole and felt over the precordium by the palpating hand (Ch 5)

**hematemesis** vomiting blood from the stomach (Ch 3)

**hemoptysis** coughing up blood from the lungs (Ch 3)

**hemostasis** the arrest of bleeding or stagnation of blood flow (Ch 7)

**hepatomegaly** enlargement of the liver (Chs 5, 12)

**Holter monitor** a portable device that continuously monitors and records the electrocardiogram, typically over an extended time period; used to assess for cardiac dysrhythmias (Ch 4)

**home medical equipment (HME)** devices designed for and used by patients whose care is being managed in the home by family members and/or nonprofessional caregivers; also called *durable medical equipment* (Ch 20)

**Hoover sign** abnormal movement of the lateral chest wall during breathing in patients with chronic obstructive pulmonary disease with severe hyperinflation (Ch 5)

**Hospital Readmissions Reduction Program (HRRP)** a federal program that penalizes hospitals for excessively high, short-term readmission rates for selected diagnoses, including COPD and pneumonia (Ch 20)

**HRmax** the highest heart rate an individual can safely achieve at peak exercise capacity (Ch 9)

**hyperbilirubinemia** an excess of bilirubin in the blood (Ch 12)

**hypercapnia** abnormal elevation of Paco$_2$ (Ch 8)

**hyperchloremia** elevation of the chloride ion concentration in the blood plasma (Ch 7)

**hyperdynamic precordium** visible beating of the heart on the chest wall; usually indicates hypertrophy of the left or right ventricles (Ch 12)

**hyperglycemia** an abnormal elevation in blood glucose levels (Chs 7, 12)

**hyperkalemia** an abnormal elevation of plasma potassium (Ch 7)

**hypernatremia** an abnormal elevation of plasma sodium (Ch 7)

**hyperoxemia** the presence of excessive blood oxygen levels (Ch 8)

**hyperresonant** as compared with normal, a louder and lower-pitched sound heard when percussing the chest wall, typically indicating an increased volume of underlying air, as in hyperinflated states and pneumothorax (Ch 5)

**hypertension** an abnormal elevation of arterial blood pressure (Ch 4)

**hyperthermia** elevation of body temperature (Ch 12)

**hypertrophy** as applied to the heart, a pathologic increase in the bulk of the myocardial fibers, typically due to a chronic increase in afterload (Ch 11)

**hyperventilation** ventilation greater than necessary to meet metabolic needs; signified by a Paco$_2$ less than 35 mm Hg in the arterial blood (Ch 8)

**hypoalbuminemia** reduced blood protein levels (Ch 7)

**hypocapnia** presence of lower than normal amounts of CO$_2$ in the blood; as applied to arterial blood, a Paco$_2$ less than 35 mm Hg (Ch 8)

**hypochloremia** an abnormal decrease in plasma chloride levels (Ch 7)

**hypoglycemia** reduced blood sugar levels (Chs 7, 12)

**hypokalemia** an abnormal decrease in serum potassium levels (Ch 7)

**hyponatremia** an abnormal decrease in serum sodium levels (Ch 7)

**hypopnea** generally refers to a reduction in the rate or depth of ventilation; as applied to diagnosis of sleep disordered breathing, a 30% or more reduction in measured airflow lasting at least 10 seconds (Ch 19)

**hypotension** an abnormal decrease in arterial blood pressure (Ch 4)

**hypothermia** an abnormal decrease in body temperature (Ch 12)

**hypotonia** decreased muscle tone (Ch 12)

**hypoventilation**   ventilation less than necessary to meet metabolic needs; signified by a $Paco_2$ greater than 45 mm Hg in the arterial blood (Ch 8)

**hypoxemia**   an abnormal reduction in the partial pressure of oxygen in the arterial blood (Ch 8)

**hypoxia**   a condition of in which oxygen levels in the tissues are inadequate to meet metabolic demands (Ch 8)

## I

**iatrogenic**   caused by treatment or diagnostic procedures (Ch 14)

**iatrogenic alkalosis**   alkalosis caused by medical intervention; most often a respiratory alkalosis caused by overly aggressive mechanical ventilation (Ch 8)

**ideal body weight**   the optimum weight of the patient as predicted from height and weight charts; also called *predicted body weight* (Ch 18)

**immunosenescence**   the age-associated decline in the immune system (Ch 13)

**impulse oscillometry (IOS)**   noninvasive method to measure airway resistance by superimposing flow oscillations on the airways during spontaneous breathing; also called the *forced oscillation technique (FOT)* (Ch 12)

**indirect calorimetry**   measurement of metabolic rate using inspired/expired gas analysis and computation of oxygen consumption ($\dot{V}O_2$) and carbon dioxide production ($\dot{V}CO_2$) (Ch 18)

**inotropic agent**   a chemical agent that affects the contractility of the heart (Ch 15)

**inspiratory capacity (IC)**   a physiologic unit of the lung defined as the sum of the tidal volume and the inspiratory reserve volume; the maximum amount of air that can be inhaled from resting FRC (Ch 9)

**inspiratory reserve volume (IRV)**   a physiologic unit of the lung defined as the maximum volume of air that can be inhaled after a normal quiet inhalation (Ch 9)

**intercostal**   referring to the muscle groups between the ribs (Ch 5)

**interrupted aortic arch syndrome**   a developmental anomaly in which the aortic arch fails to completely form (Ch 12)

**interstitial lung disease (ILD)**   respiratory disorder characterized by a dry, unproductive cough and dyspnea on exertion; x-rays usually show fibrotic infiltrates in the lung tissue, usually in the lower lobes (Ch 9)

**interventional bronchoscopy**   the art and science of medicine as related to the performance of diagnostic and invasive therapeutic procedures that require additional training beyond that required in a standard pulmonary medicine training program (Ch 17)

**interventional radiology**   the use of imaging technologies to guide and gain access to vessels and organs for therapeutic purposes (Ch 10)

**intracranial pressure (ICP)**   the level of pressure in the cranium (Ch 6)

**intimate space**   the area around the patient within 18 inches (Ch 1)

**intrapulmonary shunt ($\dot{Q}_s/\dot{Q}_t$)**   blood passing through the lung that is not exposed to ventilated alveoli (Ch 14)

**intrauterine growth retardation (IGR)**   poor growth of a fetus in utero; exists when the estimated weight is below the 10th percentile for its gestational age (Ch 12)

**intraventricular hemorrhage (IVH)**   bleeding in the lateral ventricles of the brain (grades I to III) or the tissue of the brain (grade IV) in premature infants (Ch 12)

**isolated systolic hypertension (ISH)**   elevation of only the systolic pressure (Ch 13)

## K

**Kerley B lines**   a radiographic finding on a chest x-ray of a patient in congestive heart failure; the lines are short, parallel, and 1 mm thick and start at the lung base; they originate at the pleura and extend into the lung parenchyma 1 to 2 cm; caused by engorged pleural-based lymphatic vessels (Ch 10)

**kilocalories (kcal)**   the amount of energy it takes to raise the temperature of 1 kg of water 1°C (Ch 18)

**kyphoscoliosis**   abnormal condition characterized by anteroposterior and lateral curvature of the spine (Ch 5)

**kyphosis**   abnormal condition characterized by increased anteroposterior curvature of the spine (Ch 5)

## L

**lactic acid**   the product of anaerobic metabolism (Ch 18)

**last menstrual period (LMP)**   the date of the beginning of a woman's last menstrual period before pregnancy; can be used to calculate the estimated date of confinement (Ch 12)

**late inspiratory crackles**   abnormal, fine, and discontinuous breath sounds, heard at the latter part of inhalation over the dependent lung regions, often caused by sudden opening of peripheral airways (Ch 5)

**lateral decubitus view**   a radiographic technique used to demonstrate the presence of a free-flowing pleural effusion; the patient lies on the side with the hemithorax in question, allowing for gravity to act on the effusion and layering it out along the dependent lateral chest wall (Ch 10)

**left shift**   a term used to indicate the presence of a high level of immature white cells in the circulating blood (Ch 7)

**leukocytosis**   an abnormal increase in the circulating white blood cell count (Chs 7, 12)

**leukopenia**   an abnormal decrease in the circulating white blood cell count (Chs 7, 12)

**level of consciousness**   an assessment of the extent to which someone is alert and aware of his or her surroundings, as well as his or her response to stimuli (Ch 6)

**linearity (volume, flow)**   the extent to which a gas travels in a straight, unobstructed pattern (Ch 9)

**loud $P_2$**   increased intensity of $S_2$ as a result of more forceful closure of the pulmonic valve as occurs in pulmonary hypertension (Ch 5)

**low birth weight (LBW)**   refers to infants of less than 2500 g, regardless of gestational age (Ch 12)

**lower inflection point**   considered to be the minimal PEEP that should be applied to the lung as determined using a static pressure-volume curve (Ch 14)

**lower limit of normal/upper limit of normal (LLN/ULL)**   the upper and lower limits for predicted normal values of standardized tests results, such as pulmonary function tests and laboratory values (Ch 9)

**lower motor neuron (LMN)**   motor neuron connecting the brainstem and spinal cord to muscle fibers (Ch 6)

**lumbar puncture (LP)**   puncture of the lumbar region of the spinal cord to remove and test cerebral spinal fluid (Ch 6)

**lymphadenopathy**   pertaining to a disease of the lymph nodes; refers also to the visualization of enlarged lymph nodes on radiographs (Ch 5)

**lymphocytopenia**   an abnormal decrease in the number of circulating lymphocytes (Ch 7)

**lymphocytosis**   an abnormal increase in the number of circulating lymphocytes (Ch 7)

## M

**macrocytic**   large cell size (Ch 7)

**macrophage**   a monocyte that has left the circulation and entered tissue (Ch 7)

**magnetic resonance imaging (MRI)**   a high-technology radiographic imaging technique (Ch 10)

**maximal expiratory flow-volume curve (MEFV)**   the output graph showing the relationship between maximum expiratory flow and volume (Ch 9)

**maximal inspiratory flow-volume curve (MIFV)**   the output graph showing the relationship between maximum inspiratory flow and volume (Ch 9)

**maximal voluntary ventilation (MVV)**   the volume of gas a patient can move in and out of the lung in 1 minute; value estimate based on patient performance for 15 seconds (Ch 9)

**maximum inspiratory pressure ($P_I$max)**   a maximum pressure a patient can generate during a full inspiratory effort (Ch 14)

**mean airway pressure (Paw)**   the average pressure recorded during the positive-pressure and spontaneous phases of a respiratory cycle (Ch 14)

**mean arterial pressure (MAP)**   the average pressure present in the arterial blood (Ch 15)

**meconium**   the thick tarry stool that is present in the colon of a fetus in utero (Ch 12)

**meconium aspiration syndrome (MAS)** the inhalation of meconium passed into the amniotic fluid by the fetus in utero (Ch 12)

**metabolic acidosis** nonrespiratory processes resulting in acidemia (Ch 8)

**metabolic alkalosis** nonrespiratory processes resulting in alkalemia (Ch 8)

**metabolic cart** a computer-controlled unit composed of oxygen and carbon dioxide gas analyzers and flow transducers; used to measure indirect calorimetry (Ch 18)

**metabolic equivalent of task (MET)** the ratio of metabolic rate or rate of energy consumption during a specific physical activity to a reference metabolic rate (Ch 9)

**metabolism** the body's way of transferring energy from food to the body's energy currency molecules (adenosine triphosphate) (Ch 18)

**mHealth** mobile health, which involves the use of mobile applications to enhance access to medical resources (Ch 20)

**microcytic** small cell size (Ch 7)

**micrognathia** small lower jaw (Ch 19)

**Mini-Mental State Examination (MMSE)** a brief 30-point quantitative questionnaire used to assess cognition (Ch 6)

**minute volume** ($\dot{V}_E$) the volume of air inhaled or exhaled in 1 minute (Ch 9)

**miosis** small "pinpoint" pupils usually result from pontine hemorrhage or from ingestion of narcotics or organophosphates (Chs 5, 6)

**mixed sleep apnea (MSA)** a condition characterized by a combination of both central and obstructive sleep apnea (Ch 19)

**mixed venous oxygen saturation ($S\bar{V}O_2$)** the percent saturation of mixed venous blood with oxygen; normally about 75% (Ch 14)

**mixed venous oxygen tension ($S\bar{V}O_2$)** the partial pressure of oxygen in the venous blood sample obtained from the right atrium or pulmonary artery (Ch 14)

**moderate sedation** the administration of sedation to achieve a dream-like, but arousable, state often used to facilitate selected procedures such as bronchoscopy (Ch 17)

**monitoring** the repeated or continuous observations or measurements of the patient, his or her physiologic function, and the function of life support equipment for the purpose of guiding management decisions (Ch 14)

**monocytosis** an abnormal increase in circulating monocytes (Ch 7)

**montage** the various physiologic tracings or channels that are measured as part of a polysomnographic (sleep) study (Ch 19)

**multifocal ectopic impulses** when an ectopic impulse is generated from different areas of the heart and they appear different from one another on an ECG (Ch 11)

**mydriasis** pupillary dilation that may be caused by serious brain injury or inadvertent exposure of the eyes to inhaled anticholinergics (Chs 5, 6)

## N

**nasal flaring** the dilation of the ala nasi (the openings of the nose) during inspiration; this is an attempt by the infant to decrease airway resistance and increase tidal volume (Ch 12)

**negative inotropic effect** response of the heart in which the contractility is reduced (Ch 16)

**negligence** a legal term that refers to a health care professional acting outside the standards of care that causes harm to the patient (Ch 21)

**neonatal abstinence syndrome (NAS)** the result of using drugs (especially opium-based substances) during pregnancy (Ch 12)

**neutropenia** an abnormal decrease in the circulating neutrophils (Chs 7, 12)

**neutrophilia** an abnormal increase in the circulating neutrophils (Ch 7)

**night sweats** excessive diaphoresis during sleep (Ch 3)

**nitric oxide (NO)** a soluble gas that is normally produced in the body and serves as a powerful vasodilator (Ch 18)

**nitrogen balance** when the intake of nitrogen equals excretion of nitrogen (Ch 18)

**nitrogen washout** a technique used during pulmonary function testing to determine if there is maldistribution of ventilation of gas within the lung (Ch 9)

**nonverbal communication** means of communication that involves body positioning, as well as facial and other expression and gestures but that excludes verbal clues and language (Ch 1)

**normoblasts** immature nucleated red blood cells (Ch 7)

**normochromic** RBCs with a normal complement of hemoglobin (Ch 7)

**normocytic** a form of anemia (low red blood cell count) that is somewhat common in elderly people, especially those older than 85 years (Ch 7)

**nystagmus** involuntary back-and-forth movement of the eyes (Chs 5, 6)

## O

**objective** a desired result intended to be achieved and generally related to a broader goal (Ch 21)

**objective data** information about the patient that can be measured and is not a matter of opinion (Ch 2)

**oblique views** the patient is turned 45 degrees to either the right or left, with the anterolateral portion of the chest against the film (Ch 10)

**obstructive sleep apnea** intermittent pauses in breathing for more than 10 seconds resulting from upper airway blockage during sleep (Chs 3, 19)

**obstructive ventilatory impairment** a respiratory impairment characterized by a reduction or abnormally low inspiratory and or expiratory flow pattern (Ch 9)

**oculocephalic reflex** test of brainstem function in which the head is rotated side to side and eye movement is noted (Ch 6)

**oculovestibular reflex** also known as the ice caloric or cold caloric reflex; physician instills at least 20 mL of ice water into the ear of a comatose patient; in patients with an intact brainstem, the eyes will move laterally toward the affected ear (Ch 6)

**oncotic pressure** the pressure in the vascular space created by the presence of large protein molecules that draws fluid from outside the vessels into the vasculature (Ch 18)

**orthodeoxia** hypoxemia associated with sitting upright (Ch 3)

**orthopnea** inability to breathe when in a reclining position or lying down (Ch 3)

**orthostatic hypotension** a drop in blood pressure associated with standing or sitting up (Ch 3)

**osteopenia of the premature** a bone disease in premature infants that causes weak fragile bones; it is caused by inadequate phosphorus intake (Ch 12)

**ototoxicity** a drug that is toxic to the ear (Ch 13)

**$O_2$ pulse** the ratio of oxygen consumption to heart rate (Ch 9)

**oxygen concentration indicators (OCIs)** indicators that alert the user if the oxygen concentration output drops below a certain level (Ch 20)

**oxygen consumption** the amount of oxygen consumed per minute by the body tissues (Ch 14)

**oxygen content** the amount of oxygen present in the blood; represents the oxygen combined with hemoglobin and dissolved in plasma; expressed as mL/100 mL of blood (Ch 14)

**oxygen delivery ($Do_2$)** the process of ensuring that the appropriate oxygen concentration is being delivered to the body (Ch 14)

**oxygen extraction ratio (C [a − $\dot{v}$] $O_2$/Ca$O_2$)** the portion of oxygen content in the arterial blood extracted by the tissues (Ch 14)

**oxygen transport** the amount of oxygen moved by the blood per unit of time (Ch 14)

**oxygen uptake** the amount of oxygen used by the tissues per minute (Ch 18)

**oxyhemoglobin dissociation curve (ODC)** graphic depiction of the relationship between Pa$o_2$ and the oxygen content or hemoglobin saturation (Ch 14)

## P

**pack-years** the number of packs of cigarettes smoked per day multiplied by the number of years smoked; higher pack-years are associated with greater risk for lung cancer and other lung diseases (Ch 2)

**palpation** part of a physical examination in which an anatomic structure is felt to determine its size, shape, firmness, or location (Ch 5)

**para** the number of infants a woman has delivered (Ch 12)

**paradoxic pulse** an abnormally large decrease in systolic blood pressure during inspiration (Ch 4)

**parenteral** outside the gastrointestinal tract (Ch 18)

**parenteral nutrition (PN)** feeding a patient intravenously, bypassing the gastrointestinal tract (Ch 18)

**paroxysmal nocturnal dyspnea** the sudden onset of shortness of breath during sleep (Ch 3)

**patellar reflex** reflex tested by tapping on the patellar tendon with a reflex hammer while the patient's leg hangs loosely at a right angle with the thigh; normally the lower leg jerks forward when this reflex is intact (Ch 6)

**patent ductus arteriosus (PDA)** the vessel that makes the anatomic connection between the pulmonary artery and the aorta during fetal life (Ch 12)

**patient-centered care** a model of care characterized by active involvement of patients and their families in the decision making and ongoing care planning and implementation (Ch 1)

**PC$_{20}$** the methacholine concentration at which a 20% decrease occurs in FEV$_1$ (Ch 9)

**peak expiratory flow (PEF)** the maximum flow rate achieved by the patient during the forced vital capacity maneuver (Ch 9)

**peak inspiratory pressure (PIP)** the maximum pressure attained during the inspiratory phase of mechanical ventilation (Ch 14)

**pectus carinatum** a protrusion in the sternum (Ch 5)

**pectus excavatum** a depression or inward abnormality of the sternum (Ch 5)

**pedal edema** an accumulation of fluid in the subcutaneous tissues of the ankles (Ch 5)

**percussion** tapping on the skin surface to determine characteristics of the underlying anatomic structures (Ch 5)

**periodic breathing** an irregular breathing pattern in which periods of apnea are mixed in with periods of normal breathing (Ch 12)

**peripheral cyanosis** presence of cyanosis in the digits (Ch 5)

**peripheral nervous system** the nerves and ganglia outside of the brain and spinal cord (Ch 6)

**PERRLA** abbreviation often seen in the description of a physical examination finding that indicates the pupils are equal, round, and reactive to light and accommodation (Ch 6)

**persistent vegetative state** a condition in which a patient's eyes may be open but the patient is not able to be aroused (Ch 6)

**personal space** the zone around the patient that can vary from 18 inches to 4 feet (Ch 1)

**pertinent negative** a symptom related to the system in question but denied by the patient; for example, if the patient has lung disease but denies shortness of breath, dyspnea would be a pertinent negative (Ch 2)

**pertinent positive** a symptom the patient states is present that is related to the primary problem for which the patient is seeking help (Ch 2)

**phlebostatic axis** located at the fourth intercostal space and one half the anteroposterior diameter of the chest; approximates the location of the right atrium (Ch 15)

**phlegm** mucus from the tracheobronchial tree (Ch 3)

**phrenic nerves** the spinal nerves that pace the diaphragm (Ch 6)

**physiologic dead space** the conductive airways and alveolar units that are ventilated but not perfused (Ch 14)

**phytochemicals** naturally occurring chemical compounds that are responsible for color and other properties of organic substances (Ch 18)

**plan of care** outlines the diagnostic and therapeutic modalities for a patient aimed at achieving the goal of resolving a patient's disease, symptoms, and/or discomfort (Ch 20)

**plantar reflex** a superficial reflex that is commonly assessed in comatose patients and in those with suspected injury to the lumbar IV to V or sacral I to II areas of the spinal cord; it is tested by stroking the lateral plantar aspect of the foot with the handle of a reflex hammer or thumbnail (Ch 6)

**plateau pressure** the pressure required to maintain a delivered tidal volume in a patient's lungs during a period of no gas flow (Ch 14)

**platypnea** shortness of breath in the upright position (Ch 3)

**pleural friction rub** an abnormal low-pitched, discontinuous breath sound characterized by grating of the pleural linings rubbing together (Ch 5)

**pleurisy** pain that comes from the pleural surface; usually a direct result of viral infections but has been generalized to any condition (e.g., pulmonary embolism) causing pleural pain; synonymous with *pleurodynia* (Ch 5)

**pneumoperitoneum** air in the abdomen (Ch 12)

**pneumothorax** air in the pleural space (Ch 10)

**point of maximal impulse (PMI)** the thrust of the contracting left ventricle; usually identified near the midclavicular line in the fifth intercostal space (Ch 5)

**polycythemia** an abnormal increase in the red blood cell count (Chs 7, 12)

**polycythemia vera** an uncontrolled proliferation of hematopoietic cells within the bone marrow (Ch 7)

**polysomnogram (PSG)** a sleep study used to diagnose sleep apnea and other sleep-related breathing disorders (Ch 19)

**portable oxygen concentrator (POC)** a home-fill system that facilitates ambulation (Ch 20)

**positive inotropic effect** a medication or treatment that increases cardiac contractility (Ch 16)

**positron emission tomography (PET)** a high-technology radiographic technique used to determine whether a lesion seen on a standard x-ray contains cancer cells (Ch 10)

**postanalytic error** a problem occurring after sample analysis that alters the accuracy of blood gas results (Ch 8)

**posteroanterior (PA) view** a radiographic view of the chest in which the patient is placed in the upright position and turned so that the x-ray beam travels through the patient from his or her back (posterior) to front (anterior) before striking the x-ray film cassette (Ch 10)

**postterm infants** infants born later than 42 weeks of gestational age (Ch 12)

**postural hypotension** significant decrease in blood pressure associated with changes in position (Ch 4)

**preanalytic error** problem occurring before sample analysis that can alter the accuracy of blood gas results (Ch 8)

**precordium** chest wall overlying the heart (Ch 5)

**preload** the volume of blood in the ventricle just before systole (Ch 16)

**presbycusis** the progressive loss of hearing with age (Ch 13)

**presbyopia** the loss of the ability to focus on objects held near the eye with age (Ch 13)

**pressure-volume loop** a graph designed to display the relationship between the volume inhaled and the pressure generated (Ch 14)

**preterm infants** infants born younger than 37 weeks of gestational age (Ch 12)

**privacy** the ability to keep patients and their medical information inaccessible from public view (Ch 21)

**proprioception** one's sense of position of one's body parts and strength while moving (Ch 6)

**Protected Health Information (PHI)** any information about health status, provision of health care, or payment for such services that can be linked to a specific patient and therefore must be kept private and secure (Ch 1)

**protein-energy malnutrition** loss of body protein (Ch 18)

**pseudohypertension** falsely high blood pressure in older adults because of arterial stiffness (Ch 13)

**pseudoneutropenia** a decrease in the neutrophil count associated with cells shifting from the circulatory pool to the marginated pool (Ch 7)

**pseudoneutrophilia** elevation of the neutrophil count that is the result of cells shifting from the marginated pool to the circulatory pool (Ch 7)

**ptosis** drooping of the upper eyelid (Ch 5)

**pulmonary angiography** a high-technology radiographic technique used to determine the presence of blood clots (embolisms) in the pulmonary circulation (Ch 10)

**pulmonary artery occlusion pressure (PAOP)** see *pulmonary capillary wedge pressure (PCWP)* (Ch 15)

**pulmonary artery wedge pressure (PAWP)** see *pulmonary capillary wedge pressure (PCWP)* (Ch 15)

**pulmonary capillary wedge pressure (PCWP)** also known as *pulmonary artery occlusion pressure,* the pressure measured at the tip of the pulmonary artery catheter when the balloon is inflated; an estimate of left ventricular filling pressure (Chs 15, 16)

**pulmonary interstitial emphysema (PIE)**   a diffuse form of lung injury found in neonates and infants exposed to mechanical ventilation for long time periods (Ch 12)

**pulmonary vascular resistance (PVR)**   the resistance to blood flow through the pulmonary circulation (Ch 16)

**pulse oximetry**   a monitoring technique used to estimate the oxygen saturation levels in the arterial blood (Ch 14)

**pulse pressure**   the mathematical difference between the systolic and diastolic blood pressure measurements (Chs 4, 15, 16)

**pupillary reflex**   contraction of the pupils when a light is directed at one eye (Ch 6)

### Q

**QRS complex**   central and most visually obvious part of an ECG tracing; corresponds to the depolarization of the right and left ventricles of the human heart (Ch 11)

**QT interval**   time between the start of the Q wave and the end of the T wave in an ECG that represents electrical depolarization and repolarization of the left and right ventricles (Ch 11)

### R

**radiolucent**   a term used in describing the appearance of an x-ray film in which the x-ray beam has gone unimpeded through the patient and has turned that corresponding part of the resultant film black (Ch 10)

**radionuclide lung scanning**   a technique in which a radioactive substance is introduced into the body to assess structure and function of tissues (Ch 10)

**radiopaque**   a term used in describing the appearance of an x-ray film in which the x-ray beam has been absorbed, causing the corresponding part of the resultant film to be white (Ch 10)

**rapid eye movement (REM) sleep**   the type of sleep in which dreaming is believed to occur (Ch 19)

**rapid-shallow breathing index (RSBI)**   the ratio of respiratory frequency to tidal volume (Ch 14)

**rate-pressure product**   obtained by multiplying the variables of heart rate and systolic blood pressure; used to assess the workload on the heart (Ch 16)

**reference range**   sets the boundaries for any analyte (e.g., electrolyte, blood cell, protein, enzyme) that would likely be countered in healthy subjects; this range would encompass the variability reflected in the larger, presumably healthy, population (Ch 9)

**repeatability**   when the variation is smaller than some agreed limit for multiple measurements taken under the same conditions (Ch 9)

**repolarization**   the return of a negative charge within the cell; occurs during relaxation of the myocardial cells (Ch 11)

**residual volume (RV)**   a physiologic unit of the lung determined by pulmonary function testing, which describes the volume of gas remaining in the lung after maximal exhalation (Ch 9)

**respiratory acidosis**   a decrease in pH resulting from elevation of the arterial $Pco_2$ (Ch 8)

**respiratory alkalosis**   an increase in pH from a decrease in arterial $Pco_2$ (Ch 8)

**respiratory alternans**   periods of breathing using only the chest wall muscles alternating with periods of breathing entirely by the diaphragm (Ch 5)

**respiratory distress syndrome (RDS)**   a lung disease of premature infants characterized by inadequate amounts of lung surfactant (Ch 12)

**respiratory effort–related arousal (RERA)**   an arousal from sleep that follows a 10-second or longer sequence of breaths that are characterized by increasing respiratory effort but that does not meet criteria for an apnea or hypopnea (Ch 19)

**respiratory home care**   respiratory diagnostic and/or therapeutic modalities administered in a patient's home environment (Ch 20)

**respiratory quotient (RQ)**   the ratio of carbon dioxide produced to oxygen consumed (Ch 18)

**respirometer**   a device used to measure the volume and rate of breathing (Ch 9)

**resting energy expenditure (REE)**   measure of oxygen uptake with the patient at rest (Ch 18)

**restrictive ventilatory impairment**   an abnormal condition marked with the loss of lung volumes and capacities (Ch 9)

**reticulocyte**   nucleated red blood cell (Ch 7)

**retractions**   inward movement of the skin around the chest wall during inspiration; retractions are seen in any lung disease in which the compliance of the lung is less than the compliance of the chest wall (Chs 5, 12)

**retrognathia**   a recessed or small lower jaw (Ch 19)

**return demonstration**   after being instructed on a procedure, the patient and/or caregivers are observed by the clinician doing such procedure to help ensure they are competent (Chs 1, 20)

**rhonchi**   low-pitched, discontinuous, abnormal breath sounds caused by air moving through airways with excessive secretions (Ch 5)

**RR interval**   the time elapsing between two consecutive R waves in an ECG (Ch 11)

### S

**SBAR**   situation, background, assessment, and recommendation charting (Ch 1)

**scalene**   referring to the three muscles arising from the cervical vertebrae, inserting into the first and second ribs; accessory muscles of ventilation (Ch 5)

**scoliosis**   abnormal lateral curvature of the spine (Ch 5)

**sensitivity**   the proportion of actual positive results that are correctly identified as such (e.g., the percentage of sick people who are correctly identified as having the condition) (Ch 7)

**sensorium**   general term referring to the relative state of a patient's consciousness or alertness (Ch 4)

**sensory dissociation**   one sensory system is affected, but the other one is not (Ch 6)

**serum**   the watery fluid portion of the blood (Ch 7)

**serum albumin**   the major protein fraction of blood (Ch 18)

**serum transferrin**   the protein that transports iron in the body (Ch 18)

**signs**   physical examination findings consistent with disease (Ch 2)

**silhouette sign**   a radiographic finding that occurs when the edge of a well-established object (the heart) is obliterated because there is an infiltrate in anatomic contact (Ch 10)

**sinus bradycardia**   an abnormal drop in heart rate with each beat originating in the SA node (Ch 12)

**situation, background, assessment, and recommendation charting (SBAR)**   a format of change-of-shift reporting that emphasizes selected elements of the patient's case (Ch 21)

**skinfold measurement**   method for estimating the percent of body fat (Ch 18)

**sleep apnea**   pauses in breathing of at least 10 seconds during sleep (Ch 19)

**sleep architecture**   describes the structure and pattern of sleep and encompasses several variables (Ch 19)

**sleep disordered breathing**   periods of an absence of or insufficient breathing during sleep (Ch 3, 19)

**slow vital capacity (SVC)**   a measure of the change in volume of gas in the lungs from complete inspiration to complete expiration or vice versa (Ch 9)

**slow-wave sleep**   consists of stages 3 and 4 of non–rapid eye movement sleep (Ch 19)

**snoring**   the hoarse or harsh sound that occurs when breathing is obstructed in some way during sleep (Ch 19)

**social space**   the space of 4 to 12 feet from the patient (Ch 1)

**Speak-Up initiative**   a national campaign to urge patients and their families to take a role in preventing health care errors by becoming active, involved, and informed participants on the health care team (Ch 1)

**specific conductance (Gaw/TGV)**   a measure of how well water can conduct an electrical current (Ch 9)

**specificity**   measures the proportion of negative test results that are correctly identified as such; for example, the percentage of healthy people who are correctly identified as not having the condition (Ch 7)

**spirogram**   the tracing produced by a spirograph (Ch 9)

**splenomegaly**   abnormal enlargement of the spleen (Ch 12)

**spurious**   outwardly similar or corresponding to something without having its genuine qualities (Ch 7)

**spurious polycythemia** an increase in the red blood cell count resulting from a decrease in serum (as in dehydration) (Ch 7)

**sputum** secretions from the tracheobronchial tree that are expectorated through the mouth (Ch 3)

**standard precautions** guidelines recommended by the U.S. Centers for Disease Control and Prevention to reduce the risk for transmission of blood-borne and other pathogens in hospitals; standard precautions apply to (1) blood; (2) all body fluids, secretions, and excretions, excluding sweat, regardless of whether they contain blood; (3) nonintact skin; and (4) mucous membranes (Ch 1)

**static compliance** the lung volume change per unit of pressure during a period of no gas flow (Ch 14)

**ST-elevation myocardial infarction (STEMI)** a type of "heart attack" or myocardial infarction characterized by an elevation in the ST segment (Ch 11)

**sternocleidomastoid** a form of accessory muscles of breathing located in the anterior portion of the neck (Ch 5)

**STOP-BANG analysis** a measurement tool used to classify the severity of certain sleep disorders (Ch 19)

**stridor** continuous sound heard primarily over the larynx and trachea during inhalation when upper airway obstruction is present (Ch 5)

**stroke volume (SV)** the volume of blood ejected from the ventricle during systole (Ch 16)

**ST segment** the interval between the end of the QRS complex and the T wave (Ch 11)

**subcutaneous emphysema** a crackling sound and sensation when fine beads of air are palpated in the tissues (Ch 5)

**subjective** an individual's (such as a patient's) personal perspective, feelings, beliefs, desires, or discovery (Ch 21)

**subjective data** information obtained from the patient that cannot be confirmed with objective testing (Ch 2)

**subjective, objective, assessment, and plan charting (SOAP)** a format for obtaining and recording the major elements of a patient's assessment and care plan (Ch 21)

**sudden infant death syndrome (SIDS)** a condition of unexplained death of an infant, usually seen in infants between 6 weeks and 6 months of age; the incidence of this disease is decreased by not letting the young infant sleep in a prone (face-down) position (Chs 12, 19)

**switch-in error** a specific type of error that can occur in pulmonary function tests (PFTs) (Ch 9)

**symptoms** subjective complaints by the patient (Ch 2)

**syncope** fainting or dizziness; often resulting from hypotension (Ch 3)

**systemic vascular resistance (SVR)** the amount of resistance experienced by the arterial blood as it passes through the peripheral vasculature (Ch 16)

**systolic blood pressure** the peak blood pressure in the arteries during ventricular contraction (Ch 4)

## T

**tachycardia** an abnormal increase in the heart rate (Chs 4, 12)

**tachypnea** an abnormal increase in the rate of breathing (Chs 4, 12)

**tactile fremitus** vibrations that can be felt on a patient's chest wall and that are generally caused by air moving through secretions (Ch 5)

**target** a physical structure in the x-ray machine used to direct the x-ray beam (Ch 10)

**teach-back method** a way to confirm that the clinician has explained to the patient what he or she needs to know about a procedure in a manner that the patient understands (Ch 1)

**telemetry** monitoring patient data such as vital signs at a distance and generally using wireless technology (Ch 4)

**telemonitoring** remote monitoring of a patient's health care status through the use of digital technology (Ch 20)

**tenacious** tending to stick firmly and not easily removed (Ch 3)

**term** infant an infant born between 37 and 42 weeks of gestational age (Ch 12)

**territoriality** the patient's sense that items around his or her hospital bed belong to him or her while admitted (Ch 1)

**The Joint Commission (TJC)** an organization designed to survey and improve the quality of health care organizations (Chs 20, 21)

**thoracentesis** surgical perforation of the chest wall and pleural space with a needle for diagnostic or therapeutic purposes or for the removal of a specimen for biopsy (Ch 10)

**thoracic gas volume (TGV)** technique that measures lung volume (Ch 9)

**thrombocytopenia** an abnormal decrease in the circulating platelets (Chs 7, 12)

**thrombocytosis** an abnormal increase in the number of circulating blood platelets (Chs 7, 12)

**tidal volume ($V_T$)** a physiologic unit of the lung that is the amount of gas moved in and out of the lung during relaxed, at-rest breathing (Ch 9)

**tinnitus** an auditory perception not caused by external sounds that may be described as ringing, buzzing, roaring, or chirping (Ch 13)

**total lung capacity (TLC)** a physiologic unit of the lung determined during pulmonary function testing, which describes the total amount of gas in the lungs after maximum inspiration (Ch 9)

**tracheal breath sound** tubular, loud breath sounds normally heard over the trachea (Ch 5)

**transbronchial biopsy (TBB)** a biopsy done using a bronchoscope (Ch 17)

**transient tachypnea of the newborn (TTN)** a lung disease with increased lung water in infants born by cesarean delivery (Ch 12)

**transmural pressure** the net distending pressure within the ventricle; it provides a true estimation of left ventricular end-diastolic filling because the effect of pressure around the heart is considered (Ch 15)

**transudate** when used to describe a fluid associated with a pleural effusion, with a low (<3 g/L) protein content (Ch 10)

**trepopnea** better breathing associated with a certain position (Ch 3)

## U

**upper airway resistance syndrome (UARS)** a common cause of sleep fragmentation in patients who snore (Ch 19)

**upper inflection point** the part of the curve on a static pressure-volume curve that indicates overdistention of the lung (Ch 14)

**upper motor neuron** motor neurons that originate in the motor region of the cerebral cortex or the brainstem (Ch 6)

## V

**venous return** the amount of blood returned to the right side of the heart (Ch 16)

**ventricular compliance** the ability of the ventricle to expand as blood enters from the atrium (Ch 16)

**ventricular function curves** graphs demonstrating the various stroke volumes achieved at various degrees of filling pressure (Ch 16)

**ventricular stroke work** the amount of work performed by the left ventricle during systole (Ch 16)

**very low birth weight (VLBW)** describes a newborn who weights less than the 95th percentile of weight for newborns (Ch 12)

**vesicular breath sound** a soft, muffled sound heard during auscultation over the lung parenchyma of a healthy person (Ch 5)

**vital capacity (VC)** the maximum amount of air that can be expelled after a full inspiratory effort (Ch 9)

**vocal fremitus** vibration felt by a hand placed on the chest of an individual who is speaking (Ch 5)

**volumeter** an instrument used for measuring the volume of gas (Ch 9)

**volutrauma** a lung injury that occurs from overdistention of the terminal respiratory units (Ch 14)

**$\dot{V}O_2$max** maximum oxygen consumption or uptake as measured by calorimetry (Ch 9)

## W

**wheeze** the musical sounds heard from the chest of the patient with intrathoracic airway obstruction (e.g., asthma) (Ch 5)

# INDEX

## A

a wave, in central venous pressure, 338
Abdomen, physical examination of, 92–93, 93f
Abdominal paradox, 79t, 80
Abducens nerve, 108f, 108t–109t
Abnormal ventilation-perfusion scan, 216f
Abortion, 251
Accelerated idioventricular rhythm, 243
Accessory muscles, 78–79
Accessory nerve, 108f, 108t–109t
Acetyl coenzyme A (acetyl-CoA), in metabolism, 395, 396f
Achilles reflex, 111t
Acid group (COOH), 398
Acid-base balance
  assessment of, 154–155
    base excess in, 145t, 155
    Henderson-Hasselbalch equation in, 155
    partial pressure of carbon dioxide ($Paco_2$) in, 145t, 154, 154b
    pH in, 145t, 154
    plasma bicarbonate in, 145t, 154–155
    protein intake and, 398
Acid-base imbalances
  combined, 157–158
    metabolic and respiratory alkalosis as, 158
    respiratory and metabolic acidosis as, 157
  mixed, 158–159, 158b
    metabolic acidosis and respiratory alkalosis as, 159
    metabolic alkalosis and respiratory acidosis as, 159
  simple, 155–157, 158t
    metabolic acidosis as, 156–157, 157b, 158t
    metabolic alkalosis as, 157, 157b, 158t
    respiratory acidosis as, 155–156, 156b, 158t
    respiratory alkalosis as, 156, 158t
Acidemia, 154
Acid-fast stain, 135
Acidosis
  metabolic, 156–157, 157b, 158t
    acute (uncompensated), 157, 158t
    anion gap in, 156
    Kussmaul respirations in, 157
    and respiratory acidosis, 157
    and respiratory alkalosis, 159
  respiratory, 155–156, 156b, 158t
    acute, 155
    chronic, 156

Acidosis (Continued)
    compensation for, 156, 158t
    definition of, 154
    fully compensated, 158t
    metabolic acidosis and, 157
    metabolic alkalosis and, 159
Acoustic nerve, 108t–109t
Acquired immunodeficiency syndrome (AIDS), computed tomography of, 214
Acrocyanosis, 93, 94b
Action plans, 7, 7b
Action potential, 226
Activated partial thromboplastin time (APTT), 122
Activities of daily living (ADLs)
    assessment of, in home care, 434
    instrumental, 295
Acute otitis media, fever due to, 49t
Adaptability, in culturally competent communication, 5
Adaptive equipment, for home care, 437
Adenosine triphosphate (ATP), 389–390, 390f
Admission note, 26
Advance directives, 27
Adventitious breath sounds, 85
Afferent nerve fibers, 101
Afterload, 360–361
    conditions associated with alterations in, 363t–364t
    decreased, 360
    definition of, 360
    increased, 360
    peripheral resistance in, 360–361
    systemic and pulmonary vascular resistance for, calculation of, 361, 361t, 361b
    ventricular wall stress in, 360
Ageism, 283
Age-related changes, 285–287
    in cardiovascular system, 286, 286b
    in pulmonary system, 286–287
Age-related sensory deficit, 284–285
    hearing impairment as, 284–285
    assessing for, 284
    compensating for, 285
    vision impairment as, 285
    assessing for, 285
    compensating for, 285, 285b
Aging, of organ systems, 285–289
    age-related changes in, 285–287
    in cardiovascular system, 286, 286b
    in pulmonary system, 286–287
    pulmonary defense mechanisms in, 287

Aging, of organ systems (Continued)
    immunity and, 287
    unusual presentation of illness, 287–289
      for asthma, 288, 288b
      for chronic obstructive pulmonary disease, 288
      for HIV/AIDS, 288–289, 289b
      for myocardial infarction, 288
      for pneumonia, 287–288
Air
    in arterial blood gas sample, 159t
    on radiographs, 198
Air bronchogram, 203
Air hunger, definition of, 40t
Air trapping, in critically ill patients, 302
Airway
    in critically ill infants, 273
    management problems, SOAP and, 449
Airway hyperresponsiveness and inflammation, 185–187
    bronchoprovocation testing for, 185–186, 185b
    exhaled nitric oxide ($F_ENO$) analysis for, 186–187, 186b–187b, 187f, 187t
Airway pressures, respiratory monitoring of, 304–308
    auto-positive end-expiratory pressure (auto-PEEP), 306–307
    maximum inspiratory, 301t, 306, 306b
    mean, 305
    peak inspiratory pressure (PIP), 304, 305f, 305b
    plateau, 304–305, 306f
Airway resistance ($R_{aw}$), 184, 184b
    in critically ill patients, 302, 307–308
Alanine aminotransferase (ALT), 123t, 133
Albumin, 132
    in older patients, 294
    serum, 405, 405t
Alert and oriented times three, 101
A-line, 147, 148f, 148t
Alkalemia, 154
Alkaline phosphatase (ALP), 123t, 133
Alkalosis
    metabolic, 157, 157b, 158t
      definition of, 154–155
      and respiratory acidosis, 159
      and respiratory alkalosis, 158
    respiratory, 156, 158t
      definition of, 154
      metabolic acidosis and, 159
      metabolic alkalosis and, 158
    ventilator-induced (iatrogenic), 158
Allergic reactions, 24t–25t, 26
Allow natural death (AND) order, 27

*Note:* Page numbers followed by *f* indicate figures, *t* indicate tables, and *b* indicate boxes.